THE PILL BOOK, 11th REVISED EDITION:
THE ILLUSTRATED GUIDE TO THE MOST PRESCRIBED DRUGS IN THE UNITED STATES
Illustrated with 32 pages of actual-size color photographs

With more than 14 million copies in print, THE PILL BOOK is the bestselling consumer drug reference ever, offering the most up-to-date, comprehensive information in a format designed for ease of use.

This new 11th edition of *The Pill Book* contains more profiles of commonly prescribed drugs than any other consumer reference. Compiled by a team of eminent pharmacologists, it is based on official, FDA-approved information usually available only to doctors and pharmacists, plus the latest information gathered from computer databases and online resources. It synthesizes the most important facts about each drug in a concise, readable, easy-to-understand entry.

Here are complete profiles of more than 1,800 of the most commonly prescribed drugs, including:

- Generic and brand names
- What the drug is for and how it works
- Usual dosages, and what to do if a dose is skipped
- Side effects and possible adverse reactions, highlighted for quick reference
- Interactions with other drugs and foods
- Alcohol-free and sugar-free medications
- The most popular self-injected medications and their safe handling
- Information for seniors, pregnant and breast-feeding women, and others with special needs

This completely revised and updated 11th edition contains dozens of new brand names and more than 40 important new drugs recently approved by the FDA now on sale for the first time.

THE
PILL BOOK
11th EDITION

Editor-in-Chief
HAROLD M. SILVERMAN, Pharm. D.

Production
CMD PUBLISHING
A DIVISION OF
CURRENT MEDICAL DIRECTIONS

Consultants
**DRUG INFORMATION SERVICE
ROBERT WOOD JOHNSON UNIVERSITY HOSPITAL
AND RUTGERS COLLEGE OF PHARMACY**

JUDITH I. BROWN

Digital Photography and Color Separations
**CURRENT MEDICAL DIRECTIONS
GRAPHIC SENSE**

Photography
BENN MITCHELL

**Original Creators of THE PILL BOOK
LAWRENCE D. CHILNICK
HAROLD M. SILVERMAN, Pharm. D.
GILBERT I. SIMON, Sc.D.
BERT STERN**

BANTAM BOOKS
NEW YORK • TORONTO • LONDON • SYDNEY • AUCKLAND

In Canada *Aspirin* is a registered trademark owned by Sterling Winthrop Inc.

THE PILL BOOK

A Bantam Book

PUBLISHING HISTORY

Bantam edition published June 1979
Bantam revised edition / October 1982
Bantam 3rd revised edition / March 1986
Bantam 4th revised edition / February 1990
Bantam 5th revised edition / May 1992
Bantam 6th revised edition / June 1994
Bantam 7th revised edition / June 1996
Bantam 8th revised edition / May 1998
Bantam 9th revised edition / May 2000
Bantam 10th revised edition / May 2002
Bantam 11th revised edition / May 2004
This revised edition was published simultaneously in
trade paperback and mass market paperback.

Published by Bantam Dell
A Division of Random House, Inc.
New York, New York

ISBN: 0-553-38161-X

Manufactured in the United States of America
Published simultaneously in Canada

RRC   10 9 8 7 6 5 4 3 2 1

Contents

How to Use This Book   **vii**

In an Emergency!   **xi**

The Most Commonly Prescribed Drugs in the United States, Generic and Brand Names, with Complete Descriptions of Drugs and Their Effects   **1**

Twenty Questions to Ask Your Doctor and Pharmacist About Your Prescription   **1185**

Other Points to Remember for Safe Drug Use   **1187**

Safety Tips for Self-Injectibles   **1188**

Medicine and Money   **1193**

The Top 200 Prescription Drugs in the United States   **1195**

Index
    Generic and Brand-Name Drugs   **1199**

Color Plates
    Pill Identification Charts

The purpose of this book is to provide educational information to the public concerning the majority of various types of prescription drugs that are presently used by physicians. It is not intended to be complete or exhaustive or in any respect a substitute for personal medical care. *Only a physician may prescribe these drugs and their exact dosages.*

While every effort has been made to reproduce products on the cover and insert of this book in an exact fashion, certain variations of size or color may be expected as a result of the printing process. Furthermore, pictures identified as brand-name drugs should not be confused with their generic counterparts. In any event, the reader should not rely solely upon the photographic image to identify any pills depicted herein, but should rely upon the physician's prescription as dispensed by the pharmacist.

How to Use This Book

How to Find Your Medication in *The Pill Book*

- *The Pill Book* lists most medications in alphabetic order by generic name because a medication may have many brand names but has only 1 generic name. Most generic medications produce the same therapeutic effects as their brand-name equivalents but are much less expensive. Drugs that are available generically are indicated by the G symbol.

- When a medication has 2 or more active ingredients, it is listed by the most widely known brand name. In some cases, pill profiles are listed by drug type (e.g. Sulfonylurea Antidiabetes Drugs).

- *The Pill Book* includes the names of the top 100 brand-name drugs (cross-referenced to their generic name) in alphabetic order with the pill profiles.

- Most over-the-counter (OTC) medications are not included in *The Pill Book*. For complete information on OTC medications, refer to *The Pill Book Guide to Over-the-Counter Medications*.

- All brand and generic names are listed in the Index. Brand names are indicated by boldface.

- Sugar-free and alcohol-free brand-name drugs are indicated by the S and A symbols in the beginning of each pill profile.

The Pill Book, like pills themselves, should be used with caution. Viewed properly, this book may save you money and, perhaps, your life. It contains life-size pictures of the most prescribed brand-name drugs in the U.S. *The Pill Book*'s product identification system is designed to help you check that the medication you are about to take is the one your doctor prescribed. Although many dosage forms are included, not all available forms and strengths of every medication have been shown. While every effort has been made to create accurate photographic reproductions of the products, some variations in size or color may be expected as a result of the printing process. Do not rely solely on the photographic images to identify your pills; check with your pharmacist if you have any product identification questions.

Each pill profile in *The Pill Book* contains the following information:

Generic and Brand Name: The generic name is the common name of the drug approved by the Food and Drug Administration (FDA). It is listed along with the current brand names available for each generic drug. Medications that are available in a generic form are indicated by the G symbol.

Most prescription drugs are sold in more than one dosage strength. Also, some drugs, such as oral contraceptives, come in packages containing different numbers of pills. A few manufacturers indicate these variations by adding letters or numbers to the basic drug name; for example, Loestrin 21 1.5/30 and Loestrin 21 1/20. (The numbers here refer to the number of tablets in each monthly packet, 21, and the amount of medication found in the tablets.) Other drugs come in different strengths: This is often indicated by a notation such as "DS" (double strength) or "Forte" (stronger).

The Pill Book lists generic and brand names together only where there are no differences in basic ingredients (e.g., Loestrin). However, the amount of the ingredient may vary from product to product. In most cases, the brand names and generic versions listed for each medication are interchangeable; you can use any version of the drug and expect that it will work for you. *The Pill Book* identifies within the profile those medications for which generic versions are not considered equivalent and which should not be interchanged with a brand-name product or another generic version of the same drug.

Type of Drug: Describes the general pharmacologic class of each drug: "antidepressant," "tranquilizer," "decongestant," "expectorant," and so on.

Prescribed For: All drugs are approved for some symptoms or conditions by federal authorities, but doctors also commonly prescribe drugs for other, as yet unapproved, reasons; these are also listed in *The Pill Book*. Check with your doctor if you are not sure why you have been given a certain pill.

General Information: Information on how the drug works, how long it takes for you to feel its effects, or a description of how this drug is similar to or different from other drugs.

Cautions and Warnings: This information, with key words in bold type, alerts you to important and more dangerous reactions and to physical conditions, such as heart disease, that can have serious consequences if the medication is prescribed for you.

Possible Side Effects: Side effects are generally divided into 4 categories—those that are most common, common, less common, and rare—to help you better understand what to expect from your pills. If you are not sure whether you are experiencing a drug side effect, ask your doctor.

Drug Interactions: Describes what happens when you combine your medication with other drugs and lists what should not be taken at the same time as your medication. Some interactions may be deadly. At every visit, be sure to inform your doctor of any medication you are already taking.

Food Interactions: Provides information on foods to avoid while taking your medication, whether to take your medication with meals, and other important facts.

Usual Dose: Tells you the largest and smallest doses usually prescribed. You may be given different dosage instructions by your doctor. Do not change the dosage of ANY medication you take without first calling your doctor.

Overdosage: Describes overdose symptoms and what to do if you take too much medication.

Special Information: Includes symptoms to watch for, when to call your doctor, what to do if you forget a dose of your medication, and any special instructions.

Special Populations: *Pregnancy/Breast-feeding:* For women who are or might be pregnant, and what to do if you must take a medication during the time you are nursing your baby. *Seniors:* This section presents the special facts an older adult needs to know about every drug and explains how reactions may differ from those of a younger person.

In an Emergency!

Each year over 1 million people experience drug-related poisoning in the U.S., and about 10% of those cases result in death. In fact, drug overdose is a leading cause of fatal poisoning in the U.S.

Although each of the pill profiles in *The Pill Book* has specific information on drug overdose, there are a few general rules to remember if you are faced with an accidental poisoning.

1. Make sure the victim is breathing, and call for medical help immediately.
2. Learn the phone number for your local poison control center and post it near the phone. Call the center in an emergency. When you call, be prepared to explain

   - What drug was taken and how much
   - Status of the victim (e.g., conscious, sleeping, vomiting, or having convulsions)
   - The approximate age and weight of the victim
   - Any chronic medical problems of the victim (e.g., diabetes, epilepsy, or high blood pressure), if you know them
   - What medications, if any, the victim takes regularly

3. Remove anything that might interfere with breathing. A person who is not getting enough oxygen will turn blue (the tongue or the skin under the fingernails changes color first). If this happens, lay the victim on his or her

back, open the collar, place one hand under the neck, and lift, pull, or push the victim's jaw so that it juts outward. This will open the airway between the mouth and lungs as wide as possible. Begin mouth-to-mouth resuscitation ONLY if the victim is not breathing.

4. If the victim is unconscious or having convulsions, call for medical help immediately. While waiting for the ambulance, lay the victim on his or her stomach and turn the head to one side. Should the victim throw up, this will prevent inhalation of vomit. DO NOT give an unconscious victim anything by mouth. Keep the victim warm.

5. If the victim is conscious, call for medical help and give the victim an 8-oz. glass of water to drink. This will dilute the poison.

Only a small number of poisoning victims require hospitalization. Most may be treated with simple actions or need no treatment at all.

The poison control center may tell you to make the person vomit. The best way to do this is to use ipecac syrup, which is available over-the-counter at any pharmacy. Specific instructions on how much to give infants, children, or adults are printed on the label and will also be given by your poison control center. Remember, DO NOT make the victim vomit unless you have been instructed to do so. Never make the victim vomit if the victim is unconscious, is having a convulsion, or is experiencing a painful, burning feeling in the mouth or throat.

Be Prepared

The best way to deal with a poisoning is to be prepared for it. Do the following now:

1. Write the telephone number of your local poison control center next to your other emergency phone numbers.
2. Decide which hospital you will go to, if necessary, and how you will get there.
3. Buy 1 oz. of ipecac syrup from your pharmacy. The pharmacist will tell you how to use it. Remember, this is a potent drug to be used only if directed and stored out of reach of children.
4. Learn to give mouth-to-mouth resuscitation.

Reduce the Risk of Drug-Related Poisoning

1. Keep all medications in a locked place out of the reach of young children.
2. Do not store medications in containers that previously held food.
3. Do not remove the labels from bottles so that the contents are unknown.
4. To avoid taking the wrong medication, do not take your medicine in the dark or in a dimly lit room.
5. Discard all medications when you no longer need them by flushing them down the toilet.

The Most Commonly Prescribed Drugs in the United States, Generic and Brand Names, with Complete Descriptions of Drugs and Their Effects

Generic Name

Abacavir (uh-BAK-uh-veer)

Brand Name

Ziagen

Type of Drug

Antiviral.

Prescribed For

Human immunodeficiency virus (HIV) infection.

General Information

Abacavir is a man-made nucleoside drug that inhibits the reproduction of the HIV virus. Once inside the HIV-infected cell, abacavir is transformed by enzymes into carbovir triphosphate. Carbovir triphosphate interferes with the activity of HIV reverse transcriptase, an enzyme essential to the virus' ability to reproduce. Abacavir is always given with another anti-HIV antiviral—such as didanosine, lamivudine, stavudine or zalcitabine—to achieve optimum effectiveness. Some of the drug is broken down in the liver, some passes out of the body unchanged in the urine, and some passes out of the body in the stool.

Cautions and Warnings

Stop taking this drug at the first sign of **drug allergy** or **sensitivity** (see "Special Information"). People have died from abacavir sensitivity.

People with **liver disease** should be cautious about using this drug because of the possibility that it can aggravate the condition. Some people have died from liver damage associated with abacavir.

The use of nucleoside drugs such as abacavir can very rarely cause **lactic acidosis**, a fatal metabolic disturbance.

Resistance to abacavir has developed in laboratory versions of HIV also resistant to lamivudine, didanosine, and zalcitabine. HIV that is resistant to protease inhibitors is not likely to be resistant to abacavir.

Abacavir cannot be used in infants under age 3 months.

Possible Side Effects

Because abacavir is always taken with other drugs, the side effects listed here are those of the drugs in combination.

Adults
▼ Most common: nausea, vomiting, diarrhea, and appetite loss.
▼ Common: sleep disturbances.

Children
▼ Most common: nausea, vomiting, fever, headache, diarrhea, and rash.
▼ Common: appetite loss.

Drug Interactions

• Alcohol interferes with the elimination of abacavir through the liver and can lead to a 40% increase in the amount of drug in the blood.
• Abacavir can increase blood levels of acetaminophen, amitriptyline, bumetanide, chloral hydrate, chlorpheniramine, chlorpromazine, chlorzoxazone, dapsone, doxepin, fluconazole, imipramine, ketoconazole, labetalol, lamotrigine, miconazole, morphine, naloxone, non-steroidal anti-inflammatory drugs (NSAIDs), oxazepam, promethazine, propofol, propranolol, and valproic acid.
• Cigarette smoking and clofibrate may reduce the amount of abacavir in the blood.
• Combining abacavir with isoniazid may decrease abacavir levels and increase isoniazid levels in the blood.
• Abacavir levels in the blood may be decreased if you are also taking phenobarbital, phenytoin, or T3 thyroid hormone replacement.

Food Interactions

None known.

Usual Dose

Adult (age 17 and over): 300 mg 2 times a day.
Child (age 3 months–16 years): 3.6 mg per lb. of body weight twice a day, up to a maximum of 300 mg in each dose.

Overdosage

Little is known about the effects of abacavir overdose. Overdose victims should be taken to a hospital emergency room for treatment. ALWAYS bring the prescription bottle or container.

Special Information

Stop taking this drug and call your doctor at the first sign of allergy or sensitivity. Symptoms include fever, rash, fatigue, nausea, vomiting, diarrhea, abdominal pain, sore throat, difficulty breathing, and coughing. If you continue to take abacavir and are allergic to it, more severe reactions including a life-threatening drop in blood pressure could develop in hours.

Abacavir is not a cure for HIV. People taking the drug may still develop opportunistic infections and other conditions associated with HIV infection.

People taking abacavir can still be infectious and transmit HIV to others.

The long-term effects of abacavir are not known. Report anything unusual to your doctor.

It is very important for you to take abacavir exactly as prescribed. If you forget to take a dose and remember within 2 to 3 hours, take the medication. If you forget until it is almost time for your next dose, skip the forgotten dose and continue with your regular schedule. Remember, every dose of any HIV medication you forget or skip can make it more difficult for the drugs to do their job and can also lead to the development of HIV resistant to abacavir.

Special Populations

Pregnancy/Breast-feeding

Abacavir passes into the fetal circulation. In animal studies, the drug caused low birth weight and increased the risk of stillbirth. The effect of abacavir in pregnant women is not known. When this drug is considered crucial by your doctor, its potential benefits must be carefully weighed against its risks.

It is not known if abacavir passes into breast milk. Women with HIV are advised to bottle-feed their babies to avoid transmitting the drug.

Seniors

Studies of abacavir did not include many seniors. Seniors should use this drug with caution because of the risk that normal reductions in organ function or drug interactions may affect how abacavir works in the body or increase the likelihood of side effects.

Generic Name

Acarbose (uh-CAR-bose)

Brand Name

Precose

Type of Drug

Antidiabetic.

Prescribed For

Type II (non-insulin-dependent) diabetes mellitus.

General Information

Acarbose works in a different way than other antidiabetes drugs. Acarbose interferes with enzymes in the intestine responsible for breaking down the complex carbohydrates found in starchy foods into simple sugars, including glucose. Acarbose lowers blood sugar by delaying the absorption of glucose into the blood after eating. Because it works against diabetes in this way, the blood-sugar-lowering effect of acarbose adds to that of other antidiabetes drugs. Acarbose may also be used by people who are unable to control their blood sugar by diet alone. Most of acarbose's side effects are related directly to the fact that it leaves undigested carbohydrates in the lower intestines.

Cautions and Warnings

Acarbose should not be used if you are **allergic** or **sensitive** to it.

People should not use acarbose if they have **diabetic ketoacidosis, cirrhosis, severe kidney disease, inflammatory bowel disease, ulcers of the colon, intestinal obstruction, severe digestive disease,** or **absorption diseases,** or if **intestinal gas** will be a severe problem.

Acarbose may lead to **liver inflammation.**

Possible Side Effects

▼ Most common: stomach gas (in 75% of people who take it), abdominal pain, and diarrhea. These side effects tend to improve or go away after a few weeks.

▼ Rare: liver irritation and minor abnormalities in blood tests.

Drug Interactions

• Acarbose adds to the blood-sugar-lowering effect of sulfonylureas and other antidiabetes drugs and may increase the risk of hypoglycemia (low blood sugar) associated with these drugs.

• Thiazides and other diuretics, corticosteroid anti-inflammatory drugs, phenothiazines, thyroid drugs, estrogens, oral contraceptives ("the pill"), phenytoin, nicotinic acid, stimulants, calcium channel blockers, and isoniazid may increase blood sugar levels. Your dosage of acarbose may need to be increased if you combine it with any of these drugs.

• Activated charcoal and antacids—and other drugs intended to absorb stomach contents—and digestive enzyme preparations may reduce the effectiveness of acarbose. Separate these drugs from acarbose by at least 2 hours.

• Combining acarbose and digoxin may decrease the effects of digoxin.

Food Interactions

Acarbose must be taken with the first bite of each meal.

Usual Dose

Adult: 25–100 mg with breakfast, lunch, and dinner.
Child: not recommended.

Overdosage

Acarbose overdose does not cause low blood sugar, but diarrhea, abdominal pain, and intestinal gas can be expected. Call your local poison control center for more information. If you seek treatment, ALWAYS bring the prescription bottle or container.

Special Information

As with all antidiabetes drugs, people taking acarbose must follow their doctor's instructions for diet, exercise, and blood sugar testing.

Acarbose prevents the breakdown of table sugar. If you take this drug in combination with insulin or a sulfonylurea drug, be sure to have a quick source of glucose (dextrose) with you to treat hypoglycemia (symptoms include tiredness, increased hunger, increased heart rate, sweating, and numbness in the arms and legs).

Read product labels carefully or check with your pharmacist before buying any nonprescription drug to be sure it is safe for diabetics to take with acarbose.

It is essential to take each dose of acarbose at the beginning of each meal. Since the drug works in the intestines, it has to be there at the same time as the food you are digesting.

If you forget a dose of acarbose, skip it and continue with your regular schedule. Taking a missed dose between meals will not provide any benefit.

Special Populations

Pregnancy/Breast-feeding

Animal studies of acarbose showed no effects on the fetus, but there is no information available on its effect in humans. Blood sugar control is considered essential during pregnancy and insulin is usually prescribed for that purpose. When acarbose is considered crucial by your doctor, its potential benefits must be weighed against its risks.

It is not known if acarbose passes into human breast milk. Nursing mothers who must take this drug should bottle-feed.

Seniors

Blood levels of acarbose are higher in older adults, but this is not considered important. Seniors with severe kidney disease should avoid this medication.

Accupril   *see Quinapril, page 912*

Generic Name

Acebutolol (ah-seh-BUTE-uh-lol) Ⓖ

Brand Name

Sectral

Type of Drug

Beta-adrenergic blocking agent.

Prescribed For

High blood pressure and abnormal heart rhythms.

General Information

Acebutolol hydrochloride is one of many beta-adrenergic blocking drugs, or beta blockers, that interfere with the action of a specific part of the nervous system. Beta receptors are found all over the body and affect many body functions. Beta blockers have different characteristics that can make them more suitable for certain conditions or people.

Cautions and Warnings

Do not take acebutolol if you are allergic to beta blockers.

You should be cautious about taking acebutolol if you have **asthma, severe heart failure,** a **very slow heart rate,** or **heart block** (disruption of the electrical impulses that control heart rate) because the drug may worsen these conditions.

People with **angina** taking acebutolol for high blood pressure risk aggravating their angina if they suddenly stop taking the drug. These patients should have their acebutolol dosage reduced gradually over 1 to 2 weeks.

Acebutolol should be used with caution if you have **liver or kidney disease** because your ability to eliminate this drug from your body may be impaired.

Acebutolol reduces the amount of blood pumped by the heart with each beat. This reduction in blood flow may aggravate the condition of people with **poor circulation** or **circulatory disease.**

If you are undergoing **major surgery,** your doctor may want you to stop taking acebutolol at least 2 days before surgery.

Possible Side Effects

Side effects are relatively uncommon and usually mild; normally they develop early in the course of treatment and are rarely a reason to stop taking acebutolol.

▼ Most common: impotence.

▼ Less common: unusual tiredness or weakness, slow heartbeat, heart failure (symptoms include swelling of the legs, ankles, or feet), dizziness, breathing difficulties, bronchospasm, depression, confusion, anxiety, nervousness, sleeplessness, disorientation, short-term memory loss, emotional instability, cold hands and feet, constipation, diarrhea, nausea, vomiting, upset stomach, increased sweating, urinary difficulties, cramps, blurred vision, rash, hair loss, stuffy nose, facial swelling, aggravation of lupus erythematosus (chronic condition affecting the body's connective tissue), itching, chest pain, back or joint pain, colitis, drug allergy (symptoms include fever and sore throat), and liver toxicity.

Drug Interactions

• Acebutolol may interact with surgical anesthetics to increase the risk of heart problems during surgery. Some anesthesiologists recommend gradually stopping the drug by 2 days before surgery.

• Acebutolol may interfere with the normal signs of low blood sugar and with the action of oral antidiabetes drugs.

• Acebutolol increases the blood-pressure-lowering effects of other blood-pressure-reducing agents, including clonidine, guanabenz, and reserpine; and calcium channel blockers, such as nifedipine.

• Aspirin-containing drugs, indomethacin, sulfinpyrazone, and estrogen drugs may interfere with the blood-pressure-lowering effect of acebutolol.

• Cocaine may reduce the effectiveness of all beta-blockers.

• Acebutolol may worsen the problem of cold hands and feet associated with ergot alkaloids, used to treat migraine. Gangrene is a possibility in people taking both an ergot and acebutolol.

• Acebutolol will counteract thyroid hormone replacements.

• Calcium channel blockers, flecainide, hydralazine, oral contraceptives, propafenone, haloperidol, phenothiazine

tranquilizers (molindone and others), quinolone antibacterials, and quinidine may increase the amount of acebutolol in
the bloodstream and lead to increased acebutolol effects.

• Acebutolol should not be taken within 2 weeks of taking a
monoamine oxidase inhibitor (MAOI) antidepressant.

• Cimetidine increases the amount of acebutolol absorbed
into the bloodstream from oral tablets.

• Acebutolol may interfere with the effects of some anti-
asthma drugs, including theophylline and aminophylline,
and especially ephedrine and isoproterenol.

• Combining acebutolol with phenytoin or digitalis drugs
may result in excessive slowing of the heart, possibly causing
heart block.

• If you stop smoking while taking acebutolol, your dose
may have to be reduced because your liver will break down
the drug more slowly afterward.

• Aluminum salts, barbituates, calcium salts, cholestyramine, colestipol, ampicillin, and rifampin may reduce the
effectiveness of acebutolol.

Food Interactions

None known.

Usual Dose

Adult: starting dose—400 mg a day, taken all at once or in 2
divided doses. The daily dose may be gradually increased.
Maintenance dose—400–1200 mg a day.

Senior: Older adults may respond to lower doses and
should be treated more cautiously, beginning with 200 mg a
day, increasing gradually to a maximum of 800 mg a day.

Overdosage

Symptoms of overdose include changes in heartbeat—
unusually slow, unusually fast, or irregular—severe dizziness
or fainting, breathing difficulties, bluish-colored fingernails or
palms, and seizures. The victim should be taken to a hospital
emergency room. ALWAYS bring the prescription bottle or
container.

Special Information

Acebutolol is meant to be taken continuously. When ending
acebutolol treatment, dosage should be reduced gradually
over a period of about 2 weeks. Do not stop taking this drug

unless directed to do so by your doctor: Abrupt withdrawal may cause chest pain, breathing difficulties, increased sweating, and unusually fast or irregular heartbeat.

Call your doctor at once if you develop back or joint pain, breathing difficulties, cold hands or feet, depression, rash, or changes in heartbeat. Acebutolol may produce an undesirable lowering of blood pressure, leading to dizziness or fainting; call your doctor if this happens to you. Call your doctor if you experience persistent or bothersome anxiety, diarrhea, constipation, impotence, headache, itching, nausea or vomiting, nightmares or vivid dreams, upset stomach, trouble sleeping, stuffy nose, frequent urination, unusual tiredness, or weakness.

Acebutolol may cause drowsiness, dizziness, light-headedness, or blurred vision. Be careful when driving or performing complex tasks.

It is best to take acebutolol at the same time each day. If you forget a dose, take it as soon as you remember. If you take acebutolol once a day and it is within 8 hours of your next dose, skip the dose you forgot and continue with your regular schedule. If you take acebutolol twice a day and it is within 4 hours of your next dose, skip the missed dose and continue with your regular schedule. Never take a double dose.

Special Populations

Pregnancy/Breast-feeding

Infants born to women who took a beta blocker while pregnant had lower birth weights, low blood pressure, and slow heart rates. Acebutolol should be avoided by pregnant women and women who might become pregnant while taking it.

Large amounts of acebutolol pass into breast milk. Nursing mothers taking acebutolol should bottle-feed.

Seniors

Seniors taking acebutolol may be more likely to suffer from cold hands and feet, reduced body temperature, chest pain, general feelings of ill health, sudden breathing difficulties, increased sweating, or changes in heartbeat.

Generic Name

Acetaminophen (uh-SEE-tuh-MIN-uh-fen) Ⓖ

Brand Names

Acephen	Liquiprin
Aceta	Mapap*
Acetaminophen Uniserts	Maranox
Apacet	Meda Cap/Tab
Aspirin Free Anacin	Neopap
Maximum Strength	Oraphen-PD
Aspirin Free Pain Relief	Panadol*
Childrens' Pain Reliever	Redutemp
Dapacin	Ridenol
Dynafed	Silapap
Feverall	Tapanol
Genapap*	Tempra*
Genebs	Tylenol*
Halenol	Uni-Ace
Infants' Pain Reliever	

Some products in this brand-name group are alcohol- or sugar-free. Consult your pharmacist.

Type of Drug

Antipyretic and analgesic.

Prescribed For

Relief of pain and fever for people who cannot or do not want to take aspirin or a nonsteroidal anti-inflammatory drug (NSAID). Acetaminophen may be given to children about to receive a DTP vaccination to reduce the fever and pain that commonly follow the vaccination.

General Information

Acetaminophen is generally used to relieve pain and fever associated with the common cold, flu, viral infections, or other disorders where pain or fever may occur. It is also used to relieve pain in people who are allergic to aspirin, or those who cannot take aspirin because of potential interactions with other drugs such as oral anticoagulants. It can be used to relieve pain from a variety of sources, including arthritis, headache, and tooth and periodontic pain, although it does not reduce inflammation.

Cautions and Warnings

Do not take acetaminophen if you are **allergic** or **sensitive** to it. Do not take acetaminophen for **more than 10 days in a row** (5 days for children) unless directed by your doctor. Do not take more than is prescribed or recommended on the package.

Use this drug with extreme caution if you have **kidney or liver disease** or **viral infections of the liver**. Large amounts of alcohol increase the liver toxicity of large doses or overdoses of acetaminophen. **Avoid alcohol** if you regularly take acetaminophen. Some people are more sensitive to this effect than others.

Possible Side Effects

This drug is relatively free from side effects when taken in recommended doses. For this reason it has become extremely popular, especially among those who cannot take aspirin.

▼ Rare: large doses or long-term use may cause liver damage, rash, itching, fever, lowered blood sugar, stimulation, yellowing of the skin or whites of the eyes, and/or a change in the composition of your blood.

Drug Interactions

• Acetaminophen's effects may be reduced by long-term use or large doses of barbiturate drugs, carbamazepine, phenytoin and similar drugs, izoniazid, rifampin, and sulfinpyrazone. These drugs may also increase the chances of liver toxicity if taken with acetaminophen.

• Alcoholic beverages increase the chances for liver toxicity and possible liver failure associated with acetaminophen.

Food Interactions

None known.

Usual Dose

Adult and Child (age 12 and over): 325–650 mg 4–6 times a day, or 1000 mg 3–4 times a day. Avoid taking more than 4 g (twelve 325-mg tablets) a day for long periods of time.

Child (age 11): 480 mg 4–5 times a day.
Child (age 9–10): 400 mg 4–5 times a day.
Child (age 6–8): 320 mg 4–5 times a day.
Child (age 4–5): 240 mg 4–5 times a day.
Child (age 3): 160 mg 4–5 times a day.
Child (age 1–2): 120 mg 4–5 times a day.
Child (age 4–11 months): 80 mg 4–5 times a day.
Child (under age 4 months): 40 mg 4–5 times a day.

Overdosage

Acute acetaminophen overdose may cause nausea, vomiting, sweating, appetite loss, drowsiness, confusion, abdominal tenderness, low blood pressure, abnormal heart rhythms, yellowing of the skin and whites of the eyes, and liver and kidney failure. Liver damage has occurred with 12 extra-strength tablets or 18 regular-strength tablets, but most people need larger doses—20 extra-strength or 30 regular-strength tablets—to damage their livers. Regular use of large doses for long periods—3000 to 4000 mg a day for a year—can also cause liver damage, especially if alcohol is involved. In case of overdose, induce vomiting as soon as possible with ipecac syrup—available at any pharmacy—and take the victim to a hospital emergency room. ALWAYS bring the acetaminophen bottle or container.

Special Information

Unless abused, acetaminophen is a beneficial, effective, and relatively nontoxic drug. Follow package directions and call your doctor if acetaminophen does not work in 10 days for adults or 5 days for children.

Alcoholic beverages will worsen the liver damage that acetaminophen can cause. People who take this drug on a regular basis should limit their alcohol intake.

If you forget to take a dose, take it as soon as you remember. If it is within an hour of your next dose, skip the dose you forgot and continue with your regular schedule. Do not take a double dose.

Special Populations

Pregnancy/Breast-feeding

Acetaminophen is considered safe during pregnancy when taken in usual doses. Taking continuous high doses of the drug may cause birth defects or interfere with fetal development. Three cases of congenital hip dislocation appear to have been associated with acetaminophen. Check with your doctor before taking this drug if you are or might be pregnant.

Small amounts of acetaminophen may pass into breast milk, but the drug is considered harmless to nursing infants.

Seniors

Seniors may take acetaminophen as directed by a doctor.

Generic Name

Acetazolamide (uh-sete-uh-ZOLE-uh-mide) G

Brand Names

Ak-Zol	Diamox
Dazamide	Diamox Sequels

Type of Drug

Carbonic-anhydrase inhibitor.

Prescribed For

Glaucoma and prevention or treatment of mountain sickness; also prescribed for epilepsy, including absence seizures, petit mal and grand mal epilepsy, and tonic-clonic, mixed, or partial seizures.

General Information

By blocking an enzyme in the body called carbonic anhydrase, acetazolamide produces a weak diuretic effect that helps to treat glaucoma by reducing pressure inside the eye. Acetazolamide's antiseizure properties are also produced by its effect on carbonic anhydrase, though exactly how acetazolamide prevents seizure is not well understood.

Cautions and Warnings

Do not take acetazolamide if you are **allergic** to sulfa drugs.

Do not take acetazolamide if you have **low blood sodium or potassium** or serious **kidney, liver, or Addison's disease**.

Possible Side Effects

Side effects of short-term therapy are usually minimal.

▼ Most common: nausea or vomiting; tingling feeling

Possible Side Effects *(continued)*

in the arms, legs, lips, mouth, or anus; appetite and weight loss; a metallic taste; increased frequency in urination; diarrhea; not feeling well; occasional drowsiness; and weakness. You may also experience rash, drug crystals in the urine, painful urination, low back pain, urinary difficulty, and low urine volume.

▼ Rare: Rare side effects can affect the liver, mental state, blood sugar, muscles, and senses. Contact your doctor if you experience any side effect not listed above.

Drug Interactions

• Avoid over-the-counter drug products that contain stimulants or anticholinergics, which tend to aggravate glaucoma and cardiac disease.

• Acetazolamide may increase blood concentrations of cyclosporine (used to prevent the rejection of transplanted organs).

• Acetazolamide may block or delay the absorption of primidone (prescribed for seizure).

• Avoid aspirin because it may enhance acetazolamide side effects.

• Combining diflunisal and acetazolamide can result in an excessive lowering of eye pressure.

Food Interactions

Acetazolamide may be taken with food if it upsets your stomach. Because acetazolamide can increase potassium loss, take this drug with potassium-rich foods such as bananas, citrus fruits, melons, and tomatoes.

Usual Dose

250–1000 mg a day.

Overdosage

Symptoms of overdose include drowsiness, loss of appetite, nausea, vomiting, dizziness, tingling in the hands or feet, weakness, tremors, or ringing or buzzing in the ears. In case of overdose, induce vomiting as soon as possible with ipecac syrup—available at any pharmacy—and take the victim to a hospital emergency room. ALWAYS bring the prescription bottle or container.

Special Information

Acetazolamide may cause minor drowsiness and confusion, particularly during the first 2 weeks of therapy. Be careful when driving or doing any task that requires concentration.

Call your doctor if you develop sore throat, fever, unusual bleeding or bruises, tingling in the hands or feet, rash, or unusual pains.

Acetazolamide can increase sensitivity to the sun. Avoid prolonged sun exposure and protect your eyes while taking this drug.

If you forget a dose, take it as soon as you remember. If it is almost time for your next dose, skip the dose you forgot and continue with your regular schedule. Do not take a double dose.

Special Populations

Pregnancy/Breast-feeding

High doses of this drug may cause birth defects or interfere with fetal development. When this drug is considered crucial by your doctor, its potential benefits must be carefully weighed against its risks.

Small amounts of acetazolamide may pass into breast milk. Nursing mothers who must take this drug should consider bottle-feeding.

Seniors

Seniors are more sensitive to this drug's side effects.

Aciphex   see *Proton-Pump Inhibitors,* page 906

Generic Name

Acitretin   (ah-sih-TREH-tin)

Brand Name

Soriatane

Type of Drug

Antipsoriatic.

Prescribed For

Severe psoriasis; also prescribed for a variety of other skin conditions.

General Information

Acitretin is related to vitamin A and prescription drugs such as etretinate and isotretinoin. Acitretin is produced when etretinate is broken down in the body and its effects are very similar to etretinate. The way that acitretin works is not known. Its effects are not likely to be seen until you have taken it for 2 or 3 months. Your doctor is urged to use this medication only in cases of severe psoriasis that have not responded to other treatments because of the risks associated with acitretin.

Cautions and Warnings

Women who take acitretin must not be pregnant during treatment or for 3 years after the completion of treatment. It is not known if acitretin taken by men before conception is also a risk to the fetus.

A small number of people taking this drug have developed **liver damage** including jaundice (symptoms include yellowing of the skin and whites of the eyes). Acitretin has also been associated with **hepatitis.** People with **kidney failure** have much less acitretin in their blood than people with normal kidneys. Caution is advised for people with liver or kidney damage.

Blood fat levels rise in 25% to 50% of people taking acitretin. Very large increases in triglycerides are uncommon but a few cases of **pancreatitis** (pancreas inflammation) have occurred. Your doctor should measure your blood fat levels before you start taking acitretin and monitor them weekly or biweekly until your response to the medication has been determined. People with **diabetes,** who are **obese,** or who have a **history of these conditions** are at increased risk for high blood fat levels as are people who **drink alcohol excessively**.

Drugs similar to acitretin have been associated with **pseudotumor cerebri** (increased pressure in the brain). Symptoms of pseudotumor cerebri include **visual distur-**

bances, **headache, nausea,** and **vomiting.** Report these or any unusual symptoms to your doctor at once.

People taking acitretin who had **spine or bone—including knee or ankle—problems** before starting the drug may find that their problems worsen while on the drug.

People with **diabetes** may find it more difficult to control their blood sugar while on acitretin.

Possible Side Effects

▼ Most common: hair loss or change in texture, peeling skin, and inflammation of the lips.

▼ Common: dry eyes, chills or stiffness, dry skin, fingernail problems, itching, rash, tingling in the hands or feet, increased sensory awareness, loss of some sections of skin, sticky skin, and runny nose.

▼ Less common: drying and thickening of eye tissue, eye irritation, eyebrow or eye lash loss, changes in appetite, swelling, fatigue, hot flashes, flushing, sinus irritation, headache, pain, earache, insomnia, depression, Bell's palsy, crusting of the eyelids, blurred vision, conjunctivitis (pinkeye), double vision, itchy eyes or eyelids, cataracts, swelling inside the eye, unusual sensitivity to bright light, dry mouth, nosebleeds, joint pain, and worsening of existing spinal problems.

▼ Rare: Rare side effects can occur in almost any part of the body. Contact your doctor if you experience any side effect not listed above.

Drug Interactions

• People combining acitretin and glyburide (an antidiabetic) may have unusually low blood-sugar levels. Your doctor may have to adjust your diabetic treatment program while you are taking acitretin.

• Combining acitretin with methotrexate increases the risk of liver damage.

• Acitretin reduces the effectiveness of low-progestin oral contraceptives (the "mini-pill"). If you are taking one of these contraceptives, switch to another type of birth control and use at least one other contraceptive method for at least 3 years after treatment is completed.

• Combining alcohol with acitretin produces acitretin's parent compound, etretinate. Etretinate stays in the body much longer than acitretin and may therefore affect the fetus for an even longer period of time than might acitretin. Avoid alcoholic beverages.

• Do not take a vitamin A supplement that has more than the standard minimum daily requirement (1000 mcg). Excess vitamin A plus acitretin exposes you to possible vitamin A toxicity.

• Acitretin should not be given to patients who are sensitive to parabens.

• Combining acitretin with tetracyclines may increase the risk of severe pressure on the brain.

• Notify your doctor if you are taking etretinate, isotretinoin, oral or topical tretinoin, or cyclosporine.

Food Interactions

Acitretin is best absorbed when taken with food or meals.

Usual Dose

Adult: 25–50 mg a day with your main meal. Dosage may increase after 4 weeks to 25–75 mg a day. Dosage must be individualized to your specific needs.

Child: not recommended.

Overdosage

Symptoms of acitretin overdose include vomiting, headache, and vertigo. Call your local hospital emergency room or local poison control center for more information.

Special Information

Contact your doctor at once if you become pregnant while taking acitretin or in the 3 years following treatment. The risk of birth defects persists as long as the drug is in your body. In one case, small amounts of etretinate were found in blood plasma and fatty tissue more than 5 years after treatment.

Report visual disturbances, headache, nausea, vomiting, or anything unusual to your doctor at once.

Do not drink any alcoholic beverages during acitretin treatment and for at least 2 months after treatment has been completed.

Avoid excess vitamin A (see "Drug Interactions").

Some birth control methods, including low-dose progestin contraceptives and tubal ligation may fail while taking this drug. Use at least one additional form of contraception while taking acitretin to avoid pregnancy.

You may have problems tolerating contact lenses while you are taking acitretin.

Do not donate blood while taking acitretin or for 3 years afterwards because your blood might be given to a pregnant woman.

Avoid exposure to excessive sunlight or to sunlamps because of unusual sensitivity caused by acitretin.

If you forget to take a dose of acitretin, take it with food as soon as you remember. If it is almost time for your next dose, skip the one you forgot and continue with your regular schedule. Do not take a double dose.

The full benefit of acitretin may not be seen for 2 to 3 months.

Special Populations

Pregnancy/Breast-feeding
Acitretin causes birth defects and may damage the fetus. Women who take acitretin must be sure they are not pregnant before starting therapy by using reliable contraception for at least 1 month before starting the drug and taking a pregnancy test within 1 week of starting treatment. Women must use 2 reliable contraceptive methods during treatment and for 3 years following the completion of treatment.

Acitretin may pass into breast milk. Nursing mothers who must take this drug should bottle-feed.

Seniors
Seniors have twice as much acitretin in their blood as do younger adults but may take acitretin without special precaution.

Actonel *see Bisphosphonates, page 159*

Actos *see Glitazone Antidiabetes Drugs, page 526*

Generic Name

Acyclovir (ae-SYE-kloe-vir) Ⓖ

Brand Name

Zovirax

Type of Drug

Antiviral.

Prescribed For

Serious, frequently recurring herpes simplex infections of the genitals, mucous membrane tissue, and central nervous system; herpes zoster (shingles); varicella (chickenpox); infectious mononucleosis; and viral infections including nongenital herpes simplex, herpes simplex, and cytomegalovirus (CMV) in immunocompromised patients, and varicella pneumonia.

General Information

Acyclovir is the only oral drug that reduces growth rates of the herpes virus and the related viruses, Epstein-Barr, varicella, and CMV; both oral acyclovir and oral ganciclovir work against CMV. Intravenous drugs, including acyclovir injection, may also be used for these viral infections; however, intravenous antiviral drugs are usually reserved for patients with AIDS, cancer, or otherwise compromised immune systems.

Acyclovir is selectively absorbed into cells that are infected with the herpes simplex virus, where it is converted into its active form. Acyclovir works by interfering with the reproduction of viral DNA, slowing the growth of existing viruses. It has little effect on recurrent infections. To treat both local and systemic (whole-body) symptoms acyclovir must be given by intravenous injection or taken by mouth. Local symptoms may be treated with the ointment alone. Oral acyclovir may be taken every day to reduce the number and severity of herpes attacks in people who suffer 10 or more attacks a year; it may also be used to treat intermittent attacks as they occur, but treatment must be started as soon as possible to have the greatest effect.

Cautions and Warnings

Do not use acyclovir ointment if you have had an **allergic** reaction to it or to the major component of the ointment base, polyethylene glycol. Do not apply acyclovir ointment inside the vagina because the polyethylene glycol base may cause irritation and swelling of sensitive vaginal tissue. Acyclovir ointment is not intended for use in the eye and should not be used to treat a herpes infection of the eye.

Some people develop **tenderness, swelling, or bleeding of the gums** while taking acyclovir. Regular brushing, flossing, and gum massage may help prevent these conditions.

Animal testing indicates that acyclovir may affect fertility in men. These effects may be reversible.

Possible Side Effects

Ointment

▼ Most common: mild burning, irritation, rash, and itching. These effects are more likely to occur when treating an initial herpes attack than a recurrent attack. Women are 4 times more likely to experience burning than men.

Capsules, Suspension, and Tablets

▼ Most common: dizziness, headache, diarrhea, nausea, and vomiting.

▼ Less common: appetite loss, stomach gas, constipation, fatigue, rash, not feeling well, leg pains, sore throat, a bad taste in the mouth, sleeplessness, and fever.

▼ Rare: aching joints, weakness, and tingling in the hands or feet.

Drug Interactions

• Do not apply acyclovir together with any other ointment or topical medication.

• Oral probenecid may decrease elimination of acyclovir from the body, which increases blood levels of oral or injected acyclovir, increasing the risk of side effects.

• Combining acyclovir and zidovudine (an AIDS drug—also known as AZT) may lead to severe drowsiness and lethargy.

Food Interactions

Acyclovir may be taken with food if it upsets your stomach.

Usual Dose

Capsules, Suspension, and Tablets

Adult: genital herpes attack—200 mg every 4 hours, 5 times a day for 10 days. Recurrent infections—400 mg 3 times a day or 200 mg 5 times a day for 5 days. Suppressive therapy for chronic herpes—800 mg a day, every day. Herpes zoster—800 mg 5 times a day for 7–10 days.

Child (age 2 and over): Acyclovir has been given to children in daily doses as high as 36 mg per lb. of body weight without any unusual side effects.

Child (under age 2): not recommended.

If you have kidney disease, your doctor should adjust your dose according to the degree of functional loss.

Ointment

Apply every 3 hours, 6 times a day for 7 days. Apply enough medication to cover all visible skin lesions. About ½ in. of ointment should cover about 4 sq. in. of lesions. Your doctor may prescribe a longer course of treatment to prevent the delayed formation of new lesions over the duration of an attack.

Overdosage

Overdose of oral acyclovir may lead to kidney damage due to deposits of acyclovir crystals in the kidneys. Other side effects include agitation, seizures, lethargy, and coma. The risk of experiencing toxic side effects from swallowing acyclovir ointment is quite small. In the case of overdose or accidental ingestion, call your poison control center.

Special Information

Use a finger cot or rubber glove when applying acyclovir ointment to protect against inadvertently spreading the virus. Be sure to apply the medication exactly as directed and to completely cover all lesions. Keep affected areas clean and dry. Loose-fitting clothing will reduce possible irritation of a healing lesion. If you skip several doses, or a day or more of treatment, the drug will not exert its maximum effect.

Herpes may be transmitted even if you do not have symptoms of active disease. To avoid giving the condition to a sexual partner, do not have intercourse while visible herpes lesions are present. A condom offers some protection against transmission of the herpes virus, but spermicidal products and diaphragms do not. Acyclovir alone will not prevent herpes transmission.

Women with genital herpes have an increased risk of cervical cancer. Speak with your doctor about the need for an annual Pap smear.

Call your doctor if acyclovir does not relieve your symptoms, if side effects become severe or intolerable, or if you become pregnant or want to begin breast-feeding. Check with your dentist if you notice swelling or tenderness of the gums.

Special Populations

Pregnancy/Breast-feeding
Acyclovir crosses into the circulation of the fetus. Animal studies have shown that large doses—up to 125 times the human dose—cause damage to both mother and fetus. While there is no information to indicate that acyclovir affects a human fetus, do not use it during pregnancy unless it is specifically prescribed by your doctor and the possible benefit outweighs the risk.

Acyclovir passes into breast milk in concentrations up to 4 times the concentration in blood, and it has been found in the urine of a nursing infant. Although no side effects have been found in nursing babies, mothers who must take acyclovir should consider bottle-feeding.

Seniors
Shingles attacks in people over age 50 tend to be more severe and respond best to acyclovir treatment if the drug is started within 48 to 72 hours of the appearance of the first rash. Seniors with reduced kidney function should be given a lower dose of oral acyclovir than younger adults.

Generic Name

Adapalene (uh-DAP-uh-lene)

Brand Name

Differin

Type of Drug

Anti-acne.

Prescribed For

Acne.

General Information

Adapalene is similar to a retinoid. Retinoids are compounds related to vitamin A and are used in acne treatment. When adapalene is applied to an acne lesion, it modifies several of the processes involved in skin cell function. It reduces inflammation in the acne lesion and slows the formation of the material that fills the lesion. Very little adapalene is absorbed through the skin.

Cautions and Warnings

Do not use adapalene if you are **sensitive** or **allergic** to it. If you are **sunburned,** wait until your sunburn clears before applying adapalene to your skin. **Avoid sun or sunlamp exposure** while using adapalene. If you must be in the sun, be sure to apply sunscreen or wear protective clothing over areas where you have applied adapalene. Extreme wind or cold can also be irritating to skin where adapalene has been applied.

Adapalene can **irritate the skin** if used in combination with products such as medicated or abrasive soaps or cleansers, astringents, or soaps and cosmetics with a strong drying effect. Avoid products containing sulfur, resorcinol, or salicylic acid.

Adapalene can be **highly irritating** if it gets into your eyes or if it is applied to your lips, the angles of your nose, mucous membranes, cuts, abrasions, or sunburned or damaged skin. Avoid using depilatories or waxing while using adapalene.

Possible Side Effects

▼ Most common: redness, irritation, dryness, scaling, itching, and burning are common after applying adapalene to your skin. These effects usually occur during the first 2 to 4 weeks of adapalene use and may be severe enough to cause you to stop using adapalene; call your doctor if this happens to you.

▼ Rare: skin irritation, stinging sunburn, and worsening acne.

Drug Interactions

None known.

Usual Dose

Adult and Child (age 12 and over): Wash affected areas and apply a thin layer of adapalene at bedtime.

Child (under age 12): not recommended.

Overdosage

Accidental ingestion of adapalene can cause liver toxicity and other side effects associated with swallowing large amounts of vitamin A. Swallowing adapalene gel is extremely dangerous for pregnant women, who should not take more vitamin A than is contained in their prenatal vitamins. Infants who swallow adapalene should be taken to a hospital emergency room for treatment. Ingestion of adapalene may cause symptoms such as headache, facial flushing, abdominal pain, dizziness, and weakness.

Special Information

Stop using adapalene and call your doctor if you develop a severe skin reaction or any sign of drug allergy or reaction (symptoms include rash, hives, itching, changes in complexion, and breathing difficulties or irregularities).

Adapalene may exacerbate your acne at first, but you should see improvement within 2 weeks.

If you must be in the sun, be sure to apply sunscreen or wear protective clothing over areas to which you have applied adapalene.

Using more than a thin film of adapalene does not produce better results and may be more irritating to the skin.

If you forget to apply a dose of adapalene, apply it as soon as you remember. If it is almost time for your next application of adapalene, skip the dose you forgot and continue with your regular schedule.

Special Populations

Pregnancy/Breast-feeding

Animal studies of adapalene have shown no effects on the fetus. Since the effect of adapalene on pregnant women is not known, the drug should be used only when the possible benefits outweigh the risks.

It is not known if adapalene passes into breast milk. Nursing mothers should consider bottle-feeding.

Seniors
Seniors may use this drug without special precautions.

Brand Name

Adderall

Generic Ingredients

Dextroamphetamine Sulfate + Dextroamphetamine Saccharate + Amphetamine Aspartate + Amphetamine Sulfate

Other Brand Names
Adderall XR

The information in this profile also applies to the following drug:

Generic Ingredient: Dextroamphetamine Sulfate G
Dexedrine   Dextrostat

Type of Drug
Central-nervous-system stimulant.

Prescribed For

Weight control, attention-deficit hyperactivity disorder (ADHD), and narcolepsy (uncontrollable desire to sleep).

General Information

Amphetamines are stimulants that work on the brain's feeding center. Adderall, which is a mixture of two forms of amphetamine, may be used as a short-term aid in weight reduction. It should not be taken for longer than a few months for this purpose.

Amphetamines may also be prescribed for childhood ADHD. They should be used only after a complete evaluation of the child has been done. Frequency and severity of symptoms and their appropriateness for the age of the child—not solely the presence of certain behavioral characteristics—determine whether drug therapy is required. Many experts believe that amphetamines offer only a temporary solution because they do not permanently change behavioral patterns. Psychological measures must also be taken to ensure successful treatment in the long term.

Cautions and Warnings

Amphetamines should be used with extreme caution because they are highly **addictive** and easily abused.

Do not take this drug if you are **sensitive** or **allergic** to any amphetamine or have **heart disease, high blood pressure, thyroid disease,** or **glaucoma.**

Stimulants like amphetamines are not effective for children whose symptoms are related to environmental factors or primary psychiatric conditions, including psychosis.

Possible Side Effects

▼ Common: heart palpitations, restlessness, over-stimulation, dizziness, sleeplessness, increased blood pressure, and rapid heartbeat.

▼ Less common: euphoria (feeling "high"), hallucinations, muscle spasms and tremors, headache, dry mouth, unpleasant taste in the mouth, diarrhea, constipation, upset stomach, itching, and loss of sex drive.

▼ Rare: psychotic drug reactions.

Drug Interactions

• Combining an amphetamine and a monoamine oxidase inhibitor (MAOI) drug may cause a severe increase in blood pressure as well as bleeding inside the skull. Wait at least 2 weeks after stopping an MAOI before taking an amphetamine.

• Amphetamines may reduce guanethidine's effectiveness for high blood pressure.

• Gastrointestinal acidifying agents lower the absorption of amphetamines.

• Your insulin dosage may need an adjustment if you start taking an amphetamine.

• Tricyclic antidepressants may reduce an amphetamine's effects.

• Amphetamines may decrease the effectiveness of beta blockers.

• Amphetamines may counteract the sedative effect of antihistamines.

Food Interactions

Take this drug with food if it upsets your stomach.

Usual Dose

Weight Control: 5–30 mg a day in divided doses 30–60 minutes before meals; alternately, a single, long-acting dose may be taken in the morning.

ADHD: 2.5–40 mg a day.

Narcolepsy: 5–60 mg a day.

Overdosage

Symptoms include tremors, muscle spasms, restlessness, exaggerated reflexes, rapid breathing, dry mouth, constipation, hallucinations, confusion, panic, and overaggressive behavior. These may be followed by depression, exhaustion, abnormal heart rhythms, blood pressure changes, nausea, vomiting, diarrhea, convulsions, and coma. Take the victim to a hospital emergency room immediately. ALWAYS bring the prescription bottle or container.

Special Information

When taken for weight control, this drug may gradually lose its effectiveness as the body starts breaking it down faster. Do NOT increase your dosage when this occurs. The drug must be discontinued.

To prevent this drug from interfering with sleep, take it at least 6 to 8 hours before bedtime.

Do not crush or chew the sustained-release form.

If you forget your once-daily dose, skip it and go back to your regular schedule the next day. If you take the drug 2 to 3 times a day and miss a dose, take it as soon as you remember. If it is within 3 hours of your next dose, skip the one you forgot and continue with your regular schedule. Never take a double dose.

Special Populations

Pregnancy/Breast-feeding

Use of amphetamines during the early stages of pregnancy may cause birth defects. Amphetamines also increase the risk of premature delivery and low-birth-weight infants and may cause drug withdrawal symptoms in newborns. When this drug is considered crucial by your doctor, its potential benefits must be carefully weighed against its risks.

Amphetamines pass into breast milk. Nursing mothers who must take them should bottle-feed.

Seniors
Seniors are more sensitive to this drug's effects.

Generic Name

Adefovir (ah-deh-FOE-veer)

Brand Name

Hepsera

Type of Drug

Antiviral.

Prescribed For

Chronic active hepatitis B in adults.

General Information

Hepatitis B is one of several different types of hepatitis, a viral infection of the liver. Adefovir is an antiviral drug that can reduce the amount of hepatitis B virus in the bloodstream and slow its spread to healthy liver tissue, however, it cannot cure chronic hepatitis B. People with chronic hepatitis B may develop liver cirrhosis or liver cancer and it is not known if adefovir can prevent these conditions from occurring. Like other viruses and bacteria, the hepatitis B virus can become resistant to the effects of adefovir.

Adefovir works against the hepatitis C virus in a way similar to that of certain acquired immunodeficiency syndrome (AIDS) drugs. It interferes with an enzyme called *reverse transcriptase,* which is an essential component of the viruses reproduction process. Almost half of each dose is eliminated via the urine within 24 hours of taking it.

Cautions and Warnings

Do not take adefovir if you are **sensitive** or **allergic** to it.

Adefovir can be toxic to the kidneys, especially in people who already have some **kidney problems**. Since it is eliminated from the body through the kidneys, people with **kidney disease** are often given lower doses of adefovir.

In some cases, hepatitis can become severely aggravated upon discontinuation of adefovir. Your doctor should check your liver for 12 weeks after the drug is stopped. It is possible that antiviral therapy may have to be re-started.

Adefovir has some activity against the **human immunodeficiency virus (HIV)**. An HIV blood test is recommended before starting adefovir treatment. If you are HIV positive, adefovir could make the HIV virus resistant to future antiviral drugs.

People taking adefovir can develop **liver disease, liver enlargement, fat degeneration, and lactic acidosis (potentially fatal metabolic imbalance)** This may be a reason for your doctor to stop your adefovir treatment. This occurs most frequently in obese women.

Possible Side Effects

▼ Most common: weakness and stomach pain.

▼ Common: headache and nausea.

▼ Less common: intestinal gas, diarrhea, upset stomach, abnormal liver function, cough, sore throat, sinus irritation, itching, rash, and kidney damage.

Drug Interactions

This drug was studied extensively in an attempt to predict possible drug interactions. No major interaction problems have been revealed.

• Taking drugs that can be toxic to the kidneys (such as aminoglycosides, cyclosporine, non-steroidal anti-inflammatory drugs (NSAIDs), tacrolimus, and vancomycin) together with adefovir can lead to the more rapid appearance of kidney damage.

• Ibuprofen, when taken in dosages of 800 mg 3 times a day, will increase adefovir blood levels by about 20 percent, however the importance of this finding is unknown.

Food Interactions

Adefovir may be taken without regard to food or meals.

Usual Dose

Adults: 10 mg once a day. People with kidney disease may take only 10 mg a week. The exact dosage is based on the severity of kidney disease.

Child: not recommended.

Overdosage

Gastrointestinal symptoms are the most likely outcome of an adefovir overdose. Take the victim to a hospital emergency room. ALWAYS bring the prescription bottle or container.

Special Information

Practice safe sex and safe needle use. People taking adefovir may still spread hepatitis B through sexual contact or by sharing needles. Practice safe sex using condoms and dental dams.

Do not share personal items that can have blood or body fluids on them, such as toothbrushes or razor blades.

Try to take adefovir at the same time every day.

Adefovir must be taken continuously to maintain its effectiveness. Be sure to keep enough adefovir on hand so that you do not run out of medicine.

If you take adefovir on a regular schedule and forget a dose, take it as soon as you remember. If it is almost time for your next dose, skip the forgotten dose and continue with your regular schedule. Do not take a double dose of this medicine. Call your doctor if you forget 2 or more doses in a row. Skipping or forgetting too many doses can make the hepatitis C virus resistant to adefovir.

Call your doctor at once if you feel very weak or tired, cold (especially in your arms and legs), dizzy or lightheaded, have unusual muscle pain, trouble breathing, stomach pain with nausea and vomiting, or have a fast or irregular heartbeat. These could be signs of lactic acidosis.

Call your doctor if you experience jaundice (symptoms include yellowing of the skin or whites of the eyes), appetite loss for a few days or more, lower stomach pain, nausea, dark urine, or bowel movements that are light in color. These could be signs of liver toxicity.

Special Populations

Pregnancy/Breast-feeding

Animal studies with adefovir have revealed a tendency for some birth defects when the dosage administered was more than 20 times the average human dose. There is no information on the effect of adefovir during pregnancy. The company that produces adefovir has established a registry to collect information on pregnant women who take this drug. When this drug is considered crucial by your doctor, its potential benefits may be carefully weighed against its risks.

It is not known if adefovir passes into breast milk. Nursing mothers who must take it should bottle-feed.

Seniors

Seniors may be more sensitive to adefovir's side effects because of the natural loss of kidney function that occurs with advancing age.

Advair Diskus see *Salmeterol, page 958*

Brand Name

Aggrenox

Generic Ingredients

Dipyridamole + Aspirin

Type of Drug

Antiplatelet.

Prescribed For

Prevention of recurrent stroke or transient ischemic attack (TIA)—"mini-stroke."

General Information

Stroke is often the result of a clot blocking flow in a blood vessel supplying the brain. Aggrenox helps prevent blood clot formation by reducing the "stickiness" of platelets, blood cells that stick together to form the beginnings of all clots. The combination of ingredients in Aggrenox, which achieve their antiplatelet effects in different ways, prevented 30% more strokes than aspirin in one study.

Cautions and Warnings

Do not use this drug if you are **sensitive** or **allergic** to any of its ingredients or any nonsteroidal anti-inflammatory drug (NSAID). People who have **asthma,** or **nasal polyps and a runny nose,** are likely to be sensitive to aspirin.

The aspirin in Aggrenox can cause Reye's syndrome, a severe reaction (vomiting, lethargy, and belligerence, and possibly worsening to coma) in **children under age 16.**

People with a history of **stomach ulcers or problems** should avoid Aggrenox.

People who have **angina** or have had a recent **heart attack** should be very cautious about taking this drug. It may worsen chest pain.

People with **low blood pressure, liver disease, or kidney failure** should be cautious about taking this drug.

People taking Aggrenox have a higher risk of **bleeding**.

Possible Side Effects

▼ Most common: headache, upset stomach, abdominal pain, nausea, and diarrhea.

▼ Common: pain, tiredness, and vomiting.

▼ Less common: convulsions, rectal bleeding, blood in the stool, hemorrhoids, back pain, accidental injuries, stomach bleeding, feeling unwell, weakness, fainting, memory loss, arthritis, joint or muscle pain, coughing, and respiratory infection.

▼ Rare: Rare side effects can occur in almost any part of the body. Contact your doctor if you experience any side effect not listed above.

▼ Rare: Rare side effects can occur in almost any part of the body. Contact your doctor if you experience any side effect not listed above.

Drug Interactions

• Avoid alcohol. People who take 3 or more drinks a day while using any aspirin-containing product are more likely to develop stomach ulcers or bleeding.

• Aspirin may reduce the blood-pressure-lowering effects of angiotensin-converting enzyme (ACE) inhibitor drugs, beta blockers, and diuretics.

• Aspirin blocks the effects of sulfinpyrazone and probenecid.

• Combining aspirin and acetazolamide or an NSAID can cause kidney problems.

• Aspirin can increase the blood-thinning effects of anticoagulant (blood-thinning) drugs such as warfarin. Avoid this combination.

• Aspirin can increase blood levels of oral antidiabetes drugs, methotrexate, phenytoin, or valproic acid, possibly leading to drug side effects.

• Aspirin counteracts the uric-acid-eliminating effects of probenecid and sulfinpyrazone.

• Dipyridamole increases the level of adenosine in the blood and may increase cardiovascular-related side effects. The adenosine dosage may need to be adjusted when these two drugs are combined.

• Dipyridamole may interfere with cholinesterase inhibitors used to treat myasthenia gravis.

Food Interactions

Aggrenox is best taken on an empty stomach but may be taken with food if it upsets your stomach.

Usual Dose

Adult: 1 capsule (200 mg of sustained-release dipyridamole and 25 mg of aspirin) morning and evening.

Overdosage

Symptoms include a sensation of warmth, flushing, sweating, restlessness, weakness, dizziness, low blood pressure, and rapid heartbeat. Take the victim to a hospital emergency room. ALWAYS bring the prescription bottle or container.

Special Information

Call your doctor if you experience blood in your stool or persistent diarrhea or abdominal or stomach pain.

Avoid alcohol while taking this drug.

In people taking Aggrenox, minor cuts may take longer than normal to stop bleeding.

If you forget a dose, take it as soon as you remember. If it is almost time for your next dose, skip the one you forgot and continue with your regular schedule.

Special Populations

Pregnancy/Breast-feeding

Pregnant women should avoid Aggrenox because of its aspirin content. Aspirin can cause bleeding problems in mother and fetus and result in a low-birth-weight infant. When this drug is considered crucial by your doctor, its potential benefits must be carefully weighed against its risks.

Both ingredients in Aggrenox pass into breast milk. Nursing mothers who must take this drug should bottle-feed.

Seniors

Seniors may take this drug without special precaution.

Generic Name

Albuterol (al-BUE-tuh-rawl) Ⓖ

Brand Names

AccuNeb   Ventolin*
Airet   Ventolin HFA
Proventil*   Ventolin Rotacaps
Proventil HFA   Ventolin Nebules
Proventil Repetabs   Volmax

The information in this profile also applies to the following drugs:

Generic Ingredient: Levalbuterol
Xopenex

Generic Ingredient: Pirbuterol
Maxair

Some products in this brand-name group are alcohol- or sugar-free. Consult your pharmacist.

Type of Drug

Bronchodilator.

Prescribed for

Asthma and bronchospasm.

General Information

Albuterol is similar to other bronchodilator drugs, such as metaproterenol and isoetharine, but it has a weaker effect on nerve receptors in the heart and blood vessels; therefore, it is somewhat safer for people with heart conditions. Levalbuterol is a special form of albuterol that carries a lower risk of side effects.

Cautions and Warnings

Albuterol should be used with caution by people with a history of **angina pectoris** (a condition characterized by brief attacks of chest pain), **heart disease, high blood pressure, stroke** or **seizure, diabetes, thyroid disease, prostate disease,** or **glaucoma**. Excessive use of albuterol inhalants may worsen **asthma** or other respiratory conditions, and may increase breathing difficulties rather than relieve them. In the most extreme cases, people have had heart attacks after using excessive amounts of inhalant.

Possible Side Effects

▼ Most common: restlessness, weakness, anxiety, fear, tension, sleeplessness, tremors, convulsions, dizziness, headache, flushing, appetite changes, pallor, sweating, nausea, vomiting, and muscle cramps.

▼ Less common: angina, abnormal heart rhythms, rapid heartbeat and heart palpitations, high blood pressure, not feeling well, irritability and emotional instability, nightmares, aggressive behavior, bronchitis, stuffy nose, nosebleeds, increased sputum, conjunctivitis (pinkeye), tooth discoloration, voice changes, hoarseness, and urinary difficulty.

Drug Interactions

• Albuterol's effects may be increased by monoamine oxidase inhibitors (MAOIs), tricyclic antidepressants, thyroid drugs, other bronchodilator drugs, and some antihistamines.

• The chance of cardiotoxicity may be increased in people taking both albuterol and theophylline.

• Albuterol is antagonized by beta-blocking drugs such as propranolol.

• Albuterol may antagonize the effects of blood-pressure-lowering drugs, especially methyldopa and guanethidine.

• Albuterol may reduce the amount of digoxin in the blood of people taking both drugs. Digoxin dose adjustment may be required.

Food Interactions

Albuterol tablets are more effective when taken on an empty stomach—1 hour before or 2 hours after meals—but can be taken with food if they upset your stomach.

Usual Dose

Albuterol and Pirbuterol Inhalation

Adult and Child (age 4 and over): 1–2 puffs every 4–6 hours. Asthma triggered by exercise may be prevented by taking 2 puffs 15 minutes before exercising.

Albuterol Inhalation Solution
   Adult and Child (age 12 and over): 2.5 mg 3 or 4 times a day. Dilute 0.5 ml of the 0.5% solution with 2.5 ml of sterile saline. Deliver over 5–15 minutes by nebulizer.

Levalbuterol Inhalation Solution
   Adult and Child (age 12 and over): 0.63 mg 3 times a day every 6 to 8 hours. Some people may benefit from 1.25 mg at each dose. Deliver over 5–15 minutes by nebulizer.

Albuterol Inhalation Capsules
   Adult and Child (age 4 and over): 200–400 mcg inhaled every 4–6 hours using a special Rotahaler device. Adults and adolescents (age 12 and over) may prevent asthma brought on by exercise by inhaling a single 200-mcg dose 15 minutes before exercising.

Albuterol Tablets
   Adult and Child (age 12 and over): starting dose—6–16 mg a day in divided doses. The dosage may slowly be increased to a maximum of 32 mg a day until the asthma is controlled.
   Senior: starting dose—6–8 mg a day in divided doses. Increase to the maximum daily adult dosage, if tolerated.
   Child (age 6–11): starting dose—6–8 mg a day in divided doses. Increase to a maximum daily dose of 24 mg.
   Child (age 2–5): up to 4 mg, 3 times a day.

Albuterol Sustained-Release Tablets
   Adult and Child (age 12 and over): 4–8 mg every 12 hours. Dosage may be cautiously increased to a maximum of 32 mg a day. People being switched from regular to sustained-release tablets generally take the same dosage per day, in fewer tablets—for example, a 4-mg tablet every 12 hours (1 dose) instead of a 2-mg tablet every 6 hours (2 doses).

Overdosage

Overdose of albuterol inhalation usually results in exaggerated side effects, including chest pain and high blood pressure. People who inhale too much albuterol should see a doctor. Overdose of albuterol tablets may lead to changes in heart rate, palpitations, unusual heart rhythm, chest pain, high blood pressure, fever, chills, cold sweats, nausea, vomiting, and dilation of the pupils. Convulsions, sleeplessness, anxiety, and tremors may also develop, and the victim may collapse. If the albuterol overdose was taken within the past half-hour, give the victim syrup of ipecac to induce vomiting. DO NOT GIVE IPECAC IF THE VICTIM IS UNCONSCIOUS OR CONVULSING. If symptoms have already begun to develop, the victim may need to be taken to a hospital emergency room. Call for instructions, and ALWAYS bring the prescription bottle or container.

Special Information

If you are inhaling albuterol, be sure to follow the inhalation instructions that come with the product. The drug should be inhaled during the second half of your inward breath, since this will allow it to reach deeper into your lungs. If you use more than 1 puff per dose, wait about 1–2 minutes between puffs. Do not inhale albuterol if you have food or anything else in your mouth.

Do not take more albuterol than your doctor prescribes. Taking more than you need can worsen your symptoms. If your condition worsens after taking your medicine, call your doctor at once and stop taking it.

Call your doctor immediately if you develop chest pain, palpitations, rapid heartbeat, muscle tremors, dizziness, headache, facial flushing, or urinary difficulty, or if you continue having breathing difficulties after taking the medicine.

If you forget a dose of albuterol, take it as soon as you remember. If it is almost time for your next dose, skip the one you forgot. Do not take a double dose.

Special Populations

Pregnancy/Breast-feeding

When used during childbirth, albuterol can slow or delay natural labor. It can cause rapid heartbeat and high blood sugar in the mother and rapid heartbeat and low blood sugar in the baby. Albuterol also causes birth defects in animal studies. When your doctor considers this drug crucial, its benefits must be cautiously weighed against its risks.

It is not known if albuterol passes into breast milk. Nursing mothers who must take it should consider bottle-feeding.

Seniors

Seniors are more sensitive to the effects of albuterol.

Type of Drug

Aldosterone Blockers

(al-DOH-stir-own)

Brand Names

Generic Ingredient: Eplerenone
Inspra

Generic Ingredient: Spironolactone Ⓖ
Aldactone

Prescribed For

High blood pressure, cirrhosis, and congestive heart failure
(CHF); also used for people with low blood potassium who
require a diuretic.

General Information

Aldosterone blockers limit the access of aldosterone—a hormone that helps to regulate several different body functions—from its receptor. Too much aldosterone results in
high sodium levels, which can lead to water retention and
potassium loss; it can also affect the size, shape, and function
of the heart. Aldosterone blockers are generally combined
with other medicines in the management of disease. These
drugs are useful in removing excess body fluids in conditions
associated with high aldosterone levels.

One in every ten people with high blood pressure has
excess aldosterone in their systems. In people with congestive heart failure (CHF), aldosterone levels can be 20 times
higher than normal, which can worsen their condition, making the use of aldosterone blockers an important part of their
treatment. Aldosterone blockers also help the heart return to
normal size, shape, and function in people with heart failure.
Eplerenone is broken down in the liver, primarily by an
enzyme system known as CYP3A4.

Cautions and Warnings

Do not use aldosterone blockers if you have **kidney failure** or
high blood potassium.

People with **liver disease** should be cautious about using
aldosterone blockers.

People taking an aldosterone blocker should have their potassium levels checked periodically.

Peope with diabetes who have albumin in their urine should not take aldosterone blockers.

Possible Side Effects

Eplerenone

▼ Less common: dizziness, diarrhea, fatigue, flu-like symptoms, coughing, abdominal pain, elevation of blood cholesterol and/or triglyceride levels, and albumin in the urine.

▼ Rare: painful enlargement of the breasts, impotence, and irregular menstrual cycles or deepening of the voice in women.

Spironolactone

▼ Less common: drowsiness, lethargy, headache, gastrointestinal upset, cramps and diarrhea, rash, mental confusion, fever, feeling unwell, painful enlargement of the breasts, impotence, and irregular menstrual cycles or deepening of the voice in women.

Drug Interactions

• Do not combine eplerenone with itraconazole or ketoconazole. These drugs can cause the amount of eplerenone in the blood to increase by up to 500% and may cause fatal increases in blood potassium.

• Mixing eplerenone with erythromycin, fluconazole, saquinavir, or verapamil increases the amount of eplerenone in the blood. People taking this combination must watch for signs of high blood potassium (see "Special Information") and have their blood potassium levels checked regularly.

• Combining a potassium supplement and an aldosterone blocker can lead to dangerously high blood levels of potassium. Do not use a salt-substitute or take any extra potassium unless prescribed by your doctor.

• Combining an aldosterone blocker with an ACE inhibitor drug may significantly raise blood potassium. Be sure your doctor monitors your potassium levels if you combine these drugs.

• Spironolactone may interfere with anticoagulant (blood-thinning) drugs and mitotane (an anticancer drug).

• Aspirin can interfere with the diuretic effect of spironolactone but does not alter its effect on high blood pressure or CHF.

• Combining spironolactone with alcohol, barbiturates, or narcotics can lead to dizziness or fainting when rising suddenly from a sitting or lying position.

• Combining spironolactone and a corticosteroid can lead to very low blood potassium.

• Spironolactone may alter your response to drugs used during general anesthesia.

• Lithium generally should not be combined with any diuretic.

• Combining nonsteroidal anti-inflammatory drugs (NSAIDs) such as indomethacin with aldosterone blockers can lead to severe elevations of blood potassium.

• Spironolactone may raise digoxin blood levels and increase the risk of severe digoxin side effects. Your doctor may have to adjust your digoxin dosage.

Food Interactions

Food appears to increase the amount of spironolactone absorbed into the blood. Take this drug with food at the same time every day.

Usual Dose

Eplerenone
   Adult: 50–100 mg a day.
   Child: not recommended.

Spironolactone
   Adult: Starting dosage is 50–100 mg a day in divided doses for high blood pressure; 100–200 mg a day in divided doses for high fluid levels related to other diseases; and 25 mg a day for CHF.
   Child: 1–2 mg per lb. of body weight a day.

Overdosage

Eplerenone overdose may lead to low blood pressure and high blood potassium. Spironolactone overdose may lead to drowsiness, confusion, rash, nausea, vomiting, dizziness, and diarrhea. Rarely, coma may occur in people with severe liver disease. High blood potassium may also occur, especially in people with kidney disease. Call your local poison control center or a hospital emergency room for more information. If you seek treatment, ALWAYS bring the prescription bottle or container.

Special Information

Take aldosterone blockers exactly as they are prescribed.

High blood levels of potassium associated with aldosterone blockers may cause weakness, lethargy, drowsiness, muscle pain or cramps, and muscular fatigue. Use caution while doing anything that requires intense concentration, like driving or operating machinery.

Do not use a salt substitute or take anything else that is a source of extra potassium, including many multivitamin or supplement products.

People with high blood pressure should not self-medicate with over-the-counter cough, cold, or allergy remedies containing stimulants. These drugs can raise blood pressure effectiveness and have an adverse effect on the heart.

If you forget a dose, take it as soon as you remember. If it is almost time for your next dose, skip the one you forgot and continue with your regular schedule. Do not take a double dose.

Special Populations

Pregnancy/Breast-feeding

Animal studies with eplerenone showed no effects on a developing fetus. Spironolactone crosses into the fetal circulation. When your doctor considers either of these drugs crucial, their potential benefits must be carefully weighed against their risks.

Aldosterone blockers pass into breast milk. Nursing mothers who must take aldosterone blockers should bottle-feed.

Seniors

Seniors may be more sensitive to the effects of these drugs, especially high blood-potassium levels.

Generic Name

Alitretinoin (al-ih-TRET-in-oin)

Brand Name

Panretin

Type of Drug

Retinoid.

Prescribed For

Skin lesions of Kaposi's sarcoma (KS).

General Information

Alitretinoin binds to and activates retinoid receptors in human cells. Once activated, these receptors help stimulate the body's natural mechanisms for limiting tissue growth—in this case, the growth of KS cells. KS lesions, which are primarily associated with human immunodeficiency virus (HIV), can respond to alitretinoin in as little as two weeks, but most people do not start to see results for 4 to 8 weeks or, in some cases, 14 weeks or more.

Cautions and Warnings

Do not use alitretinoin if you are **sensitive** or **allergic** to it or any ingredient in this product.

Alitretinoin is applied to individual KS lesions. It does not treat **systemic KS** or prevent **new KS lesions** from forming.

People taking **systemic KS treatment** because they have developed more than 10 new KS lesions in the past year should not use alitretinoin.

People with **swollen lymph glands, KS that affects the lungs,** or **other KS involvement** should not use alitretinoin.

Possible Side Effects

▼ Most common: rash and burning pain.

▼ Common: itchy, flaking, or peeling skin; cracking, oozing, or other skin problems; swelling; and inflammation.

▼ Less common: tingling in the area to which alitretinoin is applied.

Drug Interactions

• Do not use insect repellant products that contain DEET, a widely used chemical repellant. Alitretinoin increases DEET toxicity.

Usual Dose

Adult: Apply 2–4 times a day to KS skin lesions. Seniors should use this drug with caution.

Child: not recommended.

Overdosage

Little is known about the effects of accidental ingestion. Call your local poison control center or a hospital emergency room for information. If you seek treatment, ALWAYS bring the prescription bottle or container.

Special Information

Apply enough alitretinoin gel to cover the entire skin lesion. Allow the gel to dry for 3 to 5 minutes before covering the area with clothing.

If you use a bandage or dressing, be sure it is not tight and that air can circulate freely over the area.

Avoid applying alitretinoin to unaffected skin because it may be irritated by the drug. Avoid applying near the nose, eyes, or mouth.

Retinoids can cause unusual sensitivity to the sun. While this has not been seen with alitretinoin, you should avoid prolonged exposure to the sun or use sunscreen while taking this drug.

If you forget a dose, apply it as soon as you remember. If it is almost time for your next dose, apply the forgotten dose and then space the rest of your doses throughout the day. Continue with your regular schedule the next day.

Special Populations

Pregnancy/Breast-feeding

Alitretinoin can harm the fetus when sufficient levels of the drug are present in the mother's bloodstream, but it is not known if these levels are achieved during routine use of alitretinoin. Women who are or might be pregnant should only use this drug after discussing its potential benefits and risks with their doctors.

It is not known if alitretinoin passes into breast milk. Nursing mothers who must use alitretinoin should bottle-feed.

Seniors

There is no information on use of alitretinoin by seniors. Seniors should use it with caution.

Allegra   *see **Cetirizine**, page 216*

Allegra-D   *see **Antihistamine-Decongestant Combination Products**, page 96*

Generic Name

Allopurinol   (al-oe-PURE-in-nol) Ⓖ

Brand Name

Zyloprim

Type of Drug

Antigout medication.

Prescribed For

Gout or gouty arthritis; also prescribed for cancer, ulcers, abnormal heart rhythms in heart bypass patients, seizures, and other conditions that may be associated with too much uric acid in the body.

General Information

Unlike other antigout drugs, which affect the elimination of uric acid from the body, allopurinol acts on the system that manufactures uric acid in your body. A high level of uric acid can indicate that you have gout, psoriasis, cancer, or any of a number of other diseases. High levels of uric acid can also be caused by taking certain drugs.

In mouthwash form, allopurinol helps to prevent mouth, stomach, and intestinal ulcers caused by fluorouracil, an antineoplastic drug. Allopurinol may be given before heart bypass surgery to reduce abnormal rhythms and other surgical complications. It can be used to reduce the relapse rates of duodenal ulcers associated with *Helicobacter pylori* infection and to reduce the vomiting of blood from stomach irritation caused by nonsteroidal anti-inflammatory drugs

(NSAIDs). Allopurinol has also been used to control seizures in people for whom standard treatments are not effective.

Cautions and Warnings

Do not take this medication if you have ever developed a **severe reaction** to it. Stop taking the medication immediately and contact your doctor if you develop a **rash** or any other adverse effects while taking allopurinol. Do not start taking allopurinol again if you stopped it because of a severe reaction.

Allopurinol should be used by children only if they have high uric acid levels due to neoplastic disease or to rare metabolic conditions.

A few cases of **liver toxicity** have been associated with allopurinol; they improved when the drug was stopped. People taking allopurinol should periodically be tested for liver and kidney function. People with severely **compromised kidney function** should take a reduced dose of allopurinol.

Possible Side Effects

▼ Most common: rash associated with severe, allergic, or sensitivity reaction to allopurinol. If you develop an unusual rash or other sign of drug toxicity, stop taking this medication and contact your doctor.

▼ Less common: nausea, vomiting, diarrhea, intermittent stomach pain, effects on blood components, and drowsiness or lack of ability to concentrate.

▼ Rare: Rare side effects can occur in almost any part of the body. Contact your doctor if you experience any side effect not listed above.

Drug Interactions

• Large doses of drugs that make your urine more acidic, like megadoses of vitamin C, may increase the risk of kidney stone formation.

• Alcohol, diazoxide, mecamylamine, or pyrazinamide can increase the amount of uric acid in your blood; an increase in your allopurinol dose may be required.

• Allopurinol may increase the action of azathioprine, mercaptopurine, or cyclophosphamide and other anticancer drugs, leading to possible bleeding or infection.

• Allopurinol may prolong the effects of chloropropamide, and can lead to hypoglycemic reactions in patients with kidney disease.

• Taking allopurinol with dacarbazine, probenecid, or sulfinpyrazone may cause excessive reduction of uric acid.

• Allopurinol may interact with anticoagulant (blood-thinning) medications, reducing the rate at which the anticoagulant is broken down in the body. Dosage reduction is necessary.

• People who are susceptible to ampicillin, amoxicillin, bacampicillin, or hetacillin rash are more likely to develop such a reaction while also taking allopurinol.

• Combining a thiazide diuretic or an ACE-inhibitor (for high blood pressure or heart failure) with allopurinol increases the risk of a drug-sensitivity reaction.

• Combining vidarabine with allopurinol may increase the risk of neurotoxic effects and anemia, nausea, pain, and itching.

• Large doses of allopurinol—more than 600 mg a day—may increase the effects of and risk of toxic reactions to theophylline by interfering with its clearance from the body.

Food Interactions

Take each dose with food or a full glass of water. Drink 10 to 12 glasses of water, juices, soda, or another liquid each day to avoid the formation of crystals in your urine or kidneys.

Usual Dose

Adult and Child (age 11 and over): 100–800 mg a day, depending on disease and response.

Child (age 6–10): 200–600 mg a day.

Child (under age 6): 150 mg a day.

The dose should be reviewed periodically by your doctor to be sure that it is producing the desired therapeutic effect.

Overdosage

The expected symptoms of overdose are exaggerated side effects. Allopurinol overdose victims should be taken to a hospital. ALWAYS bring the prescription bottle or container.

Special Information

Allopurinol can make you drowsy or make it difficult to concentrate: Take care while driving a car or operating hazardous equipment.

Call your doctor at once if you develop rash, hives, itching, chills, fever, nausea, muscle aches, unusual tiredness, fever, yellowing of the whites of the eyes or skin, painful urination, blood in the urine, irritation of the eyes, or swelling of the lips or mouth.

Avoid large doses of vitamin C, which can cause the formation of kidney stones during allopurinol treatment. Be sure to drink 10 to 12 8-oz. glasses of water a day while taking this medication.

If you forget to take a dose of allopurinol, take it as soon as possible. If it is almost time for your next regular dose, double this dose. For example, if your regular dose is 100 mg and you miss a dose, take 200 mg at the next usual dose time.

Special Populations

Pregnancy/Breast-feeding

Allopurinol may cause birth defects or interfere with fetal development. Check with your doctor before taking it if you are or might be pregnant.

Allopurinol passes into breast milk. Nursing mothers who must take allopurinol should consider bottle-feeding.

Seniors

No special precautions are required. Follow your doctor's directions and report any side effects at once.

Type of Drug

Alpha Blockers

Brand Names

Generic Ingredient: Alfuzosin
Uroxatral

Generic Ingredient: Terazosin
Hytrin

Prescribed For

High blood pressure and benign prostatic hyperplasia (BPH).

General Information

Alpha blockers block nerve endings known as alpha$_1$ receptors. They reduce blood pressure by dilating (widening) and reducing pressure within the blood vessels. The maximum blood-pressure-lowering effect of terazosin is seen between 2 and 6 hours after taking a single dose. Terazosin's effect lasts for 24 hours.

In BPH, alpha blocers work by relaxing smooth muscles in the prostate and neck of the bladder. This effect is produced by blockage of alpha$_1$ receptors in the affected muscles. Despite the fact that terazosin alleviates the urinary symptoms of BPH, the drug's long-term effect on complications of BPH or the need for urinary surgery is not known. Alpha blockers are broken down in the liver.

Cautions and Warnings

Do not take alpha blockers if you are **allergic** or **sensitive** to them.

Alpha blockers may cause **dizziness and fainting**, especially after the first few doses. This is known as the "first-dose effect" and may be minimized by limiting the first dose to 1 mg at bedtime. The first-dose effect occurs in about 1% of people and may recur if the drug is stopped for a few days and then restarted.

Do not take alfuzosin if you have moderate to severe **liver disease** since this can drastically increase blood concentrations of the drug.

Alpha blockers should be taken with caution if you have **kidney disease**, since blood concentrations may be increased by 50%.

Do not take these medicines if you are already taking an alpha-blocker for either high blood pressure or prostate problems.

Terazosin may slightly reduce **cholesterol levels** and improve the high-density lipoprotein (HDL) to low-density lipoprotein (LDL) ratio, a positive step for people with blood-cholesterol problems.

Terazosin may **reduce the counts of red and white blood cells**.

People taking terazosin may experience a weight gain of about 2 pounds.

Possible Side Effects

Alfuzosin

▼ Most common: dizziness, fatigue, upper respiratory infection, and headache.

▼ Less common: pain, abdominal pain, upset stomach, constipation, nausea, impotence, bronchitis, sinusitis, sore throat, low blood pressure, dizziness, and fainting.

▼ Rare: rash, rapid heartbeat, chest pain, and painful and persistent erection.

Terazosin

▼ Most common: dizziness, weakness, and headache.

▼ Less common: Other side effects can occur in almost any part of the body. Contact your doctor if you experience any side effect not listed.

▼ Rare: depression, reduced sex drive or abnormal sexual function, fluid retention, and weight gain.

Drug Interactions

• Terazosin may interact with beta-blocking drugs to produce a higher rate of dizziness or fainting after taking the first dose of terazosin.

• The blood-pressure-lowering effect of terazosin may be reduced by indomethacin.

• When taken with other blood-pressure-lowering drugs, terazosin severely reduces blood pressure.

• The blood-pressure-lowering effect of clonidine may be reduced by terazosin.

• Antifungal drugs such as itraconazole and ketoconazole and protease inhibitors interfere with the breakdown of alfuzosin in the liver, raising the amount of drug in the blood.

• Alfuzosin moderately increases the amount of diltiazem in the blood.

Food Interactions

Alfuzosin should be taken with food to reduce its GI-irritating effect.

Usual Dose

Alfuzosin
One 10 mg tablet taken after the same meal every day. Do not crush or chew the tablets.

Terazosin
Starting dosage—1 mg at bedtime. Dosage may be increased in increments of 1–5 mg to a total of 20–40 mg a day. Terazosin may be taken once or twice a day. Dosages of 10 mg a day are generally needed to control the symptoms of BPH.

Overdosage

Symptoms may include drowsiness, poor reflexes, and very low blood pressure. Take the victim to a hospital emergency room. ALWAYS bring the prescription bottle or container.

Special Information

Take alpha blockers exactly as they are prescribed and do not stop taking it unless directed to do so by your doctor. Avoid over-the-counter drugs that contain stimulants because they may increase your blood pressure.

Alpha blockers may cause dizziness, headache, and drowsiness, especially 2 to 6 hours after taking your first dose, though these effects may persist after the first few doses. Wait 12 to 24 hours after taking the first dose before driving, operating machinery, or performing any other task that requires intense concentration. You may take alpha blockers at bedtime to minimize this problem.

Call your doctor if you develop severe dizziness, heart palpitations, or any bothersome or persistent side effect.

If you forget a dose, take it as soon as you remember. If it is almost time for your next dose, skip the forgotten dose and continue with your regular schedule. Do not take a double dose.

Special Populations

Pregnancy/Breast-feeding

Large dosages of terazosin damage the fetus in animal studies. When alpha blockers are considered crucial by your doctor, their potential benefits must be carefully weighed against their risks.

It is not known if alfuzosin or terazosin pass into breast milk. Nursing mothers who must take these drugs should consider bottle-feeding.

Seniors
Seniors may be more sensitive to the effects of terazosin.

Generic Name

Alprazolam (al-PRAY-zoe-lam) G

Brand Name

Xanax   Xanax XR

Type of Drug

Benzodiazepine tranquilizer.

Prescribed For

Anxiety, tension, fatigue, and agitation; also prescribed for irritable bowel syndrome, panic attacks, depression, and premenstrual syndrome (PMS).

General Information

Alprazolam is a member of a group of drugs known as benzodiazepines. Benzodiazepines directly affect the brain. They can relax you and make you more tranquil or sleepier, or they can slow nervous system transmissions in such a way as to act as an anticonvulsant. Many doctors prefer benzodiazepines to other drugs that can be used to similar effect because they tend to be safer, have fewer side effects, and are usually as effective, if not more so.

Cautions and Warnings

Do not take alprazolam if you know you are **sensitive** or **allergic** to it or to another benzodiazepine drug, including clonazepam.

Alprazolam can aggravate narrow-angle **glaucoma,** but you may take it if you have open-angle glaucoma.

Other conditions where alprazolam should be avoided are: severe **depression,** severe **lung disease, sleep apnea** (intermittent cessation of breathing during sleep), **liver disease, drunkenness,** and **kidney disease**. In each of these conditions, the depressive effects of alprazolam may be enhanced or could be detrimental to your overall condition.

Alprazolam should not be taken by **psychotic patients** because it is not effective for them and can trigger unusual excitement, stimulation, and rage.

Alprazolam is meant to be used for no more than 3 to 4 months in a row. Your condition should be reassessed before continuing your medicine beyond that time.

Alprazolam may be addictive. Drug withdrawal may develop if you stop taking it after only 4 weeks of regular use but is more likely after longer use. It may start with anxiety and progress to tingling in the hands or feet, sensitivity to bright light, sleep disturbances, cramps, tremors, muscle tension or twitching, poor concentration, flu-like symptoms, fatigue, appetite loss, sweating, and changes in mental state.

Possible Side Effects

▼ Most common: mild drowsiness during the first few days of therapy. Weakness and confusion may occur, especially in seniors and in those who are sickly. If these effects persist, contact your doctor.

▼ Less common: depression, lethargy, disorientation, headache, inactivity, slurred speech, stupor, dizziness, tremors, constipation, dry mouth, nausea, inability to control urination, sexual difficulties, irregular menstrual cycle, changes in heart rhythm, low blood pressure, fluid retention, blurred or double vision, itching, rash, hiccups, nervousness, inability to fall asleep, and occasional liver dysfunction. If you experience any of these symptoms, stop taking the medicine and contact your doctor immediately.

▼ Rare: Rare side effects can occur in almost any part of the body. Contact your doctor if you experience any side effect not listed above.

Drug Interactions

• Alprazolam is a central-nervous-system depressant. Avoid alcohol, other tranquilizers, narcotics, barbiturates, monoamine oxidase inhibitors (MAOIs), antihistamines, and antidepressants. Taking alprazolam with these drugs may result in excessive depression, tiredness, sleepiness, breathing difficulties, or related symptoms.

• Smoking may reduce the effectiveness of alprazolam by increasing the rate at which it is broken down by the body.

• The effects of alprazolam may be prolonged when taken together with cimetidine, oral contraceptives, disulfiram, fluoxetine, isoniazid, itraconazole, ketoconazole, metoprolol, probenecid, propoxyphene, propranolol, rifampin, and valproic acid.

• Theophylline may reduce alprazolam's sedative effects.

• If you take antacids, separate them from your alprazolam dose by at least 1 hour to prevent them from interfering with the absorption of alprazolam into the bloodstream.

• Alprazolam may raise digoxin blood levels and the chances of digoxin toxicity.

• The effect of levodopa may be decreased if it is taken together with alprazolam.

• Combining alprazolam with phenytoin may increase phenytoin blood concentrations and the chances of phenytoin toxicity.

Food Interactions

Alprazolam is best taken on an empty stomach but may be taken with food if it upsets your stomach.

Usual Dose

Adult: 0.5–6 mg a day. Dosage must be tailored to your individual needs.

Child (under age 18): not recommended.

Overdosage

Symptoms of overdose are confusion, sleepiness, poor coordination, lack of response to pain such as a pinprick, loss of reflexes, shallow breathing, low blood pressure, and coma. The victim should be taken to a hospital emergency room. ALWAYS bring the prescription bottle or container.

Special Information

Alprazolam can cause tiredness, drowsiness, inability to concentrate, or related symptoms. Be careful if you are driving, operating machinery, or performing other activities that require concentration.

Anyone taking alprazolam for more than 3 or 4 months at a time may have a drug withdrawal reaction if the medicine is stopped suddenly (see "Cautions and Warnings").

If you forget a dose of alprazolam, take it as soon as you remember. If it is almost time for your next dose, skip the dose you forgot and return to your regular schedule. Do not take a double dose. If you take Xanax XR, take your full daily dose once a day in the morning. Do not chew or crush Xanax XR tablets.

Special Populations

Pregnancy/Breast-feeding

Alprazolam may cause birth defects if taken during the first 3 months of pregnancy. You should avoid alprazolam while pregnant.

Alprazolam may pass into breast milk. Nursing mothers who must take alprazolam should bottle-feed.

Seniors

Seniors, especially those with liver or kidney disease, are more sensitive to the effects of alprazolam and generally require smaller doses to achieve the same effect.

Generic Name

Alprostadil (al-PROS-tuh-dil) Ⓖ

Brand Names

Caverject   Muse
Edex

Type of Drug

Anti-impotence agent.

Prescribed For

Erectile dysfunction; also prescribed for atherosclerosis (hardening of the arteries), gangrene, and pain due to blood vessel disease.

General Information

A male erection happens when blood flows into blood vessels and holding areas inside the penis. Problems occur when blood cannot move into the penis as it normally should. Alprostadil (prostaglandin E1 or PGE1) helps men get and keep an erection by dilating blood vessels that supply the penis and by relaxing muscles to help expand holding areas. Alprostadil also dilates other vessels and reduces platelet stickiness—which slows blood-clotting rates—and relaxes some muscle groups. Alprostadil must be injected into the tissue of the penis or inserted into the urethra.

Cautions and Warnings

Do not take alprostadil if you are **allergic** to it or to other prostaglandin drugs. Alprostadil can cause **priapism** (painful erection lasting more than 6 hours). People with diseases where priapism is a possibility—**sickle cell anemia or trait, multiple myeloma, leukemia**—those with **penile deformities,** or **penile implants, women, children,** or **those for whom sexual activity could be dangerous** should not use alprostadil.

Penile pain is common after using either form of alprostadil, although it is usually mild or moderate.

Possible Side Effects

Injection
▼ Most common: penile pain.
▼ Less common: prolonged erection; penile fibrosis (deformity); blood blister or black-and-blue marks at the injection site, usually caused by poor injection technique; penis disorders, including yeast infection, numbness, irritation, sensitivity, itching, redness, and torn skin; penile rash or swelling; headache; dizziness; fainting; respiratory infection; flu symptoms; sinus inflammation; runny or stuffed nose; cough; blood pressure changes; local pain; prostate problems; back pain; and general pain.
▼ Rare: Rare side effects can affect the penis, kidney and urinary tract, heart and blood, skin, and eyes. Contact your doctor if you experience any side effect not listed above.

Pellets
▼ Most common: penile pain.
▼ Common: urethral pain, burning or bleeding, and testicular pain.
▼ Less common: headache, dizziness, respiratory infection, flu symptoms, runny nose, sinus inflammation, low blood pressure, back pain, pelvic pain, and general pain.
▼ Rare: Rare side effects can affect the kidney and urinary tract, heart and blood, skin, and eyes. Contact your doctor if you experience any side effect not listed above.

Drug Interactions

• Alprostadil can increase the effect of anticoagulant (blood-thinning) drugs. Your doctor may have to adjust the dose of your anticoagulant.

• Alprostadil may decrease the amount of cyclosporine in your blood.

• The safety of combining alprostadil with other drugs that affect blood vessels is not known. These combinations should be used with caution.

Food Interactions

None known.

Usual Dose

Dosage must be individualized to your need and response.

Overdosage

Alprostadil overdose can lead to an extended and painful erection, as well as other side effects. Overdose victims should seek medical attention.

Special Information

Patient information leaflets are included with each alprostadil prescription. Read this information before you use your prescription.

You must be trained in proper injection technique by your doctor. Self-injection should be permitted only after your doctor has made sure you know how to do it properly.

Alprostadil begins working within 5 to 10 minutes after taking it. Dosage should be set so that your erection lasts for about 30 to 60 minutes. Use the lowest dose that works.

Special Populations

Pregnancy/Breast-feeding

This product should not be used by women. Men using alprostadil must use a condom if they have intercourse with a pregnant woman. Alprostadil passes into semen and will affect the development of a fetal heart if a condom is not worn.

Seniors

Seniors may use alprostadil without special precaution.

Altace *see Quinapril, page 913*

Amaryl *see Sulfonylurea Antidiabetes Drugs, page 1003*

Ambien *see Zolpidem, page 1178*

Generic Name

Aminolevulinic Acid (ah-MEE-noe-lev-ue-LIH-nic)

Brand Name

Levulan Kerastick

Type of Drug

Photodynamic therapy (PDT) sensitizer.

Prescribed For

Actinic keratoses.

General Information

Actinic keratoses are skin lesions that develop on sun-exposed areas of the face or hands in older adults with fair skin. Dermatologists consider them precancerous. Aminolevulinic acid solution is applied to the lesions in the doctor's office in preparation for PDT. By enhancing light sensitivity in treated skin, aminolevulinic acid increases the effectiveness of PDT, which is a form of light therapy. PDT is administered 1 day after application of this drug.

Cautions and Warnings

Aminolevulinic acid should not be applied around the **eyes** or inside the **nose** or **mouth**. Do not use this drug if you are **allergic** to it or porphyrins or have **porphyria**.

This drug causes **increased sensitivity to the sun and bright indoor lighting**. Skin reactions that may occur as a result of this sensitivity cannot be prevented by using sunscreen (see "Special Information").

Possible Side Effects

▼ Most common: scaling, crusting, itching, and changes in skin color. During PDT, which lasts for about 17 minutes, you will experience tingling, stinging, and a prickling or burning sensation in the treated lesions. These effects should begin to go away at the conclusion of PDT, though the lesions and surrounding skin will appear red. Swelling and scaling may also occur. These effects are temporary and should completely resolve within 4 weeks.

▼ Common: skin erosion and welts.

▼ Less common: pain, tenderness, swelling, skin ulcers, small blisters, oozing, loss of sensation in the area of application, scabs, and scratch marks.

Drug Interactions

• Other drugs that enhance your sensitivity to light may increase the effects of aminolevulinic acid. These drugs include griseofulvin, thiazide diuretics, sulfonylureas, phenothiazines, sulfonamides, and tetracycline medications.

Usual Dose

Aminolevulinic acid is applied to lesions in the doctor's office 14–18 hours prior to PDT.

Overdosage

Little is known about the effects of accidental ingestion, which is unlikely to occur because this drug is administered in a doctor's office.

Special Information

Only qualified medical personnel should administer this drug.

After application of the drug, avoid exposing the lesions to sunlight or bright indoor lighting for at least 40 hours. Wear a wide-brimmed hat and protective clothing during this period; sunscreen is not effective. Do not wash treated lesions until PDT has been administered.

If you experience a stinging or burning sensation, you may be able to alleviate these effects by shielding the lesions from light.

Special Populations

Pregnancy/Breast-feeding

The safety of using aminolevulinic acid during pregnancy is not known. When this drug is considered crucial by your doctor, its potential benefits must be carefully weighed against its risks.

It is not known if aminolevulinic acid passes into breast milk. Nursing mothers who must use it should consider bottle-feeding.

Seniors

Seniors may use this drug without special precaution.

Generic Name

Amiodarone (ah-mee-OE-duh-rone) G

Brand Name

Cordarone   Pacerone

Type of Drug

Antiarrhythmic.

Prescribed For

Abnormal heart rhythms.

General Information

Amiodarone should be prescribed only in situations where the abnormal rhythm is so severe as to be life-threatening and does not respond to other drug treatments. Amiodarone works by decreasing the sensitivity of heart tissue to nervous impulses within the heart. It has not been proven that people taking this drug will live longer than those with similar conditions who do not take it. Amiodarone may exert its effects 2 to 5 days after you start taking it, but often takes 1 to 3 weeks to affect your heart. Amiodarone's antiarrhythmic effects can last for weeks or months after you stop taking it.

Cautions and Warnings

Do not take amiodarone if you are **allergic** or **sensitive** to it or if you have **heart block**.

Amiodarone can cause **potentially fatal drug side effects**. At high doses, 10% or more of people taking this drug can develop potentially fatal **lung and respiratory effects,** beginning with cough and progressive breathing difficulties. **Liver damage** caused by amiodarone is usually mild. In rare cases, amiodarone has been associated with liver failure that resulted in death.

Amiodarone can cause **heart block,** a drastic slowing of electrical impulse movement between major areas of the heart, or extreme slowing of the heart rate. Amiodarone heart block occurs about as often as heart block caused by some other antiarrhythmic drugs, but its effects may last longer than those of the other drugs. Amiodarone can also **worsen existing abnormal heart rhythms** in 2% to 5% of people who take the drug. These effects can be fatal.

People taking amiodarone may develop optic nerve irritation, leading to **partial or complete loss of vision**. Most adults who take amiodarone for 6 months or more develop tiny deposits in the corneas of their eyes. These deposits may cause **blurred vision** or **halos** in up to 10% of people taking amiodarone. Some people develop dry eyes and sensitivity to bright light.

One in ten people taking amiodarone can experience **unusual sensitivity to the effects of the sun**. Use an appropriate sunscreen product and reapply it frequently.

Amiodarone can cause **thyroid abnormalities**. It may worsen an already sluggish thyroid gland in 2% to 10% of people taking the drug, and increase thyroid activity in 2% of people taking it. Amiodarone has also been associated with an increase in risk of thyroid tumors.

Antiarrhythmic drugs are less effective and cause abnormal rhythms if blood potassium is low.

Possible Side Effects

About 75% of people taking 400 mg or more of amiodarone a day develop some drug side effects. As many as 18% have to stop taking the drug because of a side effect.

Possible Side Effects *(continued)*

▼ Common: fatigue, not feeling well, tremors, unusual involuntary movements, loss of coordination, an unusual walk, muscle weakness, low blood pressure, dizziness, tingling in the hands or feet, reduced sex drive, sleeplessness, headache, nervous system problems, nausea, vomiting, constipation, appetite loss, abdominal pain, dry eyes, unusual sensitivity to bright light, and seeing halos around bright lights. Unusual sun sensitivity is the most common skin reaction to amiodarone, but people taking this drug can develop a blue skin discoloration that may not go away completely when the drug is stopped. Other skin reactions are sun rashes, hair loss, and black-and-blue spots.

▼ Rare: inflammation of the lung or fibrous deposits in the lungs, changes in thyroid function, changes in taste or smell, bloating, unusual salivation, and changes in blood clotting. Amiodarone can cause heart failure, reduced heart rate, and abnormal rhythms. Up to 9% of people taking amiodarone develop abnormalities in liver function.

Drug Interactions

• Amiodarone increases the effects of metoprolol and other beta blockers, digoxin, flecainide, fentanyl, liclocaine, procainamide, quinidine, theophylline, cyclosporine, and warfarin and other anticoagulants. These interactions can take from 2 or 3 days to several weeks to develop. The dosage of these drugs must be drastically reduced.

• Fluoroquinolones increase the effects of amiodarone, which can cause dangerous side effects.

• When amiodarone and phenytoin are taken together, both drugs can be affected. Amiodarone can be antagonized by phenytoin and other hydantoin anticonvulsants, and the effect of phenytoin can be increased by amiodarone.

• Cholestyramine interferes with the absorption of amiodarone into the bloodstream.

• Cimetidine and ritonavir interfere with the breakdown of amiodarone, leading to high drug blood levels and the increased possibility of side effects.

• Azithromycin can interfere with the effectiveness of amiodarone. This interaction may lead to dizziness and cardiac instability.

Food Interactions

Amiodarone should be taken on an empty stomach, as food delays its absorption into your bloodstream. If amiodarone upsets your stomach, however, you may take it with food.

Usual Dose

Starting dose—800–1600 mg a day, taken in 1 or 2 doses, usually for 1–3 weeks. Maintenance dose—400 mg a day. You should take the lowest effective dose in order to minimize side effects.

Overdosage

The effects of amiodarone overdose include low blood pressure, shock, slow heartbeat, and liver toxicity. Overdose victims should be taken to a hospital emergency room for treatment. ALWAYS bring the prescription bottle or container.

Special Information

Side effects are very common with amiodarone; 75% of people taking the drug will experience some drug-related problem.

Call your doctor if you develop chest pain, breathing difficulties or any other sign of changes in lung function, abnormal heartbeat, bloating in your feet or legs, tremors, fever, chills, sore throat, unusual bleeding or bruising, changes in skin color, unusual sunburn, or any other unusual side effect. See your doctor for an eye exam if your vision changes at all while taking amiodarone.

Amiodarone can make you dizzy or light-headed. Take care while driving a car or performing complex tasks.

If you take amiodarone once a day and forget to take a dose, but remember within 12 hours, take it as soon as possible. If you do not remember until later, skip the dose you forgot and continue with your regular schedule. If you take amiodarone twice a day and remember within 6 hours of your regular dose, take it as soon as you remember. Call your doctor if you forget to take 2 or more doses in a row. Do not take a double dose.

Special Populations

Pregnancy/Breast-feeding

In high doses, amiodarone has been found to be toxic to animal fetuses. Women of childbearing age should use an effective contraceptive while taking amiodarone. If you are or might be pregnant and this drug is considered crucial by your doctor, its potential benefits must be weighed against its risks.

Amiodarone passes into breast milk. Nursing mothers who must take this drug should bottle-feed.

Seniors

Dosage reduction may be needed in seniors with poor liver function.

Generic Name

Amlexanox (am-LEX-an-ox)

Brand Name

Aphthasol

Type of Drug

Skin-ulcer treatment.

Prescribed For

Canker sores in people with normal immune systems.

General Information

Amlexanox slows the production or release of factors involved in the body's inflammatory response. It aids in the healing of mouth ulcers, but the exact way that it accelerates the healing process is not known.

Cautions and Warnings

Do not use amlexanox if you are **sensitive** or **allergic** to it or to any ingredient in the paste. Stop using this drug if you develop a persistent rash or irritation.

Possible Side Effects

▼ Less common: transient pain, stinging, or burning after application.

▼ Rare: mouth irritation, diarrhea, and nausea.

Drug Interactions

None known.

Food Interactions

Do not apply amlexanox while you have any food in your mouth.

Usual Dose

Apply a small amount (¼ in.) to each mouth ulcer four times a day, preferably after breakfast, lunch, and dinner, and at bedtime.

Overdosage

Swallowing even a whole tube of amlexanox would probably cause only upset stomach, nausea, diarrhea, and vomiting. Call your local poison control center or hospital emergency room for more information.

Special Information

Begin using amlexanox as soon as possible after noticing a mouth ulcer and use it until your ulcers heal. Call your doctor if the pain does not get better or the sores do not heal after 10 days of using amlexanox.

Make sure your teeth and mouth are clean before applying amlexanox paste. Squeeze ¼ in. of the paste onto your finger and apply it to each mouth ulcer using gentle pressure.

Wash your hands immediately after using amlexanox. If you get the paste into your eyes, wash it out at once using cool water.

If you forget a dose of amlexanox, use it as soon as you remember. If it is almost time for your next dose, skip the dose you forgot and continue with your regular schedule. Do not apply more than the recommended amount at any time.

Special Populations

Pregnancy/Breast-feeding

The effect of amlexanox on pregnancy is not known; use it only after discussing the possible risks and benefits with your doctor.

Amlexanox passes into the milk of nursing animals, but its effect in humans is not known. Nursing mothers should use this drug with caution.

Seniors

Seniors may use amlexanox without special precaution.

Generic Name

Amlodipine (am-LOE-dih-pene)

Brand Name

Amvaz   Norvasc

Combination Products

Generic Ingredients: Amlodipine + Atorvastatin
Caduet

Type of Drug

Calcium channel blocker.

Prescribed For

Angina pectoris, Prinzmetal's angina, and high blood pressure; has also been studied for heart failure.

General Information

Amlodipine is one of many calcium channel blockers available in the United States. These drugs block the passage of calcium, an essential factor in muscle contraction, into the heart and smooth muscles. Such blockage interferes with the contraction of these muscles, which in turn dilates (widens) the veins and vessels that supply blood to them. This dilating effect reduces blood pressure, the amount of oxygen used by the heart muscles, and the risk of blood vessel spasm. Amlodipine is therefore useful in treating not only high blood pressure but also angina pectoris (brief attacks of chest pain), a condition related to poor oxygen supply to the heart muscles.

Amlodipine affects the movement of calcium only into muscle cells; it has no effect on calcium in the blood.

Cautions and Warnings

Amlodipine may, in rare instances, cause **low blood pressure** in some people taking it for reasons other than hypertension. This is more of a problem with other calcium channel blockers.

Amlodipine may worsen **heart failure** in some people and should be used with caution if heart failure is present.

Calcium channel blockers, alone and with aspirin, have caused **bruises, black-and-blue marks,** and **bleeding** due to an anticoagulant effect. This is mostly a problem with nifedipine but should be considered for all members of the group.

Amlodipine may cause **angina** when treatment is first started, when dosage is increased, or if the drug is rapidly withdrawn. This can be avoided by gradually reducing dosage.

Studies have shown that people taking calcium channel blockers—usually those taken several times a day, not those taken only once daily—have a greater chance of having a **heart attack** than people taking beta blockers or another medicine for the same purposes. Discuss this with your doctor to be sure you are receiving the best possible treatment.

Do not take this drug if you have had an **allergic reaction** to it in the past.

People with severe **liver disease** may require reduced dosage.

Possible Side Effects

▼ Most common: headache, dizziness or light-headedness, anxiety, nausea, swelling in the arms or legs, heart palpitations, and flushing.

▼ Less common: sleepiness, muscle weakness, cramps or abdominal discomfort, itching, rash, sexual difficulties, wheezing or shortness of breath, muscle cramps, pain, and inflammation.

▼ Rare: Rare side effects can occur in almost any part of the body. Contact your doctor if you experience any side effect not listed above.

> **Possible Side Effects** *(continued)*
>
> For side effects for Caduet, see also Statin Cholesterol-Lowering Agents, page 986.

Drug Interactions

• Amlodipine may interact with beta-blocking drugs to cause heart failure, very low blood pressure, or an increased incidence of angina.

• Amlodipine may cause unexpected blood-pressure reduction when combined with other antihypertensive drugs; however, this interaction is more likely with other calcium channel blockers.

• The combination of quinidine (prescribed for abnormal heart rhythm) and amlodipine must be used with caution because it can produce low blood pressure, very slow heart rate, abnormal heart rhythms, and swelling in the arms or legs.

• Amlodipine can increase the effects of theophylline—prescribed for asthma and other respiratory problems—and related drugs.

• Patients taking amlodipine who are given fentanyl as a short-term surgical anesthetic may experience very low blood pressure.

For drug interactions for Caduet, see also Statin Cholesterol-Lowering Drugs, page 986.

Food Interactions

None known.

Usual Dose

5–10 mg once a day. Do not stop taking amlodipine abruptly. The dosage should be gradually reduced over a period of time.

Overdosage

Overdose of amlodipine can cause nausea, weakness, dizziness, confusion, and slurred speech. Take overdose victims to a hospital emergency room, or call your local poison control center for directions. You may be asked to make the patient vomit to remove the medication from the stomach. If you go to the emergency room, ALWAYS bring the prescription bottle or container.

Special Information

Call your doctor if you develop constipation, nausea, weakness or dizziness, swelling in the hands or feet, breathing difficulties, or increased heart pains, or if other side effects are bothersome or persistent.

If you are taking amlodipine for high blood pressure, be sure to continue taking your medication even if you feel well, and follow any instructions for diet restriction or other treatments.

It is important to maintain good dental hygiene while taking amlodipine and to use extra care when using your toothbrush or dental floss because of the chance that the drug will make you more susceptible to certain infections.

If you forget a dose of amlodipine, take it as soon as you remember. If it is almost time for your next dose, skip the dose you forgot and continue with your regular schedule. Do not take a double dose.

Special Populations

Pregnancy/Breast-feeding

Animal studies of amlodipine show that it may damage a fetus. Other calcium channel blockers can be used to treat severe high blood pressure associated with pregnancy, so there is no reason for women who are or might become pregnant to take amlodipine.

It is not known if amlodipine passes into breast milk. Nursing mothers who take amlodipine should consider bottle-feeding.

Seniors

Seniors, especially those with liver disease, are more sensitive to the effects of this drug and may require reduced dosage.

Amoxil   see *Penicillin Antibiotics,* page 825

Generic Name

Amprenavir   (am-PREN-ah-vire)

Brand Name

Agenerase

The information in this profile also applies to the following drug:

Generic Ingredient: Fosamprenavir
Lexiva

Type of Drug

Protease inhibitor.

Prescribed For

Human immunodeficiency virus (HIV) infection.

General Information

Protease inhibitors revolutionized the fight against acquired immunodeficiency syndrome (AIDS) because, when combined with other drugs, they reduce the amount of HIV virus in the bloodstream to levels that are often undetectable by current methods, CD_4 cell immune system counts and viral load measurements (amount of virus in the blood). Amprenavir is taken together with other anti-HIV medications in "drug cocktails" to take advantage of different avenues of attack against the HIV virus. Fosamprenavir is rapidly and almost completely converted to amprenavir by the body and then exerts its protease inhibitor effects. It has no anti-HIV effect on its own. Triple-drug cocktails were responsible for the reduction in the AIDS death rate that began in 1996. Protease inhibitors are always taken together with 1 or 2 nucleoside antiviral drugs, such as AZT, ddI, ddC, or 3TC. Multiple drug therapy has changed the current view of HIV from a fatal disease to a manageable chronic illness.

Protease inhibitors work in a unique way, but they are not a cure for HIV infection or AIDS. When the HIV virus attacks a cell, it must be converted into viral DNA. Other drugs, known as reverse transcriptase inhibitors, interfere with this step, but they need help in fighting HIV. Protease inhibitors work at the end of the HIV reproduction process, when proteins are "cut" by a protease enzyme into strands of exactly the right size to duplicate HIV. Protease inhibitors prevent the mature HIV virus from being formed by interfering with this cutting process. Proteins that are cut incorrectly or that remain uncut are inactive.

People taking a protease inhibitor may still develop secondary infections or conditions associated with HIV disease. Because of this, it is very important for you to remain under the care of a doctor or other health care provider. The long-term effects of amprenavir are not known. You may be able to pass the HIV virus to others even if you are on triple-drug therapy.

Cautions and Warnings

Do not take amprenavir if you are **sensitive** or **allergic** to it. People allergic to **sulfa drugs** may also be allergic to amprenavir.

People with **liver disease** may require reduced dosage.

Severe and **life-threatening skin reactions** can develop in people taking amprenavir.

Amprenavir may raise your blood sugar, worsen **diabetes,** or bring out latent diabetes. Treatment with insulin or an oral diabetes drug may be required in such cases.

The risk of bleeding may be increased in people with **hemophillia** who take protease inhibitors.

Protease inhibitors can cause the redistribution of body fat, leading to **buffalo hump, breast enlargement, abnormal thinness,** or a **round, moon-shaped face.**

Possible Side Effects

Amprenavir is always taken with other drugs, so the side effects listed here are associated with multiple drug therapy rather than amprenavir taken alone.

▼ Most common: nausea, vomiting, diarrhea, mild rash, itching, high blood sugar, and high blood-triglyceride levels.

▼ Common: changes in sense of taste, and tingling in or around the mouth or in the hands or feet.

▼ Less common: depression and high blood-cholesterol levels.

▼ Rare: life-threatening rash, diabetes, and buffalo hump.

Amprenavir has been studied in children age 4 to 12 and side effects are the same as in adults.

Drug Interactions

Amprenavir can interact with many drugs. Be sure to tell your doctor about all the medications you are taking.

• Astemizole, bepridil, dihydroergotamine, ergotamine, lidocaine injection, midazolam, triazolam, ergot derivatives, tricyclic antidepressants, and quinidine should never be combined with amprenavir because of the risk of severe, life-threatening reactions.

• You may require dosage adjustments of amiodarone, lidocaine injection, warfarin, and tricyclic antidepressants when you start taking amprenavir.

• Do not combine rifampin with amprenavir because it reduces drug levels by 90%. Rifabutin reduces the amount of amprenavir in the blood by 15%.

• Combining amprenavir and sildenafil or vardenafil drastically increases the risk of sildenafil side effects including low blood pressure, visual changes, and a persistent and painful erection.

• Amprenavir can reduce the effectiveness of birth control pills. Use another means of contraception while taking amprenavir.

• Amprenavir must be taken at least 1 hour before or after antacids.

• Combining amprenavir with statin cholesterol-lowering drugs increases the risk of drug toxicity.

• Carbamazepine, phenytoin, and phenobarbital reduce the effectiveness of amprenavir.

• Other drugs that could interact with amprenavir and should be used with caution are: dapsone, erythromycin, itraconazole, alprazolam, clorazepate, diazepam, flurazepam, calcium channel blockers, delavirdine, efavirenz, nevirapine, estrogens, progestogens, corticosteroids, clozapine, carbamazepine, loratidine, and pimozide.

Food Interactions

This drug can be taken without regard to food or meals, but high-fat foods may reduce the effectiveness of amprenavir.

Usual Dose

Amprenavir Capsules

Adult and Child (age 13–16): 1200 mg (8 capsules) twice a day with other anti-HIV drugs. Adults with moderate-to-severe liver disease should take 300–450 mg twice a day.

Child (age 4–12): 9 mg per lb. 2 times a day or 6.8 mg per lb. 3 times a day with other anti-HIV drugs, up to 2400 mg a day. This dosage also applies to older children who weigh less than 110 lbs.

Child (under age 4): not recommended.

Amprenavir Oral Solution

Child (age 4–12): 10.2 mg per lb. 2 times a day or 7.7 mg per lb. 3 times a day with other anti-HIV drugs, up to 2800 mg a day. This dosage also applies to older children who weigh less than 110 lbs.

Child (under age 4): not recommended.

Fosamprenavir

Adult: First-time treatment—1,400 mg twice daily (without ritonavir); or 1,400 mg once daily with 200 mg ritonavir once daily; or 700 mg twice daily with 100 mg ritonavir twice daily. Previous treatment with another protease inhibitor—700 mg twice daily plus ritonavir 100 mg twice daily.

Child: not recommended.

Overdosage

Overdose symptoms are likely to be exaggerated side effects. Overdose victims should be taken to a hospital emergency room. ALWAYS bring the prescription bottle or container.

Special Information

Amprenavir oral solution is absorbed less efficiently than the capsules. They cannot be interchanged for each other on a milligram for milligram basis.

Tell your doctor about all other prescription and over-the-counter drugs you are taking because of the risk of drug interactions.

It is very important to take amprenavir exactly as prescribed. If you forget a dose of amprenavir, take it as soon as you remember. If you miss a dose by more than 4 hours, skip the forgotten dose and continue with your regular schedule. Never take a double dose.

Call your doctor if you have a rash, nausea, diarrhea, or vomiting, or any intolerable drug side effect.

Amprenavir capsules contain large amounts of vitamin E. Do not take a vitamin E supplement while taking this drug.

Special Populations

Pregnancy/Breast-feeding

Amprenavir caused abortions and birth defects in pregnant animals. Its effect on pregnant women is not known and the drug should be taken only after risks and possible benefits have been discussed with your doctor.

Nursing mothers who must take amprenavir should bottle-feed.

Seniors
Amprenavir was not studied in seniors. Seniors taking this drug must use caution.

Generic Name

Anagrelide (ah-NAG-rel-ide)

Brand Name

Agrylin

Type of Drug

Antiplatelet.

Prescribed For

Essential thrombocythemia (ET), to reduce blood-platelet count and the risk of excess blood clotting associated with high blood-platelet levels.

General Information

Blood platelets play an important role in the body. They help to form blood clots that "seal off" minor cuts and wounds and prevent excessive bleeding. When platelet counts are too high, as in ET, unwanted clots may form almost anywhere in the body. These clots may obstruct blood vessels, leading to leg cramps, heart attack, stroke, or other medical problems. Exactly how anagrelide reduces blood-platelet count is not known, but it may interfere with the formation of new platelets. Anagrelide is not approved for general use by children under age 16, but it has been used without apparent harm by 8 children between the ages of 8 and 17, who took it in doses up to 4 mg a day.

Cautions and Warnings

This drug should be used with caution by people who have **heart disease.**

Unusually **low blood-platelet counts** can develop in people treated with anagrelide. Platelet counts should be periodically checked while you are taking this drug; they usually rise soon after the drug is stopped.

People with **liver or kidney disease** should use this drug with caution. Anagrelide can cause liver or kidney toxicty and worsen diseases of those organs.

Possible Side Effects

▼ Most common: heart palpitations, diarrhea, abdominal pain, nausea, gas, headache, weakness, swelling, pain, dizziness, and difficulty breathing.

▼ Common: chest pain, rapid heartbeat, vomiting, upset stomach, appetite loss, rash or itching, tingling in the hands or feet, back pain, and not feeling well.

▼ Less common: fever, flu symptoms, chills, neck pain, sensitivity to bright light, abnormal heart rhythms, bleeding, heart disease, stroke, angina pain, heart failure, dizziness when rising from a sitting or lying position, flushing, migraine, fainting, depression, confusion, tiredness, high blood pressure, nervousness, memory loss, itching, skin disease, hair loss, stomach bleeding, blood in the stool, stomach irritation, vomiting, anemia, thrombocytopenia (low blood-platelet count), black-and-blue marks, swollen lymph glands, painful urination, blood in the urine, muscle and joint ache, leg cramps, runny nose, nosebleeds, lung disease, sinus inflammation, pneumonia, bronchitis, asthma, double vision, other visual difficulties, ringing or buzzing in the ears, liver inflammation, and dehydration.

Drug Interactions

• Sucralfate may interfere with the absorption of anagrelide. Do not combine these drugs.

Food Interactions

For optimal effectiveness, take anagrelide on an empty stomach.

Usual Dose

Adult: 0.5 mg 4 times a day or 1 mg twice a day, to start. After at least a week, the lowest effective dose should be sought.

Child (under age 16): not recommended.

Overdosage

Little is known about the effects of anagrelide overdose, but symptoms are likely to include a sudden drop in blood-platelet count and heart or central nervous system (CNS) side effects which could result in abnormal bleeding. Overdose victims should be taken to a hospital emergency room at once. ALWAYS bring the prescription bottle or container.

Special Information

Blood platelet counts should be checked every two days when beginning anagrelide for 1 week. Until a maintenance dose has been established, platelet counts should then be taken once a week.

Women who might become pregnant should use a reliable form of birth control while taking anagrelide.

If you forget a dose, take it as soon as possible. If it is almost time for your next dose, skip the dose you forgot and continue with your regular schedule. Call your doctor if you forget 2 or more doses in a row. Do not take a double dose.

Special Populations

Pregnancy/Breast-feeding

At high doses, anagrelide caused birth defects in animal studies. When this drug is considered crucial by your doctor, its potential benefits must be carefully weighed against its risks.

It is not known if this drug passes into breast milk. Nursing mothers who must take anagrelide should bottle-feed.

Seniors

Seniors may take anagrelide without special precaution.

Generic Name

Anakinra (an-ah-KIN-rah)

Brand Name

Kineret

Type of Drug

Immune system modulator.

Prescribed For

Moderate to severe rheumatoid arthritis in adults.

General Information

Anakinra blocks the biological activity of a substance called Interleukin-1 (IL-1), which is produced in response to inflammation. Anakinra may be prescribed together with methotrexate, azathioprine, leflunomide, sulfasalazine, or other drugs for the treatment of rheumatoid arthritis. It must be injected under the skin every day.

Cautions and Warnings

Do not use this drug if you are **sensitive** or **allergic** to it.

Serious infections and **malignancies** are possible in people using anakinra because of its ability to suppress the immune response. This may be more common in people with other conditions that predispose them to infections such as **asthma** or advanced or uncontrolled **diabetes**.

The safety and effectiveness of anakinra in people whose **immune systems** are suppressed has not been established.

Levels of some **white blood cells** may be reduced in rare cases, leading to persistent fever or pale skin color. Contact your doctor if any of these symptoms develop.

Anakinra is cleared through the kidneys. People with **severe kidney disease** may accumulate anakinra in their blood.

People taking anakinra should not receive any **live vaccines**, because the body may not be able to respond as expected to the vaccine.

Possible Side Effects

▼ Most common: infections, injection site reactions, and headache.

▼ Common: reduced white blood cell counts, nausea, and diarrhea.

▼ Less common: sinusitis, flu symptoms, and abdominal pain.

Drug Interactions

• Do not mix anakinra in the same syringe as another drug.

• Anakinra should not be used in combination with etanercept or any other TNF-blocking agent because of the increased risk of infection.

Food Interactions

None known.

Usual Dose

Adult (age 18 and over): 100 mg a day, at the same time each day, injected under the skin via pre-filled syringe. Inject the entire contents of the syringe.

Child: not recommended.

Overdosage

In animal studies, doses up to 35 times the maximum human dose have been used with no evidence of serious toxicities. Call your doctor or local poison center for more information. If you do go to a hospital emergency room, ALWAYS bring the prescription bottle or container.

Special Information

Do not use a syringe of anakinra if the contents are discolored or contain particles.

Reactions may develop at the site where anakinra is injected. Injection sites should be rotated among the thigh, abdomen, and upper arm to avoid excessive bruising or other skin damage.

If you forget a dose of anakinra, take it as soon as you remember. If you don't remember until it is almost time for your next dose, skip the dose you forgot and continue with your regular schedule.

Special Populations

Pregnancy/Breast-feeding

Animal studies at doses 100 times the human dose indicate no harm to the fetus. However, there is no information on the use of anakinra by pregnant women. When this drug is considered crucial by your doctor, its potential benefits must be weighed against its risks.

It is not known if anakinra passes into breast milk. Nursing mothers who must use anakinra should bottle-feed.

Seniors

The risk of anakinra side effects is greater in seniors because of the natural decline in kidney function.

Generic Name

Anastrozole (ah-NAS-troe-zole)

Brand Name

Arimidex

The information in this profile also applies to the following drug:

Generic Ingredient: Letrozole
Femara

Type of Drug

Aromatase inhibitor.

Prescribed For

Breast cancer in postmenopausal women.

General Information

Anastrozole is used for breast cancer that has advanced or spread despite treatment with tamoxifen, as an initial treatment for estrogen receptor positive breast cancer, or for breast cancer in which the hormone receptor status is unknown. Anastrozole reduces the amount of estradiol, an estrogenic hormone, in the blood. It does this by interfering with the action of the aromatase enzyme, an element involved in the manufacture of estradiol. Most of anastrozole is broken down in the liver.

Cautions and Warnings

Anastrozole **increases blood-cholesterol levels**.

Women with estrogen-receptor negative disease and those who did not respond at all to tamoxifen are **not likely to respond to anastrozole**.

The incidence of **benign ovarian tumors** has been shown to increase in women taking anastrozole.

Possible Side Effects

▼ Most common: weakness, nausea, headache, flushing, pain, and back pain.

Possible Side Effects *(continued)*

▼ Less common: breathing difficulties; vomiting; cough; diarrhea; constipation; abdominal pain; appetite loss; bone pain; sore throat; dizziness; rash; dry mouth; swelling in the arms, legs, or feet; pelvic pain; unexpected vaginal bleeding; depression; chest pain; and tingling in the hands or feet.

▼ Rare: Rare side effects can occur in almost any part of the body. Contact your doctor if you experience any side effect not listed above.

Drug Interactions

• Usual doses of anastrozole do not affect other medications; however, high doses of anastrozole can reduce the ability of the liver to break down certain drugs.

• Tamoxifen may reduce blood levels of anastrozole.

Food Interactions

Anastrozole may be taken with or without food.

Usual Dose

Anastrozole
    Adult: 1 mg once a day.

Letrozole
    Adult: 2.5 mg once a day.

Overdosage

Symptoms of overdose can be exaggerated side effects. Overdose victims should be taken to a hospital emergency room. ALWAYS bring the prescription bottle or container.

Special Information

Call your doctor if your side effects become severe or intolerable.

Use a condom, diaphragm, or other non-hormonal contraceptive while taking anastrozole.

If you forget a dose of anastrozole, take it as soon as you remember if it is within 12 hours of the missed dose. If it is over 12 hours, skip the missed dose and continue with your regular schedule. Call your doctor if you forget more than 2 doses in a row.

Special Populations

Pregnancy/Breast-feeding

Animal studies have shown that anastrozole can harm the fetus. Pregnant women who take anastrozole have a good chance of losing the pregnancy or harming the fetus. Conception should be prevented in women taking this drug by the use of a condom, diaphragm, or other non-hormonal contraceptive.

It is not known if anastrozole passes into breast milk. Nursing mothers who must take this drug should consider bottle-feeding.

Seniors

Seniors may take this drug without special precaution.

Type of Drug

Angiotensin II Blockers (AN-jee-oe-TEN-sin)

Brand Names

Generic Ingredient: Candesartan
Atacand

Generic Ingredients: Candesartan + Hydrochlorothiazide
Atacand HCT

Generic Ingredient: Eprosartan
Teveten

Generic Ingredients: Eprosartan + Hydrochlorothiazide
Teveten HCT

Generic Ingredient: Irbesartan
Avapro

Generic Ingredients: Irbesartan + Hydrochlorothiazide
Avalide

Generic Ingredient: Losartan Potassium
Cozaar

Generic Ingredients: Losartan Potassium + Hydrochlorothiazide
Hyzaar

Generic Ingredient: Olmesartan
Benicar

Generic Ingredients: Olmesartan + Hydrochlorothiazide
Benicar HCT

Generic Ingredient: Telmisartan
Micardis

Generic Ingredients: Telmisartan + Hydrochlorothiazide
Micardis HCT

Generic Ingredient: Valsartan
Diovan

Generic Ingredients: Valsartan + Hydrochlorothiazide
Diovan HCT

Prescribed For

High blood pressure.

General Information

These drugs work by blocking the effects of angiotensin II, a hormone found in blood vessels and other tissue. Angiotensin II plays an important role in regulating blood pressure. Unlike angiotensin-converting enzyme (ACE) inhibitors—another group of blood-pressure-lowering medication—angiotensin II (AII) blockers do not cause chronic cough. AII blockers can be used alone or with a thiazide diuretic such as hydrochlorothiazide, as in Hyzaar, Avalide, and Diovan HCT, for example. While these are single tablets, your doctor may prescribe an AII blocker and a diuretic as separate pills. Combining an AII blocker and a diuretic may reduce blood pressure twice as much as an AII blocker alone.

AII blockers may be useful in treating heart failure. Irbesartan may slow the progression of kidney disease in people with diabetes and high blood pressure.

Cautions and Warnings

Do not take an AII blocker if you are **sensitive** or **allergic** to it. You may be sensitive to one AII blocker and tolerant of another.

People being treated with diuretics may experience a sudden drop in blood pressure (symptoms include dizziness and fainting). Once your body has adjusted to a diuretic-AII blocker combination, this problem should subside.

Telmisartan is noticeably less effective in **African Americans**. Some studies indicate that losartan is less effective in African Americans, but recent research suggests that a higher drug dosage may compensate. Irbesartan and candesartan are also somewhat less effective in African Americans.

People with serious **liver disease** or **cirrhosis** should receive a lower starting dosage of losartan. Telmisartan should be used with caution by people with liver disease and related problems; alternate drug therapy should be considered. People with liver disease or cirrhosis should be cautious about taking valsartan, though no dosage adjustment is required.

Some people who take an AII blocker develop **kidney function changes** similar to those associated with ACE inhibitor drugs. Valsartan and telmisartan dosages may have to be modified in the presence of severe **kidney disease**. No adjustment is required for other AII blockers.

AII blockers have not been studied in **children under age 18**.

Possible Side Effects

AII blockers are generally very well tolerated. In clinical studies, the risk of side effects was about the same for an AII blocker as for a placebo (sugar pill).

Candesartan
▼ Common: respiratory infection.
▼ Less common: dizziness, headache, fatigue, diarrhea, nausea and vomiting, abdominal and other pain, joint pain, sinus problems, sore throat, runny nose, bronchitis, chest pain, and swollen arms or legs.
▼ Rare: Rare side effects can occur in almost any part of the body. Contact your doctor if you experience any side effect not listed above.

Eprosartan
▼ Less common: changes in urinary frequency or painful urination, dizziness, headache, sleeplessness, diarrhea, upset stomach, muscle pain or cramps, cough, sore throat, runny nose, and swelling.
▼ Rare: Rare side effects can occur in almost any part of the body. Contact your doctor if you experiece any side effect not listed above.

Possible Side Effects *(continued)*

Irbesartan
▼ Common: respiratory infection.
▼ Less common: dizziness, headache, fatigue, anxiety, nervousness, diarrhea, upset stomach, heartburn, nausea and vomiting, abdominal and other pain, accidents, cough, sinus problems, sore throat, runny nose, flu-like symptoms, swelling, chest pain, rash, rapid heart beat, and urinary infection.
▼ Rare: Rare side effects can occur in almost any part of the body. Contact your doctor if you experience any side effect not listed above.

Losartan
▼ Common: respiratory infection.
▼ Less common: dizziness, sleeplessness, diarrhea, upset stomach, heartburn, pain, muscle cramps, muscle aches, cough, stuffy nose, and sinus problems.
▼ Rare: rash, rapid heartbeat, and urinary infection. Other rare side effects can occur in almost any part of the body. Contact your doctor if you experience any side effect not listed above.

Olmesartan
▼ Less common: dizziness, diarrhea, upset stomach, heartburn, pain, muscle cramps, muscle aches, cough, stuffy nose, and sinus problems.
▼ Rare: Rare side effects can occur in almost any part of the body. Contact your doctor if you experience any side effect not listed above.

Telmisartan
▼ Common: respiratory infection.
▼ Less common: dizziness, headache, fatigue, anxiety or nervousness, diarrhea, upset stomach, heartburn, nausea and vomiting, abdominal pain, back and leg pain, muscle aches, cough, sinus irritation, sore throat, influenza, chest pain, urinary infection, swelling in the arms or legs, and high blood pressure.
▼ Rare: Rare side effects can occur in almost any part of the body. Contact your doctor if you experience any side effect not listed above.

Possible Side Effects *(continued)*

Valsartan
▼ Less common: dizziness, sleeplessness, headache, fatigue, diarrhea, upset stomach, heartburn, abdominal pain, joint pain, respiratory infection, cough, sore throat, sinus problems, runny nose, virus infection, and swelling.
▼ Rare: Rare side effects can occur in almost any part of the body. Contact your doctor if you experience any side effect not listed above.

Drug Interactions

• Telmisartan may slightly reduce warfarin blood levels, but not enough to require a change in warfarin dosage.
• Combining telmisartan and digoxin can increase digoxin blood levels by up to 50%, leading to possible drug side effects. This combination should be used with caution.
• Phenobarbital and indomethacin may reduce the effectiveness of losartan.
• Fluconazole and cimetidine may increase the effects of losartan.
• Combining an AII blocker and another blood-pressure-lowering drug, especially a diuretic, reduces blood pressure more efficiently than either drug used alone. People taking a diuretic who start an AII blocker may initially experience a rapid blood pressure drop and should start with a lower AII blocker dosage.

Food Interactions

For optimal effectiveness, take valsartan at least 1 hour before or 2 hours after meals. Other AII blockers can be taken with or without food.

Usual Dose

Candesartan
Adult: 8–32 mg once a day. Usual starting dosage is 16 mg a day.
Child: not recommended.

Eprosartan
Adult: 400–800 mg a day in one or two doses. Usual starting dosage is 600 mg.
Child: not recommended.

Irbesartan
   Adult: 150 mg once a day to start, increasing to 300 mg once a day if necessary. A lower dosage (75 mg) may be pre-scribed for people who are dehydrated or salt-depleted.
   Child: not recommended.

Losartan
   Adult: 25–50 mg once a day to start, increasing gradually up to 100 mg in 1 or 2 doses a day.
   Child: not recommended.

Olmesartan
   Adult: 20–40 mg a day. Usual starting dose is 20 mg a day.
   Child: not recommended.

Telmisartan
   Adult: 20–80 mg a day. Usual starting dosage is 40 mg a day.
   Child: not recommended.

Valsartan
   Adult: 80–320 mg once a day. Usual starting dosage is 80–160 mg a day.
   Child: not recommended.

Overdosage

Little is known about AII blocker overdose, though it could be fatal. The most likely overdose symptoms are very low blood pressure, dizziness, and rapid heartbeat. Overdose victims should be taken to a hospital emergency room. ALWAYS bring the prescription bottle or container.

Special Information

Avoid strenuous exercise and very hot weather because heavy sweating or dehydration can cause a rapid blood pres-sure drop.

   People on dialysis who take telmisartan may become dizzy or faint when rising quickly from a sitting or lying position at the beginning of treatment.

   Avoid over-the-counter diet pills, decongestants, and stim-ulants because they may contain ingredients that can raise blood pressure.

   If you take an AII blocker once a day and forget a dose, take it as soon as you remember. If it is within 8 hours of your next dose, skip the one you forgot and continue with your regular schedule. If you take an All blocker twice a day and forget a dose, take it as soon as you remember. If it is within 4 hours of your next dose, take 1 dose right away and another in 5 or 6 hours, then go back to your regular schedule. Never take a double dose.

Special Populations

Pregnancy/Breast-feeding

All blockers should not be taken during the last 6 months of pregnancy because they can cause fetal injury or death. If necessary, you should take another drug for high blood pressure if you are or might be pregnant.

It is not known if All blockers pass into breast milk, though they do in animal studies. Nursing mothers who must take an All blocker should bottle-feed.

Seniors

Seniors may take All blockers without special precautions.

Type of Drug

Antiemetics (5HT$_3$ Type)

Brand Names

Generic Ingredient: Alosetron
Lotronex

Generic Ingredient: Dolasetron
Anzemet

Generic Ingredient: Granisetron
Kytril

Generic Ingredient: Ondansetron
Zofran   Zofran ODT

Prescribed For

Nausea and vomiting caused by chemotherapy and other drugs, general anesthesia, and acetaminophen overdose. Alosetron is prescribed only for women with severe irritable bowel syndrome (IBS) whose main symptom is diarrhea; also prescribed for psychosis due to levadopa treatment, bulimia, social anxiety disorder, and itching due to morphine treatment.

General Information

These drugs prevent nausea and vomiting by interfering with a form of the neurohormone serotonin (5HT) known as $5HT_3$. They block its effects in the part of the brain that controls vomiting and in the vagus nerve in the stomach and intestines. These drugs are very effective and often work in cases in which older antiemetics have failed. Aloestrin works against IBS by blocking the action of serotonin in the intestinal system. This reduces the cramping, abdominal discomfort, urgency, and diarrhea caused by IBS. Blood concentrations of aloestrin are 30% to 50% higher in women than in men.

Cautions and Warnings

Do not take these drugs if you are **allergic** or **sensitive** to them.

Serious and possibly **fatal colitis** and serious **complications of constipation** leading to hospitalization, blood transfusions, and surgery have developed in people taking aloestrin.

People with **heart rhythm problems,** especially those taking diuretics and antiarrhythmic drugs, should be cautious about taking dolasetron.

People with **liver problems** should be cautious about taking ondansetron and should probably use another drug in this group.

These drugs should only be used when the risk of nausea and vomiting is relatively high.

Possible Side Effects

Alosetron
▼ Most common: constipation.
▼ Common: nausea and abdominal or GI discomfort or pain.

Possible Side Effects *(continued)*

▼ Less common: high blood pressure, sleep disorders, depression, abdominal gas, stomach virus infection, and hemorrhoids.

▼ Rare: abnormal heart rhythms, anxiety, sedation, abnormal dreams, acne, inflamed hair follicles, proctitis, colitis, menstrual problems, sexual dysfunction, urinary infections, frequent urination, hematoma, abnormal blood bilirubin levels, cough, throat and tonsil discomfort, breathing disorders, nasal allergies, ususual sensitivity to bright light, allergic reactions, sensing unusual tastes and odors, and ear, nose, and throat infections.

Dolasetron

▼ Common: diarrhea and headache.

▼ Less common: high or low blood pressure, abdominal pain, dizziness or light-headedness, fever or chills, and tiredness.

▼ Rare: blood in the urine; chest pain; kidney problems; painful or difficult urination; rapid heartbeat; pain; severe stomach pain with nausea or vomiting; rash; hives; itching; slow or irregular heartbeat; swollen face, feet, or lower legs; and breathing difficulties.

Granisetron

▼ Most common: headache, constipation, weakness, and low white-blood-cell count.

▼ Common: abdominal pain, diarrhea, appetite loss, chills, and anemia.

▼ Less common: stimulation, tiredness, sleeplessness, changes in sense of taste, hair loss, and low blood-platelet count.

▼ Rare: unusual muscle movements and drug sensitivity reactions.

Ondansetron

▼ Most common: headache, feeling unwell, and constipation.

▼ Common: anxiety, agitation, dizziness, drowsiness, sleepiness, diarrhea, gynecological problems, itching, urinary difficulties, abnormal heart rhythms, and low blood pressure.

Possible Side Effects *(continued)*

▼ Less common: weakness, fever or chills, dry mouth, liver inflammation, diarrhea, abdominal pain, and rash.

▼ Rare: liver failure, drug allergy, bronchial spasm, unusual tiredness or weakness, dizziness or light-headedness, rapid heartbeat, angina pain, low blood potassium, and grand mal seizures.

Drug Interactions

• Alosetron may reduce the amount of hydralazine, isoniazid, and procainamide in the blood.

• Combining rifampin and ondansetron or dolasetron may reduce the level of antiemetic in the blood.

• Blood levels of dolasetron may be increased when combined with cimetidine or atenolol for a week or more.

Food Interactions

These drugs may be taken with or without food.

Usual Dose

Alosetron
    Adult: 1 mg twice a day without food.

Dolasetron
    Adult and Child (age 17 and over): a single dose of 100 mg.
    Child (age 2–16): 0.8 mg per lb. of body weight, up to 100 mg.

Granisetron
    Adult and Child (age 17 and over): 1 mg 2 times a day.
    Child (age 2–16): 0.008 mg per lb. of body weight, up to 1 mg, 2 times a day.

Ondansetron
    Adult and Child (age 12 and over): 8 mg 2–3 times a day. People with liver failure should take no more than 8 mg a day.
    Child (age 4–11): 4 mg 3 times a day.
    Child (age 3 and under): not recommended.

Overdosage

Symptoms may include severe constipation, temporary blindness, high blood pressure, fainting, and mild headache. Call your local poison control center or a hospital emergency room for more information. If you go for treatment, ALWAYS bring the prescription bottle or container.

Special Information

Call your doctor if you develop chest tightness, wheezing, breathing difficulties, chest pain, or any bothersome or persistent side effect.

Call your doctor at once and immediately stop taking alosetron if you develop constipation or symptoms of ischemic colitis including abdominal pain, cramps, nausea, vomiting, and bloody diarrhea.

Maintain good dental hygiene while taking these drugs. Chronic dry mouth can increase the risk of tooth decay and gum disease.

If you forget a dose, take it as soon as you remember. If it is almost time for your next dose, skip the dose you forgot and continue with your regular schedule. Missing more than 1 dose may increase the risk of vomiting.

Special Populations

Pregnancy/Breast-feeding

These drugs may be associated with a slight risk of birth defects. When your doctor considers any of these drugs crucial, its potential benefits must be carefully weighed against its risks.

These drugs may pass into breast milk. Nursing mothers who must take any of these drugs should consider bottle-feeding.

Seniors

Blood levels of aloestron are 40% higher in older women.

Type of Drug

Antihistamine-Decongestant Combination Products

Brand Names

Generic Ingredients: Acrivastine + Pseudoephedrine
Semprex-D

Generic Ingredients: Azatadine + Pseudoephedrine
Trinalin Repetabs

Generic Ingredients: Brompheniramine +
Pseudoephedrine G

Brofed Liquid   Lodrane LD
Bromfed   Respahist
Bromfed-PD   Rondec
Bromfenex   Touro A & H
Bromfenex PD   ULTRAbrom
Dallergy-JR   ULTRAbrom PD
Endafed

Generic Ingredients: Dexbrompheniramine +
Pseudoephedrine
Disobrom   Drixomed
Dexaphen-SA

Generic Ingredients: Carbinoxamine +
Pseudoephedrine G

Biohist-LA   Carbodec TR
Carbiset   Cardec-S
Carbiset TR   Rondec*
Carbodec   Rondec-TR

Generic Ingredients: Chlorpheniramine Maleate +
Pseudoephedrine G

Anamine A S   Dura-Tap/PD
Anamine T.D.   Fedahist Gyrocaps
Anaplex A S   Fedahist Timecaps
Atrohist Pediatric   Histalet A
Brexin L.A.   Klerist-D
Chlorafed Timecelles   Kronofed-A
Chlorafed H.S. Timecelles   Kronofed-A Jr.
Chlordrine SR   ND Clear
Chlorphedrine SR   Novafed A
Codimal L.A.   Rescon
Colfed-A   Rescon ED
Cophene No.2   Rescon JR
Deconamine*   Rinade B.I.D.
Deconamine SR   Time-Hist
Duralex

*Generic Ingredients: Chlorpheniramine Maleate +
Phenylephrine Hydrochloride* G

Ed A-Hist	Prehist
Histor-D	

*Generic Ingredients: Chlorpheniramine Maleate +
Phenyltoloxamine + Phenylephrine Hydrochloride*

Comhist	Comhist LA

*Generic Ingredients: Chlorpheniramine Tannate +
Pseudoephedrine*

Tannate	Tanafed

*Generic Ingredients: Chlorpheniramine Tannate + Pyrilamine
Tannate + Phenylephrine Tannate* G

Atrohist Pediatric	Rynatan-S Pediatric
Rhinatate	Tanoral
R-Tannate	Triotann
R-Tannamine	Tritan
R-Tannamine Pediatric	Tri-Tannate
Rynatan	Tri-Tannate Pediatric
Rynatan Pediatric	

Generic Ingredients: Fexofenadine + Pseudoephedrine
Allegra-D

Generic Ingredients: Loratadine + Pseudoephedrine

Claritin-D 12-Hour	Claritin-D 24-Hour

*Generic Ingredients: Promethazine + Phenylephrine
Hydrochloride* G

Phenergan VC	Promethazine VC Plain
Promethazine VC	Prometh VC Plain

*Some products in this brand-name group are alcohol- or
sugar-free. Consult your pharmacist.*

Prescribed For

Sneezing, watery eyes, runny nose, itchy or scratchy throat,
nasal congestion, and other symptoms of the common cold,
allergies, and upper respiratory conditions.

General Information

The basic formula for each of these antihistamine-decongestant combinations is the same: An antihistamine is used to relieve allergy symptoms and a decongestant to treat the symptoms of either a cold or allergy.

Most of these products are taken several times a day, while others are long-acting and are taken once or twice a day. Since nothing can cure a cold or allergy, the best you can hope to achieve from a cold and allergy remedy is relief from symptoms.

Cautions and Warnings

Antihistamines in these products may cause **drowsiness**. Decongestants may cause **anxiety** and **nervousness** and may interfere with sleep.

People who are **allergic** to antihistamines or decongestants should use these products with caution.

People with narrow-angle **glaucoma, prostate disease,** certain **stomach ulcers,** and **bladder obstruction,** and those having **asthma attacks,** should not use these products.

Possible Side Effects

▼ Most common: restlessness, nervousness, sleeplessness, drowsiness, sedation, excitation, dizziness, poor coordination, and upset stomach.

▼ Less common: low blood pressure, heart palpitations, rapid heartbeat and abnormal heart rhythms, chest pain, anemia, fatigue, confusion, tremors, headache, irritability, euphoria (feeling high), tingling or heaviness in the hands, tingling in the feet or legs, blurred or double vision, convulsions, hysterical reaction, ringing or buzzing in the ears, fainting, increase or decrease in appetite, nausea, vomiting, diarrhea or constipation, frequent urination, difficulty urinating, early menstrual periods, loss of sex drive, breathing difficulties, wheezing with chest tightness, stuffed nose, itching, rash, unusual sensitivity to the sun, chills, excessive perspiration, and dry mouth, nose, or throat.

Drug Interactions

• Combining these products with alcoholic beverages, antianxiety drugs, tranquilizers, or narcotic pain relievers may lead to excessive drowsiness or difficulty concentrating.

• Avoid these products if you are taking an MAOI for depression or high blood pressure because the MAOI may cause a very rapid rise in blood pressure or increase side effects such as dry mouth and nose, blurred vision, and abnormal heart rhythms.

• The decongestant component of these products may interfere with the normal effects of blood-pressure-lowering medications and can aggravate diabetes, heart disease, hyperthyroid disease, high blood pressure, prostate disease, stomach ulcer, and urinary blockage.

• If your doctor has prescribed one of these products, do not self-medicate with an additional over-the-counter drug for the relief of cold symptoms. This combination may aggravate high blood pressure, heart disease, diabetes, or thyroid disease.

Food Interactions

These drugs are best taken on an empty stomach but may be taken with food if they upset your stomach.

Usual Dose

Dosages vary. Generally, these products are taken every 4–12 hours.

Overdosage

Symptoms of overdose are drowsiness, chills, dry mouth, fever, nausea, nervousness, irritability, rapid or irregular heartbeat, chest pain, and urinary difficulties. Most cases should be treated by inducing vomiting as soon as possible with ipecac syrup—available at any pharmacy. Then call your local poison control center for more information or take the victim to a hospital emergency room. ALWAYS bring the prescription bottle or container.

Special Information

Use extra caution while doing anything that requires concentration, such as driving a car or operating hazardous machinery.

Call your doctor if your side effects are severe or become intolerable.

If you forget to take a dose of your medication, take it as soon as you remember. If it is almost time for your next dose, skip the dose you forgot and continue with your regular schedule. Do not take a double dose.

Special Populations

Pregnancy/Breast-feeding

Animal studies suggest that some older antihistamines cause birth defects but the antihistamines in these products have not been proven harmful. If you are or might be pregnant, do not take any of these products without your doctor's knowledge.

Small amounts of antihistamine or decongestant pass into breast milk. Nursing mothers who must use these products should bottle-feed.

Seniors

Seniors are more sensitive to the side effects of these medications.

Type of Drug

Antihistamine Eyedrops

Brand Names

Generic Ingredient: Azelastine
Optivar

Generic Ingredient: Emedastine
Epivar

Generic Ingredient: Epinastine
Elestat

Generic Ingredient: Olopatadine
Patanol

Generic Ingredient: Levocabastine
Livostin

Prescribed For

Eye itching due to allergy.

General Information

Azelastine, emedastine, epinastine, and olopatadine clear conjunctivitis (pinkeye) by preventing the release of chemicals from mast cells in the eye that cause allergic symptoms. They also work to minimize the response of nerve endings to any of these allergy-causing chemicals that might be present. Livostin only affects nerve endings to minimize the allergic response.

Cautions and Warnings

Do not use antihistamine eyedrops if you are **allergic** to them.

Do not use these drugs to treat redness caused by contact lens irritation.

Possible Side Effects

Side effects are generally mild and subside as your body gets used to the medicine.

Azelastine
▼ Most common: burning or stinging sensation in the eyes, headache, and bitter taste in the mouth.
▼ Less common: asthma, pinkeye, difficulty breathing, eye pain, fatigue, flu-like symptoms, sore throat, itching, runny nose, and temporary blurring.

Emedastine
▼ Common: headache.
▼ Less common: weakness, abnormal dreams, bad taste in the mouth, blurred vision, burning or stinging sensation in the eyes, staining of the cornea, dry eyes, red eye, eye discomfort, sensation that something is in your eye, inflammation of the cornea, sinus irritation, rash, runny nose, and tearing.

Epinastine
▼ Most common: cold symptoms and upper respiratory infection.
▼ Less common: headache, runny nose, sinus irritation, cough, and sore throat.

Levocabastine
▼ Most common: mild stinging or burning in the eyes.

Possible Side Effects (continued)

▼ Common: headache.

▼ Less common: dry mouth, visual disturbances, red eyes, tearing or discharge from the eyes, eye pain or dryness, swollen eyelids, fatigue, sore throat, cough, nausea, skin rash or redness, and breathing difficulty.

Olopatadine

▼ Common: headache.

▼ Less common: changes in sense of taste, burning or stinging sensation in the eye, dry eye, sensation that something is in your eye, eye redness, inflammation of the cornea, eyelid swelling, itching, weakness, sore throat, runny nose, cold symptoms, and sinus inflammation.

Food and Drug Interactions

None known.

Usual Dose

Azelastine
1 drop twice a day in the affected eye.

Emedastine
1 drop in the affected eye up to 4 times a day.

Epinastine
Adult and Child (age 3 and over): 1 drop twice a day in the affected eye.

Levocabastine
1 drop 4 times a day.

Olopatadine
  Adult and Child (age 3 and over): 1–2 drops in each eye 2 times a day, 6–8 hours apart.
  Child (under age 3): not recommended.

Overdosage

Little is known about overdose effects of antihistamine eyedrops, but it is likely to lead to drug side effects. Accidental ingestion of either of these drugs is not likely to be severe because each bottle contains small amounts of active drug. Call your local poison center or hospital emergency room for more information. If you seek treatment, ALWAYS bring the prescription bottle or container.

Special Information

If you wear contact lenses, wait at least 15 minutes after using these medicines before putting in your lenses.

To avoid infection, do not touch the dropper tip to your finger, eyelid, or any other surface. Wait at least 5 minutes before using another eyedrop or eye ointment.

If you forget a dose, administer it as soon as you remember. If it is almost time for your next dose, skip the one you forgot and continue with your regular schedule. Do not take a double dose.

Special Populations

Pregnancy/Breast-feeding

These drugs can cause birth defects in laboratory animals but there is no information on their effect in women. When this drug is considered crucial by your doctor, its potential benefits must be carefully weighed against its risks.

Emedastine, levocabastine, and olopatadine may pass into breast milk. It is not known if azelastine or epinastine pass into breast milk. Nursing mothers who must use antihistamine eyedrops should bottle-feed.

Seniors

Seniors may use these drugs without special precaution.

Generic Name

Apraclonidine (ah-prah-KLON-ih-dene)

Brand Name

Iopidine

Type of Drug

Sympathomimetic.

Prescribed For

Post-surgical increases in eye pressure; also prescribed as additional short-term treatment in people who are using other glaucoma medicines.

General Information

Apraclonidine hydrochloride reduces both elevated and normal fluid pressure inside the eye and selectively blocks certain nerve endings without acting as a local anesthetic. The exact way it works is not known, but apraclonidine, like other drugs that reduce eye pressure, may work by decreasing the production of eye fluid. The drug starts to work within 1 hour after it is put into the eye and reaches its maximum effect in 3 to 5 hours.

Cautions and Warnings

Do not use apraclonidine if you are **allergic** to it or to clonidine. This drug can cause an allergic-like reaction, including **red eye, swelling of the lid and white of the eye, itching, burning,** and the **feeling of something in your eye**. If this happens, stop using the drug and call your doctor. Taking this drug with a **monoamine oxidase inhibitor (MAOI)** may result in severe side effects—do not combine them.

Using this medicine with other eye-pressure-lowering drugs may not provide additional benefit: Other drugs work in the same way and a further effect may not be possible.

The ability of apraclonidine to lower eye pressure decreases over time. Most **people continuously benefit for less than 1 month**.

People with **kidney or liver disease** should be monitored by their doctors while taking this medicine.

Possible Side Effects

▼ Most common: eye redness, itching, tearing, eye discomfort, lid swelling, dry mouth, feeling of something in your eye, headache, and weakness.

▼ Less common: blanching of the eye; upper lid elevation; dilated pupils; blurred vision and other eye disorders; allergic reactions; lid crusting; abnormal vision; eye pain; abdominal pain; diarrhea; stomach discomfort; vomiting; dry mouth or nose; nasal burning; runny nose; sore throat; worsening asthma; constipation and nausea; slow heartbeat; heart palpitations; abnormal heart rhythms; chest pain; fainting; swelling; difficulty sleeping; irritability; depression; reduced sex drive; pain, numbness, or tingling in the hands or feet;

Possible Side Effects *(continued)*

clammy or sweaty palms; taste changes; a feeling of having a head cold; and rash.

Drug Interactions

• Apraclonidine can reduce pulse and blood pressure. If you are also taking drugs to treat high blood pressure or other cardiovascular drugs, check your pulse and blood pressure.

• MAOI drugs can slow the breakdown of apraclonidine and increase the risk of drug side effects. This combination should be avoided.

Usual Dose

Adult: 1–2 drops in the affected eye 3 times a day.

Overdosage

Exaggerated side effects, especially those that affect the nervous system, are symptoms of overdose. Call your local poison control center for more information. ALWAYS take the prescription bottle or container with you if you go to the emergency room.

Special Information

Apraclonidine can cause dizziness and tiredness. Be careful doing anything that requires concentration, coordination, or alertness while taking this medication.

To prevent infection, do not touch the dropper tip to your finger or eyelid. Wait 5 minutes before using any other eye-drop or ointment.

If you forget a dose of apraclonidine, take it as soon as you remember. If it is almost time for your next dose, take one dose as soon as you remember and then go back to your regular schedule. Do not take a double dose.

Special Populations

Pregnancy/Breast-feeding

In animal studies, apraclonidine was toxic to embryos when given by mouth. It should be used with caution during pregnancy.

It is not known if this drug passes into breast milk, but nursing mothers should bottle-feed their babies while using it.

Seniors

Seniors may use this medicine without special precautions.

Generic Name

Aprepitant (ah-PRE-pih-tant)

Brand Name

Emend

Type of Drug

Antinauseant and antiemetic (an agent that prevents or relieves nausea and vomiting).

Prescribed For

Acute and delayed nausea and vomiting associated with chemotherapy.

General Information

Aprepitant works against nausea and vomiting by selectively inhibiting the *substance P/neurokinin 1 (NK 1)* receptor. This is a unique approach to nausea therapy and it complements other nausea therapies, such as corticosteroids and 5-HT3 receptor antagonists that should be used together with aprepitant. Aprepitant is broken down in the liver.

Cautions and Warnings

Do not take aprepitant if you are **sensitive** or **allergic** to it.

Aprepitant should be used with caution if you have **severe liver disease**. People with mild to moderate liver disease can tolerate the drug quite well.

Aprepitant is not intended for normal nausea and vomiting in those not undergoing chemotherapy treatment or for chronic continuous therapy.

Possible Side Effects

▼ Most common: fatigue, nausea, appetite loss, weakness, hiccups, and constipation or diarrhea.

▼ Common: dizziness, dehydration, heartburn, headache, and vomiting.

Possible Side Effects *(continued)*

▼ Less common: abdominal pain, fever, upset stomach, stomach pains, ringing or buzzing in the ears, mucous membrane swelling, and sleeplessness.

▼ Rare: Rare side effects can occur in almost any part of the body. Contact your doctor if you experience any side effect not listed above.

Drug Interactions

• Aprepitant is often given with cancer chemotherapy drugs that are broken down by the same enzymes. This combination might be expected to raise the amount of chemotherapeutic in the blood, but this was not a problem in clinical studies of the drug.

• Aprepitant may slow the breakdown of astemizole, cisapride, pimozide, or terfenadine, leading to serious drug side effects. Do not combine these medicines with aprepitant.

• Aprepitant increases blood levels of midazolam, increasing the chances for drug side effects. Levels of other benzodiazepine sedatives (such as alprazolam and triazolam) may rise as well.

• Aprepitant increases blood levels of corticosteroid drugs. Corticosteroid doses may need to be adjusted.

• Clarithromycin, diltiazem, itraconazole, ketoconazole, nefazodone, nelfinavir, ritonavir, and troleandomycin may raise blood levels of aprepitant, increasing the chances for drug side effects and toxicity. These drugs should be combined with caution.

• Amiodarone, carbamazepine, nevirapine, phenobarbital, phenytoin, rifampin, and St. John's wort may reduce the effectiveness of aprepitant.

• Aprepitant can increase the amount of corticosteroid drug that is absorbed into your blood. Oral dexamethasone and methylprednisolone doses should be decreased by half (oral) when combined with aprepitant.

• Blood levels of the hormones ethinyl estradiol and norethindrone—used in many oral contraceptive products—can be reduced, compromising the effectiveness of these products. Use a non-hormonal contraceptive method while taking aprepitant.

• Blood levels of aprepitant and paroxetine are both reduced by about 25% when they are combined.

• The breakdown of warfarin may be increased by aprepitant, reducing the blood thinner's effectiveness. If you take warfarin and have to use aprepitant, your doctor should closely monitor your warfarin in the 2-week period (especially days 7–10) after the beginning of each aprepitant cycle.

Food Interactions

This drug may be taken without regard to food or meals.

Usual Dose

Adult: 125 mg 1 hour before starting chemotherapy, followed by 80 mg on the two days following chemotherapy. Aprepitant should be used in combination with a corticosteroid (such as dexamethasone) and 5-HT3 receptor antagonist (such as ondansetron).

Child: not recommended.

Overdosage

There is limited information about aprepitant overdose but drowsiness and headache may occur. Overdose victims should be taken to a hospital emergency room. ALWAYS bring the prescription bottle or container.

Special Information

Aprepitant is given in a 3-day cycle. Take the first dose 1 hour before chemotherapy. Take the next two doses on the morning of the two days following your chemotherapy treatment.

Special Populations

Pregnancy/Breast-feeding

While animal studies of aprepitant revealed no adverse effects on a developing fetus, there is no information on how this drug will affect pregnant women and it should be used only if it is clearly needed. This drug should only be used during pregnancy after carefully weighing its potential benefits against its risks.

Aprepitant passes into breast milk. Nursing mothers who must take it should consider bottle-feeding while they are using it.

Seniors

Seniors may be more sensitive to the effects of aprepitant but dosage adjustments are not needed.

Aricept *see Cholinesterase Inhibitors, page 239*

Generic Name

Aripiprazole (ah-rih-PIP-rah-zole)

Brand Name

Abilify

Type of Drug

Antipsychotic.

Prescribed For

Schizophrenia; also used for bipolar disorder and other psychiatric conditions.

General Information

Aripiprazole is a new type of antipsychotic that works on serotonin and dopamine receptors in the brain. Unlike other newer antipsychotics that only decrease dopamine, it may both increase and decrease dopamine, targeting specific areas of the brain where the neurotransmitter is too plentiful or too reduced. However, the exact way it works is not known.

The effectiveness of aripiprazole was established by studying hospitalized schizophrenics for 4 to 6 weeks, and later studies also proved its effectiveness for 6 months or beyond.

Cautions and Warnings

Do not take aripiprazole if you are **sensitive** or **allergic** to it.

People with **liver or kidney disease** may have higher blood levels of aripiprazole than healthy people, but this is not a reason to adjust your drug dose.

A serious set of side effects known as **neuroleptic malignant syndrome (NMS)** may occur while taking aripiprazole. Symptoms include high fever, convulsions, difficult or fast breathing, rapid heartbeat, rapid or irregular pulse or blood pressure, increased sweating, muscle rigidity, and mental changes. NMS can be fatal and requires immediate medical attention. This condition has been associated with most antipsychotic medicines.

Tardive dyskinesia (a group of severe side effects associated with antipsychotic and other drugs) may occur while taking aripiprazole and is often considered a reason to stop taking this drug. Symptoms include lip smacking or puckering, puffing of the cheeks, rapid or worm-like movements of the tongue, uncontrolled chewing motions, and uncontrolled arm or leg movements. Symptoms can increase with the length and dosage of antipsychotic drug therapy and may become permanent. Report any of these side effects to your doctor.

Aripiprazole can cause **dizziness** or **fainting** when rising from a sitting or lying position, especially when people start taking the drug.

Seizures occur in a small number of people taking aripiprazole. It should be taken with care if you have had or are at increased risk of seizures.

Avoid exposure to **extreme heat**. Antipsychotics can upset your body's temperature-regulating mechanism.

Swallowing problems and inhaling food can be a problem with all antipsychotics, including aripiprazole.

Suicide is a danger with all psychotics. To reduce the possibility of possible overdose, people taking this drug should have no more than a 30-day supply of medication at any one time.

Possible Side Effects

In studies of aripiprazole, reported side effects were similar in people taking aripiprazole and those taking an inactive placebo medicine.

▼ Most common: headache, nausea, vomiting, constipation, anxiety, lightheadedness, tiredness, sleeplessness, and an uncontrollable feeling of restlessness.

▼ Common: weight gain, weakness, and rash.

▼ Less common: fever, tremors, runny nose, cough, blurred vision, and abnormal heart rhythms.

▼ Rare: Rare side effects can occur in almost any part of the body. Contact your doctor if you experience any side effect not listed above.

Drug Interactions

• Carbamazepine reduces blood levels of aripiprazole. If carbamazepine is added to aripiprazole treatment, the dose of aripiprazole should be doubled. Aripiprazole dosage should be reduced to normal levels when carbamazepine is stopped.

• Fluoxetine, ketoconazole, paroxetine, and quinidine increase blood levels of aripiprazole. If any of these drugs are combined with aripiprazole, the dosage of aripiprazole should be reduced in half until the other drug is stopped.

• Other drugs often associated with drug interactions (such as dextromethorphan, famotidine, lithium, omeprazole, valproate, and warfarin) are *not* a problem with aripiprazole.

Food Interactions

This drug may be taken without regard to food or meals.

Usual Dose

Adult: 10–15 mg once a day.
Child: not recommended.

Overdosage

Symptoms include tiredness and vomiting. Take the victim to a hospital emergency room. ALWAYS bring the prescription bottle or container with you.

Special Information

Aripiprazole may cause drowsiness. Use caution when doing anything that requires intense concentration, like driving or operating machinery.

Avoid alcoholic beverages while taking aripiprazole.

If you get dizzy while taking aripiprazole, avoid sudden changes in posture and avoid climbing stairs. Aripiprazole can make you more prone to heat stroke. Use caution in hot weather.

If you forget to take a dose of aripiprazole, take it as soon as you remember and continue with your regular dose on the next day. Tell your doctor or pharmacist if you forget more than one dose of aripiprazole. Do not take a double dose of this medication unless advised to do so by your doctor.

Be sure to tell your doctor about any other medicines you are taking, including over-the-counter remedies.

Special Populations

Pregnancy/Breast-feeding

This medication caused birth defects in animal studies. When this drug is considered crucial by your doctor, its potential benefits must be carefully weighed against its risks. Women who are or might be pregnant should talk with their doctor before taking aripiprazole.

Aripiprazole passes into breast milk. Nursing mothers who must take it should bottle-feed.

Seniors
Seniors eliminate 20 percent less aripiprazole than younger adults, but there is no need for dosage adjustments.

Generic Names

Aspirin, Buffered Aspirin (AS-prin) Ⓖ

Brand Names

Adprin-B	Cama Arthritis Pain Reliever
Alka-Seltzer with Aspirin	Easprin
Arthritis Pain Formula	Ecotrin
Arthritis Foundation Pain	Empirin
Reliever	Genprin
Ascriptin	Halfprin
Aspergum	Heartline
Asprimox	Magnaprin
Bayer	Norwich
Bufferin	St. Joseph Adult Chewable
Buffex	Aspirin
Buffex	ZORprin

Type of Drug

Analgesic and anti-inflammatory agent.

Prescribed For

Mild to moderate pain, fever, arthritis, and inflammation of bones, joints, or other body tissues. People who have had a stroke or transient ischemic attack (TIA)—oxygen shortage to the brain—may have aspirin prescribed to reduce the risk of having another such attack. Aspirin may also be prescribed as an anticoagulant (blood-thinning) drug in people with unstable angina and to protect against heart attack. Aspirin has a definite beneficial effect if it is taken as soon as possible after having a heart attack.

General Information

Aspirin may be the closest thing we have to a wonder drug. It has been used for more than a century for pain and fever relief and is now used for its effect on the blood as well.

Aspirin is the standard against which all other drugs are compared for relieving pain and for reducing inflammation. Chemically, aspirin is a member of the group of drugs called salicylates. Other salicylates include sodium salicylate, sodium thiosalicylate, choline salicylate, and magnesium salicylate (trilisate). These drugs are no more effective than regular aspirin, although two of them—choline salicylate and magnesium salicylate—may be a little less irritating to the stomach. They are all more expensive than aspirin.

Aspirin reduces fever by causing the blood vessels in the skin to open, allowing heat to leave the body more rapidly. Its effects on pain and inflammation are thought to be related to its ability to prevent the manufacture of complex body hormones called prostaglandins. Of all the salicylates, aspirin has the greatest effect on prostaglandin production.

Many people find that they can take buffered aspirin but not regular aspirin. The addition of antacids to aspirin can be important to people who must take large doses of aspirin for chronic arthritis or other conditions. In many cases, aspirin is the only effective drug and can be tolerated only with the antacids present.

Cautions and Warnings

People with **liver damage** should avoid aspirin. People who are **allergic** to aspirin may also be allergic to nonsteroidal anti-inflammatory drugs (NSAIDs) such as indomethacin, sulindac, ibuprofen, fenoprofen, naproxen, tolmetin, and meclofenamate sodium or to products containing tartrazine (a commonly used orange dye and food coloring). People with **asthma** and/or **nasal polyps** are more likely to be allergic to aspirin.

Alcoholic beverages may worsen the stomach irritation caused by aspirin. Alcohol increases the risk of aspirin-related ulcers.

Stop taking aspirin if you develop **dizziness, hearing loss, or ringing or buzzing in your ears**.

Reye's syndrome is a life-threatening condition characterized by vomiting and stupor or dullness and may develop in children with influenza (flu) or chickenpox that is treated with aspirin or other salicylates. Up to 30% of people who develop Reye's syndrome can die, and permanent brain damage is possible in those who survive. Because of this, authorities advise against giving children under age 16 aspirin or another salicylate, especially those with chickenpox or the flu; acetaminophen should be given instead.

Aspirin **interferes with normal blood clotting** and should therefore be avoided for 1 week **before surgery**. Ask for your surgeon or dentist's recommendation before taking aspirin for pain after surgery.

Possible Side Effects

▼ Most common: nausea, upset stomach, heartburn, loss of appetite, and loss of small amounts of blood in the stool.

▼ Less common: hives, rashes, liver damage, fever, thirst, and visual difficulties. Aspirin may contribute to the formation of stomach ulcers and bleeding. People who are allergic to aspirin and those with a history of nasal polyps, asthma, or rhinitis may experience breathing difficulty and a stuffed nose.

Drug Interactions

• People taking anticoagulant (blood-thinning) drugs should avoid aspirin because it increases the effect of the anticoagulant.

• Aspirin may increase the possibility of stomach ulcer when taken together with adrenal corticosteroids, phenylbutazone, or alcoholic beverages.

• Aspirin will counteract the uric-acid-eliminating effect of probenecid and sulfinpyrazone. Aspirin may counteract the blood-pressure-lowering effect of ACE inhibitor and beta-blocking drugs. Aspirin may also counteract the effects of some diuretics in people with severe liver disease.

• Aspirin may increase blood levels of methotrexate and of valproic acid when taken with either of these drugs, leading to increased chances of drug toxicity. Mixing aspirin and nitroglycerin tablets may lead to an unexpected drop in blood pressure.

• Do not take aspirin with an NSAID. There is no benefit to the combination, and the chance of side effects—especially stomach irritation—is vastly increased.

• Large aspirin doses (2000 mg a day or more) can lower blood sugar. This can be a problem in people with diabetes who take insulin or oral antidiabetes drugs to control their condition.

Food Interactions

Because aspirin can cause upset stomach and bleeding, take each dose with food, milk, or a glass of water.

Usual Dose

Adult: aches, pains, and fever—325–650 mg every 4 hours. Arthritis and rheumatic conditions—up to 5200 mg a day in divided doses. Rheumatic fever, up to 7800 mg a day in divided doses. To prevent heart attack, stroke, or TIA—325 mg every 2 days or 80–160 mg a day.

Child (under age 16): not recommended because of the risk of Reye's syndrome (see "Cautions and Warnings").

Overdosage

Aspirin may be lethal for adults in overdoses of 30 regular-strength tablets—325 mg each—or 20 maximum-strength tablets—500 mg. Aspirin may be lethal for children in overdoses of 12 regular-strength tablets or 8 maximum-strength tablets.

Symptoms of mild overdose are rapid and deep breathing, nausea, vomiting, dizziness, ringing or buzzing in the ears, flushing, sweating, thirst, headache, drowsiness, diarrhea, and rapid heartbeat.

Severe overdose may cause fever, excitement, confusion, convulsions, liver or kidney failure, coma, and bleeding.

The initial treatment of aspirin overdose involves inducing vomiting to remove any drug remaining in the stomach. Further treatment depends on how the situation develops and what must be done to maintain the patient. Do not induce vomiting until you have spoken with your doctor or poison control center. If in doubt, go to a hospital emergency room. ALWAYS bring the aspirin bottle or container.

Special Information

Contact your doctor if you develop continuous stomach pain or ringing or buzzing in the ears.

Do not use an aspirin product if it has a strong odor of vinegar. This is an indication that the product has started to break down in the bottle.

Do not crush or chew a sustained-release preparation of aspirin.

If you forget to take a dose of aspirin, take it as soon as you remember. If it is almost time for your next dose, skip the dose you forgot and continue with your regular schedule. Do not take a double dose.

Special Populations

Pregnancy/Breast-feeding

Check with your doctor before taking any aspirin-containing product during pregnancy. Aspirin may cause bleeding problems in the fetus during the last 2 weeks of pregnancy. Taking aspirin during the last 3 months of pregnancy may extend the length of pregnancy, prolong labor, and lead to a low-birth-weight infant. It can also cause bleeding in the mother before, during, or after delivery. Anemia may also result from taking aspirin during pregnancy.

Aspirin passes into breast milk, but has not caused any problems in nursing babies. Nursing mothers should speak to their doctors before using aspirin.

Seniors

Aspirin, especially in larger doses that a senior may take for arthritis and rheumatic conditions, may be irritating to the stomach. Seniors with liver disease should not use aspirin.

Generic Name

Atazanavir Sulfate (at-ah-ZAN-ah-veer)

Brand Name

Reyataz

Type of Drug

Protease inhibitor.

Prescribed For

Advanced human immunodeficiency virus (HIV) infection.

General Information

Atazanavir is a member of the group of anti-HIV drugs called protease inhibitors, which is an important part of the multidrug cocktail responsible for gains in the fight against acquired immunodeficiency syndrome (AIDS). These drugs work at the end of the HIV reproduction process, when an enzyme known as protease "cuts" proteins into strands of exactly the correct size to duplicate HIV. Protease inhibitors prevent the mature HIV virus from being formed by inhibiting this cutting process. Proteins cut to the wrong length or remain uncut are inactive.

Protease inhibitors are always taken with 1 or 2 nucleoside antiviral drugs such as zidovudine (AZT), didanosine (ddI), zalcitabine (ddC), tenofovir, or lamivudine (3TC). Protease inhibitors have revolutionized HIV management because, when taken with other antivirals, they reduce the amount of HIV virus in the bloodstream to levels that are often undetectable by current methods such as CD4 cell (immune system cell) counts and viral load (amount of virus in the blood) measurements. Multiple-drug therapy has changed the view of HIV from a fatal disease to a manageable chronic illness.

This drug is broken down in the liver. People with moderate or severe liver disease may have more atazanavir in their blood stream and require a lower dose of this medicine.

Cautions and Warnings

Do not take this drug if you are **sensitive** or **allergic** to it.

If a serious **toxic reaction** occurs while taking atazanavir, you should stop taking it until your doctor can determine the cause or until the reaction resolves itself. Then treatment can be resumed.

This drug can cause jaundice (yellow discoloration of the skin or whites of the eyes). Use caution if you have moderate **liver disease**. People with severe **liver disease** should not take atazanavir sulfate.

Atazanavir may **raise blood sugar** levels, worsen diabetes, or trigger latent diabetes. People with diabetes who take atazanavir may need to adjust the dosage of their antidiabetes medication.

HIV virus may become **resistant** to atazanavir or other protease inhibitors. For this reason it is essential that you take atazanavir exactly according to your doctor's directions.

People with hemophilia have experienced bleeding while taking this drug.

Atazanavir may cause the redistribution or accumulation of body fat, leading to **buffalo hump, breast enlargement, abnormal thinness,** or a **round, moon-shaped face**.

Possible Side Effects

Most side effects are mild. Other side effects become more prominent when atazanavir is taken together with antiretroviral drugs; these include weakness, muscle pain, and mouth ulcers.

▼ Most common: nausea and headache.

▼ Common: vomiting, diarrhea, abdominal pain, rash, infection, headache, drowsiness, insomnia, and jaundice (yellow discoloration of the skin or whites of the eyes).

▼ Less common: fever, pain, fatigue, back pain, fat accumulation, joint pain, depression, sleeplessness, dizziness, coughing, and tingling or other unusual sensation in the arms, hands, legs or feet.

▼ Rare: Rare side effects can occur in almost any part of the body. Contact your doctor if you experience any side effect not listed above.

Drug Interactions

• Rifampin, proton pump inhibitors, and St. John's wort substantially reduce atazanavir blood levels. Do not combine these drugs.

• Cimetidine, famotidine, and ranitidine can also reduce atazanavir blood levels. Separate these drugs from atazanavir by at least 12 hours.

• Both atazanavir and indinavir cause elevated levels of bilirubin in the blood. Do not combine these medicines.

• Atazanavir increases levels of cisapride, ergot drugs, irinotecan (an anticancer drug), midazolam, pimozide, and triazolam leading to potentially serious drug toxicities. These drugs should not be combined with atazanavir.

• Combining atazanavir with the antibiotic clarithromycin may lead to an increased chance of clarithromycin-related cardiac toxicity. Clarithromycin dose should be halved.

• Atazanavir may increase side effects of the statin-type blood cholesterol drugs. Do not take this drug with atorvastatin, lovastatin, or simvastatin. Other statins may not be as affected because of how they are broken down in the body.

• If you also take didanosine or use antacids, take atazanavir with food, 1 hour before or 2 hours after you take didanosine or antacid.

• If you must take efavirenz and atazanavir, your doctor should also be prescribing ritonavir to increase the effectiveness of atazanavir.

• Atazanavir can increase blood levels of the hormones in oral contraceptive pills. Your doctor should prescribe the lowest effective dose product to avoid undesirable hormone side effects.

• Atazanavir may raise blood levels of amiodarone, calcium channel blockers, cyclosporine, lidocaine, quinidine, rifabutin, sirolimus, tacrolimus, tricyclic-type antidepressants, and warfarin. It may be necessary for your doctor to reduce drug dosage by as much as half to avoid drug side effects if you start taking atazanavir.

• Protease inhibitors, including atazanavir, may drastically increase sildenafil, vardenafil, and taldenafil blood levels, increasing the risk of side effects including low blood pressure, visual changes, and persistent, painful erection. A lower dose may be required.

Food Interactions

Take atazanavir within 2 hours after a full meal. The amount of atazanavir absorbed into the blood is vastly reduced when it is taken on an empty stomach, thus negating its antiviral effects.

Usual Dose

Adult: 400 mg daily, within 2 hours after a meal. Patients with moderate liver disease should take only 300 mg a day.

Child (under age 16): consult your doctor.

Overdosage

A drug overdose may cause cardiac problems. Take the victim to a hospital emergency room for evaluation and treatment. ALWAYS bring the prescription bottle or container.

Special Information

Atazanavir does not cure HIV infection or AIDS. It will not prevent you from transmitting the HIV virus to another person; you must still practice safe sex. You may still develop opportunistic infections or other illnesses associated with advanced HIV disease. The long-term effects of this drug are not known.

Call your doctor if you become dizzy or lightheaded. This could be a sign that the drug is affecting your heart.

Take this medication exactly according to your doctor's instructions. Skipping doses of atazanavir increases the risk that you will become resistant to the drug. It should be taken after meals with your nucleoside antiviral drug. If you forget a dose of atazanavir, take it as soon as you remember and continue with your regular schedule. Do not take a double dose.

Special Populations

Pregnancy/Breast-feeding

While animal studies of atazanavir reveal minor damage to the fetus at double the human dosage, this drug should only be used during pregnancy after carefully weighing its potential benefits against its risks. The company making atazanavir has established a registry to gather information on pregnant women who take this drug.

It is not known if atazanavir passes into breast milk. Nursing mothers with HIV should always bottle-feed, regardless of whether they take this drug, to avoid transmitting the virus to their child.

Seniors

Seniors can take this drug without special precaution.

Generic Name

Atenolol (ah-TEN-uh-lol) G

Brand Name

Tenormin

Combination Products

Generic Ingredients: Atenolol + Chlorthalidone G
Tenoretic

Type of Drug

Beta-adrenergic blocking agent.

Prescribed For

High blood pressure, abnormal heart rhythms, angina pectoris, prevention of second heart attack and migraine, alcohol withdrawal, stage fright and other anxieties, and bleeding from the esophagus.

General Information

Atenolol is one of many beta-adrenergic blocking drugs, or beta blockers, that interfere with the action of a specific part of the nervous system. Beta receptors are found all over the body and affect many body functions. Each beta blocker has particular characteristics that may make it more suitable for certain conditions or people.

Cautions and Warnings

Do not take atenolol if you are allergic to beta blockers.

People with **angina** who take atenolol for high blood pressure risk aggravating their angina if they suddenly stop taking the drug. These people should have their drug dosage reduced gradually over 1 to 2 weeks.

Atenolol should be used with caution if you have **liver or kidney disease,** because your ability to eliminate this drug from your body may be impaired.

Atenolol reduces the amount of blood the heart pumps. This reduction in blood flow may aggravate the condition of people with **poor circulation** or **circulatory disease**.

If you are undergoing **major surgery,** your doctor may want you to stop taking atenolol at least 2 days before surgery.

If you have **pheochromocytoma,** use atenolol with caution.

Possible Side Effects

Side effects are relatively uncommon and usually mild; they usually develop early in the course of treatment and are rarely a reason to stop taking atenolol.

▼ Most common: impotence.

▼ Less common: unusual tiredness or weakness, slow heartbeat, heart failure (symptoms include swelling of the legs, ankles, or feet), dizziness, breathing difficulties, bronchospasm, depression, confusion, anxiety, nervousness, sleeplessness, disorientation,

---

Possible Side Effects (continued)

short-term memory loss, emotional instability, cold hands and feet, constipation, diarrhea, nausea, vomiting, upset stomach, increased sweating, urinary difficulties, cramps, blurred vision, rash, hair loss, stuffy nose, facial swelling, aggravation of lupus erythematosus (chronic condition affecting the body's connective tissue), itching, chest pain, back or joint pain, colitis, drug allergy (symptoms include fever and sore throat), and liver toxicity.

Drug Interactions

• Atenolol may interact with surgical anesthetics to increase the risk of heart problems during surgery. Some anesthesiologists recommend gradually stopping the drug by 2 days before surgery.

• Atenolol may interfere with the normal signs of low blood sugar and with oral antidiabetic drugs.

• Atenolol increases the blood-pressure-lowering effects of other blood-pressure-reducing agents, including clonidine, guanabenz, and reserpine; and calcium channel blockers, such as nifedipine.

• Aspirin-containing drugs, indomethacin, sulfinpyrazone, and estrogen drugs may interfere with the blood-pressure-lowering effect of atenolol.

• Cocaine may reduce the effectiveness of all beta blockers.

• Atenolol may worsen the problem of cold hands and feet associated with taking ergot alkaloids, used to treat migraine. Gangrene is a possibility in people taking both an ergot and atenolol.

• Atenolol will counteract thyroid hormone replacements.

• Calcium channel blockers, flecainide, hydralazine, oral contraceptives, propafenone, haloperidol, phenothiazine tranquilizers—molindone and others—quinolone antibacterials, and quinidine may increase the amount of atenolol in the bloodstream and lead to increased atenolol effects.

• Atenolol should not be taken within 2 weeks of taking a monoamine oxidase inhibitor (MAOI) antidepressant.

• Cimetidine increases the amount of atenolol absorbed into the bloodstream from oral tablets.

• Atenolol may interfere with the effectiveness of some antiasthma drugs, including theophylline and aminophylline, and especially ephedrine and isoproterenol.

• Combining atenolol with phenytoin or digitalis drugs may result in excessive slowing of the heart, possibly causing heart block (disruption of the electrical impulses that control heart rate).

• If you stop smoking while taking atenolol, your dose may have to be reduced because your liver will break down the drug more slowly.

• Aluminum salts, barbituates, calcium salts, cholestyramine, colestipol, ampicillin, and rifampin may reduce the effectiveness of atenolol.

Food Interactions

None known.

Usual Dose

Adult: starting dose—50 mg a day, increased gradually up to 200 mg. Maintenance dose—50–200 mg once a day. People with kidney disease may need only 50 mg every other day. Older adults should be treated more cautiously and may need a lower dose.

Overdosage

Symptoms of overdose include changes in heartbeat—unusually slow, unusually fast, or irregular—severe dizziness or fainting, breathing difficulties, bluish-colored fingernails or palms, and seizures. Heart failure and shock may also result from an overdose of atenolol. The victim should be taken to a hospital emergency room. ALWAYS bring the prescription bottle or container.

Special Information

Atenolol is meant to be taken continuously. When ending atenolol treatment, dosage should be reduced gradually over a period of about 2 weeks. Do not stop taking this drug unless directed to do so by your doctor: Abrupt withdrawal may cause chest pain, breathing difficulties, increased sweating, and unusually fast or irregular heartbeat.

Call your doctor at once if you develop back or joint pain, breathing difficulties, cold hands or feet, depression, rash, or changes in heartbeat. Atenolol may produce an undesirable lowering of blood pressure, leading to dizziness or fainting; call your doctor if this happens. Call your doctor if you experience persistent or bothersome anxiety, diarrhea, constipation, impotence, headache, itching, nausea or vomiting, nightmares or vivid dreams, upset stomach, insomnia, stuffy nose, frequent urination, unusual tiredness, or weakness.

Atenolol may cause drowsiness, light-headedness, dizziness, or blurred vision. Be careful when driving or performing complex tasks.

It is best to take atenolol at the same time each day. If you forget a dose, take it as soon as you remember. If you take atenolol once a day and it is within 8 hours of your next dose, skip the dose you forgot and continue with your regular schedule. If you take atenolol twice a day and it is within 4 hours of your next dose, skip the one you forgot and continue with your regular schedule. Never take a double dose.

Special Populations

Pregnancy/Breast-feeding

Infants born to women who took a beta blocker while pregnant had lower birth weights, low blood pressure, and reduced heart rates. Atenolol should be avoided by pregnant women and women who might become pregnant while taking it.

Atenolol passes into breast milk. Nursing mothers should avoid taking atenolol.

Seniors

Seniors taking atenolol may be more likely to suffer from cold hands and feet, reduced body temperature, chest pain, general feelings of ill health, sudden breathing difficulties, increased sweating, or changes in heartbeat.

Generic Name

Atomoxetine (ah-tom-OX-eh-teen)

Brand Name

Strattera

Type of Drug

Selective norepinephrine reuptake inhibitor.

Prescribed For

Attention deficit hyperactivity disorder (ADHD).

General Information

Atomoxetine is the first of a new class of treatments for attention deficit hyperactivity disorder (ADHD). This drug may be used by children, teenagers, and adults. Unlike other medicines used for ADHD, it is not a stimulant and does not carry many of the liabilities associated with other drugs.

Cautions and Warnings

Do not take atomoxetine if you are **sensitive** or **allergic** to it.

Separate atomoxetine from any **MAO inhibitor** drug by at least 2 weeks. Serious, sometimes fatal, symptoms including **body temperature elevations, rigidity, muscle stiffness, rapid changes of vital signs or mental status** (including extreme agitation progressing to delirium and coma) may occur.

Atomoxetine can increase blood pressure and heart rate. People with **high blood pressure, rapid heartbeat, and cardiovascular or cerebrovascular disease** should use it with caution.

People with **liver disease** may require a lower dosage of atomoxetine. People with moderate liver disease should take half of the regular dose and those with severe liver disease should take one-quarter of the regular dose.

People taking atomoxetine may feel **dizzy** or **faint** when rising quickly from a sitting or lying position.

Atomoxetine can worsen **narrow angle glaucoma**.

Children taking atomoxetine may not grow or gain weight as quickly as those who don't take it. It is not known if the drug affects final height or weight.

Possible Side Effects

Children

In clinical studies, drug side effects were similar to those reported by people taking an inactive placebo.

▼ Most common: headache, upper abdominal pain, vomiting, and coughing.

Possible Side Effects *(continued)*

▼ Common: dizziness, tiredness, and irritability.

▼ Less common: constipation, upset stomach, runny nose, appetite loss, weight loss, crying mood swings, and skin rash.

Adults

▼ Most common: dry mouth, headache, nausea, and sleeplessness.

▼ Common: urinary hesitation or difficulty urinating, constipation, upset stomach, tiredness or fatigue, sinus infection, appetite loss, dizziness, sleeping problems, painful menstruation, erectile dysfunction, and reduced sex drive or other sexual concerns.

▼ Less common: heart palpitation, abdominal gas, fever and chills, weight loss, abnormal dreams, sinus headache, tingling in the hands or feet, muscle ache, impotence, delayed onset of menstruation, irregular or other menstrual issues, prostate irritation, skin rash, increased sweating, and hot flushes.

▼ Rare: sleeplessness, chest pain, and heart palpitations.

Drug Interactions

• Atomoxetine increases the effects of albuterol, causing high blood pressure and rapid heartbeat. Dosage adjustments may be required.

• Fluoxetine, paroxetine, and quinidine substantially increase the amount of atomoxetine in the blood. Atomoxetine dosages adjustements may be necessary.

• Atomoxetine raises blood pressure and should be given with caution to people who are already taking medicines that raise blood pressure. It may counter the effects of some drugs used to treat high blood pressure.

Food Interactions

Atomoxetine may be taken without regard to food or meals.

Usual Dose

Adult and Child (155 lbs. and over): 40–80 mg a day in a single or divided dose. Maximum dose is 100 mg a day. Divided doses should be taken in the morning and late afternoon or early evening.

Child (age 6 and over and less than 155 lbs.): Starting dose—0.23 mg per lb. of body weight. Dose can be gradually increased up to 0.55 mg per lb. as a single dose in the morning or 2 doses, one in the morning and the second in the late afternoon or early evening. The maximum daily dose is 100 mg.

Overdosage

Little is known about the effects of atomoxetine overdose. Call your local poison control center or a hospital emergency room for information. If you seek treatment, ALWAYS bring the prescription bottle or container.

Special Information

If you forget a dose of atomoxetine, take it as soon as you remember. If it is almost time for your next dose, skip the one you forgot and continue with your regular schedule. Do not take a double dose of atomoxetine.

Use caution while driving or operating machinery when you start taking atomoxetine until you can determine how it will affect your abilities.

Special Populations

Pregnancy/Breast-feeding

Animal studies show that atomoxetine may affect a developing fetus. When this drug is considered crucial by your doctor, its potential benefits must be carefully weighed against its risks.

Atomoxetine may pass into breast milk. Nursing mothers who must take this drug should bottle-feed.

Seniors

Atomoxetine has not been studied in older adults.

Generic Name

Atovaquone (ah-TOE-vuh-quone)

Brand Name

Mepron Ⓢ

Type of Drug

Anti-infective.

Prescribed For

Pneumocystis carinii pneumonia (PCP).

General Information

Atovaquone is an anti-infective with specific activity against PCP, an infection commonly associated with AIDS. It is used in people who cannot take trimethoprim and sulfamethoxazole. In studies comparing atovaquone with trimethoprim-sulfamethoxazole, approximately 60% of people with PCP improved on each drug. However, more people died of PCP and other infections while being treated with atovaquone. Of those who died, most had less atovaquone in their bloodstream than those who lived. In studies comparing oral atovaquone with intravenous pentamidine for treating PCP in people with AIDS, both drugs were equally effective, at 14%. Again, there was a direct correlation between the amount of atovaquone in the blood and survival. The drug stays in the body for several days and is eliminated through the liver.

Cautions and Warnings

Do not take atovaquone if you are or may be **allergic** to it or to any of the product's components.

This drug has not been studied for PCP prevention or for severe PCP, or in those who are failing on TMP-SMZ.

Atovaquone only works against PCP. People with PCP who have bacterial, viral, fungal, or other infections of the lung may continue to worsen despite atovaquone therapy. If this happens, it may be a sign that another kind of infecting organism is the cause. Additional medicine will be necessary.

Since atovaquone absorption is so strongly influenced by high-fat foods, **people who cannot eat enough** may not be able to absorb enough medicine, and may have to take intravenous treatments of other PCP anti-infectives while taking atovaquone.

Possible Side Effects

Overall, only 4% to 7% of people stopped taking the drug because of side effects, a much smaller percentage than occurs with other PCP treatments.

▼ Most common: rash, nausea, diarrhea, headache, vomiting, fever, sleeplessness, weakness, itching, oral fungal infections, abdominal pain, upset stomach, appetite loss, constipation, cough, dizziness, pain, increased sweating, anxiety, sinus inflammation, and runny nose.

▼ Less common: changes in sense of taste, low blood sugar, and low blood pressure.

Drug Interactions

• Atovaquone may increase blood levels of warfarin, oral antidiabetes drugs, digoxin, and other drugs that bind strongly to blood proteins.

• Rifampin and rifabutin may reduce blood levels of atovaquone, possibly diminishing its effectiveness.

• Taking atovaquone with TMP-SMZ has resulted in reduced blood levels of TMP-SMZ. This should not reduce TMP-SMZ's effectiveness.

• Taking atovaquone with zidovudine (AZT) drastically reduces the rate at which zidovudine is eliminated from the body. For most people, this is not a problem.

Food Interactions

Take atovaquone with food or meals to improve drug absorption. A high-fat meal can increase the amount absorbed by 300%.

Usual Dose

For prevention, 1500 mg daily with food.
For treatment, 750 mg 2 times a day for 3 weeks, taken with food.

Overdosage

Little is known about the effects of atovaquone overdose; symptoms are likely to be exaggerated drug side effects. No life-threatening experiences have been reported. Call your local poison control center or hospital emergency room for more information. If you go to the hospital, ALWAYS bring the prescription bottle or container.

Special Information

Taking atovaquone regularly and with food is essential to the drug's effectiveness. If you cannot eat 2 meals a day, your doctor may have to prescribe another PCP treatment.

Call your doctor if you develop any persistent or bothersome side effects.

If you forget a dose, take it as soon as you remember. If it is almost time for your next dose, space your remaining doses equally throughout the rest of the day so that you can still take a total daily dose of 1500 mg, or 2 tsp.

Special Populations

Pregnancy/Breast-feeding

In animal studies, atovaquone has affected fetal development. If you are pregnant this drug should be used only if the potential risks and benefits have been carefully weighed by you and your doctor.

Atovaquone is likely to pass into breast milk because of its affinity for body fat. Nursing mothers should bottle-feed while taking atovaquone.

Seniors

This drug has not been tested systematically in people over age 65. Seniors, especially those with kidney, heart, or liver disease, may be more sensitive to atovaquone side effects.

Augmentin ES see *Penicillin Antibiotics*, page 825

Brand Name

Auralgan Otic

Generic Ingredients

Antipyrine + Benzocaine + Glycerin Ⓖ

Other Brand Names

Allergen Ear Drops   Otocalm Ear
Auroto Otic

Type of Drug

Analgesic.

Prescribed For

Earache.

General Information

Auralgan contains benzocaine, a local anesthetic that deadens nerves inside the ear that transmit painful impulses; antipyrine, an analgesic that provides additional pain relief; and glycerin, which absorbs any water present in the ear. This drug is often used to treat painful conditions caused by water in the ear canal, such as "swimmer's ear."

Cautions and Warnings

Do not use the product if you are **allergic** to any of its ingredients.

Possible Side Effects

▼ Most common: local irritation.

Drug Interactions

• Do not use other ear medications at the same time as Auralgan.

Usual Dose

Place drops of Auralgan in the ear canal until the canal is filled. Saturate a piece of cotton with Auralgan, and put it in the ear canal to keep the drug from leaking out. Leave the drug in the ear for several minutes. Repeat 3–4 times a day.

Overdosage

Auralgan overdose is not likely to cause serious effects. In the case of overdose or accidental ingestion, call your local poison control center.

Special Information

Before using the product, warm the medicine bottle to body temperature by holding it in your hand for several minutes. Do not warm the bottle to a temperature above normal body temperature. Protect the bottle from light.

Call your doctor if you develop a burning or itching sensation or if the pain does not go away after 2 to 4 days of treatment.

If you forget a dose of Auralgan, take it as soon as you remember. If it is almost time for your next dose, skip the dose you forgot and continue with your regular schedule.

Special Populations

Pregnancy/Breast-feeding

The safety of using Auralgan Otic during pregnancy is not known. When this medication is considered crucial by your doctor, its potential benefits must be carefully weighed against its risks.

It is not known if the ingredients in Auralgan Otic pass into breast milk. Nursing mothers who take this medication should watch their infants for drug-related side effects.

Seniors

Seniors may use this product without restriction.

Avandia see *Glitazone Antidiabetes Drugs,* page 526

Avapro see *Angiotensin II Blockers,* page 84

Generic Name

Azithromycin (uh-ZIH-throe-MYE-sin)

Brand Name

Zithromax

Type of Drug

Macrolide antibiotic.

Prescribed For

Upper and lower respiratory tract infections, skin infections, sexually transmitted diseases (STDs), middle ear infections, tonsillitis, and pharyngitis.

General Information

Azithromycin is an azalide antibiotic, a subgroup of the macrolides. Macrolide drugs are either bactericidal (bacteria-killing) or bacteriostatic (inhibiting bacterial growth) depending on the organism in question and amount of antibiotic present.

Cautions and Warnings

Do not take azithromycin if you are **allergic** to it or any macrolide antibiotic.

Azithromycin is excreted primarily through the liver. People with **liver disease or damage** should consult their doctors. Those on long-term therapy with this drug should have periodic blood tests.

Colitis (bowel inflammation), ranging from mild to life-threatening, has been associated with all antibiotics (see "Possible Side Effects").

Azithromycin is considered appropriate only for the treatment of more mild forms of pneumonia in non-hospitalized patients. People with other underlying conditions, those who are **immune-compromised,** and those who contract pneumonia in a hospital or other institutional setting probably should be treated with other antibiotics.

Possible Side Effects

Most side effects are mild and go away once you stop taking azithromycin.

▼ Most common: nausea, vomiting, abdominal pain, and diarrhea. Colitis (symptoms include severe abdominal cramps and severe, persistent, and possibly bloody diarrhea) may develop.

▼ Less common: heart palpitations, chest pain, hairy tongue, vaginal irritation, stomach upset, gas, dizziness, headache, tiredness, unusual sun sensitivity, rash, itching, and swelling.

Drug Interactions

• Pimozide should not be taken by anyone also taking a macrolide antibiotic. Two people died while taking this combination.

• Antacid products containing aluminum magnesium may delay the absorption of azithromycin into the blood. Separate your antacid dose from azithromycin by at least 1 hour.

• All macrolide antibiotics increase blood levels of cyclosporine and may cause kidney damage.

• Combining azithromycin and a statin cholesterol-lowering drug increases the risk of developing a painful and potentially fatal condition involving severe muscle degeneration.

Food Interactions

It is important to take azithromycin liquid on an empty stomach, 1 hour before or 2 hours after meals. Tablets may be taken with or without food.

Usual Dose

Respiratory Tract Infections, Skin Infections, and STDs
    Adult (age 16 and over): 500 mg as a single dose for 3 days, or 500 mg as a single dose on day 1, then 250 mg once a day on days 2–5 of treatment. STDs are treated with a single dose of 1000–2000 mg.

Middle Ear Infections
    Child (age 6 months and over): 100–500 mg a day for 3 days, or 100–500 mg on day 1, then 50–250 mg on days 2–5 of treatment. Actual dose depends on body weight.

Tonsillitis and Sore Throat
    Child (age 2 and over): 100–500 mg a day for 5 days. Actual dose depends on body weight.

Overdosage

Overdose may cause severe side effects, especially nausea, vomiting, stomach cramps, and diarrhea. Call your local poison control center or hospital emergency room for more information. If you seek treatment, ALWAYS bring the prescription bottle or container.

Special Information

Call your doctor if you develop nausea, vomiting, diarrhea, stomach cramps, or severe abdominal pain. Stop taking this drug and immediately call your doctor if you experience breathing difficulties, chest pain, hives, rash, itching, mouth sores, or unusual sensitivity to light.

It is crucial that you follow your doctor's directions on how to take the drug and how many days to take it—even if you feel well sooner. This drug's effectiveness may be severely reduced otherwise. Taking azithromycin at the same time each day may help you remember your medication.

If you forget a dose of azithromycin, take it as soon as you remember. If it is almost time for your next dose, skip the dose you forgot and go back to your regular schedule.

Special Populations

Pregnancy/Breast-feeding
It is not known if azithromycin passes into the fetal circulation. This medication should be taken by pregnant women only if it is clearly needed.

It is not known if azithromycin passes into breast milk, but other macrolide antibiotics do. Nursing mothers who must take this drug should bottle-feed.

Seniors
Seniors with liver disease should use caution. Seniors who have pneumonia or are especially sickly or debilitated probably should be treated with other medications.

Generic Name

Baclofen (BAK-loe-fen) G

Brand Name

Lioresal

Type of Drug

Skeletal muscle relaxant.

Prescribed For

Muscle spasms associated with multiple sclerosis (MS), spinal cord injury or disease, or other nervous system conditions; may also be used to treat trigeminal neuralgia (tic douloureux), and hiccups.

General Information

Baclofen may work by interfering with nervous system reflexes at the spinal cord, although it may also have some effect outside the spinal cord. Baclofen is chemically similar to a natural nerve transmitter known as GABA; baclofen's effect on muscle spasm may be related to its effect on GABA nerve receptors.

Cautions and Warnings

Do not take baclofen if you are **allergic** or sensitive to it. It should not be taken for muscle spasm resulting from **rheumatic disease, stroke, cerebral palsy,** or **Parkinson's disease** because its benefit in these situations has not been proven. The condition of people with **epilepsy** or **psychotic disorders** may worsen while taking baclofen.

About 4% of women with MS who take baclofen for less than 1 year develop **ovarian cysts** that usually disappear on their own. This is within the normal range for all women—1% to 5%—for developing ovarian cysts.

Baclofen is excreted primarily through the kidneys, so patients with **kidney disease** or **impaired kidney function** should use baclofen with caution.

Abruptly stopping baclofen can lead to **hallucinations** and **seizure**. Dosage should always be gradually reduced, except in cases of severe side effects.

Possible Side Effects

Baclofen may affect lab tests for liver function and can raise blood sugar levels.

▼ Most common: drowsiness, low blood pressure, weakness, dizziness, light-headedness, nausea and vomiting, headache, and sleeplessness.

▼ Less common: frequent urination, fatigue or lethargy, confusion, euphoria, excitement, depression, hallucinations, tingling in the hands or feet, muscle pain, ringing or buzzing in the ears, coordination difficulties, tremors, rigidity, weakness, loss of muscle tone, unusual eye movement and other muscle-control problems, double vision, pinpoint or wide-open pupils, breathing difficulties, heart palpitations, dry mouth, appetite loss, changes in sense of taste, abdominal pain, diarrhea, bed-wetting, difficulty urinating, painful urination, impotence, blood in the urine, rash, itching, swelling of the ankle, excessive sweating, weight gain, and stuffy nose.

▼ Rare: slurred speech, blurred vision, seizure, fainting, chest pain, and testing positive for blood in the stool.

Drug Interactions

• Avoid alcoholic beverages and other nervous system depressants while taking baclofen.

• Combining a monoamine oxidase inhibitor (MAOI) antidepressant with baclofen may cause drowsiness, nervous system depression, and low blood pressure.

• Combining a tricyclic antidepressant with baclofen may lead to severe muscle weakness.

• Baclofen may increase blood sugar. Diabetics may need to increase their dosage of antidiabetic drugs to account for this effect.

• Combining blood-pressure-lowering drugs with baclofen may lead to dizziness or fainting due to severe lowering of blood pressure.

Food Interactions

This drug may be taken without regard to food or meals.

Usual Dose

Adult and Child: 5 mg 3 times a day for 3 days, gradually increased every 3 days until the desired effect is achieved, usually at 40–80 mg a day. People with kidney disease require lower doses.

Overdosage

Symptoms of baclofen overdose include vomiting, loss of muscle tone, twitching, convulsions, pinpoint or wide-open pupils, drowsiness, blurred or double vision, breathing difficulties, seizure, and coma. Overdose victims should be taken to a hospital emergency room for treatment. ALWAYS bring the prescription bottle or container.

Special Information

Baclofen is a nervous system depressant. Take care when driving or doing anything that requires concentration and physical coordination.

Call your doctor if you develop a frequent urge to urinate, painful urination, constipation, nausea, headache, sleeplessness, or persistent confusion.

Do not stop taking baclofen on your own. Abruptly stopping this drug may lead to hallucinations or seizure.

Your pharmacist may prepare a baclofen liquid. This mixture should be kept in the refrigerator and must be thrown away after 1 month.

If you forget a dose of baclofen and remember within 1 hour of your scheduled time, take it immediately. If you do not remember until more than 1 hour later or if you forget it completely, skip the dose you forgot and continue with your regular schedule. Do not take a double dose.

Special Populations

Pregnancy/Breast-feeding

Baclofen increases the chances of certain birth defects in lab animals. Pregnant women should only take baclofen after carefully weighing its possible benefits against its risks with their doctor.

Baclofen taken by mouth passes into breast milk. Nursing mothers who must take this drug should bottle-feed or receive the drug by injection directly into the spinal cord, because baclofen administered by injection does not pass into breast milk.

Seniors

Seniors may be more sensitive to nervous system side effects including hallucinations, depression, drowsiness, and confusion.

Bactroban see *Mupirocin*, page 735

Generic Name

Becaplermin (beh-CAP-ler-min)

Brand Name

Regranex

Type of Drug

Human growth factor.

Prescribed For

Diabetic foot and leg wounds.

General Information

Becaplermin is a type of human growth factor produced in a laboratory. While it is not a substitute for good wound care, becaplermin can stimulate wound tissue to heal faster. Studies of the drug have produced mixed results. In some studies, people using becaplermin were 1½ to 2 times more likely to have complete healing of their wounds. In another study, the results with becaplermin were the same as those with good wound care alone.

Cautions and Warnings

Do not use becaplermin if you are **sensitive** or **allergic** to it.

Becaplermin should not be used to **speed the healing** of wounds that are healing by themselves.

Becaplermin should not be applied to **skin cancer** or **tumors** or **exposed bones, joints, tendons, or ligaments** because its effect on these body structures is not known.

Becaplermin should not be used for wounds that extend to **subcutaneous tissue**.

Possible Side Effects

People treated with becaplermin plus wound care had a slightly larger risk of developing a rash than those who received wound care alone.

Drug Interactions

None known.

Usual Dose

Adult and Child (age 16 and over): Apply a thin layer to the wound and leave in place for 12 hours. Then, remove the becaplermin bandage, rinse the wound, and cover it with a plain saline-soaked bandage for the rest of the day. Continue this process until the wound has healed completely.

Child (under age 16): not recommended.

Overdosage

Little is known about the effects of accidental ingestion. Call your local poison control center or a hospital emergency room for information.

Special Information

Call your doctor if your wound worsens or is irritated by becaplermin.

Wash your hands before applying becaplermin.

Do not allow the tip of the becaplermin tube to touch any surface, including the wound being treated.

Your doctor should reassess your treatment if the wound is not 30% smaller in 10 weeks and completely healed in 20 weeks.

Applying more becaplermin than recommended will not make your wound heal better or faster.

If you forget a dose, apply it as soon as you remember. If it is almost time for your next dose, skip the missed dose and continue with your regular schedule.

Special Populations

Pregnancy/Breast-feeding

The safety of using becaplermin during pregnancy is not known. The drug should only be used during pregnancy if it is absolutely necessary.

It is not known if becaplermin passes into breast milk. Nursing mothers who must take this drug should bottle-feed.

Seniors

Seniors may take this drug without special precautions.

Generic Name

Benazepril (ben-AY-zuh-pril)

Brand Name

Lotensin

Combination Products

Generic Ingredients: Benazepril + Hydrochlorothiazide
Lotensin HCT

Type of Drug

Angiotensin-converting enzyme (ACE) inhibitor.

Prescribed For

High blood pressure.

General Information

Benazepril hydrochloride and other ACE inhibitors prevent the conversion of a hormone called angiotensin I to another hormone called angiotensin II, a potent blood-vessel constrictor. Preventing this conversion relaxes blood vessels, thus reducing blood pressure and relieving symptoms of heart failure. Benazepril also affects the production of other hormones and enzymes that participate in the regulation of blood-vessel dilation. Benazepril starts working in 1 hour and continues to work for about 24 hours.

Some people who start taking benazepril after they are already on a diuretic (agent that increases urination) experience a rapid drop in blood pressure after their first dose or when their dosage is increased. To prevent this from happening, your doctor may tell you to stop taking your diuretic 2 or 3 days before starting benazepril, or to increase your salt intake during that time. The diuretic may then be restarted gradually.

Cautions and Warnings

Do not take benazepril if you have had an **allergic reaction** to it in the past.

Benazepril occasionally causes **very low blood pressure**.

Benazepril may affect **kidney function**. Your doctor should check your urine for protein content during the first few months of treatment. Dosage adjustment is necessary if you have reduced kidney function.

Benazepril can affect white-blood-cell counts, possibly increasing your susceptibility to **infection**. Your doctor should monitor your blood counts periodically.

Benazepril can cause serious injury or death to the fetus if taken during pregnancy. Pregnant women should not take benazepril.

Possible Side Effects

▼ Most common: dizziness, tiredness, headache, nausea, and chronic cough. The cough usually goes away a few days after you stop taking the medication.

▼ Rare: Rare side effects can occur in almost any part of the body. Contact your doctor if you develop any side effect not listed above.

Drug Interactions

• Combining 325 mg a day or more of aspirin with benazepril carries a higher risk of death than taking lower doses (less than 160 mg a day). People taking aspirin to prevent a heart attack should use the lower dose.

• The blood-pressure-lowering effect of benazepril is additive with diuretics and beta blockers. Any other drug that causes a rapid drop in blood pressure should be used with caution if you are taking benazepril.

• Benazepril may increase blood-potassium levels, especially if taken with Dyazide or other potassium-sparing diuretics.

• Benazepril may increase the effect of lithium; this combination should be used with caution.

• Antacids and benazepril should be taken at least 2 hours apart.

• Capsaicin may trigger or aggravate the cough associated with benazepril therapy.

• Indomethacin may reduce the blood-pressure-lowering effects of benazepril.

• Phenothiazine tranquilizers and antivomiting drugs may increase the effects of benazepril.

• Combining allopurinol and benazepril increases the risk of side effects.

• Benazepril increases blood levels of digoxin, which may increase the chance of digoxin-related side effects.

Food Interactions

You may take benazepril with food if it upsets your stomach.

Usual Dose

20–40 mg a day as a single dose or in 2 equally divided doses. People with poor kidney function may need less medication.

Overdosage

The principal effect of benazepril overdose is a rapid drop in blood pressure, as evidenced by dizziness or fainting. Take the overdose victim to a hospital emergency room immediately. ALWAYS bring the prescription bottle or container.

Special Information

Benazepril can cause swelling of the face, lips, hands, and feet. This swelling can also affect the larynx (throat) and tongue and interfere with breathing. If this happens, go to a hospital at once. Call your doctor if you develop a sore throat, mouth sores, abnormal heartbeat, sudden difficulty breathing, chest pain, persistent rash, or loss of taste perception.

You may get dizzy if you rise to your feet too quickly from a sitting or lying position.

Avoid strenuous exercise or very hot weather because heavy sweating or dehydration can cause a rapid drop in blood pressure.

While taking benazepril, avoid over-the-counter diet pills, decongestants, and other stimulants that can raise blood pressure.

If you take benazepril once a day and forget a dose, take it as soon as you remember. If it is within 8 hours of your next dose, skip the dose you forgot and continue with your regular schedule. If you take benazepril twice a day and miss a dose, take the missed dose right away. If it is within 4 hours of your next dose, take 1 dose immediately and another in 5 or 6 hours, and then go back to your regular schedule. Never take a double dose.

Special Populations

Pregnancy/Breast-feeding

ACE inhibitors can cause fetal injury or death. Women who are or might become pregnant should not take ACE inhibitors. If you become pregnant, stop taking the medication and call your doctor immediately.

Small amounts of benazepril pass into breast milk. Nursing mothers who must take this drug should consider bottle-feeding.

Seniors

Seniors may be more sensitive to the effects of this drug due to age-related losses in kidney or liver function.

Generic Name

Bepridil (bep-RIH-dil)

Brand Name

Vascor

Type of Drug

Calcium channel blocker.

Prescribed For

Angina pectoris.

General Information

Bepridil hydrochloride is one of many calcium channel blockers available in the U.S. These drugs block the passage of calcium, an essential factor in muscle contraction, into the heart and smooth muscles. Such blockage of calcium interferes with the contraction of these muscles, which in turn dilates (widens) the veins and vessels that supply blood to them. This dilating effect reduces blood pressure, the amount of oxygen used by the heart muscles, and the risk of blood vessel spasm. Bepridil is therefore useful in treating not only high blood pressure but also angina pectoris (brief attacks of chest pain), a condition related to poor oxygen supply to the heart muscles.

Bepridil affects the movement of calcium only into muscle cells; it has no effect on calcium in the blood.

Cautions and Warnings

Do not take this drug if you have had an **allergic reaction** to it.

Bepridil should be used with extreme caution if you have a history of problems related to **heart rhythm**. It has caused serious derangement of heart rhythm and has affected white-blood-cell counts; therefore, it is usually reserved only for people who do not respond to other treatments.

Low blood pressure may occur, especially in people also taking a beta blocker.

Use bepridil with caution if you have **heart failure,** since the drug can worsen the condition. Bepridil may cause **angina** when treatment is first started, when the dosage is increased, or if the drug is rapidly withdrawn. This can be avoided by reducing the dosage gradually.

Studies have shown that people taking calcium channel blockers—usually those taken several times a day, not those taken only once daily—have a greater chance of having a **heart attack** than do people taking beta blockers or other medications for the same purposes. Discuss this with your doctor to be sure you are receiving the best possible treatment.

Calcium channel blockers can affect **blood platelets,** leading to possible bruising, black-and-blue marks, and bleeding.

People with **kidney problems** or serious **liver disorders** may require dosage adjustments.

Possible Side Effects

▼ Most common: diarrhea, nausea, and light-headedness.

▼ Less common: abnormal heart rhythms; very slow or very rapid heartbeat; breathing difficulties; coughing or wheezing, which may be signs of lung congestion or heart failure; constipation; headache; and unusual tiredness or weakness.

▼ Rare: low blood pressure, fainting, and swelling in the ankles, feet, or legs. Other rare side effects can occur in almost any part of the body. Contact your doctor if you experience any side effect not listed above.

Drug Interactions

• Bepridil may interact with beta-blocking drugs to cause heart failure, very low blood pressure, or an increased incidence of angina. However, many people have taken these drugs together with no problem.

• Bepridil may, in rare instances, increase the effects of anticoagulant (blood-thinning) drugs.

• Some calcium channel blockers may increase the amount of digoxin in the blood, but this interaction does not occur with bepridil.

• Bepridil should not be taken with ritonavir or sparfloxacin.

Food Interactions

Taking bepridil with food has a minor effect on the absorption of the drug. You may take it with food if it upsets your stomach.

Usual Dose

200–400 mg a day. Do not stop taking this drug abruptly: The dosage should be gradually reduced over a period of time.

Overdosage

Bepridil overdose can cause nausea, dizziness, weakness, drowsiness, confusion, slurred speech, very low blood pressure, reduced heart efficiency, and unusual heart rhythms. Overdose victims should be taken to a hospital emergency room. ALWAYS bring the prescription bottle or container.

Special Information

Call your doctor if you develop swelling in the arms or legs, breathing difficulties, abnormal heartbeat, increased heart pain, dizziness, constipation, nausea, light-headedness, or very low blood pressure.

If you forget to take a dose of bepridil, take it as soon as you remember. If it is almost time for your next dose, skip the dose you forgot and continue with your regular schedule. Do not take a double dose.

Special Populations

Pregnancy/Breast-feeding

Very high doses of bepridil affect the development of animal fetuses. Women who are or might be pregnant should take it only with their doctor's approval. When this drug is considered crucial by your doctor, its potential benefits must be carefully weighed against its risks.

Bepridil passes into breast milk. If you must take bepridil, you should consider the potential effect on your infant before nursing.

Seniors

Older adults are likely to have reduction in kidney or liver function and may require dosage adjustments. Seniors require more frequent monitoring by their doctors after treatment has started.

Generic Name

Betaine (BEE-tane)

Brand Name

Cystadane

Type of Drug

Homocysteine antagonist.

Prescribed For

Homocysteinuria.

General Information

Homocysteinuria is a group of 3 disorders of the metabolism characterized by too much homocysteine in the blood and urine. People with this problem tend to have skeletal problems, problems with the lens of the eye, and blood-clotting problems that can cause chest pain or heart attack. Virtually all people treated with betaine experience a decrease of homocysteine in their blood. When used together with other homocysteinuria treatments, including folate and vitamins B_{12} and B_6, betaine's effect has been additive to those treatments. Betaine starts working in several days and has been used for several years with no loss of effect. Most patients treated with betaine have been children. The effects of homocysteinuria can be devastating in children and include developmental problems, lethargy, seizures, and eye problems.

Cautions and Warnings

None known.

Possible Side Effects

Side effects, which are uncommon, include nausea, upset stomach, diarrhea, choking if the powder is inhaled, and bad odors. Reported psychological changes from betaine are questionable.

Drug Interactions

None known. Betaine has been used successfully together with folate and vitamins B_{12} and B_6.

Food Interactions

Betaine should be taken with food.

Usual Dose

Adult and Child: 3 g twice a day. Dosage for children under age 3 may be started at about 50 mg per lb. a day and then increased in weekly 50-mg steps. Dosage should be

increased in all patients until homocysteine is either undetectable in the blood or present in small amounts; doses up
to 20 g a day have been required. Carefully measure all doses
with the scoop provided. Each level scoopful is equal to 1 g of
betaine.

Overdosage

Little is known about the effects of betaine overdose. People
have been safely and successfully treated at doses up to 20 g
a day. Call your poison control center or a hospital emergency room for more information.

Special Information

Shake the bottle lightly before removing the cap to loosen
the powder. Protect the powder from moisture.

Mix each dose with 4 to 6 oz. of water until it dissolves
completely, then drink it at once.

Do not use the product if the final solution is either not
clear or colored, or if the powder does not completely dissolve.

If you forget a dose, take it as soon as you remember. If it is
almost time for your next dose, skip the dose you forgot and
continue with your regular schedule. Tell your doctor about
any missed doses.

Special Populations

Pregnancy/Breast-feeding
The safety of using betaine during pregnancy is not known.
This drug should only be used during pregnancy if it is
absolutely necessary.

It is not known if betaine passes into breast milk. Nursing
mothers who must take this drug should consider bottle-
feeding.

Seniors
Seniors may use this drug without special precaution.

Generic Name

Betaxolol (bay-TAX-uh-lol) Ⓖ

Brand Names

Betoptic   Betoptic S

The information in this profile also applies to the following drugs:

Generic Ingredient: Carteolol
Ocupress

Generic Ingredient: Levobunolol Ⓖ
AK Beta   Betagan

Generic Ingredient: Levobetaxolol
Betaxon

Generic Ingredient: Metipranolol Ⓖ
Optipranolol

Generic Ingredient: Timolol Ⓖ
Betimol   Timoptic-XE
Timoptic

Type of Drug

Beta-adrenergic blocking agent.

Prescribed For

High blood pressure and glaucoma.

General Information

Betaxolol hydrochloride is one of many beta-adrenergic blocking drugs, or beta blockers, which interfere with the action of a specific part of the nervous system. Beta receptors are found all over the body and affect many body functions. Each beta blocker has particular characteristics that make it more suitable for certain conditions or people. Beta-blocker eyedrops reduce ocular pressure (pressure inside the eye) by slowing the production of eye fluids and by slightly increasing the rate at which these fluids flow through and leave the eye. Small amounts of these drugs are absorbed into the general blood circulation after they are instilled in the eye and may affect areas of the body other than the eye.

Cautions and Warnings

You should be cautious about taking betaxolol if you have **asthma, chronic bronchitis, emphysema, severe heart failure,** a **very slow heart rate,** or **heart block** (disruption of the electrical impulses that control heart rate) because the drug may aggravate these conditions.

People with **angina** risk aggravating their angina if they suddenly stop taking the drug. These people should have their beta-blocker eyedrops dosage reduced gradually over 1 to 2 weeks.

Liver or kidney problems may reduce your ability to eliminate beta-blocker eyedrops from your body.

Beta-blocker eyedrops may mask the physical signs of **low blood sugar**. People with **type 1 diabetes** and those subject to **hypoglycemia** should use beta-blocker eyedrops with caution.

Beta-blocker eyedrops may reduce the amount of blood your heart pumps with each beat. This reduction in blood flow may aggravate the condition of people with **poor circulation** or **circulatory disease**.

If you are undergoing **major surgery,** your doctor may want you to stop using beta-blocker eyedrops at least 2 days before surgery.

Betaxolol eyedrops should be avoided by people who cannot take oral beta-blocking drugs such as propranolol.

Possible Side Effects

Side effects are relatively uncommon and usually mild.

▼ Less common: unusual tiredness or weakness, slow heartbeat, heart failure, dizziness, breathing difficulties, bronchospasm, depression, confusion, anxiety, nervousness, sleeplessness, disorientation, short-term memory loss, emotional instability, cold hands and feet, constipation, diarrhea, nausea, vomiting, upset stomach, increased sweating, urinary difficulties, cramps, blurred vision, rash, hair loss, stuffy nose, facial swelling, aggravation of lupus erythematosus, itching, chest pain, back or joint pain, colitis, drug allergy (symptoms include fever and sore throat), and liver toxicity.

Drug Interactions

• Beta-blocker eyedrops may interact with surgical anesthetics to increase the risk of heart problems during surgery. Some anesthesiologists recommend gradually stopping the drug by 2 days before surgery.

• Beta-blocker eyedrops increase the blood-pressure-lowering effects of other blood-pressure-reducing agents, including clonidine, guanabenz, and reserpine, and calcium channel blockers, such as nifedipine.

• Combining beta-blocker eyedrops and oral beta blockers will increase the effects of each drug. These drugs should be combined cautiously.

• Cocaine may reduce the effectiveness of all beta-blocker eyedrops.

• Betaxolol will counteract thyroid hormone replacements.

• Calcium channel blockers, flecainide, hydralazine, oral contraceptives, propafenone, haloperidol, phenothiazine tranquilizers—molindone and others—quinolone antibacterials, and quinidine may increase the amount of beta-blocker eyedrops in the bloodstream and lead to a slowed heart rate.

• Betaxolol should not be taken within 2 weeks of taking a monoamine oxidase inhibitor (MAOI) antidepressant.

• Combining betaxolol with phenytoin or digitalis drugs can result in excessive slowing of the heart, possibly causing heart block.

• If you use other glaucoma eye medications, separate your doses to avoid physically combining them.

• Small amounts of beta-blocker eyedrops are absorbed into the bloodstream and may interact with other drugs in the same way as oral beta blockers, although this is unlikely.

Food Interactions

None known.

Usual Dose

1 drop in the affected eye twice a day.

Overdosage

Symptoms of overdose are changes in heartbeat—unusually slow, unusually fast, or irregular—severe dizziness or fainting, breathing difficulties, bluish-colored fingernails or palms, low blood pressure, heart failure, shock, and seizures. The victim should be taken to a hospital emergency room. ALWAYS bring the prescription bottle or container with you.

Special Information

Call your doctor at once if you develop back or joint pain, breathing difficulties, cold hands or feet, depression, rash, or

changes in heartbeat. Beta-blocker eyedrops may produce an undesirable lowering of blood pressure, leading to dizziness or fainting; call your doctor if this happens to you. Also call your doctor if you experience persistent or bothersome anxiety, diarrhea, constipation, impotence, headache, itching, nausea or vomiting, nightmares or vivid dreams, upset stomach, trouble sleeping, stuffy nose, frequent urination, unusual tiredness, or weakness.

If you forget a dose of beta-blocker eyedrops, administer it as soon as you remember. If it is almost time for your next dose, skip the dose you forgot and continue with your regular schedule. Do not take a double dose.

Special Populations

Pregnancy/Breast-feeding
Some beta-blockers pass into breast milk. Nursing mothers taking beta-blocker eyedrops should consider bottle-feeding.

Seniors
Seniors may require less of the drug to achieve results. Seniors taking beta-blocker eyedrops may be more likely to suffer from cold hands and feet, reduced body temperature, chest pain, general feelings of ill health, sudden breathing difficulties, increased sweating, or changes in heartbeat.

Bextra see *Celecoxib, page 206*

Biaxin see *Clarithromycin, page 250*

Biaxin XL see *Clarithromycin, page 250*

Generic Name
Bicalutamide (bye-kal-UTE-uh-mide)

Brand Name
Casodex

The information in this profile also applies to the following drug:

Generic Ingredient: Nilutamide
Nilandron

Type of Drug

Antiandrogen.

Prescribed For

Prostate cancer.

General Information

Antiandrogens are prescribed together with another hormone product for prostate cancer. Bicalutamide competes with testosterone and other natural androgens (male hormones) by binding to the same places in body tissue where androgens normally bind. Prostate cancer is androgen sensitive and responds to treatments that counteract the effects of androgen or remove the sources of androgen.

Cautions and Warnings

Do not take this drug if you are **allergic** to it or any ingredient in the product. People taking this medication may develop severe **liver injury**. People with **liver disease** may be at greater risk for serious side effects. Almost 40% of men taking bicalutamide as single therapy for prostate cancer develop **breast pain and enlargement**. Bicalutamide may **reduce sperm count**.

Two of every 100 people taking nilutamide develop **interstitial pneumonitis** (symptoms include cough, chest pain, fever, and breathing difficulties). People with **lung disease** and Asians may be at greater risk.

Isolated cases of **aplastic anemia** (a potentially fatal blood disorder) have been reported in people taking nilutamide, but the relationship between the drug and the disease is not established.

Possible Side Effects

▼ Most common: hot flashes, hot flushes, general pain, headache, weakness, back pain, nausea, constipation, sleeplessness, breathing difficulties, and swollen

---

Possible Side Effects *(continued)*

breasts. Nilutamide—difficulty seeing in the dark and loss of testicle function.

▼ Common: diarrhea and pelvic pain.

▼ Less common: vomiting, abdominal pains, chest pain, flu symptoms, high blood pressure, swelling in the ankles or lower legs, high blood sugar, weight loss, dizziness, tingling in the hands or feet, sweating, rash, nighttime urination, blood in the urine, urinary or other infection, loss of libido, impotence, breast pain, painful urination, anemia, and bone pain.

▼ Rare: Rare side effects can occur in almost any part of the body. Contact your doctor if you experience any side effect not listed above.

Drug Interactions

• Bicalutamide and nilutamide increase the effect of oral anticoagulant (blood-thinning) drugs such as warfarin. Dosage adjustment may be necessary.

• Nilutamide may increase the risk of the potentially serious side effects of phenytoin or theophylline.

Food Interactions

None known.

Usual Dose

Bicalutamide
    Adult: 50 mg once a day, morning or night.

Nilutamide
    Adult: 300 mg a day, reduced to 150 mg a day after 30 days.

Overdosage

Symptoms of overdose include slow breathing, poor muscle coordination, reduced activity, teariness, appetite loss, vomiting, and tiredness. Overdose victims should be taken to a hospital emergency room. ALWAYS bring the prescription bottle or container.

Special Information

Report anything unusual to your doctor, especially pain or tenderness in the upper right abdomen, yellowing of skin or whites of eyes, severe itching, dark urine, persistent appetite loss, and unexplained flu symptoms. These may be signs of severe liver toxicity. Also report any breathing difficulties, cough, chest pain, or fever.

Up to half of people taking nilutamide can take from a few seconds to a few minutes to adapt to darkness. This can be a problem especially when driving at night or through tunnels. Wearing tinted glasses will minimize this effect.

Bicalutamide should be taken at the same time each day for best results. If you forget a dose of bicalutamide, take it as soon as you remember. If it is almost time for your next dose, skip the dose you forgot and continue with your regular schedule. Call your doctor if you forget to take more than 1 dose.

Special Populations

Pregnancy/Breast-feeding
Antiandrogens are not intended for use by women.

Seniors
Seniors may take this drug without special precaution.

Generic Name

Bisoprolol (bye-SOPE-roe-lol) G

Brand Name
Zebeta

Combination Products

Generic Ingredients: Bisoprolol + Hydrochlorothiazide G
Ziac

The information in this profile also applies to the following drug:

Generic Ingredient: Betaxolol G
Kerlone

Type of Drug
Beta-adrenergic blocking agent.

Prescribed For

High blood pressure, angina pectoris, and abnormal heart rhythms.

General Information

Bisoprolol fumarate is one of many beta-adrenergic blocking drugs, or beta blockers, which interfere with the action of a specific part of the nervous system. Beta receptors are found all over the body and affect many body functions. Each beta blocker has particular characteristics that make it more suitable for certain conditions or people. Hydrochlorothiazide is a diuretic that lowers blood pressure.

Cautions and Warnings

People with **angina** who take bisoprolol for high blood pressure risk aggravating their angina if they suddenly stop taking the drug. These people should have their dosage reduced gradually over 1 to 2 weeks.

Bisoprolol should be used with caution if you have **liver or kidney disease,** because your ability to eliminate the drug from your body may be impaired.

People with **chronic bronchitis** or **emphysema** should use bisoprolol with caution.

Bisoprolol reduces the amount of blood pumped by the heart with each beat. This blood flow reduction may aggravate the condition of people with **poor circulation** or **circulatory disease**.

If you are undergoing **major surgery,** your doctor may want you to stop taking bisoprolol at least 2 days before surgery.

Possible Side Effects

Side effects are relatively uncommon and usually mild.

▼ Most common: impotence.

▼ Less common: unusual tiredness or weakness, slow heartbeat, heart failure, dizziness, breathing difficulties, bronchospasm, depression, confusion, anxiety, nervousness, sleeplessness, disorientation, short-term memory loss, emotional instability, cold hands and feet, constipation, diarrhea, nausea, vomiting, upset stomach, increased sweating, urinary difficulties,

Possible Side Effects *(continued)*

cramps, blurred vision, rash, hair loss, stuffy nose, facial swelling, aggravation of lupus erythematosus, itching, chest pain, back or joint pain, colitis, drug allergy (symptoms include fever and sore throat), and liver toxicity.

Drug Interactions

• Bisoprolol may interact with surgical anesthetics to increase the risk of heart problems during surgery. Some anesthesiologists recommend gradually stopping the drug by 2 days before surgery.

• Bisoprolol may interfere with the normal signs of low blood sugar and with the action of oral antidiabetes drugs.

• Bisoprolol increases the blood-pressure-lowering effects of other blood-pressure-reducing agents, including clonidine, guanabenz, and reserpine, and calcium channel blockers, such as nifedipine.

• Aspirin-containing drugs, indomethacin, sulfinpyrazone, and estrogen drugs may interfere with the blood-pressure-lowering effect of bisoprolol.

• Cocaine may reduce the effectiveness of all beta blockers.

• Bisoprolol may worsen the problem of cold hands and feet associated with taking ergot alkaloids, used to treat migraine. Gangrene is possible in people taking both an ergot and bisoprolol.

• Bisoprolol will counteract thyroid hormone replacements.

• Calcium channel blockers, flecainide, hydralazine, oral contraceptives, propafenone, haloperidol, phenothiazine tranquilizers—molindone and others—quinolone antibacterials, and quinidine may increase the amount of bisoprolol in the bloodstream and lead to increased bisoprolol effects.

• Bisoprolol should not be taken within 2 weeks of taking a monoamine oxidase inhibitor (MAOI) antidepressant.

• Cimetidine increases the amount of bisoprolol absorbed into the bloodstream from oral tablets.

• Bisoprolol may lessen the effectiveness of some anti-asthma drugs, including theophylline and aminophylline, and especially ephedrine and isoproterenol.

• Combining bisoprolol with phenytoin or digitalis drugs may result in excessive slowing of the heart, possibly causing heart block.

• Smoking makes the liver break this drug down more quickly. If you stop smoking while taking bisoprolol, your daily dose may have to be reduced.

Food Interactions

This drug may be taken without regard to food or meals.

Usual Dose

Bisoprolol
    Adult: starting dose—5 mg once daily. The daily dose may be gradually increased up to 20 mg. Maintenance dose—5–10 mg once daily. People with kidney or liver disease may need only 2.5 mg a day to start. Seniors should be treated cautiously; they may respond to lower doses.

Betaxolol
    Adult: starting dose—10 mg once daily for high blood pressure. The daily dose may be gradually increased up to 20 mg a day over 2 weeks, and other blood pressure medications may be added if needed. People with kidney disease may need only 5 mg a day to start. Seniors should be treated cautiously; they may respond to lower doses.

Overdosage

Symptoms of overdose include changes in heartbeat—unusually slow, unusually fast, or irregular—severe dizziness or fainting, breathing difficulties, bluish fingernails or palms, low blood pressure, heart failure, shock, and seizures. The victim should be taken to a hospital emergency room. ALWAYS bring the prescription bottle or container.

Special Information

Do not stop taking bisoprolol unless directed to do so by your doctor. It is meant for continuous use. Abrupt withdrawal may cause chest pain, breathing difficulties, increased sweating, and unusually fast or irregular heartbeat. Dosage should be reduced gradually over a period of about 2 weeks when bisoprolol treatment is stopped.

    Call your doctor at once if you develop back or joint pain, breathing difficulties, cold hands or feet, depression, rash, or

changes in heartbeat. Bisoprolol may produce an undesirable lowering of blood pressure, leading to dizziness or fainting; call your doctor if this happens to you. Also call your doctor if you experience persistent or bothersome anxiety, diarrhea, constipation, impotence, headache, itching, nausea or vomiting, nightmares or vivid dreams, upset stomach, trouble sleeping, stuffed nose, frequent urination, unusual tiredness, or weakness.

Bisoprolol may cause drowsiness, dizziness, blurred vision, or light-headedness. Be careful when driving or performing complex tasks.

It is best to take bisoprolol at the same time every day. If you forget a dose, take it as soon as you remember. If it is within 8 hours of your next dose, skip the dose you forgot and continue with your regular schedule. Do not take a double dose.

Special Populations

Pregnancy/Breast-feeding

Infants born to women who took a beta blocker while pregnant had lower birth weights, low blood pressure, and reduced heart rates. Bisoprolol should be avoided by pregnant women and women who might become pregnant while taking it.

It is not known if bisoprolol passes into breast milk. Nursing mothers taking bisoprolol should bottle-feed.

Seniors

Seniors taking bisoprolol may be more likely to suffer from cold hands and feet, reduced body temperature, chest pain, general feelings of ill health, sudden breathing difficulties, increased sweating, or changes in heartbeat.

Type of Drug

Bisphosphonates (bis-FOS-fuh-nates)

Brand Names

Generic Ingredient: Alendronate
Fosamax

Generic Ingredient: Etidronate
Didronel

Generic Ingredient: Ibandronate
Bonviva

Generic Ingredient: Risedronate
Actonel

Generic Ingredient: Tiludronate
Skelid

Prescribed For

Prevention and treatment of osteoporosis (a condition characterized by loss of bone mass due to calcium depletion) in postmenopausal women and in older men; Paget's disease of bone, and high blood calcium associated with high dosages of corticosteroid treatments and cancer.

General Information

Bisphosphonates have been used for many years to treat a variety of conditions associated with low bone mass caused by calcium depletion. They work on cells called *osteoclasts* that normally break down bone tissue, making bones stronger by preventing loss of bone mass. In osteoporosis, bones become weak and brittle, increasing the risk of spine, hip, and other bone fractures that are a major cause of death and disability in older women. Etidronate has been used occasionally in children, but these drugs generally are not considered safe for use in children.

Cautions and Warnings

Do not use any bisphosphonate if you are **sensitive** or **allergic** to it.

Do not use bisphosphonates if you have severe **kidney disease** or active **stomach or intestinal disease** such as difficulty swallowing, ulcers, or stomach irritation.

It is not known if **men with osteoporosis** benefit from taking a bisphosphonate.

Bisphosphonates can cause **low blood calcium** and should not be used by people whose blood calcium is already low.

Do not use ibandronate if you cannot stand or sit upright for at least 60 minutes.

Possible Side Effects

Side effects are generally mild and similar to those reported by people taking an inactive placebo.

Alendronate
▼ Most common: pain.
▼ Common: abdominal pain and discomfort, gas, stomach ulcers, and back pain.
▼ Less common: upset stomach, constipation, diarrhea, nausea, difficulty swallowing, muscle pain, headache, flu-like symptoms, accidents, and swelling in the arms or legs.
▼ Rare: vomiting and changes in taste.

Etidronate
▼ Most common: fever.
▼ Common: nausea, excess fluids, and flu-like symptoms.
▼ Less common: convulsions, constipation, inflammation of the lining of the mouth, changes in liver function, low blood levels of magnesium or phosphate, breathing difficulties, and changes in sense of taste.
▼ Rare: allergic reactions.

Pamidronate
▼ Most common: fever.
▼ Common: anorexia, low blood levels of calcium, magnesium, phosphate, and potassium; and fatigue.
▼ Less common: psychosis, constipation, nausea, and vomiting.
▼ Rare: irregular heartbeat, high blood pressure, sleeplessness, abdominal pain, diarrhea, and runny nose.

Ibandronate
▼ Most common: upper respiratory infection, back pain, bronchitis, and upset stomach.
▼ Common: arm or leg pain, muscle pain, headache, pneumonia, and urinary infections.
▼ Less common: dizziness, fainting, pain due to nerve lesions, weakness, allergic reactions, diarrhea, vomiting, dental problems, stomach pain, low blood cholesterol, joint problems, arthritis, and sore throat.

Possible Side Effects (continued)

▼ Rare: eye problems have occurred with other drugs in this group but not with ibandronate. Contact your doctor if anything unusual develops.

Risedronate

▼ Most common: headache, diarrhea, abdominal pain, rash, and severe joint pain.

▼ Common: chest pain, dizziness, swelling in the arms or legs, constipation, nausea, sinus irritation, and bone pain.

▼ Less common: leg cramps, weakness, bronchitis, poor vision in one eye, dry eyes, ringing or buzzing in the ears, parathyroid gland problems, infection, rash and other skin problems, tooth problems, and vitamin D deficiency.

▼ Rare: fatigue.

Tiludronate

▼ Most common: diarrhea and nausea.

▼ Common: headache, upset stomach, respiratory infection, runny nose, fluid in the lungs, and sinus irritation.

▼ Less common: vomiting, dizziness, tingling in the hands or feet, coughing, sore throat, gas, aches and pains, cataracts, eye redness, glaucoma, rash, skin disorders, tooth problems, swelling, infection, vitamin D deficiency, and muscle aches.

▼ Rare: tiredness, high blood pressure, fainting, appetite loss, constipation, abdominal pain, and sleeplessness.

Drug Interactions

• Antacids, calcium, and iron containing supplements and foods can interfere with the absorption of bisphosphonates. Separate doses of these drugs and foods and a bisphosphonate by at least 30 minutes.

• Separate doses of tiludonate and aluminum-containing antacids by 1 hour.

• Combining alendronate and aspirin or other nonsteroidal anti-inflammatory drugs (NSAIDs) or other anti-inflammatory drugs can increase the risk of developing stomach or intestinal side effects.

• Aspirin can interfere with the absorption of tiludronate.

• Indomethacin can increase the amount of tiludronate absorbed into the blood by 2 to 4 times.

• Bisphosphonates may increase the GI-irritating effects of aspirin, ibuprofen, and other NSAID drugs.

• Drugs that reduce the amount of stomach acid including ranitidine, cimetidine, and omeprazole may increase the amount of ibandronate in the blood, but the degree of increase is not clinically important.

• Bisphosphonates reduce the ability of teriparatide to build new bone. Teriparatide alone produces better improvements in bone density than either a bisphosphonate alone or taking the two drugs together.

Food Interactions

Take these medicines with plain water. Food and drink—even mineral water, orange juice, or coffee—interfere with the absorption of these drugs. Take alendronate or risedronate every morning at least 30 minutes before eating, drinking, or taking other medications. Etidronate should be taken on an empty stomach 2 hours before a meal. Ibandronate should be taken as soon as you wake up and 1 hour before you eat or take any other medications, vitamins, or supplements. Tiludronate should be taken when you first wake up; wait 4 hours before eating breakfast.

Usual Dose

Alendronate
    Adult: 10–40 mg a day.
    Child: not recommended.

Etidronate
    Adult: up to 4.5 mg per lb. a day to start, gradually increasing to no more than 9 mg per lb. per day.
    Child: not recommended.

Ibandronate
    Adult: 2.5 mg a day.
    Child: not recommended.

Pamidronate
    Adult: 30–90 mg a day.
    Child: not recommended.

Risedronate
    Adult: 30 mg a day.
    Child: not recommended.

Tiludronate
    Adult: 480 mg (2 tablets) a day.
    Child: not recommended.

Overdosage

Little is known about the effects of bisphosphonate overdose. Very low blood calcium is the most serious symptom and requires emergency treatment. Other symptoms include upset stomach, heartburn, ulcer, and irritation of the esophagus. Milk or antacids may reverse these effects. These drugs can irritate the esophagus. Do not let the victim lie down and do not make him vomit. Overdose victims should be taken to a hospital emergency room. ALWAYS bring the prescription bottle or container.

Special Information

Food interferes with the effectiveness of these drugs. Carefully follow the directions in "Food Interactions" above.

Do not suck on any of these tablets or allow them to dissolve in your mouth because they can cause mouth sores.

To reduce the risk of stomach and throat irritation, do not lie down for at least 30 minutes after taking alendronate or risedronate. Do not lie down for 60 minutes after taking ibandronate.

Separate doses of calcium, iron, and vitamin D supplements from those of a bisphosphonate by at least 2 hours.

If you forget a dose, take it as soon as you remember. If it is almost time for your next dose, skip the dose you forgot and continue with your regular schedule. If you forget a morning dose and take it later in the day, you must still follow the instructions in "Food Interactions" about avoiding food.

Special Populations

Pregnancy/Breast-feeding

Bisphosphonates cause abnormal bone development in animal fetuses and are toxic to pregnant animals. When any of these drugs is considered crucial by your doctor, its potential benefits must be carefully weighed against its risks.

It is not known if bisphosphonates pass into breast milk. Since these drugs affect bone formation, nursing mothers who must take a bisphosphonate should bottle-feed.

Seniors

Seniors may use these drugs without special restriction.

Generic Name

Bitolterol (bye-TOL-ter-ol)

Brand Name

Tornalate

The information in this profile also applies to the following drug:

Generic Ingredient: Foromoterol
Foradil Aerolizer

Type of Drug

Bronchodilator.

Prescribed For

Asthma and bronchospasm.

General Information

Bitolterol mesylate is currently available only as an inhalant, but may be taken with other medications to control your asthma. The drug starts working 3 to 4 minutes after it is taken and continues to work for 5 to 8 hours. It can be used as necessary to treat asthma attacks or on a regular basis to prevent them. Formoterol cannot be used to treat an acute asthma attack; it is used as a part of asthma prevention.

Cautions and Warnings

Bitolterol should be used with caution by people with a history of **angina pectoris** (a condition characterized by brief attacks of chest pain), **heart disease, high blood pressure, stroke, seizures, diabetes, prostate disease,** or **glaucoma.**

Using excessive amounts of bitolterol can lead to increased **breathing difficulties,** rather than relief. In the most extreme cases, people have had **heart attacks** after using excessive amounts of inhalant.

Possible Side Effects

▼ Most common: tremors, cough, and dry or sore throat.

▼ Common: restlessness, weakness, anxiety, shakiness and nervousness, tension, sleeplessness, dizziness and fainting, headache, pallor, sweating, nausea, vomiting, and muscle cramps.

▼ Less common: light-headedness, angina, abnormal heart rhythm, heart palpitations, breathing difficulties, bronchospasm, and flushing.

▼ Rare: abnormalities in liver tests, white-blood-cell counts, and tests for urine protein. The importance of these reactions is not known.

Drug Interactions

• Bitolterol's effects may be enhanced by monoamine oxidase inhibitor (MAOI) antidepressants, thyroid drugs, other bronchodilators, and some antihistamines.

• Bitolterol is antagonized by beta-blocking drugs, such as propranolol, and tricyclic antidepressants.

• Bitolterol may antagonize the effects of blood-pressure-lowering drugs, especially reserpine, methyldopa, and guanethidine.

• The risk of heart damage may be increased in people taking both bitolterol and theophylline.

Food Interactions

None known.

Usual Dose

Bitolterol

Adult and Child (age 12 and over): to treat an attack—2 inhalations at an interval of at least 1–3 minutes, followed by a third inhalation, if needed. To prevent an attack—2 inhalations every 8 hours. Do not take more than 3 puffs in 6 hours or 2 every 4 hours.

Formoterol

Adult and Child (age 5 and over): Inhale 12 mcg (1 capsule) every 12 hours using the inhaler that comes with the drug.

Overdosage

Bitolterol overdose can result in exaggerated side effects, including chest pain and high blood pressure, although the pressure can drop to a low level after a short period of elevation. People who inhale too much bitolterol should see a doctor or go to a hospital emergency room.

Special Information

The drug should be inhaled during the second half of your inward breath. This will allow the medication to reach more deeply into your lungs.

Be sure to follow your doctor's directions for the use of bitolterol. Using more than you need can lead to drug tolerance and actually worsen your symptoms. If your condition worsens after taking bitolterol, stop taking it and call your doctor at once.

Call your doctor at once if you develop chest pains, rapid heartbeat, palpitations, muscle tremors, dizziness, headache, or facial flushing, or if you still have trouble breathing after using the medication.

If a dose of bitolterol is forgotten, take it as soon as you remember. If it is almost time for your next dose, skip the dose you forgot and continue with your regular schedule. Do not take a double dose.

Special Populations

Pregnancy/Breast-feeding

Bitolterol is widely used to treat pregnant women with asthma, even though there are no studies to support this practice. The potential benefit of using this medication must be carefully weighed against its risks.

It is not known if bitolterol passes into breast milk. Nursing mothers who take this may want to consider bottle-feeding.

Seniors

Seniors may be more sensitive to the effects of this drug. Follow your doctor's directions and report any side effects at once.

Generic Name

Bosentan (boh-SEN-tan)

Brand Name

Tracleer

Type of Drug

Endothelin receptor antagonist.

Prescribed For

Pulmonary arterial hypertension.

General Information

Bosentan is the first drug to lower blood pressure by working on the endothelin system. Endothelin is a hormone that plays an important role in maintaining blood pressure. It is normally found in blood vessels, but endothelin levels are very high in the blood and lungs of people with pulmonary arterial hypertension. People with this condition have high blood pressure, trouble breathing, and get very tired even when walking or doing other moderate exercising. Pulmonary arterial hypertension can be fatal.

Cautions and Warnings

Bosentan can cause **liver injury**. People taking this drug should have their liver enzymes checked regularly. Enzyme increases can be a sign of liver injury and may be a reason to stop taking bosentan.

Bosentan is broken down in the liver. People with **liver damage** should take it with caution.

Bosentan causes a reduction in **red blood cells,** leading to anemia. Larger doses of bosentan cause a greater loss of red blood cells.

Possible Side Effects

▼ Most common: headache and sore throat and nose.

▼ Common: flushing, abnormal liver function, leg swelling, low blood pressure, and heart palpitations.

▼ Less common: upset stomach, swelling, itching, anemia, and tiredness.

Drug Interactions

• Cyclosporine, used to prevent transplant rejection, increases blood levels of bosentan. Do not combine these drugs.

• Mixing glyburide, an antidiabetes drug, with bosentan increases the risk of elevated liver enzyme levels. Do not combine these drugs.

• Ketoconazole greatly increases blood levels of bosentan by slowing its breakdown in the liver.

• Combining bosentan with a statin-type cholesterol-lowering drug such as simvastatin, lovastatin, or atorvastatin reduces the amount of statin drug in the blood. Dose increases may be needed.

• Bosentan can reduce the amount of warfarin in the blood by about ⅓. Changes in warfarin dosage may be needed.

Food Interactions

None known.

Usual Dose

Adult (age 18 and over): 62.5 mg 2 times a day for 4 weeks, then 125 mg 2 times a day.

Child: not recommended.

Overdosage

Massive overdose may result in severe lowering of blood pressure, requiring emergency attention. However, people have taken as much as 2400 mg at one time or 2000 mg a day of bosentan for 2 months with no major problems. The most common effects associated with overdosage are headache, low blood pressure, increased heart rate, and nausea and vomiting. Overdose victims should be taken to a hospital emergency room for treatment. ALWAYS bring the prescription bottle or container.

Special Information

Do not stop taking this drug without gradually reducing the dosage as instructed by your doctor.

If you forget to take a dose of bosentan, take it as soon as you remember. If it is almost time for your next dose, skip the dose you forgot and continue with your regular schedule.

Contact your doctor at once if you develop severe itching, yellowing of the skin or eyes, or tiredness.

Special Populations

Pregnancy/Breast-feeding

Bosentan is very likely to cause major birth defects and should not be taken by pregnant women. Women must be sure they are not pregnant before beginning bosentan treatment.

Women should also use non-hormone contraceptives while on the drug. Hormone-based contraceptives such as birth control pills, injections, and implants may not work in women taking bosentan.

It is not known if bosentan passes into breast milk. Nursing mothers should bottle-feed.

Seniors

It is not known if seniors respond differently to bosentan than younger adults.

Type of Drug

Bowel Anti-Inflammatory Drugs (5-ASA Type)

Brand Names

Generic Ingredient: Mesalamine

Asacol	Rowasa
Canasa	Pentasa

Generic Ingredient: Balsalazide
Colazal

Generic Ingredient: Olsalazine
Dipentum

Prescribed For

Ulcerative colitis; rectal products prescribed for distal ulcerative colitis, proctitis, and proctosigmoiditis.

General Information

Chemical cousins of aspirin, these bowel anti-inflammatory drugs (5-ASA type) are used to treat symptoms of bowel inflammation. No one knows exactly how they work, but they are believed to have a local effect on the bowel. The tablet forms are made to delay drug release until they reach the colon. Little of the drug is absorbed into the blood; 70% to 90% remains in the colon.

Cautions and Warnings

Bowel anti-inflammatories may **worsen colitis** or cause **cramping,** sudden **abdominal pain**, bloody **diarrhea, fever, headache,** or **rash**. Stop taking the drug at once and call your doctor if any of these symptoms develop.

People who are **allergic** to any of these drugs or to aspirin should not use this drug. Although people who are sensitive or allergic to sulfasalazine have generally been able to tolerate mesalamine—which is an active agent in sulfasalazine—they should be cautious.

Some people taking mesalamine have developed kidney problems. People who have or have had **kidney disease** should be cautious about using these drugs. All people taking mesalamine should have kidney function tests before and during drug therapy.

Possible Side Effects

Bowel anti-inflammatories are generally well tolerated. Tablets and capsules have the most side effects, suppositories the least.

Tablets

▼ Most common: abdominal pain, cramps, or discomfort; stomach rumbling; and generalized pain.

▼ Common: headache, constipation, diarrhea, upset stomach, vomiting, muscle weakness, dizziness, fever, runny nose, rash, skin spots, achy joints, back pain, and stiff muscles.

▼ Less common: worsening of colitis, gas, chills, sweating, feeling unwell, tiredness, acne, itching, arthritis, chest pain, pinkeye, painful menstruation, swelling, and flu-like symptoms.

▼ Rare: sleeplessness, hair loss, and urinary burning or infection. Other rare side effects can occur in almost any part of the body. Contact your doctor if you experience any side effect not listed above.

Possible Side Effects *(continued)*

Capsules
▼ Less common: abdominal pain, cramps, or discomfort; diarrhea; nausea; headache; rash; and skin spots.
▼ Rare: worsening of colitis, constipation, gas, vomiting, dizziness, fever, sleeplessness, sweating, feeling unwell, tiredness, itching, acne, achy joints, leg or joint pain, muscle aches, pinkeye, swelling, and hair loss. Other rare side effects can occur in almost any part of the body. Contact your doctor if you experience any side effect not listed above.

Suppositories
▼ Common: headache.
▼ Less common: abdominal pain, cramps, or discomfort; diarrhea or frequent stools; worsening of colitis; flatulence or gas; upset stomach; nausea; rectal pain, soreness, or burning; muscle aches or weakness; joint pain; dizziness; dry mouth; fever; sore throat; cold symptoms; acne; rash; skin spots; and swelling.

Rectal Suspension
▼ Common: abdominal pain, cramps, or discomfort; gas; nausea; headache; and flu-like symptoms.
▼ Less common: bloating; diarrhea; hemorrhoids; pain on enema insertion; rectal pain, soreness, or burning; dizziness; fever; feeling unwell; tiredness; cold symptoms; sore throat; itching; rash; skin spots; back pain; leg pain; and joint pain.
▼ Rare: constipation, muscle weakness, sleeplessness, swelling, hair loss, and urinary burning or infection.

Drug Interactions

None known.

Food Interactions

Take the tablets and capsules products with food.

Usual Dose

Balsalazide
    Tablets: 2250 mg 3 times a day for 8 weeks.

Mesalamine
  Tablets: 800 mg 3 times a day for 6 weeks.
  Capsules: 1000 mg 4 times a day for up to 8 weeks.
  Suppositories: 1 500-mg suppository 2 times a day for 3–6 weeks. Retain the suppository for 1–3 hours for maximum benefit.
  Rectal Suspension: 1 bottle of suspension taken as an enema at bedtime every night for 3–6 weeks. The enema liquid should be retained for about 8 hours.

Olsalazine
  Tablets: 1000 mg a day in two divided doses.

Overdosage

Symptoms are likely to include: ringing or buzzing in the ears, fainting or dizziness, headache, lethargy, confusion, drowsiness, sweating, rapid breathing, vomiting, and diarrhea. In case of overdose, call your local poison control center or hospital emergency room. You may be told to induce vomiting with ipecac syrup—available at any pharmacy—before taking the victim to the emergency room. If you seek treatment, ALWAYS bring the prescription bottle or container.

Special Information

The tablets and capsules must be swallowed whole. Call your doctor if they are visible in your stool. When using suppositories, handle them as little as possible to prevent melting.

Call your doctor if you develop chest pain, breathing or urinary difficulties, fever, unusual bleeding or bruising, worsening of colitis, or any bothersome or persistent side effects.

If you forget to administer a dose, do so as soon as you remember. If you take a tablet or capsule and it is within 4 hours of your next dose, skip the dose you forgot and continue with your regular schedule. If you take the suppositories or rectal solution and you do not remember until it is almost time for the next dose, skip the one you forgot and continue with your regular schedule. Do not take a double dose.

Special Populations

Pregnancy/Breast-feeding
Bowel anti-inflammatories can pass into the fetal circulation. When your doctor considers these drugs crucial, their potential benefits must be carefully weighed against their risks.

Small amounts of these drugs can pass into breast milk. Nursing mothers who must take these drugs should consider bottle-feeding.

Seniors
Seniors may use these drugs without special restriction.

Generic Name

Brimonidine (brim-ON-ih-dene) G

Brand Name

Alphagan   Alphagan P

Type of Drug

Alpha agonist.

Prescribed For

Glaucoma and ocular hypertension (high pressure inside the eye).

General Information

Brimonidine tartrate stimulates alpha-2 receptors in the eye and lowers pressure there. The maximum effect occurs 2 hours after the drops are administered. Brimonidine reduces the amount of aqueous humor (liquid) produced inside the eye and increases the rate at which fluid flows out of the eyeball. That portion of brimonidine that finds its way into the bloodstream is broken down by the liver.

Cautions and Warnings

Do not use this drug if you are **sensitive** or **allergic** to it.

People with **kidney or liver disease** should use this drug with caution. People with **cardiovascular disease** should exercise caution with this medication because it can affect blood pressure. It should be used with caution in people with **depression, cerebral or coronary insufficiency, Raynaud's dis-**

ease, and **dizziness or fainting** when rising from a sitting or lying position.

Brimonidine's effectiveness may decrease over time. Your doctor should check your eye pressure periodically to make sure the drug is still working.

Possible Side Effects

▼ Most common: dry mouth; redness, burning, and stinging of the eye; headache; blurred vision; sensation of something in the eye; drowsiness; and eye allergy and itching.

▼ Common: staining or erosion of the cornea, unusual sensitivity to bright light, eyelid redness or swelling, eye pain or ache, dry eye, respiratory symptoms, dizziness, eye irritation, upset stomach, weakness, abnormal vision, and muscle pain.

▼ Less common: crusty deposit on the eyelid, eye bleeding, abnormal taste sensation, sleeplessness, eye discharge, high blood pressure, anxiety, heart palpitations, dry nose, and fainting.

Drug Interactions

• Brimonidine may enhance the effects of alcohol, barbiturates, sedatives, anesthetics, beta-blocking drugs, blood-pressure-lowering drugs, and cardiac glycosides.

• Tricyclic antidepressants can increase the breakdown of brimonidine.

• Do not combine brimonidine with MAO inhibitors.

Usual Dose

Adult: 1 drop in the affected eye every 8 hours, 3 times a day.

Overdosage

Little is known about the effects of accidental ingestion. Victims should be taken to a hospital emergency room for treatment. ALWAYS bring the prescription bottle or container.

Special Information

If you wear soft contact lenses, wait at least 15 minutes between the time you put the drops in your eye and when you put your lenses in.

To prevent possible infection, do not allow the dropper to touch your fingers, eyelids, or any surface. Wait at least 5 minutes before using any other eyedrops.

Brimonidine may make you drowsy. Be careful while driving or doing anything else that requires concentration while you are taking this drug.

It is important that brimonidine be used according to your doctor's directions. If you forget to administer a dose of brimonidine, do so as soon as you remember. If it is almost time for your next dose, skip the dose you forgot and continue with your regular schedule. Do not take a double dose.

Special Populations

Pregnancy/Breast-feeding

A small amount of brimonidine may pass into the circulation of the fetus. Pregnant women should use this drug with care.

It is not known if this drug passes into breast milk. Nursing mothers who must use this drug should consider bottle-feeding.

Seniors

Seniors may use brimonidine without special precaution.

Generic Name

Bupropion (bue-PROE-pee-on) G

Brand Names

Wellbutrin   Wellbutrin XL
Wellbutrin SR   Zyban

Type of Drug

Antidepressant and smoking deterrent.

Prescribed For

Depression and nicotine addiction.

General Information

Bupropion hydrochloride is usually used for severe or major depression only after other drugs have failed because of the risk of seizure with bupropion. It is chemically different from other antidepressants and is similar to diethylpropion, an appetite suppressant. Bupropion may work as a smoking deterrent by acting on key hormone systems in the brain. Studies of bupropion in smoking cessation found that people taking 150 to 300 mg a day of the drug were able to stop smoking for 4 weeks of the 7-week study. The people in these studies were not depressed. Bupropion is not likely to work until you have taken it for 3 to 4 weeks. The drug clears your system about 2 weeks after you stop taking it.

Cautions and Warnings

People with **seizure disorders,** people who have had a seizure in the past, and people with **bulimia** or **anorexia nervosa** should be very careful about taking bupropion because they are at a higher risk of having a seizure. About 4 in 1,000 people taking bupropion in dosages up to 450 mg a day develop a seizure. This is about 4 times the seizure rate associated with other antidepressants. The risk of developing a seizure increases by about 10 times with dosages between 450 and 600 mg a day. About half of the people who developed a seizure on bupropion had a risk factor such as a history of head injury, a previous seizure, or a nervous system tumor, or were taking another drug associated with increased seizure risk.

People with unstable **heart disease** or those who have had a recent **heart attack** should take this drug with caution because of possible side effects.

Many people taking bupropion experience some **restlessness, agitation, anxiety,** and **sleeplessness,** especially soon after they start taking the drug. Some even require sleeping pills to counter this effect, and others find the stimulation so severe that they have to stop taking bupropion.

People taking bupropion may experience **hallucinations, delusions,** or **psychotic episodes**. Dosage reduction or drug withdrawal is usually necessary to manage these reactions.

One-quarter of those who take bupropion **lose their appetite** and 5 or more lbs. of body weight. People who have lost weight due to their depression should be cautious about taking bupropion.

People switching from bupropion to a **monoamine oxidase inhibitor (MAOI) antidepressant,** or vice versa, should allow at least 2 weeks to pass between stopping one drug and starting the other.

People with **kidney or liver disease** require less bupropion at the beginning of treatment. Dosage should be increased cautiously.

An antidepressant other than bupropion should be seriously considered for people with a history of drug abuse because of the mild stimulation bupropion causes. These people may require larger-than-usual dosages, but they are still susceptible to seizures at these higher dosages.

Suicide is always a risk in severely depressed people, who should only have minimal quantities of medication in their possession.

Possible Side Effects

About 10% of people stop taking bupropion due to side effects.

▼ Most common: dry mouth; dizziness; rapid heartbeat; headache, including migraine; excessive sweating; nausea; vomiting; constipation; appetite loss; weight changes; sedation; agitation; sleeplessness; and tremors.

▼ Less common: upset stomach, diarrhea, increased appetite, menstrual complaints, impotence, urinary difficulties, slowness of movement, salivation, muscle spasms, warmth, uncontrolled muscle movement, compulsion to move around or change positions, abnormal heart rhythms, blood-pressure changes, heart palpitations, fainting, itching, redness and rash, confusion, hostility, loss of concentration, reduced sex drive, anxiety, delusions, euphoria (feeling high), fatigue, joint pain, fever or chills, respiratory infection, and visual, taste, and hearing disturbances.

Many other side effects have been reported with bupropion, but their link to the drug is not well established.

Drug Interactions

• Carbamazepine may reduce blood concentrations of bupropion.

• People taking both bupropion and levodopa experience increased side effects. People taking levodopa should have their bupropion dosage increased gradually.

• Ritonavir may significantly increase bupropion blood levels and the risk of side effects.

• Phenelzine (an MAOI) increases the risk of bupropion side effects. Allow at least 2 weeks to pass between stopping an MAOI and starting bupropion.

• Don't mix bupropion with other drugs that increase the risk of seizures—including tricyclic antidepressants, haloperidol, lithium, loxapine, molindone, phenothiazine tranquilizers, and thioxanthene tranquilizers.

• Combining bupropion with a nicotine replacement drug can cause high blood pressure.

• Combining bupropion with warfarin can increase the risk of side effects.

• Do not combine Wellbutrin and Zyban, as they contain the same active ingredient.

Food Interactions

Bupropion may be taken with food if it upsets your stomach.

Usual Dose

Depression
   Adult: 200–450 mg a day divided into 3 or 4 daily doses; normal daily dosage is 300 mg.
   Child (under age 18): not recommended.

Smoking Cessation
   Adult: 150 mg twice a day. Begin treatment while you are still smoking.
   Child (under age 18): not recommended.

Overdosage

Symptoms of overdose are likely to include severe side effects, such as seizures—present in $\frac{1}{3}$ of overdoses—hallucinations, loss of consciousness, and abnormal heart rhythms. Overdose victims should be taken to a hospital emergency room at once. ALWAYS bring the prescription bottle or container.

Special Information

Do not stop taking bupropion without your doctor's knowledge. Suddenly stopping the drug may cause withdrawal reactions and side effects.

   Call your doctor if you experience agitation or excitement, restlessness, confusion, difficulty sleeping, fast or abnormal heart rhythm, severe headache, seizure, rash, fainting, or any unusual or persistent side effect.

To reduce the risk of a seizure, take bupropion in 3 or 4 equal doses each day. Total daily dosage should not exceed 450 mg; single doses should not exceed 150 mg.

Bupropion may make you tired, dizzy, or light-headed. Be careful when driving or doing any task that requires concentration.

Alcohol, tranquilizers, and other nervous-system depressants increase the depressant effects of this drug. Alcohol also increases the risk of a seizure.

If you forget a dose, take it as soon as you remember. If it is almost time for your next dose, take 1 dose as soon as you remember and another in 3 or 4 hours, then go back to your regular schedule. Do not take a double dose.

Special Populations

Pregnancy/Breast-feeding

The safety of using bupropion during pregnancy is not known. When your doctor considers this drug crucial, its potential benefits must be carefully weighed against its risks. Pregnant women trying to quit smoking should use non-drug methods until their pregnancy is completed.

Bupropion passes into breast milk. Nursing mothers who must use bupropion should bottle-feed.

Seniors

Seniors with reduced kidney or liver function may require reduced dosage.

Generic Name

Buspirone (bue-SPYE-rone) G

Brand Name

BuSpar   BuSpar Dividose

Type of Drug

Minor tranquilizer and antianxiety drug.

Prescribed For

Anxiety; also prescribed for the aches, pains, fatigue, and cramps of premenstrual syndrome (PMS).

General Information

Buspirone hydrochloride has a potent antianxiety effect. It is approved by the Food and Drug Administration (FDA) for short-term relief of anxiety, but it may apparently be used safely for more than 4 weeks. The exact way in which bus-pirone works is not known, but it seems to lack the addiction dangers associated with other antianxiety drugs, including benzodiazepines. It neither severely depresses the nervous system nor acts as an anticonvulsant or muscle relaxant, as other antianxiety drugs do. Minor improvement will be apparent after only 7 to 10 days of drug treatment, but the maximum effect does not occur for 3 or 4 weeks.

Cautions and Warnings

Do not take buspirone if you are **allergic** to it.

Buspirone should be used cautiously by people with **liver or kidney disease**.

Buspirone does not have any antipsychotic effect and should not be taken for symptoms of **psychosis**.

Although buspirone has not shown a potential for **drug abuse,** you should be aware of this possibility.

Possible Side Effects

▼ Most common: dizziness, nausea, headache, fatigue, nervousness, light-headedness, and excitement.

▼ Common: heart palpitations, muscle aches and pains, tremors, rash, sweating, and clamminess.

▼ Less common: sleeplessness, chest pain, rapid heartbeat, low blood pressure, fainting, stroke, heart attack, heart failure, dream disturbances, difficulty concentrating, euphoria (feeling high), anger or hostility, depression, depersonalization or disassociation, fearfulness, loss of interest, hallucinations, suicidal tendencies, claustrophobia, stupor, slurred speech, intolerance to noise, and intolerance to cold temperatures.

▼ Rare: Rare side effects can occur in almost any part of the body. Contact your doctor if you experience any side effect not listed above.

Drug Interactions

• Combining buspirone with a monoamine oxidase inhibitor (MAOI) antidepressant may produce severe hypertension and may be dangerous.

• The effects of combining buspirone with other drugs that work in the central nervous system (CNS) are not known. Do not take other tranquilizers or antianxiety or psychoactive drugs with buspirone unless prescribed by a doctor familiar with your complete medical history.

• Erythromycin, itraconazole, and nefazodone may increase blood levels of buspirone. When used in combination, your buspirone dosage may need to be adjusted.

• Buspirone may increase the side effects of haloperidol.

• Studies show that buspirone is not affected by alcohol, but this combination should still be used with caution because buspirone causes drowsiness and dizziness.

• The combination of buspirone and trazodone may cause liver inflammation.

Food Interactions

This drug may be taken either with or without food, but for the most consistent results, always take your dose at the same time of day in the same way—that is, with or without food.

Usual Dose

Starting dosage—5 mg 3 times a day. Dosage may be increased gradually to 60 mg a day.

Overdosage

Symptoms of overdose are nausea, vomiting, dizziness, drowsiness, pinpointed pupils, and upset stomach. The overdose victim should be taken to a hospital emergency room. ALWAYS bring the prescription bottle or container.

Special Information

Buspirone may cause nervous-system depression, drowsiness, and dizziness. Be careful while driving or operating hazardous equipment. Avoid other CNS drugs and alcoholic beverages because they will enhance buspirone's effects.

Contact your doctor if you become restless, develop uncontrolled or repeated movements of the head, face, or neck, or have any intolerable side effects. About 1 in 10 people stop taking buspirone because of side effects.

If you forget a dose, take it as soon as you remember. If it is almost time for your next dose, skip the dose you forgot and go back to your regular schedule. Do not take a double dose.

Special Populations

Pregnancy/Breast-feeding

Though buspirone has not been found to cause birth defects, be sure to inform your doctor if you are or might be pregnant while taking this drug. When this drug is considered crucial by your doctor, its potential benefits must be carefully weighed against its risks.

It is not known how much buspirone passes into breast milk. Nursing mothers who must take this drug should consider bottle-feeding.

Seniors

Several hundred seniors participated in drug evaluation studies without any unusual problems. However, the effect of this drug in seniors is not well known, and special problems may surface, particularly in those with kidney or liver disease.

Generic Name

Butenafine (bue-TEN-uh-fene)

Brand Name

Mentax   Mentax-TC

Type of Drug

Antifungal.

Prescribed For

Athlete's foot, jock itch, and ringworm.

General Information

Butenafine hydrochloride works by blocking the natural synthesis of a chemical—ergosterol—essential to the cell membrane (outer skin) of the fungus cell. Butenafine may actually kill the fungus if enough of it is present. Some butenafine is absorbed into the bloodstream.

Cautions and Warnings

Do not use butenafine if you are **sensitive** or **allergic** to it.

Possible Side Effects

▼ Common: rash, burning, stinging, worsening of the infection, swelling, irritation, and itching.

Drug Interactions

When you apply butenafine to the skin, do not combine it with any other medication.

Usual Dose

Adult and Child (age 12 and over): Apply enough to cover the affected area and surrounding skin once a day for 2–4 weeks, or twice a day for one week. Wash your hands after each application.

Child (under age 12): not recommended.

Overdosage

Little is known about the effects of accidental ingestion. Call your local poison control center or hospital emergency room for more information.

Special Information

This drug may irritate sensitive skin. Call your doctor if this happens—another medication may be more appropriate. Also call your doctor if you experience redness, itching, burning, blistering, swelling, or oozing.

Athlete's foot is relatively common and may be caused by a number of different kinds of fungi. Do not use this drug without your doctor's knowledge.

Butenafine is to be applied only to your skin. It should not be applied to other areas, including the eyes, nose, mouth, or vagina.

Do not bandage the area where the medication has been applied unless otherwise directed by your doctor.

If you apply the cream after bathing, be sure that your feet are completely dry, especially the areas between your toes. Do not wear socks made from wool or synthetic material or shoes that do not have adequate ventilation.

As is often the case when using an anti-infective, your symptoms may begin to improve before you have completed the full course of treatment. Be sure to use all of the medication as directed. If you are taking butenafine for jock itch or ringworm, wear loose-fitting clothing and keep the area cool and dry.

Call your doctor if the condition does not improve after 4 weeks of using the cream.

Special Populations

Pregnancy/Breast-feeding

Butenafine should only be used during pregnancy if absolutely necessary.

It is not known if this drug passes into breast milk. Nursing mothers who must use this drug should consider bottle-feeding.

Seniors

Seniors may use this medication without special precaution.

Generic Name

Calcitonin (kal-sih-TONE-in)

Brand Names

Calcimar   Miacalcin

Type of Drug

Peptide hormone.

Prescribed For

Osteoporosis (condition characterized by loss of bone mass due to depletion of minerals, especially calcium) in post-menopausal women.

General Information

Calcitonin helps to strengthen bone by adding more calcium to it and slowing the natural process by which bone is broken down. The calcitonin used in this drug is essentially identical to human calcitonin except that it is more potent. It is a synthetic version of the natural calcitonin found in salmon. Calcitonin can increase bone density and reduce the risk of fractures of the vertebrae (bones that comprise the spinal column), which are associated with back pain and loss of height. Calcitonin has been available for years as an injection, but the development of the nasal spray makes the drug easier to use.

Cautions and Warnings

Do not use this drug if you are **sensitive** or **allergic** to it. Although **serious allergic reactions** were reported with the injectable form, none have occurred with the nasal spray.

Changes in the **tissues lining of your nose** are possible with long-term use of this product. An initial and then periodic nasal examinations are recommended.

Possible Side Effects

▼ Most common: stuffy nose, runny nose, and other nasal symptoms; and back pain.

▼ Less common: joint pain, nosebleed, and headache.

Food and Drug Interactions

None known.

Usual Dose

Adult: 1 spray (200 IU) a day.

Child: Information is lacking on the use of this drug in children.

Overdosage

Little is known about the effects of calcitonin overdose or accidental ingestion. Nausea and vomiting have been reported after high doses. Call your local poison control center for more information. Overdose victims should be taken to a hospital emergency room. ALWAYS bring the prescription bottle or container.

Special Information

Alternate nostrils daily when using the nasal spray.

Before you take your first dose, you must activate the pump. Hold the bottle upright and press the two white arms toward the bottle 6 times until a faint spray is emitted. Once this occurs, the pump is activated and ready for use. It is not necessary to reactivate the pump every day.

If you forget to administer a dose of the nasal spray, do so as soon as you remember. If it is almost time for the next dose, skip the dose you forgot and continue with your regular schedule. Call your doctor if you forget 2 or more doses.

Call your doctor if you develop severe nose irritation or any unusual or intolerable symptom. Follow your doctor's recommendations regarding calcium and vitamin D supplements. This drug is not intended to replace the need for dietary calcium.

Special Populations

Pregnancy/Breast-feeding

Calcitonin does not cross into the fetal circulation, though animal studies have associated the injectable form of the drug with low birth weight. This drug is recommended for use during pregnancy only if its possible benefits outweigh its risks.

It is not known if calcitonin passes into breast milk, though animal studies have shown that it reduces the amount of milk produced. Nursing mothers who must use calcitonin should consider bottle-feeding.

Seniors

Seniors may use this product without special precaution.

Generic Name

Capecitabine (cape-SE-tah-been)

Brand Name

Xeloda

Type of Drug

Antimetabolite.

Prescribed For

Breast cancer and colorectal cancer that has metastasized (spread) to other parts of the body.

General Information

Capecitabine is prescribed for people whose breast cancer or colorectal cancer has metastasized despite previous cancer treatment. This drug is converted in the body to 5-FU, a widely used anticancer agent. Unlike some anticancer medications, capecitabine can be taken by mouth and has relatively few serious side effects.

Cautions and Warnings

People who are **allergic** or **sensitive** to 5-FU should not take capecitabine.

People with **liver or kidney disease** should be carefully monitored by their doctors because capecitabine's effect on these conditions is not known.

Capecitabine may **reduce fertility**.

Capecitabine use is associated with **heart and blood vessel disease**.

Capecitabine may cause severe **diarrhea**. Call your doctor if you experience symptoms (see "Special Information").

Possible Side Effects

▼ Most common: diarrhea, constipation, nausea, vomiting, mouth sores, abdominal pain, hand-and-foot syndrome (see "Special Information"), inflammation of the skin, tingling or pain in the hands or feet, fatigue, loss of appetite, low blood-cell counts, eye irritation, and fever.

▼ Common: upset stomach, nail problems, headache, dizziness, sleeplessness, dehydration, swelling, muscle aches, and pain in the arms or legs.

Less common and rare side effects can affect the stomach and intestines, skin, nervous system, lungs and respiratory system, heart and blood vessels, blood, urinary and reproductive tracts, liver, and other organs.

Other side effects can occur in almost any part of the body. Contact your doctor if you experience any side effect not listed above.

Drug Interactions

• Combining antacids and capecitabine can increase the amount of drug absorbed by about 20%. Separate doses of antacids and capecitabine by 2 hours.

• Leucovorin (a drug used in cancer treatment) increases the side effects of 5-FU. This combination has caused death in several seniors.

• Combining capecitabine with warfarin or phenytoin can increase the risk of side effects.

Food Interactions

Capecitabine should be taken within 30 minutes of a meal to avoid stomach problems.

Usual Dose

Adult (age 18 and over): 3000–5600 mg a day, depending on height and weight, in 2 doses. Capecitabine is used in 3-week cycles: 2 weeks on the drug, followed by 1 week off. Dosage may be reduced by 50% in people who experience severe side effects.

Child (under age 18): not recommended.

Overdosage

Symptoms include nausea, vomiting, diarrhea, bleeding and reduced blood-cell counts, and stomach irritation. Overdose victims should be taken to a hospital emergency room. ALWAYS bring the prescription bottle or container.

Special Information

Stop taking capecitabine and call your doctor if you have 4 to 6 more bowel movements a day than normal, vomit 2 to 5 times in 1 day, or become very nauseous. Depending on the severity of your symptoms, your doctor may reduce your dosage.

Capecitabine has caused hand-and-foot syndrome. Symptoms of this condition include numbness, tingling, pain, swelling, redness, skin loss and blistering of the hands or feet. Stop taking the drug and call your doctor if you experience any of these symptoms.

People who develop stomatitis (symptoms include swelling, pain, or sores in the area of the mouth or tongue) should stop taking the drug and call their doctors at once.

Call your doctor, but do not stop taking the drug, if you develop a fever of 100.5°F or higher or other signs of infection.

If you forget a dose, take it as soon as you remember. If it is almost time for your next dose, take 1 dose right away and space the remaining daily dosage evenly throughout the day. Go back to your regular schedule the next morning. Call your doctor if you miss more than 2 doses in a row.

Special Populations

Pregnancy/Breast-feeding

Capecitabine can harm the fetus. Its potential benefits must be carefully weighed against its risks when capecitabine is considered crucial by your doctor. Effective contraception is absolutely necessary while taking this drug.

It is not known if capecitabine passes into breast milk. Nursing mothers who must take this drug should bottle-feed.

Seniors

Seniors may be more sensitive to side effects, especially diarrhea and other stomach problems.

Generic Name

Captopril (KAP-toe-pril) G

Brand Name

Capoten

Combination Products

Generic Ingredients: Captopril + Hydrochlorothiazide G
Capozide

Type of Drug

Angiotensin-converting enzyme (ACE) inhibitor; antihypertensive.

Prescribed For

High blood pressure and congestive heart failure; also used to treat and prevent diabetic kidney disease and high blood pressure associated with other medical conditions, such as scleroderma and Takayasu's disease. Captopril combined with the diuretic hydrochlorothiazide is used to treat high blood pressure.

General Information

Captopril and other ACE inhibitors work by preventing the conversion of a hormone called angiotensin I to another hormone called angiotensin II, a potent blood-vessel constrictor. Preventing this conversion relaxes blood vessels, helps to reduce blood pressure, and relieves the symptoms of heart failure. Captopril also affects the production of other hormones and enzymes that participate in the regulation of blood-vessel dilation. Captopril usually begins working about 1 hour after it is taken.

People who are already taking a diuretic (an agent that increases urination) may experience a rapid blood-pressure drop after their first dose of captopril or when their captopril dose is increased. To prevent this, your doctor may tell you to stop taking your diuretic or to increase your salt intake 2 or 3 days before starting captopril. The diuretic may then be restarted gradually.

In addition to its labeled uses, captopril has been studied in the diagnosis of certain kidney diseases and of primary aldosteronism, and in the treatment of rheumatoid arthritis, swelling and fluid accumulation, Bartter's syndrome, Raynaud's disease, and post-heart-attack treatment when the function of the left ventricle is affected.

Cautions and Warnings

Do not take captopril if you are **allergic** to it.

Although not common, captopril may cause **very low blood pressure**. It may also affect your **kidneys,** especially if you have congestive **heart failure**. Your doctor should check your urine for protein content during the first few months of captopril treatment. Captopril may cause a decline in kidney function. Dosage adjustment of captopril is necessary if you have reduced kidney function because the drug is generally eliminated from the body via the kidneys.

Captopril may affect white-blood-cell counts, possibly increasing your susceptibility to **infection**. Your doctor should monitor your blood counts periodically.

Captopril can cause serious injury or death to the fetus if taken during pregnancy. Pregnant women should not take captopril.

Possible Side Effects

▼ Most common: rash, itching, and cough that usually goes away a few days after you stop taking the drug.

▼ Less common: dizziness, tiredness, sleep disturbances, headache, tingling in hands or feet, chest pain, heart palpitations, feeling unwell, abdominal pain, nausea, vomiting, diarrhea, constipation, appetite loss, dry mouth, breathing difficulties, and hair loss.

▼ Rare: Rare side effects can occur in almost any part of the body. Contact your doctor if you experience any side effect not listed above.

Drug Interactions

• The blood-pressure-lowering effect of captopril is additive with diuretic drugs and beta blockers. Any other drug that causes a rapid blood-pressure drop should be used with caution if you are taking captopril.

• Combining 325 mg of aspirin a day with captopril carries a higher risk of death than taking lower doses (less than 160 mg a day). People taking aspirin to prevent a heart attack should use the lower dose.

• Captopril may increase blood-potassium levels, especially when taken with Dyazide or other potassium-sparing diuretics.

• Captopril may increase the effects of lithium; this combination should be used with caution.

• Antacids and captopril should be taken at least 2 hours apart.

• Capsaicin may trigger or aggravate the cough associated with captopril.

• Indomethacin may reduce the blood-pressure-lowering effect of captopril.

• Phenothiazine tranquilizers and antivomiting agents may increase the effects of captopril.

• Probenecid increases this drug's effect as well as the chance of side effects.

• The combination of allopurinol and captopril increases the chance of an adverse drug reaction.

• Captopril may increase blood levels of digoxin, which may increase the chance of digoxin-related side effects.

Food Interactions

Captopril should be taken on an empty stomach, at least 1 hour before or 2 hours after a meal.

Usual Dose

Adult: 25 mg 2 or 3 times a day to start. Dosage may be increased to 450 mg a day in divided doses, if needed. Dosage must be tailored to your needs. People with poor kidney function must take lower doses.

Child: approximately 0.15 mg per lb. of body weight, 3 times a day.

Overdosage

The principal effect of captopril overdose is a rapid drop in blood pressure, which may lead to dizziness or fainting. Take the overdose victim to a hospital emergency room immediately. ALWAYS bring the prescription bottle or container.

Special Information

Captopril may cause swelling of the face, lips, hands, and feet. This swelling may also affect the larynx (throat) and tongue and interfere with breathing. If this happens, go to a hospital emergency room at once. Call your doctor if you develop a sore throat, mouth sores, abnormal heartbeat, chest pain, a persistent rash, or losses in the sense of taste.

You may get dizzy if you rise to your feet too quickly from a sitting or lying position.

Avoid strenuous exercise or very hot weather because heavy sweating or dehydration may lead to a rapid drop in blood pressure.

Avoid over-the-counter stimulants that can raise blood pressure while taking captopril, including diet pills and decongestants.

If you forget to take a dose of captopril, take it as soon as you remember. If it is within 4 hours of your next dose, take 1 dose immediately and another in 5 or 6 hours, then go back to your regular schedule. Do not take a double dose.

Special Populations

Pregnancy/Breast-feeding

ACE inhibitors can cause fetal injury or death. Women who are or might be pregnant should not take ACE inhibitors. If you become pregnant, stop taking captopril and call your doctor immediately.

Small amounts of captopril pass into breast milk. Nursing mothers who must take this drug should consider bottle-feeding.

Seniors

Seniors may be more sensitive to the effects of captopril due to age-related declines in kidney or liver function.

Generic Name

Carbamazepine (car-bam-A-zuh-pene) G

Brand Names

Atretol   Tegretol
Carbatrol   Tegretol-XR
Epitol   Teril

Type of Drug

Anticonvulsant.

Prescribed For

Seizure disorders as well as trigeminal and other neuralgias; also used to treat severe pain; psychiatric disorders including depression, bipolar disorder, intermittent explosive disorder, post-traumatic stress disorder, psychotic disorders, and schizophrenia; withdrawal from alcohol, cocaine, or benzodiazepine-type drugs; restless leg syndrome; hereditary and non-hereditary chorea in children; and diabetes insipidus.

General Information

Carbamazepine was first approved for relief of the severe pain of trigeminal neuralgia. Over the years, it has gained wide use in seizure control, especially in people whose seizures are uncontrolled with phenytoin, phenobarbital, or primidone, or who have suffered severe side effects from these drugs. Carbamazepine is not a simple pain reliever and should not be taken for everyday aches and pains. It is associated with potentially fatal side effects.

Cautions and Warnings

Carbamazepine should not be used if you have had **bone marrow depression** or if you are **sensitive** or **allergic** to this drug or any tricyclic antidepressant.

   Monoamine oxidase inhibitor (MAOI) antidepressants should be discontinued 2 weeks before starting carbamazepine.

   Carbamazepine may cause severe, **possibly life-threatening blood reactions**. People who have had blood reactions to other drugs are at particular risk for another reaction with carbamazepine. Your doctor should have a complete blood count done before you start taking this drug and repeat these tests weekly during the first 3 months of treatment, and then every month for the next 2 to 3 years. Unexplained fever or infection may be a sign of a blood reaction.

Severe, **possibly fatal skin reactions** have developed in a few people taking carbamazepine.

Carbamazepine may aggravate **glaucoma** and should be used with caution by people with this condition. This drug may activate underlying **psychosis,** confusion, or agitation, especially in older adults.

Possible Side Effects

▼ Most common: dizziness, drowsiness, unsteadiness, nausea, and vomiting. Other common side effects are blurred or double vision, confusion, hostility, headache, and severe water retention.

▼ Less common: mood and behavioral changes, especially in children. Hives, itching, rash, and other allergic reactions may also occur.

▼ Rare: Rare side effects can affect your breathing, speech, emotions, liver function, urinary function, and many other parts of the body. Contact your doctor if you experience any side effect not listed above.

Drug Interactions

• Carbamazepine blood levels may be increased by cimetidine, danazol, diltiazem, isoniazid, propoxyphene, erythromycin-type antibiotics (except azithromycin), fluoxetine, fluvoxamine, levetiracetam, mexiletine, nicotinamide, quetiapine, troleandomycin, or verapamil, leading to possible carbamazepine toxicity.

• Carbamazepine may reduce the effectiveness of oral contraceptives and cause breakthrough bleeding.

• Charcoal tablets or powder, phenobarbital and other barbiturates, phenytoin, and primidone may decrease the absorption of carbamazepine. Levels of phenobarbital, a breakdown product of primidone, may be increased by combining primidone and carbamazepine.

• Carbamazepine reduces the effects of acetaminophen, the anticoagulant (blood thinner) warfarin, and theophylline (prescribed for asthma). Increased dosage of these drugs may be necessary. Other drugs counteracted by carbamazepine are bupropion, cyclosporine, dacarbazine, digitalis drugs, disopyramide, doxycycline, haloperidol, levothyroxine, and quinidine.

• Combining carbamazepine and other antiseizure drugs, including felbamate, hydantoins, succinimides, and valproic acid, may cause unpredictable results. Combination treatments to control seizures must be customized to each person.

• Combining carbamazepine and lithium may increase nervous system side effects.

Food Interactions

Take carbamazepine with food if it causes stomach upset.

Usual Dose

Adult and Child (age 13 and over): 400–1200 mg a day, depending on the condition. Usual maintenance dose is 400–800 mg a day in 2 divided doses.

Child (age 6–12): 200–1000 mg a day, or 10–15 mg per lb. of body weight a day, divided into 3–4 equal doses. Do not exceed 1000 mg a day.

Dosage varies according to form. Liquid carbamazepine must be taken 3 times a day, regular carbamazepine tablets twice a day, and sustained-release tablets once daily. Never change your dosage schedule without first checking with your doctor.

Overdosage

Carbamazepine is a potentially lethal drug. Overdose symptoms appear in 1 to 3 hours. These include irregularity or difficulty in breathing, rapid heartbeat, changes in blood pressure, shock, loss of consciousness or coma, convulsions, muscle twitching, restlessness, uncontrolled body movements, drooping eyelids, psychotic mood changes, nausea, vomiting, and reduced urination. Induce vomiting right away with ipecac syrup—available at any pharmacy. Then take the victim to a hospital emergency room. ALWAYS bring the prescription bottle or container.

Special Information

Carbamazepine may cause dizziness and drowsiness. Take care while driving or doing any task that requires concentration.

Call your doctor at once if you experience yellowing of the skin or whites of the eyes, unusual bleeding or bruising, abdominal pain, pale stools, dark urine, impotence, mood changes, nervous system symptoms, swelling, fever, chills, sore throat, or mouth sores. These may be signs of a potentially fatal drug reaction.

If you forget a dose, skip it and go back to your regular schedule. If you miss more than 1 dose in a day, call your doctor. Do not stop taking this drug without first consulting your doctor.

Special Populations

Pregnancy/Breast-feeding

Carbamazepine caused birth defects in animal studies. Seizure disorder itself also increases the risk of birth defects. Pregnant women should take carbamazepine only after discussing with their doctors its potential benefits and risks.

Carbamazepine passes into breast milk. Nursing mothers who must take carbamazepine should bottle-feed.

Seniors

Seniors taking this drug are more likely to develop heart problems, psychosis, confusion, or agitation.

Type of Drug

Carbonic-Anhydrase Inhibitors, Eyedrops (kar-BON-ik an-HYE-drase)

Brand Names

Generic Ingredient: Dorzolamide
Trusopt

Generic Ingredient: Brinzolamide
Azopt

Prescribed For

Glaucoma.

General Information

These drugs are similar to acetazolamide, a carbonic-anhydrase inhibitor taken by mouth. Carbonic anhydrase is an enzyme found in many parts of the body, including the eyes. By blocking the effects of this enzyme, dorzolamide and brinzolamide slow the production of fluid inside the eye, reducing pressure there. This effect is useful in treating glaucoma because the disease is characterized by elevated eye pressure.

Cautions and Warnings

Do not use these drugs if you are **sensitive** or **allergic** to it or to other sulfa drugs. Small amounts of these drugs enter the bloodstream. Rarely, people using them experience **side effects or allergies associated with sulfa drugs**.

These drugs have not been studied in people with very **poor kidney or liver function**. Since these drugs are eliminated via the kidneys, people with impaired kidney function should use an alternate glaucoma medication.

Possible Side Effects

Dorzolamide

▼ Most common: eye burning, stinging, or discomfort and a bitter taste in the mouth immediately after administering the eyedrops.

▼ Less common: allergic reactions, blurred vision, tearing, dry eye, and increased sensitivity to bright light.

▼ Rare: headache, nausea, weakness, tiredness, rash, and kidney stones. Dorzolamide can cause the same types of side effects as other sulfa drugs, but this is very unlikely. Report any unusual symptoms to your doctor.

Brinzolamide

▼ Common: blurred vision and a bitter, sour, or unusual taste in the mouth.

▼ Less common: eyelid inflammation; rash; dry eye; sensation of something in the eye; headache; eye redness, itching, discharge, or pain; and runny nose.

▼ Rare: allergic reactions, hair loss, chest pain, pinkeye, diarrhea, nausea, sore throat, tearing, itchy rash, double vision, dizziness, dry mouth, breathing difficulties, upset stomach, tired eyes, kidney pain, cornea problems, and formation of a crust or sticky sensation around the eyelid. Brinzolamide can cause the same types of side effects as other sulfa drugs, but this is very unlikely. Report any unusual symptoms to your doctor.

Drug Interactions

• If you are using more than 1 eyedrop product, separate doses of these drugs by at least 10 minutes.

Usual Dose

Adult: 1 drop in the affected eye 3 times a day.

Overdosage

Accidental ingestion of a bottle of dorzolamide or brinzolamide may affect blood levels of potassium and other electrolytes. The victim should be taken to a hospital emergency room. ALWAYS bring the prescription bottle or container.

Special Information

Call your doctor and stop using your eyedrops if you develop any unusual eye reaction or condition, including swollen eyelids and pinkeye.

Vision may be temporarily blurred when using the eyedrops. Use caution when driving or operating machinery.

If you wear soft contact lenses, take them out before using the eyedrops and put them back in 15 minutes after a dose.

To prevent infection, do not allow the eyedropper tip to touch your fingers, eyelids, or any surface. Wait at least 10 minutes before using any other eyedrops.

If you forget to administer a dose, do so as soon as you remember. If it is almost time for your next dose, skip the one you forgot and continue with your regular schedule. Do not take a double dose.

Special Populations

Pregnancy/Breast-feeding

Very high dosages of dorzolamide or brinzolamide caused birth defects in animal studies. While the risks of using these drugs during pregnancy are small in people, pregnant women should use dorzolamide or brinzolamide only after discussing its potential benefits and risks with their doctors.

It is not known if these drugs pass into breast milk. Nursing mothers who must use either drug should bottle-feed.

Seniors

Seniors may be more sensitive to side effects.

Generic Name

Carteolol (car-TEE-uh-lol) G

Brand Names

Cartrol

Type of Drug

Beta-adrenergic blocking agent.

Prescribed For

High blood pressure and angina pectoris.

General Information

Carteolol hydrochloride is one of many beta-adrenergic blocking drugs, or beta blockers, that interfere with the action of a specific part of the nervous system. Beta receptors are found all over the body and affect many body functions. Each beta blocker has particular characteristics that make it more suitable for certain conditions or people.

Cautions and Warnings

You should be cautious about taking carteolol if you have **asthma, severe heart failure,** a **very slow heart rate,** or **heart block** (disruption of the electrical impulses that control heart rate) because the drug may aggravate these conditions.

People with **angina** who take carteolol for high blood pressure risk aggravating their angina if they suddenly stop taking the drug. These people should have their drug dosage reduced gradually over 1 to 2 weeks.

Carteolol should be used with caution if you have **liver or kidney disease** because the ability to eliminate the drug from your body may be impaired. Carteolol should also be used with caution in people who have **bronchial asthma** or **non-allergic bronchospasm** (such as chronic bronchitis or emphysema).

Carteolol reduces the amount of blood pumped by the heart with each beat. This reduction in blood flow may aggravate the condition of people with **poor circulation** or **circulatory disease.**

If you are undergoing **major surgery,** your doctor may want you to stop taking carteolol at least 2 days before surgery.

Use carteolol with caution if you have **diabetes** or **thyroid problems.**

Possible Side Effects

Side effects are relatively uncommon and usually mild.

▼ Most common: impotence.

▼ Less common: unusual tiredness or weakness, slow heartbeat, heart failure, dizziness, breathing difficulties, bronchospasm, depression, anxiety, nervousness, sleeplessness, disorientation, short-term memory loss, emotional instability, cold hands and feet, constipation, diarrhea, nausea, vomiting, upset stomach, increased eating, sweating, urinary difficulties, cramps, blurred vision, rash, hair loss, stuffy nose, facial swelling, aggravation of lupus erythematosus, itching, chest pain, back or joint pain, colitis, and drug allergy (symptoms include fever and sore throat).

Drug Interactions

• Carteolol may interact with surgical anesthetics to increase the risk of heart problems during surgery. Some anesthesiologists recommend gradually stopping the drug by 2 days before surgery.

• Carteolol may interfere with the normal signs of low blood sugar and with the action of oral antidiabetes drugs.

• Carteolol increases the blood-pressure-lowering effects of other blood-pressure-reducing agents, including clonidine, guanabenz, and reserpine, as well as calcium channel blockers, such as nifedipine.

• Aspirin-containing drugs, indomethacin, sulfinpyrazone, and estrogen drugs may interfere with the blood-pressure-lowering effect of carteolol.

• Cocaine may reduce the effectiveness of all beta blockers.

• Carteolol may worsen the problem of cold hands and feet associated with ergot alkaloids, used to treat migraine. Gangrene is a possibility in people taking both an ergot and carteolol.

• Carteolol will counteract thyroid hormone replacements.

• Calcium channel blockers, flecainide, hydralazine, oral contraceptives, propafenone, haloperidol, phenothiazine tranquilizers—molindone and others—quinolone antibacterials, and quinidine may increase the amount of carteolol in the bloodstream and lead to increased carteolol effects.

• Carteolol should not be taken within 2 weeks of taking a monoamine oxidase inhibitor (MAOI) antidepressant.

• Cimetidine increases the amount of carteolol absorbed into the bloodstream from oral tablets.

• Carteolol may reduce the effect of some antiasthma drugs, including theophylline and aminophylline, and especially ephedrine and isoproterenol.

• Combining carteolol with phenytoin or digitalis drugs may result in excessive slowing of the heart, possibly causing heart block.

• If you stop smoking while taking carteolol, your dose may have to be reduced because your liver will break down the drug more slowly afterward.

Food Interactions

None known.

Usual Dose

2.5–10 mg once a day. People with poor kidney function may need to take their dose as infrequently as once every 72 hours.

Overdosage

Symptoms of overdose include changes in heartbeat— unusually slow, unusually fast, or irregular—severe dizziness or fainting, breathing difficulties, bluish-colored fingernails or palms, and seizures. Low blood pressure and bronchospasm may also occur. The victim should be taken to a hospital emergency room. ALWAYS bring the prescription bottle or container.

Special Information

Carteolol should be taken continuously. When ending carteolol treatment, dosage should be lowered gradually over a period of about 2 weeks. Do not stop taking this drug unless directed to do so by your doctor. Abrupt withdrawal may cause chest pain, breathing difficulties, increased sweating, and unusually fast or irregular heartbeat.

Call your doctor at once if you develop back or joint pain, breathing difficulties, cold hands or feet, depression, rash, or

changes in heartbeat. This drug may produce an undesirable lowering of blood pressure, leading to dizziness or fainting; call your doctor if this happens to you. Call your doctor if you experience persistent or bothersome anxiety, diarrhea, constipation, impotence, headache, itching, nausea or vomiting, nightmares or vivid dreams, upset stomach, trouble sleeping, stuffy nose, frequent urination, unusual tiredness, or weakness.

Carteolol can cause drowsiness, light-headedness, dizziness, or blurred vision. Be careful when driving or performing complex tasks.

It is best to take carteolol at the same time each day. If you forget a dose of carteolol tablets, take it as soon as you remember. If you take carteolol once a day and it is within 8 hours of your next dose, skip the dose you forgot and continue with your regular schedule. If you take carteolol twice a day and it is within 4 hours of your next dose, skip the one you forgot and continue with your regular schedule. Never take a double dose.

Special Populations

Pregnancy/Breast-feeding

Infants born to women who took a beta blocker while pregnant had lower birth weights, low blood pressure, and reduced heart rates. Carteolol should be avoided by pregnant women and women who might become pregnant while taking it.

It is not known if carteolol passes into breast milk. Nursing mothers taking carteolol should bottle-feed.

Seniors

Seniors may require less of the drug to achieve results. Seniors taking carteolol may be more likely to suffer from cold hands and feet, reduced body temperature, chest pain, general feelings of ill health, sudden breathing difficulties, increased sweating, or changes in heartbeat.

Generic Name

Carvedilol (car-VAY-dih-lol)

Brand Name

Coreg

Type of Drug

Alpha-beta-adrenergic blocker.

Prescribed For

Heart failure, high blood pressure, angina pain, and cardiomyopathy.

General Information

Carvedilol was the first beta blocker approved for heart failure. It is also the only beta blocker approved for severe heart failure.

Carvedilol blocks both the alpha- and beta-adrenergic portions of the central nervous system. This dual action reduces the amount of blood pumped with each heartbeat and also decreases the risk of tachycardia (very rapid heartbeat). Carvedilol's beta-blocking effects begin within an hour of taking the first dose; maximum blood pressure lowering occurs after 1 or 2 weeks. The drug also causes blood vessels to dilate (widen), allowing the heart to pump blood more efficiently.

Cautions and Warnings

Carvedilol should not be taken by patients with **bronchial disease,** such as chronic bronchitis, emphysema, or asthma.

In studies, carvedilol caused mild and reversible **liver injury** in about 1 of every 100 people who took it. Those with severe liver disease should not take this medication. Call your doctor at once if you develop signs of liver damage (symptoms include severe itching, dark-colored urine, flu-like symptoms, appetite loss, and yellowing of the skin or whites of the eyes).

Check with your doctor about continuing carvedilol if you are to receive **general anesthesia;** heart function that is depressed by anesthetics can worsen if carvedilol is used at the same time.

Carvedilol can mask signs of **low blood sugar** and may increase the effects of insulin or oral antidiabetes drugs, making it more difficult to recover from the effects of low blood sugar.

Carvedilol can mask symptoms of an **overactive thyroid gland.** Abruptly stopping carvedilol can trigger an attack of hyperthyroidism.

Possible Side Effects

Most side effects are considered mild or moderate.

▼ Most common: dizziness, sleepiness or sleepless-ness, diarrhea, abdominal pain, slow heartbeat, dizziness when rising from a sitting or lying position, swelling of the hands or feet, sore throat, breathing difficulties, tired-ness, back pain, urinary infection, viral infection, high blood-triglyceride levels, and low blood-platelet counts.

▼ Less common: extra heartbeats; palpitations; blood-pressure changes; fainting; reduced blood supply to the arms and legs (symptoms include aches, cramps, pain, or tiredness on walking, or pain in the foot, thigh, hip, or buttocks); tingling in the hands or feet; reduced sensa-tion; depression; nervousness; constipation; gas; liver irritation; cough; impotence and reduced sex drive in men; itching; rash; visual difficulties; ringing or buzzing in the ears; high blood cholesterol, sugar, or uric acid; anemia; weakness; hot flushes; leg cramps; dry mouth; not feeling well; sweating; and muscle ache.

▼ Rare: Rare side effects can affect the heart, mental status, the respiratory tract, the urinary tract, and the kid-ney. It can also cause hair loss, weight gain, and sugar in the urine.

Drug Interactions

• Carvedilol increases the effects of insulin and oral antidi-abetes drugs. People taking this combination must monitor their blood sugar levels regularly. Call your doctor if there is any change from your normal pattern.

• Carvedilol increases the effects of verapamil, diltiazem, and similar calcium-channel blocking drugs.

• SSRIs may increase the effects of carvedilol.

• Carvedilol increases the blood-pressure-lowering effect of clonidine. People taking this combination may need less clonidine to control their pressure.

• Carvedilol increases the amount of digoxin in the blood by about 15%. Your digoxin dosage may have to be adjusted.

• Cimetidine increases the amount of carvedilol absorbed into the blood by about 30%, but the importance of this inter-action is not clear.

• Rifampin reduces the amount of carvedilol in the blood by about 70%. Dosage adjustment is necessary.

Food Interactions

Take carvedilol with food to reduce the risk of dizziness or fainting.

Usual Dose

Heart Failure
    Adult: 3.125 mg 2 times a day for 2 weeks. Dose may be doubled every 2 weeks to the highest level tolerated. Maximum daily dosage is 25 mg 2 times a day in people weighing less than 187 lbs., and 50 mg twice a day in people who weigh more.

High Blood Pressure and Cardiomyopathy
    Adult: 6.25 mg twice a day to start, increased to 25 mg twice a day if needed.
    Senior: Seniors may require smaller doses than younger adults.
    Child: not recommended.

Overdosage

Overdose may lead to very low blood pressure (symptoms include dizziness and fainting), slow heartbeat and other cardiac symptoms including shock and heart attack, breathing difficulties, bronchial spasm, vomiting, periods of unconsciousness, and seizures. Overdose victims must be taken to a hospital emergency room. ALWAYS bring the prescription bottle or container.

Special Information

Carvedilol should be taken continuously. Do not stop taking it without your doctor's knowledge, because abrupt withdrawal may cause chest pain, breathing difficulties, increased sweating, and unusually fast or irregular heartbeat. The dose should be gradually reduced over a period of about 2 weeks.

People taking carvedilol may become dizzy or faint when rising quickly from a sitting or lying position. If this happens to you, sit or lie down until you feel better. Carvedilol can also cause drowsiness, light-headedness, or blurred vision. Be careful when driving or doing any task that requires concentration.

Contact lens wearers are more likely to experience dry eyes with carvedilol.

It is best to take carvedilol at the same time each day. If you forget a dose, take it as soon as you remember. If it is within

4 hours of your next dose, skip the dose you forgot and continue with your regular schedule. Do not take a double dose.

Special Populations

Pregnancy/Breast-feeding

Animal studies indicate that carvedilol passes into the fetal bloodstream and may interfere with pregnancy. When this drug is considered crucial by your doctor, its potential benefits must be carefully weighed against its risks.

It is not known if carvedilol passes into human breast milk, though it passes into rat breast milk. Beta-blocking drugs like carvedilol may affect babies' hearts. Nursing mothers who must take this drug should bottle-feed.

Seniors

Seniors are more likely to develop dizziness and may require reduced dosage.

Cefzil   *see Cephalosporin Antibiotics, page 211*

Celebrex   *see Celecoxib, below*

Generic Name

Celecoxib   (sel-eh-KOX-ib)

Brand Name

Celebrex

The information in this profile also applies to the following drug:

Generic Ingredient: Valdecoxib
Bextra

Type of Drug

Cyclooxygenase-2 (COX-2) inhibitor NSAID (non-steroidal anti-inflammatory drug).

Prescribed For

Osteoarthritis and rheumatoid arthritis, acute pain, familial adenomatous polyposis (FAP), and menstrual pain.

General Information

Traditional NSAIDs work primarily by blocking the effects of COX-2, a body enzyme that plays an important role in regulating pain and inflammation. But these NSAIDs also have an unwanted effect: They interfere with cyclooxygenase-1 (COX-1), a related enzyme that helps to maintain the stomach's protective lining. NSAIDs that block the effects of this enzyme may produce side effects such as stomach irritation, gas, and stomach ulcers.

COX-2 inhibitors such as celecoxib are a new class of NSAIDs that work about as well as the older NSAIDs. In fact, both 200 mg a day and 400 mg a day of celecoxib work as well as naproxen 500 mg twice a day. They interfere primarily with COX-2, leaving the stomach-protecting COX-1 relatively unaffected. This means that COX-2 inhibitor NSAIDs can relieve pain and inflammation just like traditional NSAIDs but are less likely to cause gastrointestinal (GI) side effects. Another advantage of celecoxib is that it does not cause thinning of the blood or affect blood platelets as can happen with older NSAIDs. Celecoxib is broken down in the liver.

African Americans absorb about 40% more celecoxib than Caucasians; its importance is unclear. Celecoxib is the first drug proven effective in reducing the number of intestinal polyps in people with the rare genetic disorder FAP.

Cautions and Warnings

Do not take celecoxib if you are **sensitive** or **allergic** to it or to sulfa drugs. NSAIDs should not be taken by people with **asthma** or by those who have had an **allergic reaction to aspirin or another NSAID**. They can develop a group of symptoms (runny nose with or without nasal polyps and a severe bronchial spasm) known as the aspirin triad.

NSAIDs can cause **GI bleeding and ulcers** and **stomach perforation**. This can occur at any time, with or without warning, in people who take NSAIDs regularly. Celecoxib should be used with caution by people who have had **stomach ulcers** or **GI bleeding**. Minor upper GI problems, such as upset stomach, are common and may occur at any time during NSAID therapy. People who develop bleeding or ulcers and continue NSAID treatment should be aware of the risk of developing more serious side effects. Risk of GI bleeding and ulcers is increased with longer duration of therapy as well as treatment with oral corticosteroids and anticoagulants, smoking, alcoholism, older age, and general poor health.

Celecoxib has not been studied in people with severe kidney disease. They should not use this drug unless their doctors closely monitor their kidney function.

Celecoxib can cause **liver irritation** and should be used with caution by people with **hepatitis** or **cirrhosis**. People with moderate liver disease can have twice as much celecoxib in their blood and require a reduced dosage. The effect of celecoxib in people with severe liver failure is not known.

Possible Side Effects

Side effects are similar to those of traditional NSAIDs. Stomach and intestinal side effects are about half as common.

▼ Most common: headache.

▼ Common: diarrhea, upset stomach, sinus irritation, and respiratory infection.

▼ Less common: abdominal pain, gas, nausea, back pain, swelling in the legs or arms, accidental injuries, sleeplessness, dizziness, sore throat, runny nose, and rash.

▼ Rare: Rare side effects can occur in almost any part of the body. Contact your doctor if you experience any side effect not listed above.

Drug Interactions

• Alcohol may increase the risk of serious GI-related side effects. Avoid alcohol.

• Combining celecoxib with an aluminum and magnesium antacid slightly reduces the amount of drug absorbed. Separate doses of these antacids and celecoxib by 1 to 2 hours.

• Fluconazole and lithium may raise celecoxib blood levels and increase the risk of side effects.

• While celecoxib may be combined with low dosages of aspirin, taking these drugs together can increase the risk of stomach or intestinal ulcers or other complications. The ulcer risk associated with this combination is less than that posed by single-drug therapy with a traditional NSAID.

• Celecoxib can reduce the blood-pressure-lowering effect of angiotensin-converting enzyme (ACE) inhibitors and diuretic drugs. This combination can also increase the risk of kidney damage after chronic celecoxib use.

• Celecoxib may affect lithium blood levels.

• NSAIDs can reduce the effect of furosemide and thiazide-type diuretics.

Food Interactions

Celecoxib can be taken without regard to food or meals. For optimal effectiveness, avoid taking this drug with high-fat meals.

Usual Dose

Celecoxib
   Adult (age 18 and over): Arthritis—100–200 mg once or twice a day. FAP—400 mg twice a day.
   Child (under age 18): not recommended.

Valdecoxib
   Adult (age 18 and over): 10–20 mg once or twice a day.
   Child (under age 18): not recommended.

Overdosage

Symptoms include lethargy, drowsiness, nausea, vomiting, and stomach pain. Stomach or intestinal bleeding or severe allergic reactions can occur. High blood pressure, kidney failure, breathing difficulties, and coma are rare.

The victim should be taken to a hospital emergency room. ALWAYS bring the prescription bottle or container.

Special Information

Call your doctor if you develop rash, itching, unexplained weight gain, nausea, fatigue, jaundice (yellowing of the skin or whites of the eyes), flu-like symptoms, lethargy, swelling, black stools, severe stomach pain, persistent headache, or any bothersome or persistent side effect.

If you forget a dose and remember within 1 or 2 hours of your scheduled time, take it right away. If you do not remember until later, skip the forgotten dose and continue with your regular schedule.

Special Populations

Pregnancy/Breast-feeding

Celecoxib has caused birth defects in animal studies. Any NSAID may affect fetal heart development during the second half of pregnancy. Pregnant women should not take celecoxib without their doctor's approval. When this drug is considered crucial by your doctor, its potential benefits must be carefully weighed against its risks.

NSAIDs may pass into breast milk. There is a possibility that a nursing mother taking celecoxib could affect her baby's heart or cardiovascular system. Nursing mothers who must take this drug should bottle-feed.

Seniors

Generally, seniors can take this drug without special precaution. Those who weigh less than 110 lbs. should begin with the lowest possible dosage.

Celexa   see Selective Serotonin Reuptake Inhibitors (SSRIs), page 965

Type of Drug

Cephalosporin Antibiotics

(CEF-uh-loe-SPOR-in)

Brand Name

Generic Ingredient: Cefaclor G
Ceclor   Ceclor Pulvules
Ceclor CD

Generic Ingredient: Cefadroxil G
Duricef

Generic Ingredient: Cefdinir
Omnicef

Generic Ingredient: Cefditoren Pivoxil
Spectracef

Generic Ingredient: Cefixime
Suprax

Generic Ingredient: Cefpodoxime Proxetil G
Vantin

Generic Ingredient: Cefprozil
Cefzil

Generic Ingredient: Ceftibuten
Cedax

Generic Ingredient: Cefuroxime Axetil G
Ceftin

Generic Ingredient: Cephalexin G
Keflet   Panixine Disperdose
Keflex

Generic Ingredient: Cephalexin Hydrochloride
Keftab

Generic Ingredient: Cephradine G
Anspor   Velosef

Generic Ingredient: Loracarbef
Lorabid

Prescribed For

Bacterial infections.

General Information

These antibiotics are related to cephalosporin C, which is similar to penicillin and is isolated from the *Cephalosporium acremonium* fungus. Of the more than 20 different antibiotic drugs derived from cephalosporin C, only those that are taken by mouth are included in *The Pill Book*. Injectable drugs are not discussed. Most common infections can be treated with these antibiotics, but they are not interchangeable. Your doctor must select the appropriate antibiotic for a particular infection.

Cautions and Warnings

Up to 15% of people **allergic** to penicillin may also be allergic to cephalosporins. The most common cephalosporin allergic reaction is a hive-like condition with redness over large areas of the body. Other sensitivity reactions include rash, fever, and joint aches or pain. Such reactions generally begin after a few days of taking the antibiotic and resolve within a few days after the antibiotic is stopped.

Prolonged or repeated use of a cephalosporin may lead to a **secondary infection** not susceptible to the antibiotic.

Occasionally, people taking a cephalosporin develop **colitis**. Call your doctor if you develop severe diarrhea while taking one of these drugs.

People with **poor kidney function** may require less medicine to treat their infections. Rarely, people taking a cephalosporin have had a **seizure,** especially those with kidney disease where the dose was not reduced.

Some injectable cephalosporins have caused **blood-clotting problems**. This has not occurred in people taking an oral drug.

Rarely, severe **anemia** occurs in people taking cephalosporin antibiotics. Report any signs of anemia (such as pale skin color, weakness, tiredness, difficulty breathing, and abnormal heart rhythms) to your doctor.

Cefprozil oral suspension contains phenylalanine and cannot be taken by people with **phenylketonuria (PKU disease)**.

Possible Side Effects

Most side effects are mild.

▼ Most common: diarrhea, headache, abdominal pain, constipation, gas, upset stomach, nausea, vomiting, itching, and rash.

▼ Less common: dizziness, tiredness, weakness, tingling in the hands or feet, confusion, appetite loss, changes in taste perception, and genital and anal itching. Colitis may develop.

Cefaclor may cause serum sickness (symptoms include fever, joint pain, and rash).

Cephalosporins may cause changes in blood cells, kidney problems, liver inflammation, and jaundice, but these side effects are rarely a problem with oral cephalosporins.

Drug Interactions

• Antacids can reduce the amounts of cefaclor, cefdinir, cefditoren pivoxil, and cefpodoxime in the blood. Do not take antacids within 2 hours of these antibiotics.

• Cimetidine, famotidine, ranitidine, or nizatidine can reduce the effectiveness of cefpodoxime, cefditoren pivoxil, and cefuroxime—do not combine these drugs.

• Iron and iron-fortified foods may interfere with the absorption of cefdinir. Separate your iron dose from the antibiotic by at least 2 hours. Iron-fortified infant formula does not produce this effect.

• Probenecid may increase blood levels of some cephalosporins.

• Potent (loop-type) diuretics can lead to kidney damage if mixed with a cephalosporin antibiotic.

• Drinking alcohol with or within 72 hours of some injectable cephalosporins can lead to a severe reaction. This reaction has not occurred with oral cephalosporins.

• Combining warfarin and some injectable cephalosporins can lead to unexpected bleeding. This reaction has not occurred with oral cephalosporins.

Food Interactions

Generally, cephalosporins may be taken with food or milk if they upset your stomach. Cefditoren pivoxil should be taken with a meal. Food increases the absorption of cefpodoxime and cefuroxime.

Usual Dose

Cefaclor
   Adult: 250 mg every 8 hours, or 375–500 mg every 12 hours.
   Child: 9 mg per lb. of body weight a day, in 2–3 equal doses.

Cefadroxil
   Adult: 1–2 g a day, in 1–2 doses.
   Child: 13 mg per lb. of body weight a day, in 1–2 doses.

Cefdinir
   Adult and Child (age 13 and over): 600 mg a day, in 1–2 doses.
   Child (age 6 months–12 years): 6½ mg per lb. of body weight a day in 1–2 doses.

Cefditoren
   Adult (age 12 and over): 200–400 mg twice a day for 10 days.

Cefixime
  Adult: 400 mg a day, in 1–2 doses.
  Child: 3.5 mg per lb. of body weight a day, in 1–2 doses.

Cefpodoxime
  Adult and Child (age 13 and over): 200–400 mg a day, in 1–2 doses.
  Child (age 5 months–12 years): 5 mg per lb. of body weight a day in 1–2 doses. Maximum daily dose for middle-ear infections is 400 mg; 200 mg for sore throat or tonsillitis.

Cefprozil
  Adult (age 13 and over): 500–1000 mg a day.
  Child (age 6 months–12 years): 7–13 mg per lb. of body weight a day in 1–2 doses.

Ceftibuten
  Adult and Child (age 12 and over): 400 mg once a day for 10 days.
  Child: 4 mg per lb. of body weight, up to 400 mg, once a day.

Cefuroxime
  Adult and Child (age 13 and over): 250–1000 mg a day in 1–2 doses.
  Child (age 3 months–12 years): tablets—125–250 mg every 12 hours. Liquid—9–13 mg per lb. of body weight every 12 hours.

Cephalexin
  Adult: 1000–4000 mg a day in divided doses, usually 250 mg every 6 hours, or 500 mg every 12 hours.
  Child: 11–23 mg per lb. of body weight a day in divided doses. The dose may be increased to 46 mg per lb. of body weight for middle-ear infections.

Cephradine
  Adult: 250–1000 mg every 6–12 hours.
  Child (age 9 months and over): 11–45 mg per lb. of body weight a day, in 2–4 doses. Dosage should not exceed 4 g per day.

Loracarbef
  Adult and Child (age 13 and over): 200–400 mg every 12–24 hours.

Child (age 6 months–12 years): 7–13 mg per lb. of body weight a day in 2 doses.

Overdosage

Common symptoms of overdose are nausea, vomiting, and upset stomach. These can often be treated with milk or antacid. Cephalosporin overdoses are generally not serious; contact a hospital emergency room or local poison control center for more information. If you seek treatment, ALWAYS bring the prescription bottle or container.

Special Information

Call your doctor if you develop severe abdominal cramps or diarrhea. Stop taking this drug and immediately call your doctor if you experience fever, chest tightness, breathing difficulties, redness, muscle aches, or swelling.

You must take the full course of treatment prescribed—even if you feel better in 2 or 3 days—to obtain the maximum benefit from any antibiotic.

Proper diagnosis is key to the effectiveness of an antibiotic: Do not take any antibiotic without consulting your doctor.

All cephalosporins may cause false results for certain urine tests for sugar. Cefuroxime may cause false results for blood sugar. Diabetics taking cephradine should not change their diet or diabetes medication without consulting their doctor.

If you miss a dose that you take once a day, take it as soon as you remember. If it is almost time for your next dose, take the dose you forgot right away and your next one 10 to 12 hours later. Then go back to your regular schedule. If you take the medication 2 times a day, take the dose you forgot right away and the next dose 5 to 6 hours later. Then go back to your regular schedule. If you take the medication 3 or more times a day, take the dose you missed right away and your next dose 2 to 4 hours later. Then go back to your regular schedule.

Most cephalosporin liquids must be kept in the refrigerator to maintain their strength. Only cefixime liquid does not require refrigeration. All of the liquid cephalosporins have a very limited shelf life. Do not keep any of these liquids beyond the 10 days to 2 weeks specified on the label. Follow your pharmacist's storage instructions.

Special Populations

Pregnancy/Breast-feeding

These drugs are considered relatively safe during pregnancy, though small amounts pass into the fetus. Little information is available about the newer members of the group. Also, cephalosporins pass more quickly out of the bodies of pregnant women. Cephalosporins should be taken during pregnancy only if the benefit outweighs the risk.

Small amounts of most cephalosporin antibiotics pass into breast milk. Nursing mothers who must take a cephalosporin should bottle-feed.

Seniors

Seniors may require a lower dosage because of reduced kidney function.

Generic Name

Cetirizine (seh-TERE-ih-zene)

Brand Name

Zyrtec   Zyrtec-D

The information in this profile also applies to the following drugs:

Generic Ingredient: Azelastine
Astelin

Generic Ingredient: Fexofenadine
Allegra

Type of Drug

Antihistamine.

Prescribed For

Azelastine: runny nose, sneezing, nasal itching, and post-nasal drip. Cetirizine: stuffy and runny nose, itchy eyes, and scratchy throat caused by seasonal and year-round allergy, and for other symptoms of allergy such as rash, itching, and hives; also prescribed for chronic itching and for asthma. Fexofenadine:

sneezing, stuffy and runny nose, scratchy throat and mouth, and itchy, watery, and red eyes caused by seasonal allergies.

General Information

Antihistamines generally work by blocking the release of histamine (a chemical released by body tissue during an allergic reaction) from the cell at the H_1 histamine receptor site, drying up secretions of the nose, throat, and eyes. Cetirizine causes less sedation than older antihistamines and appears to be just as effective.

Cautions and Warnings

Do not take cetirizine if you are **allergic** or **sensitive** to it.

People with **kidney disease** should receive reduced dosage of cetirizine.

Possible Side Effects

▼ Common: headache, drowsiness, fatigue, dry mouth, bitter taste in the mouth (azelastine), and dizziness.

▼ Less common: nosebleeds, nausea, nervousness, upset stomach, sore throat, cough, stuffy nose, sneezing, and changes in bowel habits.

Drug Interactions

• Cimetidine may increase the level of azelastine in the blood.

• Cetirizine is less likely than other antihistamines to interact with drugs.

Food Interactions

Take cetirizine on an empty stomach, 1 hour before or 2 hours after meals; it may be taken with food or milk if it upsets your stomach.

Usual Dose

Azelastine Nasal Spray

Adult and Child (age 12 and over): 2 sprays in each nostril twice a day.

Child (age 5–11): 1 spray in each nostril twice a day.

Cetirizine
Adult and Child (age 6 and over): 5–10 mg once a day depending on symptoms. Reduce dosage in people with kidney disease.
Child (age 2–5): 2.5–5 mg a day.

Fexofenadine
Adult (age 12 and over): 60 mg twice a day or 180 mg once a day. People with kidney disease should take 60 mg a day.
Child (age 6–11): 30 mg twice a day.

Overdosage

Drug overdose is likely to cause severe side effects. Overdose victims should be given ipecac syrup—available at any pharmacy—to make them vomit and be taken to a hospital emergency room. ALWAYS bring the prescription bottle or container.

Special Information

Report sore throat, unusual bleeding, bruising, tiredness, weakness, or any other unusual side effect to your doctor. Do not combine this drug with alcohol or other nervous system depressants. Do not put azelastine nasal solution into your eyes.

If you forget to take a dose of cetirizine, take it as soon as you remember. If it is almost time for your next dose, skip the one you forgot and continue with your regular schedule. Do not take a double dose.

Special Populations

Pregnancy/Breast-feeding
Oral antihistamines are generally considered safe for use during pregnancy. But do not take any antihistamine without your doctor's knowledge if you are or might become pregnant—especially during the last 3 months of pregnancy, because newborns may have severe reactions to antihistamines.

Small amounts of antihistamine pass into breast milk. Nursing mothers who must take cetirizine should bottle-feed.

Seniors
Antihistamines are more likely to cause dizziness, sleepiness, and confusion in seniors. Dosage reduction may be recommended.

Generic Name

Cevimeline (seh-VIM-ih-lene) Ⓖ

Brand Name

Evoxac

Type of Drug

Cholinergic.

Prescribed For

Dry mouth in people with Sjögren's syndrome.

General Information

Sjögren's syndrome is a group of symptoms related to a lack of bodily secretions. People with this condition have very dry eyes and mucous membranes, facial lesions, and neck swelling. It often occurs in menopausal woman and is often associated with rheumatoid arthritis, poor blood circulation in the legs, and tooth decay. Cevimeline increases secretions in the mouth by binding to specific nervous system receptors and causing the release of more saliva.

Cautions and Warnings

Do not take cevimeline if you are **sensitive** or **allergic** to it. This drug may make breathing more difficult and worsen **lung conditions** such as asthma, chronic bronchitis, or chronic obstructive pulmonary disease (COPD).

Eye conditions like **glaucoma** or **inflammation of the iris** may be worsened by cevimeline.

Cevimeline may affect the heart, and some people with **severe heart disease**, including those with a history of severe angina or a heart attack, may not be able to compensate for this effect.

Cevimeline may worsen **gallstones** and **kidney stones** and should be avoided by people with a history of these conditions.

Possible Side Effects

▼ Most common: excessive sweating, headache, nausea, sinus irritation, respiratory infection, runny nose, and diarrhea.

Possible Side Effects *(continued)*

▼ Common: upset stomach, abdominal pains, urinary infection, coughing, and sore throat.

▼ Less common: vomiting, back pain, injury, rash, conjunctivitis (pinkeye), dizziness, bronchitis, severe joint pain, fatigue, bone pain, sleeplessness, hot flushes, excess salivation, chills, and anxiety.

▼ Rare: frequent urination, weakness, flushing. Other rare side effects can occur in almost any part of the body. Contact your doctor if you experience any side effect not listed above.

Drug Interactions

• Mixing cevimeline with a beta blocker can lead to heart rhythm disturbances.

• Cevimeline may interfere with the effects of anticholinergics, found in some medications for abdominal or stomach spasms or cramps.

• Cholinergics such as bethanechol, donepezil, physostigmine, pilocarpine, and pyridostigmine can add to the effects of cevimeline.

• Some drugs may interfere with the breakdown of cevimeline in the liver, increasing the chance of drug side effects. These include amiodarone, celecoxib, chlorpheniramine, cimetidine, ciprofloxacin, clarithromycin, clomipramine, cocaine, diltiazem, erythromycin, fluconazole, fluoxetine, halofantrine, indinavir, itraconazole, ketoconazole, methadone, mibefradil, nelfinavir, paroxetine, quinidine, ranitidine, ritonavir, saquinavir, and terbinafine.

Food Interactions

Grapefruit juice may interfere with the breakdown of cevimeline in the liver, increasing the chance of drug side effects. Food interferes with the absorption of cevimeline into the bloodstream. Take this drug on an empty stomach.

Usual Dose

30 mg three times a day. The safety of using cevimeline in children is not known.

Overdosage

Overdose symptoms can include exaggerated drug side effects including headache, visual difficulty, excess tearing and/or sweating, breathing difficulty, stomach or intestinal spasms, nausea, vomiting, diarrhea, changes in heart rhythm, blood pressure changes, shock, mental confusion, and tremors. Overdose victims should be taken to a hospital emergency room. ALWAYS bring the prescription bottle or container.

Special Information

Cevimeline may cause blurred vision, possibly interfering with driving or performing tasks that require reliable vision, especially at night or in low light.

If you sweat excessively while taking cevimeline, be sure to drink a lot of water. Excessive sweating can lead to dehydration.

If you miss a dose, take it as soon as you remember. If it is almost time for your next dose, skip the missed dose and continue with your regular schedule. Do not take a double dose.

Special Populations

Pregnancy/Breast-feeding

Pregnant women should take cevimeline only if it is considered crucial by your doctor, since its effect on the developing fetus is not known.

It is not known if cevimeline passes into breast milk, but nursing mothers who must take this drug should consider bottle-feeding.

Seniors

Older adults should be cautious about using this drug because of its possible effects on the kidney, liver, and heart, and on other diseases or medications.

Generic Name

Chlordiazepoxide (klor-dye-az-uh-POX-ide) Ⓖ

Brand Names

Librium

Type of Drug

Benzodiazepine tranquilizer.

Prescribed For

Anxiety, tension, fatigue, agitation, and withdrawal symptoms of alcoholism; also prescribed for irritable bowel syndrome and panic attacks.

General Information

Chlordiazepoxide is a member of the group of drugs known as benzodiazepines.

Benzodiazepines work by a direct effect on the brain. They can relax you and make you more tranquil or sleepier, or they can slow nervous system transmissions in such a way as to act as an anticonvulsant. Many doctors prefer benzodiazepines to other drugs that can be used to similar effect because they tend to be safer, have fewer side effects, and are usually as effective, if not more so.

Cautions and Warnings

Do not take chlordiazepoxide if you know you are **sensitive** or **allergic** to it or another member of the group, including clonazepam.

Chlordiazepoxide can aggravate narrow-angle **glaucoma**, but you may take it if you have open-angle glaucoma.

Other conditions in which chlordiazepoxide should be used with caution are severe **depression**, severe **lung disease, sleep apnea** (intermittent cessation of breathing during sleep), **liver disease, drunkenness,** and **kidney disease.**

Chlordiazepoxide should not be taken by **psychotic patients** because it is not effective for them and can trigger unusual excitement, stimulation, and rage.

Chlordiazepoxide is not intended for more than 3 to 4 months of continuous use. Your condition should be reassessed before continuing chlordiazepoxide beyond that time.

Chlordiazepoxide may be **addictive**. Drug withdrawal may develop if you stop taking it after only 4 weeks of regular use, but is more likely after longer use. It may start with anxiety and progress to tingling in the hands or feet, sensitivity to bright light, sleep disturbances, cramps, tremors, muscle tension or twitching, poor concentration, flu symptoms, fatigue, appetite loss, sweating, and changes in mental state.

Dosage of chlordiazepoxide should be decreased gradually over 4–8 weeks after **prolonged use.**

Possible Side Effects

Weakness and confusion may occur, especially in seniors and in those who are sickly.

▼ Most common: mild drowsiness during the first few days of therapy.

▼ Less common: depression, lethargy, disorientation, headache, inactivity, slurred speech, stupor, dizziness, tremor, constipation, dry mouth, nausea, inability to control urination, sexual difficulties, irregular menstrual cycle, changes in heart rhythm, low blood pressure, fluid retention, blurred or double vision, itching, rash, hiccups, nervousness, inability to fall asleep, and occasional liver dysfunction. If you experience any of these symptoms, stop taking the medicine and contact your doctor immediately.

▼ Rare: Rare side effects can occur in almost any part of the body. Contact your doctor if you experience any side effect not listed above.

Drug Interactions

• Chlordiazepoxide is a central-nervous-system depressant. Avoid alcohol, other tranquilizers, narcotics, barbiturates, monoamine oxidase inhibitors (MAOIs), antihistamines, and antidepressants. Taking chlordiazepoxide with these drugs may result in excessive depression, tiredness, sleepiness, breathing difficulties, or related symptoms.

• Smoking may reduce the effectiveness of chlordiazepoxide by increasing the rate at which it is broken down by the body.

• The effects of chlordiazepoxide may be prolonged when it is taken with cimetidine, oral contraceptives, disulfiram, fluoxetine, isoniazid, ketoconazole, metoprolol, probenecid, propoxyphene, propranolol, rifampin, or valproic acid.

• Theophylline may reduce chlordiazepoxide's sedative effects.

• If you take antacids, separate them by at least 1 hour from your chlordiazepoxide dose to prevent them from interfering with the passage of chlordiazepoxide into the bloodstream.

• Chlordiazepoxide may increase blood levels of digoxin and the chances for digoxin toxicity.

• Levodopa's effectiveness may be reduced by chlordiazepoxide.

• Phenytoin blood concentrations may be increased when taken with chlordiazepoxide, resulting in possible phenytoin toxicity.

Food Interactions

Chlordiazepoxide is best taken on an empty stomach but may be taken with food if it upsets your stomach.

Usual Dose

Adult: 5–100 mg a day. This range is due to individual response related to age, weight, disease severity, and other characteristics.

Child (age 6 and over): may be given if deemed appropriate by a doctor. Starting dose—5 mg 2–4 times a day. Maintenance dose—up to 30 mg a day for some children, but must be individualized to obtain maximum benefit.

Child (under age 6): not recommended.

Overdosage

Symptoms of overdose are confusion, sleepiness, poor coordination, lack of response to pain such as a pin prick, loss of reflexes, shallow breathing, low blood pressure, and coma. The victim should be taken to a hospital emergency room. ALWAYS bring the prescription bottle or container.

Special Information

Chlordiazepoxide can cause tiredness, drowsiness, inability to concentrate, or similar symptoms. Be careful if you are driving, operating machinery, or performing other activities that require concentration.

If you forget a dose of chlordiazepoxide, take it as soon as you remember. If it is almost time for your next dose, skip the dose you forgot and continue with your regular schedule. Do not take a double dose.

Special Populations

Pregnancy/Breast-feeding

Chlordiazepoxide may cause birth defects if taken during the first 3 months of pregnancy. Avoid chlordiazepoxide while pregnant.

Chlordiazepoxide may pass into breast milk. Nursing mothers who must take chlordiazepoxide should bottle-feed.

Seniors

Seniors, especially those with liver or kidney disease, are more sensitive to the effects of chlordiazepoxide and generally require smaller doses to achieve the same effect.

Generic Name

Chlorpheniramine Maleate

(KLOR-fen-ERE-uh-mene MAL-ee-ate) G

Brand Names

Chlor-Phen   Pro-Hist-8
Chlor-Trimeton

The information in this profile also applies to the following drugs:

Generic Ingredient: Azatadine Maleate
Optimine

Generic Ingredient: Cyproheptadine Hydrochloride G
Periactin

Generic Ingredient: Dexchlorpheniramine Maleate G
Mylaramine   Polarmine Repetabs

Generic Ingredient: Tripelennamine Hydrochloride G
PBZ   PBZ-SR

Type of Drug

Antihistamine.

Prescribed For

Stuffy and runny nose, itchy eyes, and scratchy throat caused by seasonal allergy, and other symptoms of allergy such as rash, itching, and hives.

General Information

Antihistamines generally work by blocking the release of histamine (a chemical released by body tissue during an allergic reaction) from body cells at the H_1 histamine receptor site, drying up secretions of the nose, throat, and eyes.

Cautions and Warnings

Do not use this drug if you are **allergic** to it.

Use chlorpheniramine maleate with care if you have a history of **thyroid disease, heart disease, high blood pressure,** or **diabetes.** This drug should be avoided or used with extreme care if you have narrow-angle **glaucoma, stomach ulcer** or other **stomach problems, enlarged prostate,** or **problems passing urine.** It should not be used by people who have **deep-breathing problems** such as asthma, emphysema, or chronic bronchitis.

Possible Side Effects

▼ Less common: rash or itching, sensitivity to bright light, increased sweating, chills, lowered blood pressure, headache, rapid heartbeat, sleeplessness, dizziness, disturbed coordination, confusion, restlessness, nervousness, irritability, euphoria (feeling "high"), tingling in the hands or feet, blurred or double vision, ringing in the ears, upset stomach, appetite loss, nausea, vomiting, constipation, diarrhea, urinary difficulties, chest tightness, wheezing, stuffy nose, and dryness of the mouth, nose, or throat. Young children may also develop nervousness, irritability, tension, and anxiety.

Drug Interactions

• Chlorpheniramine maleate should not be taken with a monoamine oxidase inhibitor (MAOI) antidepressant, because the combination may cause severe side effects.

• The effects of tranquilizers, benzodiazepines such as diazepan, sedatives, and sleeping medications will be increased when any of these drugs is combined with chlorpheniramine maleate. It is extremely important for your doctor to know if you are taking any other medication with chlorpheniramine maleate so that the dosage of that medication can be properly adjusted.

• Anticholinergics may cause an increase in side effects of chlorpheniramine maleate.

• Be extremely cautious when drinking alcoholic beverages while taking this drug, which enhances the intoxicating and sedating effects of alcohol.

Food Interactions

You may take this drug with food if it upsets your stomach.

Usual Dose

Azatadine
1–2 mg twice a day.

Chlorpheniramine
  Adult and Child (age 13 and over): 4–mg tablet every 4–6 hours; do not take more than 24 mg a day.
  Child (age 6–12): 2-mg tablet every 4–6 hours; do not take more than 12 mg a day.
  Child (age 2–5): 1 mg every 4–6 hours; do not take more than 4 mg a day.

Chlorpheniramine, Sustained-Release
  Adult and Child (age 13 and over): 8–12 mg at bedtime, or every 8–12 hours during the day.
  Child (age 6–12): 8 mg during the day or at bedtime.
  Child (under age 6): not recommended.

Cyproheptadine
  Adult and Child (age 15 and over): do not exceed 32 mg a day.
  Child (age 7–14): 4 mg 2–3 times a day; do not exceed 16 mg a day.
  Child (age 2–6): 2 mg 2–3 times a day; do not exceed 12 mg a day.

Dexchlorpheniramine
  Adult and Child (age 12 and over): 2 mg every 4–6 hours.
  Child (age 6–11): 1 mg every 4–6 hours.

Child (age 2–5): 0.5 mg every 4–6 hours.

Dexchlorpheniramine, Sustained-Release
  Adult and Child (age 12 and over): 4–6 mg every 8–10 hours and at bedtime.
  Child (age 6–11): 4 mg once a day and at bedtime.
  Child (under age 6): not recommended.

Tripelennamine
  Adult and Child (age 12 and over): 25–50 mg every 4–6 hours; do not take more than 600 mg a day. Adults may take up to 3 100-mg, sustained-release tablets a day, although this much is not usually needed.
  Child (under age 12): 2 mg per lb. of body weight a day in divided doses; no more than 300 mg should be given a day.

Overdosage

Symptoms of overdose include depression or stimulation, especially in children; dry mouth; fixed or dilated pupils; flushing of the skin; upset stomach; unsteadiness; and convulsions. Overdose victims should be made to vomit as soon as possible with ipecac syrup—available at any pharmacy—to remove excess drug from the stomach. Take the victim to a hospital emergency room immediately if the victim is unconscious or if you cannot induce vomiting. ALWAYS bring the prescription bottle or container.

Special Information

This drug may cause tiredness or loss of concentration: Be extremely cautious when driving or doing anything that requires close attention.

If you forget a dose of this drug, take it as soon as you remember. If it is almost time for your next dose, skip the one you forgot and continue with your regular schedule. Do not take a double dose.

Special Populations

Pregnancy/Breast-feeding
Animal studies have shown that some antihistamines may cause birth defects. Do not take any antihistamine without your doctor's knowledge if you are or might be pregnant—especially during the last 3 months of pregnancy, because newborns may have severe reactions to antihistamines.

Small amounts of some antihistamines pass into breast milk. Nursing mothers who must take chlorpheniramine maleate should bottle-feed.

Seniors
Seniors are more sensitive to antihistamine side effects. Dosage reduction may be needed.

Generic Name

Chlorpromazine (klor-PROE-muh-zene) Ⓖ

Brand Name

Sonazine
Thorazine*

Thorazine Spansules

The information in this profile also applies to the following drugs:

Generic Ingredient: Fluphenazine Hydrochloride Ⓖ
Permitil   Prolixin

Generic Ingredient: Mesoridazine Besylate
Serentil Ⓢ

Generic Ingredient: Thioridazine Hydrochloride Ⓖ
Mellaril   Mellaril-S

Generic Ingredient: Trifluoperazine Hydrochloride Ⓖ
Stelazine

Some products in this brand-name group are alcohol- or sugar-free. Consult your pharmacist.

Type of Drug

Phenothiazine antipsychotic.

Prescribed For

Psychotic disorders, moderate to severe depression with anxiety, agitation or aggressiveness in disturbed children, intractable pain, and senility; may also be used to relieve nausea, vomiting, hiccups, restlessness, acute intermittant porphyria, and apprehension before surgery or other procedures.

General Information

Chlorpromazine and other phenothiazines act upon a portion of the brain called the hypothalamus. Phenothiazines affect parts of the hypothalamus that control metabolism, body temperature, alertness, muscle tone, hormone balance, and vomiting. Chlorpromazine is available in suppositories and as liquid for those who have trouble swallowing tablets.

Cautions and Warnings

Chlorpromazine may depress the **cough reflex**. People have accidentally choked to death because the cough reflex failed to protect them. Because of its effect in reducing vomiting, chlorpromazine may obscure symptoms of disease or toxicity due to overdose of another drug.

Do not take chlorpromazine if you are **allergic** to it or any phenothiazine drug. Do not take it if you have very **low blood pressure, Parkinson's disease,** or **blood, liver, kidney, or heart disease**.

Use chlorpromazine under your doctor's strict supervision if you have **glaucoma, epilepsy, ulcers,** or **urinary difficulties**.

Avoid exposure to **extreme heat,** because this drug may upset your body's temperature-control mechanism. Do not allow the liquid forms of this drug to come in contact with your skin, because they are highly irritating.

Chlorpromazine may cause unusually high or low levels of cholesterol.

Possible Side Effects

▼ Most common: drowsiness, especially during the first or second week of therapy. If drowsiness becomes troublesome, contact your doctor.

▼ Less common: changes in blood components including anemias, raised or lowered blood pressure, abnormal heart rate, heart attack, sensitivity to light, and faintness or dizziness.

▼ Rare: Rare side effects can occur in almost any part of the body. Contact your doctor if you experience any side effect not listed in this section.

Jaundice (symptoms include yellowing of the whites of the eyes or skin) may appear; when it does it is usually within the first 2 to 4 weeks of treatment. Normally it

Possible Side Effects *(continued)*

goes away when the drug is discontinued, but there have been cases when it has not.

Phenothiazines may produce extrapyramidal side effects, including spasm of the neck muscles, rolling back of the eyes, convulsions, difficulty swallowing, and symptoms associated with Parkinson's disease. These side effects seem very serious but usually disappear after the drug has been withdrawn; however, symtoms affecting the face, tongue, or jaw may persist for as long as several years, especially in older adults with a history of brain damage. Chlorpromazine may cause an unusual increase in psychotic symptoms or may cause paranoid reactions, tiredness, lethargy, restlessness, hyperactivity, confusion at night, bizarre dreams, sleeplessness, depression, and euphoria (feeling high).

Drug Interactions

• Be cautious about taking chlorpromazine with barbiturates, alcohol, sleeping pills, narcotics or other tranquilizers, or any other drug that may produce a depressive effect.

• Aluminum antacids may reduce the effectiveness of phenothiazine drugs.

• Chlorpromazine may reduce the effectiveness of bromocriptine and appetite suppressants.

• Anticholinergic drugs may reduce the effectiveness of chlorpromazine and increase the chance of side effects.

• Phenothiazine drugs may counter the blood-pressure-lowering effect of guanethidine.

• Taking lithium together with a phenothiazine drug may lead to disorientation, loss of consciousness, or uncontrolled muscle movements.

• Combining propranolol and a phenothiazine drug may lead to unusually low blood pressure.

• Combining tricyclic antidepressants with a phenothiazine drug can lead to antidepressant side effects.

• Chlorpromazine may reduce the effectiveness of epinephrine and norepinephrine.

Food Interactions

Take liquid chlorpromazine with fruit juice or other liquids. You may also take it with food if it upsets your stomach.

Usual Dose

Adult: 30–1000 mg or more a day, individualized according to your disease and response.

Child (age 6 months and over): 0.25 mg per lb. of body weight every 4–6 hours, up to 200 mg or more a day, depending on disease, age, and response.

Overdosage

Overdose symptoms include depression, extreme weakness, tiredness, lowered blood pressure, agitation, restlessness, uncontrolled muscle spasms, convulsions, fever, dry mouth, abnormal heart rhythms, and coma. The victim should be taken to a hospital emergency room immediately. ALWAYS bring the prescription bottle or container.

Special Information

Call your doctor at once if you develop sore throat, fever, rash, weakness, visual problems, tremors, muscle movements or twitching, yellowing of the skin or whites of the eyes, or darkening of the urine.

This drug may cause drowsiness. Use caution when driving or operating hazardous equipment. Avoid alcoholic beverages.

Chlorpromazine may cause unusual sensitivity to the sun and may turn your urine reddish-brown to pink.

If dizziness occurs, avoid rising quickly from a sitting or lying position and avoid climbing stairs. Use caution in hot weather, because this drug may make you more prone to heat stroke.

If you are using sustained-release capsules, do not chew them or break them: Swallow them whole. Liquid forms of phenothiazines must be protected from light. Do not take them out of their opaque bottles.

If you take chlorpromazine more than once a day and forget to take a dose, take it right away if you remember within an hour. If you do not remember within an hour, skip the dose you forgot and continue with your regular schedule. If you take 1 dose a day and forget a dose, skip the dose you forgot and continue your regular schedule the next day. Never take a double dose.

Special Populations

Pregnancy/Breast-feeding

Infants born to women taking this drug have experienced side effects—including jaundice and nervous system effects. Check with your doctor about taking chlorpromazine if you are or might be pregnant.

This drug may pass into breast milk. Consider bottle-feeding if you must take chlorpromazine.

Seniors

Seniors are more sensitive to the effects of this drug and usually achieve desired results with lower dosages. Some experts feel that seniors should receive ½ to ¼ the usual adult dose.

Generic Name

Chlorzoxazone (klor-ZOX-uh-zone) G

Brand Names

Paraflex   Remular-S
Parafon Forte DSC   Strifon Forte DSC

Type of Drug

Skeletal muscle relaxant.

Prescribed For

Pain and spasm of muscular conditions, including strain, sprain, bruising, and lower back problems.

General Information

Chlorzoxazone works primarily on the spinal cord level and on the brain, acting as a mild sedative. This results in fewer spasms, less pain, and greater mobility. Chlorzoxazone provides only temporary relief and is not a substitute for other types of therapy, such as rest, surgery, and physical therapy.

Cautions and Warnings

Do not take chlorzoxazone if you are **allergic** to it or if you have a condition known as **porphyria**.

People with **poor liver or kidney function** should take this drug with caution because serious liver toxicity has rarely occured in people using chlorzoxazone.

Chlorzoxazone may interact with other drugs that cause nervous system depression (see "Drug Interactions").

Because it is possible to become **dependent** on this drug, people with a history of substance abuse should take chlorzoxazone with caution.

Possible Side Effects

▼ Most common: dizziness, drowsiness, and light-headedness.

▼ Less common: headache, stimulation, stomach cramps or pain, diarrhea, constipation, heartburn, nausea, and vomiting.

▼ Rare: internal bleeding, liver problems, severe allergic reactions and breathing problems. Contact your doctor if you experience any unlisted side effect.

Drug Interactions

• The depressive effects of chlorzoxazone may be enhanced by taking it with alcohol, tranquilizers, sleeping pills, or other nervous system depressants. Avoid these combinations.

Food Interactions

Take this drug with food if it upsets your stomach. The tablets may be crushed and mixed with food.

Usual Dose

Adult: 250–750 mg 3–4 times a day.
Child: 125–500 mg 3–4 times a day.

Do not take more medication than is prescribed.

Overdosage

Early signs of chlorzoxazone overdose may include nausea, vomiting, diarrhea, drowsiness, dizziness, light-headedness, and headache. Victims may also feel sluggish or sickly and lose the ability to move their muscles. Breathing may become slow or irregular, and blood pressure may drop. Contact a doctor immediately or go to a hospital emergency room for treatment. ALWAYS bring the prescription bottle or container.

Special Information

Chlorzoxazone may make you drowsy or reduce your ability to concentrate. Be extremely careful while driving or operating hazardous equipment. Avoid alcoholic beverages.

Chlorzoxazone may turn your urine orange to purple-red; this is not dangerous.

Call your doctor if you develop drowsiness, weakness, an allergic reaction, breathing difficulties, black or tarry stools, vomiting of material that resembles coffee grounds, liver problems, or any other severe or bothersome side effect.

If you miss a dose of chlorzoxazone by more than an hour, skip the dose you forgot and continue with your regular schedule. Do not take a double dose.

Special Populations

Pregnancy/Breast-feeding

As with all drugs, chlorzoxazone should not be used without their doctor's approval by pregnant women and women who might become pregnant.

It is not known if chlorzoxazone passes into breast milk. Nursing mothers should consider bottle-feeding.

Seniors

Seniors, especially those with severe liver disease, are more sensitive to the effects of chlorzoxazone.

Generic Name

Cholestyramine (kol-es-TYE-rah-meen) [G]

Brand Names

LoCHOLEST Prevalite
LoCHOLEST Light
Prevalite

Questran
Questran Light

The information in this profile also applies to the following drugs:

Generic Ingredient: Colesevelam
Welchol

Generic Ingredient: Colestipol
Colestid

Type of Drug

Anti-hyperlipidemic (blood-fat reducer).

Prescribed For

High blood-cholesterol levels; generalized itching associated with bile duct obstruction—cholestyramine only; colitis; digitalis or thyroid overdose; and pesticide poisoning.

General Information

Cholestyramine resin lowers blood-cholesterol levels by absorbing bile acids in the bowel. Since the body uses cholesterol to make the bile acids—needed to digest fat—fat digestion can only continue by making more bile acid from blood cholesterol. This results in lower blood-cholesterol levels 4 to 7 days after starting cholestyramine.

Cholestyramine works entirely within the bowel and is never absorbed into the bloodstream. Though usually given 3 to 4 times a day, there appears to be no advantage to taking it more often than 2 times a day. The cholesterol-lowering effect of cholestyramine may be increased when it is taken with an HMG-CoA inhibitor or nicotinic acid. In some kinds of hyperlipidemia, colestipol may be more effective in lowering total blood cholesterol than clofibrate.

Cautions and Warnings

Do not use cholestyramine if you are **sensitive** to it or if your **bile duct is blocked**. The powder form should not be taken dry; doing so may result in the inhalation of powder into your lungs or a clogged esophagus.

Cholestyramine may cause or worsen **constipation** and **hemorrhoids**. Most constipation is mild but some people may need to stop the medication or take less of it.

Possible Side Effects

▼ Most common: constipation, which may be severe and result in bowel impaction. Hemorrhoids may be worsened.

▼ Less common: abdominal pain and bloating, and bleeding disorders or black-and-blue marks due to inter-

Possible Side Effects *(continued)*

ference with the absorption of vitamin K, a necessary fac-tor in the blood clotting process. One person developed night-blindness because the medication interfered withvitamin A absorption into the blood. Other side effects include belching, gas, nausea, vomiting, diarrhea, heartburn, and appetite loss. Your stool may have an unusual appearance because of a high fat level.

▼ Rare: Rare side effects can affect your mouth, stomach and intestines, muscles and joints, mental status, urinary tract, and breathing. Contact your doctor if you experience any side effect not listed above.

Drug Interactions

• Cholestyramine interferes with the absorption of virtually all oral drugs, including acetaminophen, amiodarone, aspirin, cephalexin, chenodiol, clindamycin, clofibrate, corticosteroids, diclofenac, iron, digitalis drugs, furosemide, gemfibrozil, glipizide, hydrocortisone, imipramine (an antidepressant), methyldopa, mycophenolate, nicotinic acid, penicillin, phenobarbital, phenytoin, piroxicam, propranolol, tetracycline, thiazide diuretics, thyroid drugs, tolbutamide, trimethoprim, warfarin and other anticoagulant (blood-thinning) drugs, and vitamins A, D, E, and K. Take other medications at least 1 hour before or 4 to 6 hours after taking cholestyramine.

Food Interactions

Take this medication before meals. It may be mixed with soda, water, juice, cereal, or pulpy fruits, such as applesauce or crushed pineapple. Cholestyramine bars should be thoroughly chewed and taken with plenty of fluids.

Usual Dose

Cholestyramine: 4 g (1 packet) taken 1–2 times a day or up to 6 times a day.

Colesevelam: 6 tablets once a day or in 2 divided doses.

Colestipol: 5–30 g (1–6 packets) once a day or in divided doses.

Overdosage

The most severe effect of overdose is obstruction of the GI tract. Take the overdose victim to a hospital emergency room. ALWAYS bring the prescription bottle or container.

Special Information

Do not swallow the granules or powder in their dry form. Prepare each packet of powder by mixing it with soup, cereal, or pulpy fruit or by adding the powder to a 6-oz. glass of liquid, such as a carbonated beverage. If some of the drug sticks to the sides of the glass, rinse it with liquid and drink the remainder.

Constipation, gas, nausea, and heartburn may occur and then disappear with continued use of this medication. Call your doctor if these side effects persist or if you develop unusual problems such as bleeding from the gums or rectum.

If you miss a dose of cholestyramine, skip it and continue with your regular schedule. Do not take a double dose.

Special Populations

Pregnancy/Breast-feeding

While cholestyramine does not affect the fetus directly, it may prevent the absorption of vitamins A, D, and E and other nutrients essential to the fetus' proper development—even when you take a prenatal vitamin supplement. When this drug is considered crucial by your doctor, its potential benefits must be carefully weighed against its risks.

Cholestyramine is not absorbed into the body. However, reduced absorption of vitamins A, D, and E and other nutrients may make your milk less nutritious. Nursing mothers who must take cholestyramine should bottle-feed.

Seniors

Seniors are more likely to experience side effects, especially those relating to the bowel.

Type of Drug

Cholinesterase Inhibitors

(KO-lin-ESS-tuh-rase)

Brand Names

Generic Ingredient: Donepezil
Aricept

Generic Ingredient: Galantamine
Reminyl

Generic Ingredient: Rivastigmine
Exelon

Generic Ingredient: Tacrine
Cognex

Prescribed For

Alzheimer's disease.

General Information

Cholinesterase inhibitors work by increasing the function of certain receptors in the brain that are stimulated by the hormone acetylcholine. They do this by interfering with *cholinesterase*, the enzyme that breaks down acetylcholine. People with Alzheimer's disease (degenerative condition of the central nervous system) develop a shortage of this brain chemical early in the disease. There is no evidence that cholinesterase inhibitors reverse the degenerative effects of Alzheimer's, but they may slow the rate at which the disease worsens.

Cautions and Warnings

Do not take these drugs if you are **sensitive** or **allergic** to them.

Cholinesterase inhibitors must be discontinued before **surgery** because it increases the effects of anesthetic drugs.

People with **heart disease** should use cholinesterase inhibitors with caution because they may slow heart rate and cause fainting.

Cholinesterase inhibitors may be expected to cause increased stomach acid production and increased activity of the GI tract. Possible complications include **ulcers** or **bleeding**. Alcohol and nonsteroidal anti-inflammatory drugs (NSAIDs) such as aspirin or ibuprofen may worsen this effect. Using cholinesterase inhibitors may also lead to **urinary blockage,** increase the risk of generalized **seizures,** and worsen **asthma or other pulmonary diseases**.

People with severe **liver dysfunction** should not take galantamine or tacrine.

Possible Side Effects

People taking cholinesterase inhibitors generally experience side effects at about the same rate as those taking a placebo (sugar pill).

▼ Most common: headache, general pain, accidents, nausea, diarrhea, sleeplessness, and dizziness.

▼ Common: tiredness, vomiting, appetite loss, and muscle cramps.

▼ Less common: arthritis, depression, abnormal dreams, fainting, black and blue marks, and weight loss.

▼ Rare: Rare side effects can occur in almost any part of the body. Contact your doctor if you experience any side effect not listed above.

Drug Interactions

• Cholinesterase inhibitors interfere with anticholinergic drugs (often prescribed for stomach disorders).

• Cholinesterase inhibitors can be expected to increase the effects of cevimeline, surgical anesthetic drugs and drugs that irritate the stomach and intestines, such as aspirin, ibuprofen, and other NSAIDs.

• The breakdown of cholinesterase inhibitors (except rivastigmine) in the liver can be slowed by ketoconazole, itraconazole, quinidine, delavirdine, indinavir, nelfinavir, ritonavir, saquinavir, amiodarone, cimetidine, ciprofloxacin, norfloxacin, clarithromycin, diltiazem, erythromycin, fluconazole, fluvoxamine, celecoxib, chlorpheniramine, clomipramine, cocaine, doxorubicin, fluoxetine, halofantrine, haloperidol, levopromazine, methadone, mibefradil, paroxetine, ranitidine, terbinafine, mifepristone, nefazodone, and grapefruit juice.

• The breakdown of cholinesterase inhibitors (except rivastigmine) in the liver can be increased by efavirenz, nevi-

rapine, barbiturates, carbamazepine, corticosteroids, phenytoin, pioglitazone, troglitazone, and rifampin.

Food Interactions

Donepezil can be taken with or without food.

Galantamine and rivastigmine should be taken with morning and evening meals.

Food reduces the absorption of tacrine into the blood. It is
best taken on an empty stomach, but you can take it with
food if it upsets your stomach.

Usual Dose

Donepezil
  Adult: 5 or 10 mg once a day.

Galantamine
  Adult: 8–32 mg a day, divided into 2 doses.

Rivastigmine
  Adult: 3–12 mg a day, divided into 2 doses.

Tacrine
  Adult: 40–160 mg a day, divided into 4 doses.

Overdosage

Cholinesterase inhibitor overdose can be very serious. Symptoms include severe nausea, vomiting, salivation, sweating,
slow heart rate, low blood pressure, slow breathing rate, convulsions, muscle weakness, and collapse. Take the overdose
victim to a hospital emergency room at once. ALWAYS bring
the prescription bottle or container.

Special Information

Donepezil should be taken just before bedtime.

Follow the special package directions for rivastigmine solution.

Tobacco or nicotine use increases the rate at which tacrine
and rivastigmine are cleared from the body.

If you forget a dose and take your medication once a day,
take it as soon as you remember. If it is almost time for your
next dose, skip the dose you forgot and continue with the
regular schedule. If you take your medication 2 or more times
a day, take your dose as soon as you remember. If it is almost
time for your next dose, skip the dose you forgot and continue with your regular schedule. Do not take a double dose.

Special Populations

Pregnancy/Breast-feeding

One animal study of a cholinesterase inhibitor indicated a small risk of birth defects. When your doctor considers this drug crucial, its potential benefits must be carefully weighed against its risks.

It is not known if cholinesterase inhibitors pass into breast milk. Nursing mothers who must take this drug should consider bottle-feeding.

Seniors

Seniors with moderate kidney function loss should not take galantamine. Dosage adjustments are not needed for donepezil, tacrine, or rivastigmine.

Generic Name

Ciclopirox (sye-kloe-PERE-ox)

Brand Names

Loprox   Penlac Nail Lacquer

Type of Drug

Antifungal.

Prescribed For

Fungus and yeast infections of the nails and skin, including athlete's foot and candida.

General Information

Ciclopirox slows the growth of a variety of fungus organisms and yeasts and kills many others. The drug penetrates the skin, hair, hair follicles, and sweat glands. Cicloprox nail lacquer is used for toenail and fingernail fungus infections.

Cautions and Warnings

Do not use this product if you are **allergic** to it.

Possible Side Effects

▼ Common: burning, itching, and stinging at the application site.

Drug Interactions

None known.

Usual Dose

Cream/Lotion: Massage into cleansed affected skin and surrounding area twice a day.

Nail Lacquer: Apply to infected nails once a day.

Overdosage

Accidental ingestion may cause nausea and upset stomach. Call your local poison control center or hospital for more information.

Special Information

This product can be expected to relieve symptoms within the first week of use. Follow your doctor's directions for the complete 2- to 4-week course of treatment with the cream or lotion to gain maximum benefit. The nail lacquer may be used for up to 48 weeks. Stopping the medication too soon can lead to a relapse.

When using ciclopirox nail lacquer, do not apply it to any skin other than that which surrounds the infected nails because of possible irritation. Do not apply nail polish or any other nail lacquer to infected nails while you are using this product.

Avoid using cicloprox nail lacquer near an open flame since the product is flammable.

Call your doctor if the affected area burns, stings, or becomes red after you use this product, or if your symptoms do not clear up after 4 weeks of treatment; by then it is unlikely that the cream will be effective.

If you forget a dose of ciclopirox, apply it as soon as you remember. Do not apply more than prescribed to make up for the missed dose.

Special Populations

Pregnancy/Breast-feeding

Ciclopirox may pass to the fetus in very small amounts. In animal studies, high doses of ciclopirox given by mouth did not harm the fetus. As with all drugs, caution should be exercised when using ciclopirox during pregnancy.

It is unknown if ciclopirox passes into breast milk. Nursing mothers who must use this drug should consider bottle-feeding.

Seniors

Seniors may use this drug without special restriction.

Generic Name

Cilostazol (sil-oe-STAY-zol)

Brand Name

Pletal

Type of Drug

Antiplatelet.

Prescribed For

Intermittent claudication.

General Information

In intermittent claudication, leg muscles go into spasm due to reduced blood flow. This occurs when plaque buildup narrows blood vessels leading to the calf or other leg muscles. People with this condition often develop leg pain after walking only a short distance. Cilostazol prevents blood platelets from "clumping together" to begin the process of forming a blood clot, which can further obstruct arteries and worsen intermittent claudication. This drug is broken down in the liver.

Cautions and Warnings

Do not take this drug if you are **sensitive** or **allergic** to it.

People with **congestive heart failure** (CHF) should not take cilostazol. Some studies indicate that long-term use of this drug may cause **cardiovascular** problems.

Possible Side Effects

The risk of side effects increases with dosage.

▼ Most common: headache, infection, abdominal pain, abnormal stool, and diarrhea.

▼ Common: heart palpitations, rapid heartbeat, dizziness, upset stomach, nausea, sore throat, runny nose, back pain, and swelling in the arms or legs.

▼ Less common: gas, cough, fainting, and muscle aches.

▼ Rare: Rare side effects can occur in almost any part of the body. Contact your doctor if you experience any side effect not listed above.

Drug Interactions

• Avoid mixing cilostazol with ketoconazole, itraconazole, fluconazole, miconazole, fluvoxamine, fluoxetine, nefazodone, or sertraline because this interaction may slow the breakdown of cilostazol, prolonging its effects. Cilostazol dosage is reduced by 50% when it is combined with any of these drugs.

• Aspirin can increase the anticoagulant (blood-thinning) effect of cilostazol, but this combination has not caused serious bleeding problems. There is no information on the effect of combining cilostazol and other antiplatelet or anticoagulant drugs. Cilostazol dosage is reduced by 50% when it is combined with any of these drugs.

• Diltiazem increases cilostazol blood levels by about 50%. Cilostazol dosage is reduced by 50% when it is combined with diltiazem.

• Erythromycin and similar antibiotics increase cilostazol blood levels. Take half the regular dose of cilostazol when combining it with any of these drugs.

• Combining cilostazol and omeprazole increases the effects of cilostazol. Cilostazol dosage is reduced by 50% when it is combined with omeprazole.

• Smoking reduces the effectiveness of cilostazol by causing the liver to break it down faster.

Food Interactions

Take this drug on an empty stomach at least 30 minutes before or 2 hours after meals. Do not drink grapefruit juice at any time while taking cilostazol because it can interfere with the breakdown of the drug.

Usual Dose

Adult: 100 mg twice a day. 50 mg twice a day when combined other drugs that may increase the effect of cilostazol.
Child: not recommended.

Overdosage

Symptoms of overdose are likely to be the most common side effects. Overdose victims should be taken to a hospital emergency room. ALWAYS bring the prescription bottle or container.

Special Information

Several weeks of cilostazol treatment may be necessary before you notice any improvement in symptoms. Maximum benefit usually occurs after 12 weeks.

If you forget a dose, take it as soon as you remember. If it is almost time for your next dose, skip the forgotten dose and continue with your regular schedule. Do not take a double dose.

Special Populations

Pregnancy/Breast-feeding

Animal studies suggest that cilostazol may harm the fetus, but there is no information on the effect of cilostazol in pregnant women. When this drug is considered crucial by your doctor, its potential benefits must be carefully weighed against its risks.

Cilostazol may pass into breast milk. Nursing mothers who must take this drug should bottle-feed.

Seniors

Seniors can take this drug without special precaution.

Generic Name

Cimetidine (sih-MET-ih-dene) [G]

Brand Names

Tagamet   Tagamet HB [S]

Type of Drug

Histamine H$_2$ antagonist.

Prescribed For

Ulcers of the stomach and duodenum (upper intestine); also used for upset stomach, gastroesophageal reflux disease (GERD), benign stomach ulcer, bleeding in the stomach and duodenum, colorectal cancer, prevention of stress ulcer, hyperparathyroidism, fungal infections of the hair and scalp, herpes virus infection, excessive hairiness in women, chronic itching of unknown cause, skin reactions, warts, acetaminophen overdose, and other conditions characterized by the production of large amounts of gastric fluids. Cimetidine may be prescribed to stop the production of stomach acid during surgery. The non-prescription version is recommended for heartburn and stomach gas.

General Information

Histamine H$_2$ antagonists work by turning off the system that produces stomach acid and other secretions. Cimetidine is effective in treating the symptoms of ulcer and preventing complications of the disease, although an ulcer that does not respond to another histamine H$_2$ antagonist will probably not respond to cimetidine. Histamine H$_2$ antagonists differ only in their potency. Cimetidine is the least potent; 1000 mg are roughly equal to 300 mg of either nizatidine or ranitidine, or 40 mg of famotidine. These drugs are roughly equal in their ability to treat ulcer disease and their risk of side effects.

Cautions and Warnings

Do not take cimetidine if you have had an **allergic reaction** to it or any histamine H$_2$ antagonist. Cimetidine has a mild antiandrogen effect, which probably causes the painful, swollen breasts that some people experience after taking this drug for a month or more.

People with **kidney or liver disease** should take cimetidine with caution because it is broken down in the liver and passes out of the body through the kidneys.

The fact that symptoms are alleviated by cimetidine does not preclude the possibility of **stomach cancer**, which can have symptoms similar to other gastrointestinal (GI) disorders. Make sure your doctor screens for possible malignancy.

Some people—mostly the very ill—experience confusion, agitation, psychosis, hallucinations, depression, anxiety, or

disorientation, usually within 2 or 3 days of starting cimetidine. Normally these symptoms stop 3 to 4 days after discontinuing the drug. Call your doctor if this happens to you.

Possible Side Effects

Serious side effects are uncommon.

▼ Most common: mild diarrhea, dizziness, rash,
painful breast swelling, nausea and vomiting, headache,
confusion, drowsiness, hallucinations, and impotence.

▼ Less common: liver inflammation, peeling or red and
swollen rash, breathing difficulties, tingling in the hands
or feet, delirious feelings, and oozing from the nipples.

▼ Rare: Cimetidine may affect white blood cells or
blood platelets. Some symptoms of these effects are
unusual bleeding or bruising, unusual tiredness, and
weakness. Other rare side effects are inflammation of the
pancreas, hair loss (reversible), abnormal heart rhythms,
heart attack, reversible muscle or joint pains, and
reversible drug reactions.

Drug Interactions

• Separate cimetidine from antacid doses by about 3 hours
to avoid reducing cimetidine's effectiveness. Other drugs that
may reduce the absorption of cimetidine are metoclopramide
and anticholinergic drugs, including trihexyphenidyl hydrochloride, oxybutynin, and benztropine mesylate.

• Cigarette smoking reverses the healing effect cimetidine
has on ulcers.

• Cimetidine may increase the side effects of a variety of
drugs, possibly leading to drug toxicity. These drugs include
alcohol; aminophylline; oral antidiabetes drugs; benzodiazepine tranquilizers and sleeping pills, except lorazepam,
oxazepam, and temazepam; caffeine; calcium channel blockers; carbamazepine; carmustine; chloroquine; flecainide; fluorouracil; labetalol; lidocaine; metoprolol; metronidazole;
moricizine; mexiletine; narcotic pain relievers; ondansetron;
pentoxifylline; phenytoin; procainamide; propafenone; propranolol; quinine; quinidine; tacrine; theophylline drugs,
except dyphylline; triamterene; tricyclic antidepressants; valproic acid; and warfarin (a blood-thinner).

• Drugs whose absorption may be decreased by cimetidine are iron, indomethacin, fluconazole, ketoconazole, and tetracycline antibiotics.

• Enteric-coated tablets should not be taken with cimetidine. The change in stomach acidity causes the tablets to disintegrate prematurely in the stomach.

• Cimetidine may decrease the effects of digoxin and tocainide.

Food Interactions

None known.

Usual Dose

Adult: 400–800 mg at bedtime; 300 mg 4 times a day with meals and at bedtime, or 400 mg 2 times a day. To treat GERD—400 mg 4 times a day. Do not exceed 2400 mg a day. Users of Tagamet HB should not take more than 400 mg a day. Smaller doses may be as effective for seniors or those with impaired kidney function.

Overdosage

Little is known about the effects of cimetidine overdose, but victims may experience exaggerated side effects. Two deaths have occurred. Your local poison control center may advise giving ipecac syrup—available at any pharmacy—to induce vomiting and remove any drug remaining in the stomach. Victims who have definite symptoms should be taken to a hospital emergency room. ALWAYS bring the prescription bottle or container.

Special Information

Take cimetidine exactly as directed and follow your doctor's instructions regarding diet and other treatment in order to get the maximum benefit from the drug.

Cigarettes are associated with stomach ulcers and reduce cimetidine's effectiveness.

Call your doctor at once if you develop any unusual side effects such as bleeding or bruising, tiredness, diarrhea, dizziness, rash, or hallucinations. Black, tarry stools or vomiting material that resembles coffee grounds may indicate your ulcer is bleeding.

If you miss a dose of cimetidine, take it as soon as possible. If it is almost time for your next dose, skip the dose you forgot and continue with your regular schedule. Do not take a double dose.

Special Populations

Pregnancy/Breast-feeding
Animal studies reveal no damage to the fetus, although cimetidine does pass into the fetal blood. When this drug is considered crucial by your doctor, its potential benefits must be carefully weighed against its risks.

Large amounts of cimetidine pass into breast milk. Nursing mothers who must take this drug should bottle-feed.

Seniors
Seniors may need less medication due to loss of kidney function and be more susceptible to side effects, especially confusion and other nervous system effects (see "Cautions and Warnings").

Cipro *see Fluoroquinolone Anti-Infectives, page 495*

Clarinex *see Loratadine, page 651*

Generic Name

Clarithromycin (klah-rith-roe-MYE-sin)

Brand Name

Biaxin   Biaxin XL
Biaxin Filmtabs

Type of Drug

Macrolide antibiotic.

Prescribed For

Mild to moderate infections of the upper and lower respiratory tract, tonsillitis, pharyngitis, middle ear infections, and for duodenal ulcers; also used for skin and other infections including membrane attack complex (MAC).

General Information

Clarithromycin and other macrolide antibiotics are either bactericidal (bacteria-killing) or bacteriostatic (inhibiting bacterial growth), depending on the organism in question and amount of antibiotic present. In ulcer disease, clarithromycin is used to fight *Helicobacter pylori* infection, which is present in almost all ulcers and most cases of stomach inflammation.

Cautions and Warnings

Do not take clarithromycin if you are **allergic** to it or any macrolide antibiotic.

Clarithromycin is primarily eliminated from the body through the liver and kidneys. People with severe **kidney disease** may require dose adjustments. Liver disease generally does not call for an adjustment.

Colitis (bowel inflammation) has been associated with all antibiotics (see "Possible Side Effects").

Possible Side Effects

Most side effects are mild and go away once you stop taking clarithromycin.

▼ Most common: nausea, upset stomach, changes in sense of taste, headache, diarrhea, abdominal pain, vomiting, and rash in children. Colitis (symptoms include severe abdominal cramps and severe, persistent, and possibly bloody diarrhea) may develop.

▼ Rare: serious abnormal heart rhythms.

Drug Interactions

• Clarithromycin may increase the anticoagulant (blood-thinning) effects of warfarin in people who take it regularly, especially older adults. This combination requires careful monitoring by your doctor.

• Do not combine clarithromycin with astemizole or terfenadine.

• Combining clarithromycin and omeprazole raises the amount of both drugs in the blood.

• Combining clarithromycin and rifabutin or rifampin can interfere with the antibiotic's effect and increase the risk of intestinal side effects.

• Combining clarithromycin and ranitidine bismuth-sulfate (for ulcers) can raise the amount of both drugs in the blood, but these effects are not considered important.

• Clarithromycin can increase the effects of alprazolam, diazepam, midazolam, and triazolam, causing excessive central nervous system (CNS) depression.

• Clarithromycin increases the effects of buspirone and can lead to buspirone side effects.

• Clarithromycin can raise blood levels of carbamazepine. People combining these drugs should be checked by their doctors for changes in blood-carbamazepine levels.

• Two deaths have been reported in people combining clarithromycin and pimozide. Pimozide should not be used by people taking a macrolide antibiotic.

• Clarithromycin may raise blood levels of theophylline, possibly leading to a theophylline overdose. It can also increase the effects of caffeine.

• Combining clarithromycin and digoxin, cyclosporine, ergot alkaloids, or tacrolimus may lead to serious side effects.

• Combining clarithromycin and a statin cholesterol-lowering drug increases the risk of developing a painful and potentially fatal condition involving severe muscle degeneration.

• Fluconazole increases the amount of clarithromycin in the blood.

• Combining zidovudine (an AIDS drug—also known as AZT) and clarithromycin may affect the amount of zidovudine in the bloodstream.

Food Interactions

Clarithromycin can be taken without regard to food or meals.

Usual Dose

Adult: infections—250–500 mg every 12 hours for 7–14 days. Dosage must be reduced in people with severe kidney disease. Ulcer—500 mg 3 times a day plus 40 mg omeprazole in the morning or ranitidine bismuth citrate 400 mg twice a day for 14 days, then omeprazole 20 mg every morning or ranitidine bismuth citrate 400 mg twice a day, for 15–28 days.

Child (age 6 months and older): infections—3.4 mg per lb. of body weight every 12 hours, up to 250–500 mg a dose, depending on the offending organism, for 10 days.

Overdosage

Overdose may cause severe side effects, especially nausea, vomiting, stomach cramps, and diarrhea. Call your local poison control center or hospital emergency room for more information. If you seek treatment, ALWAYS bring the prescription bottle or container.

Special Information

Call your doctor if you develop nausea, vomiting, diarrhea, stomach cramps, or severe abdominal pain. Stop taking this medication and immediately call your doctor if you experience breathing difficulties, chest pain, hives, rash, itching, mouth sores, or unusual sensitivity to light.

Clarithromycin suspension must be shaken well before each dose. Do not store it in the refrigerator.

Clarithromycin may be gentler on the digestive tract than erythromycin.

Remember to complete the full course of treatment exactly as prescribed, even if you feel well sooner. Clarithromycin's effectiveness may be severely reduced otherwise.

Take clarithromycin at the same time each day. If you forget a dose, take it as soon as you remember. If it is within 4 hours of your next dose, skip the one you forgot and go back to your regular schedule.

Special Populations

Pregnancy/Breast-feeding

Clarithromycin affected the fetus in animal studies. When this drug is considered crucial by your doctor, its potential benefits must be carefully weighed against its risks.

It is not known if clarithromycin passes into breast milk, but other macrolide antibiotics do. Nursing mothers who must take this drug should bottle-feed.

Seniors

Seniors with severe kidney disease require a dosage adjustment.

Generic Name

Clemastine (KLEH-mas-tene) Ⓖ

Brand Name

Tavist

The information in this profile also applies to the following drug:

Generic Ingredients: Acetaminophen + Clemastine + Pseudoephedrine
Travist

Type of Drug

Antihistamine.

Prescribed For

Sneezing, stuffy and runny nose, itchy eyes, and scratchy throat caused by seasonal allergy and for other symptoms of allergy such as rash, itching, and hives.

General Information

Antihistamines generally work by blocking the release of histamine (a chemical released by body tissue during an allergic reaction) from cells at the H_1 histamine receptor site, drying up secretions of the nose, throat, and eyes. Clemastine fumarate is less sedating than most antihistamines, but not less sedating than astemizole, cetirizine, or loratadine.

Cautions and Warnings

Clemastine should not be taken if you are **allergic** to it. People with **asthma** or other **deep-breathing problems, glaucoma, stomach ulcers** or other **stomach problems,** and **hyperthyroidism** should avoid clemastine because its side effects can aggravate these problems.

Possible Side Effects

▼ Most common: drowsiness, headache, weakness, nervousness, stomach upset, nausea, vomiting, cough,

---

Possible Side Effects *(continued)*

stuffy nose, changes in bowel habits, sore throat, nosebleeds, and dry mouth, nose, or throat.
▼ Less common: hair loss, allergic reaction (symptoms include rash, itching, hives, and breathing difficulties), depression, sleeplessness, menstrual irregularities,
muscle aches, sweating, tingling in the hands or feet, frequent urination, visual disturbances, and ringing or
buzzing in the ears.

Drug Interactions

• Combining clemastine with alcohol, tranquilizers, sleeping pills, or other nervous system depressants may increase
the depressant effects of clemastine. Do not combine these
drugs.

• The effects of oral anticoagulant (blood-thinning) drugs
may be decreased by clemastine. Do not take this combination without your doctor's knowledge.

• Monoamine oxidase inhibitor (MAOI) antidepressants
may increase the drying and other effects of clemastine. This
combination can also worsen urinary difficulties.

• When taking antihistamines on a regular basis, notify
your doctor if you are taking large amounts of aspirin. Effects
of too much aspirin may be masked by the antihistamine.

Food Interactions

Clemastine is best taken on an empty stomach at least 1 hour
before or 2 hours after eating; it may be taken with food if it
upsets your stomach.

Usual Dose

Adult and Child (age 12 and over): 1.34 mg 2 times a day up
to 8.04 mg of the syrup or 2.68 mg of the tablets in 24 hours.

Child (age 6–12) (syrup only): 67 mg 2 times a day or up to
4.02 mg a day.

Overdosage

Overdose is likely to cause severe side effects. Overdose victims should be given ipecac syrup—available at any pharmacy—to induce vomiting and should then be taken to a hospital emergency room for treatment. ALWAYS bring the
prescription bottle or container.

Special Information

Clemastine may make it difficult for you to concentrate or perform complex tasks such as driving a car. Be sure to report any unusual side effects to your doctor.

If you forget to take a dose of clemastine, take it as soon as you remember. If it is almost time for your next dose, skip the one you forgot and continue with your regular schedule. Do not take a double dose.

Special Populations

Pregnancy/Breast-feeding

Do not take any antihistamines without your doctor's knowledge if you are or might be pregnant—especially during the last 3 months of pregnancy, because newborns may have severe reactions to antihistamines.

Small amounts of clemastine pass into breast milk. Nursing mothers who must take clemastine should bottle-feed.

Seniors

Seniors are more sensitive to side effects.

Generic Name

Clindamycin (klin-duh-MYE-sin) G

Brand Name

Cleocin	Clindagel
Cleocin T	ClindaMax
Clinda-Derm	Clindets

Type of Drug

Antibiotic.

Prescribed For

Bacterial infections. The vaginal cream is used to treat bacterial vaginosis. Topical clindamycin is used to treat acne and rosacea.

General Information

Clindamycin is one of the few oral drugs that is effective against anaerobic bacteria, which grow only in the absence of oxygen and are often found in infected wounds, lung abscesses, abdominal infections, and infections of the female genital tract. It also works against bacteria usually treated by penicillin or erythromycin. Clindamycin may be useful for treating certain skin or soft tissue infections. It kills the bacteria that frequently cause acne.

Cautions and Warnings

Do not take clindamycin if you are **allergic** to it or lincomycin, another antibiotic.

People with **asthma** or a history of **allergies** should use clindamycin capsules with caution.

Clindamycin can cause a severe intestinal irritation called **colitis,** which can be fatal. Signs of colitis are diarrhea, blood in the stool, and abdominal cramps. Any form of this drug, including products applied to the skin and the vaginal cream, can provoke colitis. Because of this, clindamycin should be reserved for serious infections or those that cannot be treated with other drugs.

Clindamycin should be used with caution if you have **gastrointestinal disease, kidney** or **liver disease**.

Possible Side Effects

Capsules
▼ Most common: stomach pain; nausea; vomiting; diarrhea, in up to 20 percent of people; and pain when swallowing.
▼ Less common: itching; rash; signs of serious drug sensitivity, such as difficulties in breathing, and yellowing of the skin or the whites of the eyes; colitis (see "Cautions and Warnings"); effects on blood components; and joint pain.

Topical Lotion
▼ Most common: dry skin, redness, burning, peeling, oily skin, and itching.
▼ Less common: diarrhea, abdominal pain, upset stomach and colitis (see "Cautions and Warnings").

Vaginal Cream
▼ Most common: cervicitis, vaginitis, and irritation.
▼ Less common: nausea, vomiting, diarrhea, constipation, abdominal pain, dizziness, headache, vertigo, and colitis (see "Cautions and Warnings").

Drug Interactions

- Do not combine clindamycin and erythromycin.
- The absorption of clindamycin capsules into the blood-stream is delayed by Kaolin-Pectin Suspension (prescribed for diarrhea). Separate these drugs by at least 1 hour.

Food Interactions

Take the oral medication with a full glass of water or with food to prevent irritation of the stomach and intestine.

Usual Dose

Capsules
   Adult: 150–450 mg every 6 hours.
   Child: 3.5–11 mg per lb. of body weight a day, in 3–4 doses. For severe infections, at least 37.5 mg 3 times a day, regardless of weight.

Topical Lotion
Apply enough to cover the affected area(s) with a thin coat twice a day.

Vaginal Cream
Insert 1 applicator's worth at bedtime for 7 consecutive days.

Overdosage

Clindamycin overdose may lead to severe diarrhea and other drug side effects. Do not treat this diarrhea on your own. Call your local poison center for information. ALWAYS take the prescription bottle or container with you if you go to an emergency room for treatment.

Special Information

Prolonged or unsupervised use of clindamycin may lead to secondary infections from susceptible organisms, such as fungi. Take this drug for the full course of therapy as indicated by your physician.

If you develop severe diarrhea or abdominal pain, call your doctor at once. Call your doctor immediately if you experience breathing difficulties or janudice (yellowing of the skin or whites of the eyes).

Women using the vaginal cream should not have vaginal intercourse until treatment is complete.

If you miss a dose of oral clindamycin, take it as soon as you remember. If it is almost time for your next dose of clindamycin, double that dose and go back to your regular dosage schedule.

Special Populations

Pregnancy/Breast-feeding
This drug crosses into fetal blood circulation. When the drug is considered crucial by your doctor, its potential benefits must be carefully weighed against its risks.

Clindamycin passes into breast milk. Nursing mothers who must take oral clindamycin should consider bottle-feeding.

Seniors
Seniors with other illnesses may be unable to tolerate diarrhea and other clindamycin side effects.

Generic Name

Clofibrate (cloe-FIH-brate) G

Brand Name

Atromid-S

Type of Drug

Anti-hyperlipidemic (blood-fat reducer).

Prescribed For

High blood levels of triglycerides; also prescribed for high cholesterol and low-density lipoprotein (LDL) cholesterol levels and for diabetes insipidus.

General Information

Clofibrate reduces cholesterol and triglyceride levels by interfering with the body's production of these blood fats and increasing the rate at which they are broken down. Less predictable and effective than other cholesterol-lowering medications, it is usually prescribed for people whose blood fats remain high despite changes in diet, weight control, and exercise, and who are at risk for pancreatitis. People with high cholesterol and low triglycerides should not take clofibrate because it is most effective in lowering triglycerides.

Cautions and Warnings

Clofibrate should be used with caution if you are **allergic** to it or have **cirrhosis of the liver, heart disease, kidney disease, gallstones** (clofibrate users have twice the risk of developing gallstones), **liver disease,** an **underactive thyroid,** or stomach **ulcer**.

People with **kidney disease** require dosage adjustments.

Clofibrate does not reduce the risk of a fatal heart attack. A 1978 study suggests that taking clofibrate regularly for many years increases the risk of dying from noncardiac causes, but this has not been confirmed by more recent research. Another clofibrate study shows an increase in side effects, including abnormal heart rhythms and intermittent leg pains due to blood-vessel spasm. Clofibrate should be used only by people whose other efforts to reduce their triglyceride or cholesterol levels have failed.

Possible Side Effects

▼ Most common: nausea.

▼ Less common: vomiting; loose stools; upset stomach; gas; abdominal pain; liver enlargement; gastric irritation; mouth sores; headache; dizziness; tiredness; cramped muscles; aching and weakness; rash; itching; brittle hair or hair loss; abnormal heart rhythms; blood clots in the lungs or veins; gallstones, especially in people who have taken clofibrate for a long time; decreased sex drive; and impotence.

If you suffer from angina pectoris (a condition characterized by brief attacks of chest pain), clofibrate may increase or decrease this pain. It may cause you to produce smaller quantities of urine and has been associated with blood or protein in the urine, painful urination, tiredness, weakness, drowsiness, and mildly increased appetite and weight gain. Some experts claim that clofibrate causes stomach ulcer, stomach bleeding, arthritis-like symptoms, uncontrollable muscle spasm, increased perspiration, blurred vision, breast enlargement, and effects on the blood.

Drug Interactions

• Your anticoagulant (blood thinner) dosage may have to be reduced by up to 50% if you start taking clofibrate. It is essential that your doctor know that you are taking both drugs so that the proper dosage adjustments can be made.

• Combining clofibrate and a statin cholesterol-lowering drug may lead to skeletal muscle destruction.

• Clofibrate may increase the effects of oral antidiabetics and any drug used to treat diabetes insipidus including carbamazepine, chlorpropamide, desmopressin, diuretics, and hormone replacement products.

Food Interactions

This drug may be taken with food or milk to prevent upset stomach.

Usual Dose

2000 mg a day in divided doses.

Overdosage

Symptoms are most likely to be severe side effects. Take the overdose victim to a hospital emergency room. ALWAYS bring the prescription bottle or container.

Special Information

Call your doctor if you develop chest pain, breathing difficulties, abnormal heart rates, severe stomach pain with nausea and vomiting, fever and chills, sore throat, swelling of the legs, weight gain, blood in the urine, changes in urinary habits, or any bothersome or persistent side effect.

Follow the diet recommended by your doctor. Limit alcohol consumption.

Clofibrate should be stored at room temperature in a dry place—not in a bathroom medicine cabinet—to protect this drug's gelatin covering.

Regular blood counts and liver function tests are necessary to be sure that clofibrate is still working. Testing also may uncover possible side effects.

If you forget a dose of clofibrate, take it as soon as you remember. If it is almost time for your next dose, skip the one you forgot and continue with your regular schedule. Do not take a double dose.

Special Populations

Pregnancy/Breast-feeding

Pregnant women should not take clofibrate because large amounts of this drug pass into the bloodstream of the fetus.

If you are planning to become pregnant, stop taking clofibrate several months before trying to conceive.

Clofibrate passes into breast milk. Nursing mothers who
must take clofibrate should bottle-feed.

Seniors

Seniors with loss of kidney function may require dosage
adjustments.

Generic Name

Clonazepam (klon-A-zeh-pam) G

Brand Name

Klonopin

Type of Drug

Anticonvulsant.

Prescribed For

Petit mal and other seizure; also prescribed for panic attacks,
periodic leg movements during sleep, speaking difficulty
associated with Parkinson's disease, acute manic episodes,
nerve pain, and schizophrenia.

General Information

Clonazepam is a benzodiazepine drug. Clonazepam is not
used as a sedative or hypnotic. It is used only for the uses
described above in people who have not responded to other
drug treatments. Tolerance to the effects of clonazepam commonly develops within about 3 months of use. Your doctor
may raise your clonazepam dosage periodically to maintain
the drug's effect.

Cautions and Warnings

Do not take clonazepam if you are **sensitive** or **allergic** to it or
any other benzodiazepine.

When stopping clonazepam treatments, the drug must be
discontinued gradually. Abrupt discontinuance of clonazepam may lead to drug **withdrawal symptoms** including
severe seizures, tremors, abdominal or muscle cramps, vomiting, and increased sweating.

Use clonazepam with caution if you have a chronic **respiratory illness**, since the drug tends to increase salivation and other respiratory secretions and can make breathing more labored. Avoid using clonazepam if you have severe **depression**, severe **lung disease**, **sleep apnea** (intermittent cessation of breathing during sleep), **liver disease**, **alcoholism**, or **kidney disease**. These conditions may exacerbate the depressive effects of benzodiazepines, and such effects may be detrimental to your overall condition.

Clonazepam can aggravate **narrow-angle glaucoma**, but if you have open-angle glaucoma, you may take it.

Possible Side Effects

▼ Most common: drowsiness, poor muscle control, and behavioral changes.

▼ Rare: Rare side effects can occur in almost any part of the body but are most likely to affect mental function, stomach and intestines, urinary function, blood, and liver. Contact your doctor if you experience any side effect not listed above.

Drug Interactions

• The depressant effects of clonazepam are increased by tranquilizers, sleeping pills, narcotic pain relievers, antihistamines, alcohol, monoamine oxidase inhibitors (MAOIs), tricyclic antidepressants, and other anticonvulsants.

• Mixing valproic acid and clonazepam may produce severe petit mal seizures.

• Smoking, phenobarbital, phenytoin, carbamazapine, and rifampin may reduce clonazepam's effectiveness.

• Clonazepam may increase the requirement for other anticonvulsant drugs in people who suffer from multiple types of seizures.

• The effects of clonazepam may be prolonged when it is taken with cimetidine, oral contraceptives, disulfiram, fluoxetine, isoniazid, ketoconazole, metoprolol, probenecid, propoxyphene, propranolol, or valproic acid.

• Theophylline may reduce clonazepam's sedative effects.

• Separate antacids from your clonazepam dose by at least 1 hour to prevent them from interfering with clonazepam being absorbed into the bloodstream.

- Clonazepam may increase blood levels of digoxin and the risk of digoxin toxicity.
- Clonazepam may decrease the effect of levodopa.

Food Interactions

Clonazepam is best taken on an empty stomach but may be taken with food if it upsets your stomach.

Usual Dose

Adult and Child (age 10 and over): starting dose—0.5 mg 3 times a day. The dose is increased by 0.5–1 mg every 3 days until seizures are controlled or side effects develop. The maximum daily dose is 20 mg. Other uses for clonazepam involve doses from 0.5–16 mg a day, depending on the condition and its severity.

Child (under age 10, or below 66 lbs.): starting dose—0.004–0.013 mg per lb. of body weight a day in divided doses. Dosage can be increased gradually to a maximum of 0.045–0.09 mg per lb. of body weight.

Clonazepam dosage must be reduced in people with impaired kidney function.

Overdosage

Overdose may cause confusion, coma, poor reflexes, sleepiness, low blood pressure, labored breathing, and other depressive effects. If the overdose is discovered within a few minutes and the victim is still conscious, it may be helpful to induce vomiting with ipecac syrup—available at any pharmacy. Overdose victims must be taken to a hospital emergency room. ALWAYS bring the prescription bottle or container.

Special Information

Clonazepam may interfere with your ability to drive or perform other complex tasks because it can cause drowsiness and difficulty in concentrating.

Your doctor should perform periodic blood counts and liver function tests while you are taking this drug to check for possible side effects.

Do not suddenly stop taking clonazepam—severe seizures may result. The dosage must be discontinued gradually by your doctor.

If you miss a dose by 1 hour or less, take it right away. Otherwise, skip the dose you forgot and go back to your regular schedule. Do not take a double dose.

Carry identification or wear a bracelet indicating that you have a seizure disorder for which you take clonazepam.

Special Populations

Pregnancy/Breast-feeding

Clonazepam crosses into the fetal circulation and can affect the fetus. Women who are or might be pregnant should avoid it. When the drug is considered crucial by your doctor, its potential benefits must be carefully weighed against its risks.

Some reports suggest a strong link between anticonvulsant drugs and birth defects, though most of the information pertains to phenytoin and phenobarbital, not clonazepam. It is also possible that the epileptic condition itself or genetic factors common to people with seizure disorders may figure in the higher incidence of birth defects.

Clonazepam may pass into breast milk. Nursing mothers who must take this drug should bottle-feed.

Seniors

Seniors, especially those with liver or kidney disease, are more sensitive to the effects of this drug—especially dizziness and drowsiness—and may require smaller doses.

Generic Name

Clonidine (KLAH-nih-dene) Ⓖ

Brand Names

Catapres	Catapres-TTS-2
Catapres-TTS-1	Catapres-TTS-3

Type of Drug

Alpha receptor stimulant.

Prescribed For

High blood pressure, including hypertensive emergency (diastolic blood pressure over 120); also used for excess sweating, childhood growth delay, attention-deficit hyperactivity disorder (ADHD), Tourette's syndrome, restless leg syndrome, schizophrenic psychosis, migraine, ulcerative colitis, painful or difficult menstruation, flushing related to menopause, diagnosis of pheochromocytoma (adrenal gland tumor), kidney poisoning associated with cyclosporine, diabetic diarrhea, smoking cessation, methadone and opiate detoxification, withdrawal from alcohol and benzodiazepines such as Valium, nerve pain following herpes attack, and allergic reactions in the presence of asthma triggered by external sources. Clonidine by epidural injection has been used to treat cancer pain.

General Information

Clonidine stimulates nerve endings in the brain called alpha-adrenergic receptors. It reduces blood pressure by dilating (widening) blood vessels. Clonidine works quickly, decreasing blood pressure within 1 hour. The other uses of clonidine relate to its stimulation of alpha receptors throughout the body.

Cautions and Warnings

Do not take clonidine if you are **allergic** to it. People who have had a stroke or recent **heart attack** or who have **cardiac insufficiency** or **chronic kidney failure** should avoid clonidine.

Some people develop a **tolerance** of their clonidine dosage. If this happens, your blood pressure may increase and your doctor may prescribe a higher dose.

Never stop taking clonidine without your doctor's knowledge. If you **abruptly stop taking clonidine,** you may experience an unusual **increase in blood pressure** accompanied by **agitation, headache, nervousness** and severe reactions, possibly **death**. Restarting clonidine therapy or taking another antihypertensive can reverse these effects.

Clonidine may cause **degeneration of the retina**. See your eye doctor for regular check-ups if you are taking this drug.

If you require **surgery,** your doctor will continue your clonidine therapy until about 4 hours before surgery and resume it as soon as possible afterward.

People who develop **skin sensitivity** (symptoms include rash, itching, and swelling) to Catapres-TTS, the transdermal patch form of clonidine, may experience the same reactions with oral clonidine.

Possible Side Effects

Tablets

▼ Most common: dry mouth, drowsiness, dizziness, constipation, and sedation.

▼ Common: headache and fatigue. These effects tend to diminish within 4 to 6 weeks.

▼ Less common: appetite loss, swelling or pain in the glands of the throat, nausea, vomiting, weight gain, blood-sugar elevation, breast pain or enlargement, worsening of congestive heart failure, heart palpitations, rapid heartbeat, dizziness when rising quickly from a sitting or lying position, painful blood-vessel spasm, abnormal heart rhythms, electrocardiogram changes, feeling unwell, changes in dream patterns, nightmares, difficulty sleeping, hallucinations, delirium, anxiety, depression, nervousness, restlessness, headache, rash, hives, thinning or loss of scalp hair, difficult or painful urination, nighttime urination, retaining urine, decrease or loss of sex drive, weakness, muscle or joint pain, leg cramps, increased alcohol sensitivity, dryness and burning of the eyes, dry nose, loss of color, and fever.

Transdermal Patch

▼ Most common: dry mouth and drowsiness.

▼ Less common: constipation, nausea, changes in sense of taste, dry throat, fatigue, headache, lethargy, changes in sleep patterns, nervousness, dizziness, impotence, sexual difficulties, and mild skin reactions including itching, swelling, contact dermatitis, discoloration, burning, peeling, throbbing, white patches, and generalized rash. Rashes of the face and tongue have also occurred but cannot be specifically tied to transdermal clonidine.

Drug Interactions

• Avoid alcohol, barbiturates, sedatives, and tranquilizers because they increase the depressive effects of clonidine.

• Tricyclic and other antidepressants, appetite suppressants, estrogens, stimulants, indomethacin and other nonsteroidal anti-inflammatory drugs (NSAIDs), and prazosin may counteract the effects of clonidine.

• Combining clonidine and a beta blocker may increase the severity of a drug-withdrawal reaction and rebound high blood pressure and may cause blood pressure to rise.

• Combining verapamil and clonidine may lead to very low blood pressure and atrioventricular (AV) block (abnormality in heartbeat patterns).

• Clonidine may reduce the therapeutic effects of levadopa.

Food Interactions

The tablets are best taken on an empty stomach but may be taken with food if they upset your stomach.

Usual Dose

Tablets

Adult: high blood pressure—100 mcg twice a day to start; may be raised by 100 mcg a day until maximum control is achieved. Take no more than 2400 mcg a day. Other uses—100–900 mcg a day, or up to 0.8 mcg per lb. of body weight in divided doses. Seniors should start with a lower dose and increase more slowly.

Child: 50–400 mcg orally twice a day.

Transdermal Patch

Adult: 100 mcg delivered daily from a patch applied once every 7 days. Up to two 300-mcg patches may be needed to control blood pressure. Transdermal dosage exceeding 600 mcg a day has not been shown to increase effectiveness.

Child: not recommended.

Overdosage

Symptoms of overdose are slow heartbeat, central nervous system (CNS) depression, very slow breathing or no breathing, low body temperature, pinpoint pupils, seizures, lethargy, agitation, irritability, nausea, vomiting, abnormal heart rhythms, mild increases in blood pressure followed by a rapid drop in blood pressure, dizziness, weakness, loss of reflexes, and vomiting. Victims should be taken to a hospital emergency room immediately. ALWAYS bring the prescription bottle or container.

Special Information

Clonidine causes drowsiness in about a third of people who take it. Be extremely careful while driving or performing any task that requires concentration. This effect is prominent during the first few weeks of clonidine therapy and then tends to decrease.

Do not take over-the-counter cough and cold medications unless directed by your doctor.

Call your doctor if you become depressed or have vivid dreams or nightmares while taking clonidine, or if you develop swelling in your feet or legs, paleness or coldness in your fingertips or toes, or any persistent or bothersome side effect.

Apply the transdermal patch to a hairless area of skin such as the upper arm or torso. Use a different skin site each time. If the patch becomes loose, apply the supplied adhesive directly over it. If the patch falls off before 7 days are up, apply a new one. Do not remove the patch while bathing.

If you forget a dose of oral clonidine, take it as soon as possible and then go back to your regular schedule. If you miss 2 or more consecutive doses, consult your doctor; missed doses may cause blood pressure increases and severe adverse effects. Do not take a double dose.

Special Populations

Pregnancy/Breast-feeding
Clonidine passes into the fetal bloodstream. Animal studies show that clonidine may damage the fetus in doses as low as ⅓ the maximum dose. Women who are or might be pregnant should only take clonidine after talking with their doctor about its risks and possible benefits.

Clonidine passes into breast milk. Nursing mothers who must take this drug should bottle-feed.

Seniors
Seniors are more susceptible to the effects of this drug and should begin with lower doses.

Generic Name

Clopidogrel (kloe-PID-oe-grel)

Brand Name

Plavix

Type of Drug

Antiplatelet.

Prescribed For

Heart attack and stroke prevention; blood thinning after placement of a vascular stent.

General Information

Artery-clogging blood clots are often the cause of heart attacks and strokes. Clopidogrel reduces the risk of both by helping prevent blood-clot formation. This drug thins the blood by making platelets—the cells that aggregate to form clots—less "sticky." It starts working in as little as 2 hours after taking a single tablet. The drug's blood-thinning effect lasts until inactivated platelets are replaced by the body. Studies suggest that clopidogrel is more effective than aspirin in preventing heart attack and stroke in people at risk. People taking clopidogrel after stent surgery usually take it for a relatively short period. Those taking it to pre-vent a heart attack or stroke must take it for life.

Cautions and Warnings

Do not take this drug if you are **sensitive** or **allergic** to it or ticlopidine, a related antiplatelet. These drugs can rarely cause a rapid drop in white-blood-cell count.

People with **bleeding ulcers, brain hemorrhages,** or **other bleeding problems** should use clopidogrel with caution.

People with **liver problems** should use clopidogrel with caution.

Possible Side Effects

▼ Most common: rash and other skin problems.

Possible Side Effects *(continued)*

▼ Common: chest pain, accidents, flu-like symptoms, pain, headache, dizziness, abdominal pain, upset stomach, joint pain, back pain, black-and-blue marks, and respiratory infection.

▼ Less common: tiredness, swollen arms or legs, high blood pressure, diarrhea, nausea, bleeding, nosebleeds, breathing difficulties, runny nose, coughing, bronchitis, high blood cholesterol, urinary infection, and depression.

▼ Rare: bleeding in the brain and stomach ulcer.

Drug Interactions

• Clopidogrel may interfere with the body's ability to break down fluvastatin, nonsteroidal anti-inflammatory drugs (NSAIDs), phenytoin, tamoxifen, tolbutamide, torsamide, and warfarin.

• Combining clopidogrel and NSAIDs may increase blood loss and bleeding in the stomach and intestines.

• Do not combine clopidogrel and other antiplatelet drugs or the anticoagulant (blood thinner) warfarin unless you are under your doctor's direct supervision. This interaction may prevent normal blood clotting and lead to severe bleeding problems.

Food Interactions

Clopidogrel may be taken without regard to food or meals.

Usual Dose

Adult: 75 mg a day.

Overdosage

Little is known about the effects of clopidogrel overdose aside from reduced blood clotting. Overdose victims should be taken to a hospital emergency room. ALWAYS bring the prescription bottle or container.

Special Information

Minor cuts may take longer to stop bleeding during treatment with clopidogrel. If you are having surgery, make sure your doctor knows you are taking clopidogrel. You may have to stop taking the drug 1 week before surgery.

If you forget a dose, take it as soon as you remember. If it is almost time for your next dose, skip the forgotten dose and continue with your regular schedule.

Special Populations

Pregnancy/Breast-feeding

The safety of using clopidogrel during pregnancy is not known. Other antiplatelet drugs, like aspirin, are not used during pregnancy due to their possible effects on mother and fetus. When this drug is considered crucial by your doctor, its benefits must be carefully weighed against its risks.

Clopidogrel may pass into breast milk. Nursing mothers who must take this drug should bottle-feed.

Seniors

Seniors may take this drug without special precaution.

Generic Name

Clorazepate (klor-AZ-uh-pate) G

Brand Names

Gen-Xene   Tranxene-SD
Tranxene   Tranxene T-Tab

Type of Drug

Benzodiazepine tranquilizer.

Prescribed For

Anxiety, tension, fatigue, and agitation; symptoms of acute alcohol withdrawal; also prescribed for irritable bowel syndrome and panic attacks.

General Information

Clorazepate dipotassium is a benzodiazepine. Benzodiazepines directly affect the brain. They can relax you and make you more tranquil or sleepier, or they can slow nervous system transmissions in such a way as to act as an anticonvulsant. Many doctors prefer benzodiazepines to other drugs that can be used to similar effect because they tend to be safer, have fewer side effects, and usually work as well, if not better.

Cautions and Warnings

Do not take clorazepate if you know you are **sensitive** or **allergic** to it or to another benzodiazepine drug, including clonazepam.

Clorazepate can aggravate narrow-angle **glaucoma**, but you may take it if you have open-angle glaucoma.

Other conditions in which clorazepate should be avoided are: severe **depression**, severe **lung disease**, **sleep apnea** (intermittent cessation of breathing during sleep), **liver disease**, **drunkenness**, and **kidney disease**. In each of these conditions, the depressive effects of clorazepate may be enhanced or could be detrimental to your overall condition.

Clorazepate should not be taken by **psychotic patients** because it is not effective for them and can trigger unusual excitement, stimulation, and rage.

Clorazepate is not intended to be used for more than 3 to 4 months at a time. Your doctor should reassess your condition before continuing your prescription beyond that time.

Clorazepate may be **addictive**. Drug withdrawal may develop if you stop taking it after only 4 weeks of regular use but is more likely after longer use. It may start with anxiety and progress to tingling in the hands or feet, sensitivity to bright light, sleep disturbances, cramps, tremors, muscle tension or twitching, poor concentration, flu symptoms, fatigue, appetite loss, sweating, and changes in mental state.

Possible Side Effects

Weakness and confusion may occur, especially in seniors and in those who are more sickly.

▼ Most common: mild drowsiness during the first few days of therapy.

▼ Less common: confusion, depression, lethargy, disorientation, headache, inactivity, slurred speech, stupor, dizziness, tremors, constipation, dry mouth, nausea, inability to control urination, sexual difficulties, irregular menstrual cycle, changes in heart rhythm, low blood pressure, fluid retention, blurred or double vision, itching, rash, hiccups, nervousness, inability to fall asleep, and occasional liver and kidney dysfunction. If you have any of these symptoms, stop taking the medicine and contact your doctor immediately.

Possible Side Effects *(continued)*

▼ Rare: Rare side effects can affect your heart, stomach and intestines, urinary tract, blood, muscles and joints. Contact your doctor if you experience any side effects not listed above.

Drug Interactions

• Clorazepate is a central-nervous-system depressant. Don't mix it with alcohol, other tranquilizers, narcotics, barbiturates, monoamine oxidase inhibitors (MAOIs), antihistamines, and antidepressants. Taking clorazepate with these drugs may result in excessive depression, tiredness, sleepiness, breathing difficulties, or related symptoms.

• Smoking may reduce clorazepate's effectiveness by increasing the rate at which it is broken down by the body.

• Clorazepate's effects may be prolonged when it is mixed with cimetidine, oral contraceptives, disulfiram, fluoxetine, isoniazid, ketoconazole, metoprolol, probenecid, propoxyphene, propranolol, rifampin, or valproic acid. Theophylline may reduce clorazepate's sedative effects.

• If you take antacids, separate them from your clorazepate dose by at least 1 hour to prevent them from interfering with the absorption of clorazepate into the bloodstream.

• Clorazepate may increase blood levels of digoxin and the chances of digoxin toxicity.

• The effect of levodopa may be decreased if it is taken together with clorazepate.

• Combining clorazepate with phenytoin may increase phenytoin blood concentrations and the chances of phenytoin toxicity.

Food Interactions

Clorazepate is best taken on an empty stomach, but it may be taken with food if it upsets your stomach.

Usual Dose

Immediate-Release

Adult and Child (age 9 and over): 15–60 mg daily. The average dose is 30 mg in divided quantities, but dosage must be adjusted to individual response for maximum effect. Maximum recommended daily dose is 90 mg.

Child (under age 9): not recommended.

Sustained-Release

Adult: The sustained-release form of clorazepate may be given as a single dose, either 11.25 or 22.5 mg, once every 24 hours. Sustained-release tablets are not recommended for the initial dosage.

Child: not recommended.

Overdosage

Symptoms of overdose are confusion, sleepiness, poor coordination, lack of response to pain such as a pin prick, loss of reflexes, shallow breathing, low blood pressure, and coma. The victim should be taken to a hospital emergency room. ALWAYS bring the prescription bottle or container.

Special Information

Clorazepate can cause tiredness, drowsiness, inability to concentrate, or similar symptoms. Be careful if you are driving, operating machinery, or performing other activities that require concentration.

People taking clorazepate for more than 3 or 4 months at a time may develop drug withdrawal reactions if the medication is stopped suddenly (see "Cautions and Warnings").

If you forget a dose of clorazepate, take it as soon as you remember. If it is almost time for your next dose, skip the dose you forgot and continue with your regular schedule. Do not take a double dose.

Special Populations

Pregnancy/Breast-feeding

Clorazepate may cause birth defects if taken during the first 3 months of pregnancy. Avoid this drug if you are or might be pregnant.

Clorazepate may pass into breast milk. Nursing mothers who must take clorazepate should bottle-feed.

Seniors

Seniors, especially those with liver or kidney disease, are more sensitive to the effects of clorazepate and generally require smaller doses to achieve the same effect.

Generic Name

Clotrimazole (kloe-TRIM-uh-zole) [G]

Brand Names

Fungoid   Mycelex
Lotrimin

The information in this profile also applies to the following drug:

Generic Ingredient: Sertaconazole
Ertaczo Cream

Type of Drug

Antifungal.

Prescribed For

Fungus infections of the mouth, skin, and vaginal tract.

General Information

Clotrimazole is useful against a variety of fungus organisms that other drugs do not affect. The exact way in which clotrimazole works is unknown. Sertaconazole is used for athlete's foot in people age 12 and older with compromised immune systems.

Cautions and Warnings

If clotrimazole causes local **itching** or **irritation,** stop using it. Do not use clotrimazole in your **eyes**. Proper diagnosis is essential for effective treatment. Do not use this product without first consulting your doctor.

Possible Side Effects

Side effects are infrequent and usually mild.
Cream and Solution
▼ Most common: redness, stinging, blistering, peeling, itching, and swelling of local areas.

Vaginal Tablets
▼ Most common: mild burning, rash, mild cramps, frequent urination, and burning or itching in a sexual partner.

Possible Side Effects *(continued)*

Lozenges
▼ Most common: stomach cramps or pain, diarrhea, nausea, and vomiting.

Drug Interactions

None known.

Food Interactions

The oral form of clotrimazole is best taken on an empty stomach, at least 1 hour before or 2 hours after meals. However, you may take it with food as long as you allow the lozenge to dissolve in your mouth.

Usual Dose

Topical Cream and Solution: Apply to affected areas morning and night for 7 consecutive days or as needed.

Vaginal Cream: 1 applicator's worth at bedtime for 3–7 consecutive days.

Vaginal Tablet: 1 tablet inserted into the vagina at bedtime for 7 days, or 2 tablets a day for 3–7 consecutive days.

Lozenge: 1 lozenge 5 times a day for 2 weeks or more.

Overdosage

Little is known about the effects of clotrimazole overdose or accidental ingestion. Call your local poison control center for more information.

Special Information

If treating a vaginal infection, you should refrain from sexual activity. Call your doctor if burning or itching develops or if the condition does not improve within 7 days.

If you are using the vaginal cream, you may want to wear a sanitary napkin to avoid staining your clothing. Do not use a tampon during treatment.

Dissolve the lozenge slowly in the mouth.

This medicine must be taken on consecutive days. If you forget a dose of oral clotrimazole, take it as soon as you remember. Do not double your dose.

When using clotrimazole for skin infections, do not cover the area with any kind of bandage unless directed to do so by your doctor.

Special Populations

Pregnancy/Breast-feeding

Women who are or might be pregnant should talk to their doctors about the medication's risks and benefits. Women who are in the first 3 months of pregnancy should use this drug only if directed to do so by their doctors. If you are pregnant, your doctor may want you to insert vaginal tablets by hand rather than use a vaginal applicator.

It is unknown whether the drug passes into breast milk. Use with caution or discontinue breast feeding during treatment.

Seniors

Seniors may use this medication without special restriction.

Generic Name

Clozapine (KLOE-zuh-pene) G

Brand Name

Clozaril

Type of Drug

Antipsychotic.

Prescribed For

Severe schizophrenia.

General Information

Clozapine is a unique antipsychotic that has the capacity to treat people who do not respond to or cannot tolerate other drugs. It works by a mechanism that differs from those of other antipsychotic drugs.

A very small number of people who take clozapine develop a rapid drop in their white-blood-cell count, known as agranulocytosis. This effect usually reverses itself when the drug is stopped, but the drug must be stopped AS SOON AS IT IS DIS-

COVERED. An unusually large number of people who have developed clozapine agranulocytosis in the U.S. are of Eastern European Jewish descent, but the association is not very strong. Most cases of agranulocytosis occur between week 4 and week 10 of treatment. It is essential that blood samples be taken approximately every week and for 4 weeks after the drug is stopped to watch for this effect. Because of the risk of agranulocytosis, clozapine should not be tried until at least 2 other antipsychotic medicines have failed.

Some people taking antipsychotic drugs develop tardive dyskinesia, a potentially irreversible condition marked by uncontrollable movements. Tardive dyskinesia has not been seen in patients taking clozapine, a major advantage of this drug over other antipsychotic medicines. However, there is still a risk that this set of symptoms could occur with clozapine.

Cautions and Warnings

Women, seniors, people with **serious illnesses,** those who are **emaciated,** those with a history of **diseases affecting the white blood cells,** or those who are taking **other medication that could affect white blood cells** may be more susceptible to clozapine agranulocytosis.

About 5% of people taking the drug experience a **seizure** in the first year of treatment. Seizure is most likely to occur at higher drug doses.

People with **heart disease** should be carefully monitored while on clozapine because of possible cardiac risks.

Clozapine has been associated with obesity, high cholesterol, and diabetes.

A serious set of side effects, known as **neuroleptic malignant syndrome (NMS),** includes a high fever and has been associated with clozapine when it is used together with lithium or other drugs. The symptoms that constitute NMS include muscle rigidity, mental changes, irregular pulse or blood pressure, increased sweating, and abnormal heart rhythm. NMS is potentially fatal and requires immediate medical attention.

Use this drug with caution if you have **glaucoma, prostate problems,** or **liver, kidney, or heart disease**.

Clozapine may interfere with mental or physical abilities because of the **sedation** it usually causes during the first few weeks of treatment.

Possible Side Effects

▼ Most common: rapid heartbeat, low blood pressure, dizziness, fainting, drowsiness or sedation, salivation, and constipation.

▼ Less common: headache, tremor, sleep disturbance, restlessness, slow muscle motions, absence of movement, agitation, convulsions, rigidity, restlessness, confusion, sweating, dry mouth, visual disturbances, high blood pressure, nausea, vomiting, heartburn or abdominal discomfort, fever, and weight gain.

▼ Rare: agranulocytosis (symptoms include fever with or without chills, sore throat, and sores or white spots on the lips or mouth, tardive dyskinesia (symptoms include lip smacking or puckering, puffing of the cheeks, rapid or wormlike tongue movement, uncontrolled chewing motions, and uncontrolled arm and leg movements), and NMS (see "Cautions and Warnings"). Other rare side effects can occur in almost any part of the body. Contact your doctor if you experience any side effect not listed above.

Drug Interactions

• Clozapine's anticholinergic effects—blurred vision, dry mouth, and confusion—may be enhanced by interaction with other anticholinergics, such as tricyclic antidepressants like amitriptyline.

• Drugs that reduce blood pressure may enhance the blood-pressure-lowering effects of clozapine.

• Alcohol and other nervous system depressants, including benzodiazepines and other antianxiety drugs, may enhance clozapine's sedative action. At least 1 person has died as a result of combining diazepam and clozapine.

• Combination oral contraceptives may increase blood levels of clozapine leading to toxic side effects. Women starting on a combination contraceptive may need to have their clozapine dose adjusted.

• Clozapine may increase blood levels of digoxin, warfarin, heparin, and phenytoin.

• The combination of lithium and clozapine may cause seizures, confusion, and NMS (see "Cautions and Warnings").

• Cigarette smoking may alter clozapine dosage requirements.

Food Interactions

None known.

Usual Dose

Starting dose—25 mg 2 times a day. Maintenance dose—generally, 300–450 mg a day. Dosage may be increased gradually to a daily maximum of 900 mg if required.

Overdosage

Symptoms of overdose are delirium, drowsiness, changes in heart rhythm, unusual excitement, nervousness, restlessness, hallucinations, excessive salivation, dizziness or fainting, slow or irregular breathing, and coma. Overdose victims must be taken to a hospital emergency room immediately. ALWAYS bring the prescription bottle or container.

Special Information

Clozapine may cause a fever during the first few weeks of treatment. Generally, the fever is not important, but it may occasionally be necessary to stop treatment due to persistent fever, a decision that would be made by your doctor.

Regular blood tests are necessary to monitor blood composition for any changes that might be caused by clozapine.

Call your doctor at once if you develop lethargy or weakness, a flu-like infection, sore throat, feelings of ill health, fever, sweating, muscle rigidity, mental changes, irregular pulse or blood pressure, mouth ulcers, or dry mouth that lasts for more than 2 weeks. Dry mouth, a common side effect of clozapine, may be countered by using gum, candy, ice, or a saliva substitute such as Orex or Moi-Stir.

Do not stop taking clozapine without your doctor's knowledge and approval, because a gradual dosage reduction may be necessary to prevent side effects.

Avoid alcohol or any other nervous system depressant while taking clozapine.

Some of the side effects of clozapine—drowsiness, blurred vision, or seizures—may interfere with the performance of complex tasks like driving or operating hazardous equipment.

While taking clozapine, rapidly rising from a sitting or lying position may cause you to become dizzy or faint.

If you take clozapine twice a day and forget a dose, take it as soon as you remember. If it is almost time for your next dose, take 1 dose as soon as you remember and another in 5 or 6 hours, then go back to your regular schedule. If you take clozapine 3 times a day and forget a dose, take it as soon as you remember. If it is almost time for your next dose, take 1 dose as soon as you remember and another in 3 or 4 hours, then go back to your regular schedule. Never take a double dose.

Special Populations

Pregnancy/Breast-feeding

This drug should be used during pregnancy only if your doctor determines that it is absolutely necessary.

Clozapine may pass into breast milk. Nursing mothers who must take this drug should bottle-feed.

Seniors

Seniors may be more sensitive to the side effects of clozapine, such as dizziness on rapidly rising from a sitting or lying position, confusion, and excitability. Older men are also more likely to have prostate problems, a reason to be cautious with clozapine.

Generic Name

Codeine (KOE-deen) G

Brand Name

Only available in generic form.

The information in this profile also applies to the following drugs:

Generic Ingredient: Fentanyl G
Actiq Lozenge on a Stick   Fentanyl Oralet (Lozenge)
Duragesic (Patch)

Generic Ingredient: Oxycodone Hydrochloride G
Endocodone   OxyFAST
M-Oxy   OxyIR
OxyContin   Percolone
Oxydose   Roxicodone

Type of Drug

Narcotic.

Prescribed For

Mild to moderate pain, and cough.

General Information

Codeine relieves pain and suppresses cough. The pain-relieving effect of 30 to 60 mg of codeine is equal to approximately 650 mg, or 2 tablets, of aspirin. Codeine may be less effective than aspirin for pain associated with inflammation because aspirin reduces inflammation and codeine does not. Codeine suppresses the cough reflex but does not cure the underlying cause of the cough. Other narcotic cough suppressants are stronger pain relievers, but codeine remains the best cough medication available.

Fentanyl is a potent pain reliever that can be substituted for other narcotic drugs. The patch form, which must be replaced about every 3 days, delivers fentanyl to the bloodstream at a steady rate. The lozenge has a shorter length of action than any other narcotic pain reliever, which make them useful when given to children before surgery because it provides doctors with the flexibility to obtain maximum benefit with minimal side effects. The lozenge on a stick is used for breakthrough cancer pain as a booster for people already taking narcotic pain relievers. These forms should only be used under controlled circumstances because of the risk of side effects or overdose. Low dosages of fentanyl relieve pain—larger amounts cause loss of consciousness and breathing difficulties.

Oxycodone is a narcotic used to control moderate to severe pain. Most people take it together with aspirin (Percodan) or acetaminophen (Percocet), but it can be used by itself. This is a potent pain reliever that carries a risk of addiction with continued use.

Cautions and Warnings

Do not take narcotics if you are **allergic** or **sensitive** to them. Use narcotics with extreme caution if you suffer from **asthma or other breathing problems**. Long-term use of narcotics may cause drug dependence or **addiction**. Narcotics may make it difficult to monitor the progress of people who have suffered **head injuries** and **acute abdominal conditions**.

Possible Side Effects

▼ Most common: light-headedness, dizziness, sleepiness, nausea, vomiting, appetite loss, and sweating. If these occur, ask your doctor about lowering your dosage. Most of these side effects disappear if you lie down.

▼ Less common: euphoria (feeling "high"), headache, agitation, uncoordinated muscle movement, minor hallucinations, disorientation and visual disturbances, dry mouth, constipation, flushing of the face, rapid heartbeat, palpitations, faintness, urinary difficulties or hesitancy, reduced sex drive or impotence, itching, rash, anemia, lowered or raised blood sugar, and yellowing of the skin or whites of the eyes. Narcotic analgesics may aggravate convulsions in those who have had them.

More serious side effects of codeine are shallow breathing or breathing difficulties.

Drug Interactions

• Avoid combining narcotics with alcohol, sleeping medications, tranquilizers, or other depressant drugs.
• Combining a narcotic pain reliever with any other medication that lowers blood pressure can lead to excessive blood-pressure lowering. Avoid this combination.
• Combining cimetidine with a narcotic pain reliever may cause confusion, disorientation, breathing difficulties, and seizure.

Food Interactions

Codeine may be taken with food to reduce upset stomach. The fentanyl patch may be used without regard to food.

Usual Dose

Codeine
Adult: 15–60 mg every 4–6 hours for relief of pain; 10–20 mg every few hours as needed to suppress cough.

Child: 1 mg per lb. of body weight every 4–6 hours for relief of pain; 2.5–10 mg every 4–6 hours to suppress cough.

Fentanyl Lozenge and Lozenge on a Stick
   Adult and Child: 200–1600 mcg. Dosage may be repeated up to 4 times daily. Allow the lozenge to dissolve in your mouth. DO NOT CHEW.

Fentanyl Patch
Apply to a clean and non-irritated patch of skin as directed, usually once every 3 days.

Oxycodone
   Adult: 10–30 mg every 4 hours as needed. OxyContin should be swallowed whole and not broken.
   Child: not recommended.

Overdosage

Symptoms include breathing difficulties or slowing of respiration, extreme tiredness progressing to stupor and then coma, pinpointed pupils, no response to pain stimulation, cold and clammy skin, slowing of heartbeat, lowering of blood pressure, convulsions, and cardiac arrest. The victim should be taken to a hospital emergency room immediately. ALWAYS bring the prescription bottle or container.

Special Information

Codeine is a respiratory depressant and affects the central nervous system (CNS), producing sleepiness, tiredness, or inability to concentrate. Be careful when driving or doing any task that requires concentration. Avoid alcohol.

   Call your doctor if you develop breathing difficulties, constipation, dry mouth, or any bothersome or persistent side effect.

   Apply the fentanyl patch only to non-irritated skin on a flat surface of the upper body. Hair at the application site should be clipped or cut, not shaved, before applying the patch. Do not use oils, soaps, lotions, alcohol, or anything else that might irritate the skin before applying the patch.

   If you forget a dose of codeine, take it as soon as you remember. If it is almost time for your next dose, skip the one you forgot and continue with your regular schedule. Never take a double dose.

Special Populations

Pregnancy/Breast-feeding

Narcotics pass into the fetal circulation. Excessive use of them during pregnancy may cause drug dependence in newborns. Narcotics may also cause breathing difficulties in infants during delivery. Animal studies show that codeine may cause fetal harm. If given to a pregnant woman before cesarean section, fentanyl may cause drowsiness in newborns. When either of these drugs is considered crucial by your doctor, its potential benefits must be carefully weighed against its risks.

Narcotics pass into breast milk. Nursing mothers who must take codeine should bottle-feed.

Seniors

Seniors are more likely to be sensitive to side effects and should be treated with the smallest effective dosage.

Generic Name

Colchicine (KOLE-chih-sene) [G]

Brand Name

Only available in generic form.

Type of Drug

Antigout.

Prescribed For

Gouty arthritis; also prescribed for Mediterranean fever; chronic progressive multiple sclerosis; cirrhosis of the liver; biliary cirrhosis; Behçet's disease; pseudogout (a condition caused by calcium deposits); amyloidosis; very low blood-platelet count (also known as ITP); skin reactions, including scleroderma, psoriasis, and other conditions; and nerve disability associated with chronic progressive multiple sclerosis.

General Information

While no one knows exactly how colchicine works, it appears to help people with gout by reducing the inflammatory response to uric acid crystals that form inside joints and by interfering with the body's mechanism for making uric acid. Unlike drugs that affect uric acid levels, colchicine does not block the progression of gout to chronic gouty arthritis; it will, however, relieve the pain of acute attacks and lessen the frequency and severity of attacks. It has no effect on other kinds of pain.

Cautions and Warnings

Do not use colchicine if you suffer from any serious **blood, kidney, liver, stomach,** or **cardiac condition**.

Vomiting, abdominal pain, diarrhea, nausea, kidney damage, and **blood in the urine** may occur with colchicine, especially at maximum doses. This can worsen existing gastrointestinal (GI) or other conditions. Stop taking the medication and call your doctor if you develop one of these symptoms.

The **weakness** that people develop while taking colchicine is frequently related to high levels of colchicine in the blood caused by poor kidney function and improves without treatment 3 to 4 weeks after the drug is stopped. This reaction is often mistaken for other conditions.

Periodic **blood counts** should be done if you are taking colchicine for long periods of time.

Colchicine interferes with the absorption of vitamin B_{12} by affecting the lining of the GI tract.

Colchicine may affect the process of **sperm** generation in men.

The safety and effectiveness for **use by children** have not been established.

Possible Side Effects

▼ Common: vomiting, diarrhea, and abdominal pain may occur if you take maximum doses of colchicine for an acute gout attack. You may also experience severe diarrhea, kidney and blood-vessel damage, blood in the urine, and reduced urination.

▼ Less common: hair loss, rash, appetite loss, and muscle and nerve weakness.

Rare: with long-term colchicine therapy—reduced white-blood-cell and platelet counts, nerve inflammation, blood-clotting problems, rash, and other reactions. Colchicine may interfere with sperm formation.

Drug Interactions

• Colchicine interferes with the absorption of vitamin B_{12}.

• Colchicine may increase sensitivity to central-nervous-system depressants, such as tranquilizers and alcohol.

• The following drugs may reduce colchicine's effectiveness: anticancer drugs, bumetanide, diazoxide, thiazide diuretics, ethacrynic acid, furosemide, mecamylamine, pyrazinamide, and triamterene.

• Taking phenylbutazone with colchicine increases the risk of side effects.

Food Interactions

None known.

Usual Dose

Acute Gout Attack: 1–1.2 mg. This dose may be followed by 0.5–1.2 mg every 1–2 hours until pain is relieved or nausea, vomiting, or diarrhea occurs. The total dose needed to control pain and inflammation during an attack varies from 4–8 mg.

Gout Prevention: 0.5–1.8 mg daily. In mild cases, 0.5 mg or 0.6 mg may be taken 3–4 days a week.

Familial Mediterranean Fever: 1–3 mg a day.

Cirrhosis of the Liver: 1 mg a day for 5 days each week.

Biliary Cirrhosis: 0.6 mg 2 times a day.

Amyloidosis: 0.5 mg 1–2 times a day.

Behçet's Disease: 0.5–1.5 mg a day.

Pseudogout: 0.6 mg 2 times a day.

ITP: 1.2–1.8 mg a day for 2 weeks or more.

Scleroderma: 1 mg a day.

Other Skin Disorders: up to 1.8 mg a day, depending on the specific condition.

Overdosage

The lethal dose is estimated at 65 mg, although people have died after taking as little as 7 mg at once. Usually 1 to 3 days pass between the time that an overdose is taken and symptoms begin. Overdose symptoms start with nausea, vomiting, stomach pain, diarrhea—which may be severe and bloody—and burning sensations in the throat or stomach or on the skin. If you think you are experiencing overdose symptoms, contact your doctor immediately, or go to a hospital emergency room. ALWAYS bring the prescription bottle or container.

Special Information

Call your doctor if you develop rash, sore throat, fever, unusual bleeding or bruising, tiredness, or numbness or tingling. Seniors are more likely to develop drug side effects and should use this drug with caution.

Stop taking maximum doses of colchicine as soon as gout pain is relieved and reduce your dose to a maintenance level if your doctor has prescribed it for gout prevention. Stop taking the drug entirely and contact your doctor at the first sign of nausea, vomiting, stomach pain, or diarrhea.

If you forget a dose of colchicine, take it as soon as possible. If it is almost time for your next dose, skip the dose you forgot and continue with your regular schedule. Do not take a double dose.

Special Populations

Pregnancy/Breast-feeding

Colchicine can harm the fetus. Pregnant women should not take it unless the potential benefits clearly outweigh the risks.

It is not known if colchicine passes into breast milk. No problems with nursing infants are known, but nursing mothers who must take colchicine should consider bottle-feeding.

Seniors

Seniors are more likely to develop side effects and should use colchicine with caution.

Combivent see *Ipratropium*, page 585

Type of Drug

Contraceptives

Brand Names

Generic Ingredients: Low-Dose Estrogen + Low-Dose Progestin (Single-Phase Combination)

Alesse   Lessina
Aviane   Levlite

Generic Ingredients: Low-Dose Estrogen + Intermediate-Dose Progestin (Single-Phase Combination)

Cryselle	Loestrin Fe 1/20
Levlen	Microgestin Fe 1/20
Levora	Nordette
Lo/Ovral	Portia
Low-Ogestrel	Yasmin
Loestrin 21 1/20	

Generic Ingredients: Low-Dose Estrogen + High-Dose Progestin (Single-Phase Combination)

Demulen 1/35	Loestrin Fe 1.5/30
Kariva	Microgestin Fe 1/20
Loestrin 1/20	Microgestin Fe 1.5/30
Loestrin 21 1.5/30	Mircette
Loestrin Fe 1/20	Zovia 1/35E

Generic Ingredients: Intermediate-Dose Estrogen + Low-Dose Progestin (Single-Phase Combination)

Ortho-Cyclen	Sprintec

Generic Ingredients: Intermediate-Dose Estrogen and Intermediate-Dose Progestin (Single-Phase Combination)

Necon 1/50	Ortho-Novum 1/50
Norinyl 1 + 50	

Generic Ingredients: Intermediate-Dose Estrogen + High-Dose Progestin (Single-Phase Combination)

Apri	Nortrel 1/35
Demulen 1/50	Ortho-Cept
Desogen	Ortho-Novum 1/35
Necon 1/35	Zovia 1/50E
Norinyl 1 + 35	

Generic Ingredients: High-Dose Estrogen + High-Dose Progestin (Single-Phase Combination)

Demulen 1/50	Ovcon-50
Ogestrel	Ovral

Generic Ingredients: High-Dose Estrogen + Low-Dose Progestin (Single-Phase Combination)

Brevicon	Nortrel 0.5/35

Modicon   Ovcon-35
Neocon 0.5/35

Generic Ingredients: High-Dose Estrogen + Intermediate-Dose Progestin (2-Phase Combination)
Necon 10/11   Ortho-Novum 10/11

Generic Ingredients: Low-Dose Estrogen + Low-Dose Progestin (3-Phase Combination)
Ortho Tri-Cyclen Lo

Generic Ingredients: Low-Dose Estrogen + High-Dose Progestin (3-Phase Combination)
Cyclessa   Estrostep Fe
Estrostep 21

Generic Ingredients: Intermediate-Dose Estrogen + Low-Dose Progestin (3-Phase Combination)
Enpresse   Tri-Norinyl
Ortho Tri-Cyclen   Triphasil
Tri-Levlen   Trivora

Generic Ingredients: High-Dose Estrogen + Intermediate-Dose Progestin (3-Phase Combination)
Necon 7/7/7   Ortho-Novum 7/7/7

Generic Ingredient: Low-Dose Progestin (Mini-Pill)
Ovrette

Generic Ingredient: High-Dose Progestin (Mini-Pill)
Camila   Nor-Q.D.
Errin   Nora-BE
Jolivette   Ortho–Micronor

Generic Ingredients: Low-Dose Estrogen + Low-Dose Progestin (Patch)
OrthoEvra

Generic Ingredients: Low-Dose Estrogen + Low-Dose Progestin (Vaginal Ring)
NuvaRing

Generic Ingredient: Progestin (Implant)
Norplant II

Generic Ingredient: Progestin (Intrauterine Insert)
Mirena   Progestasert

Generic Ingredient: High-Dose Progestin (Emergency Contraceptive)
Plan B

Generic Ingredients: High-Dose Progestin + High-Dose Estrogen (Emergency Contraceptive)
Preven

Prescribed For

Prevention of pregnancy, endometriosis, excessive menstruation, and cyclic withdrawal bleeding. Ortho Tri-Cyclen and Estrostep may be prescribed for moderate acne in women over age 15.

General Information

Oral contraceptives ("the pill") are synthetic hormones containing either progestin or a progestin-estrogen combination. These drugs are similar to natural female hormones, which cannot be used as contraceptives because very large dosages would be required. Synthetic hormones are more potent and are effective at smaller dosages. Oral contraceptives work by preventing sperm from reaching the unfertilized egg, preventing the implantation of a fertilized egg in the uterus, or preventing ovulation (the release of an unfertilized egg from the ovaries). They prevent acne by balancing hormone levels.

When properly used, oral contraceptives can be 97% to 99% effective at preventing pregnancy. These products vary in their effectiveness and in the amount and type of estrogen or progestin used. The side effects of these drugs tend to increase with the amount of hormone they contain. While low hormone dosages are preferred, contraceptives with the smallest amounts of estrogen may be less effective in some women than others.

Single-phase products provide constant levels of estrogen and progestin throughout the entire month-long pill cycle. In 2-phase combinations, the amount of estrogen remains at a steady low level throughout the cycle, while progestin levels increase and then decrease. This variation in progestin allows normal changes to take place in the uterus. Three-phase products are meant to simulate the normal hormone cycle and reduce breakthrough bleeding. Throughout the cycle, estrogen levels remain the same while those of progestin change to create a 3-part wave pattern. The amount of estrogen in 3-phase products is considered low. Breakthrough bleeding may occur with the older combination products from day 8 through 16 of the cycle.

The mini-pill, a progestin-only product, may cause irregular menstrual cycles and may be less effective than estrogen-progestin combinations. Mini-pills may be recommended to older women or women who should avoid estrogens (see "Cautions and Warnings").

The contraceptive patch releases small amounts of progestin and estrogen continuously over 3 weeks. The medication is absorbed into the blood vessels just below the skin. The patch works in the same way as contraceptive pills do.

The vaginal ring releases small amounts of etonogestrel, a progestin, and estradiol, an estrogen, in the vaginal canal over 3 weeks. The combination prevents pregnancy in the same way as combination pills do.

Most oral contraceptives are designed to simulate a normal menstrual cycle. By not taking the pills 1 week out of the month, you continue to have your regular period. In fact, these products are often used to stabilize a woman's period. One product, Seasonale, comes in an 84-pill packet and is taken once a day for 3 months. This means you will only have your period once every 3 months.

Levonorgestrel, a progestin, is used in implants that provide effective contraception for up to 5 years after surgical implantation under the skin of the upper arm or inside the uterus. Levonorgestrel implants should be replaced at least once every 5 years. They can be removed at any time, reversing the contraceptive effect. The progestin intrauterine inserts provide effective contraception for about 1 year. The implant and intrauterine systems contain the same hormone found in the mini-pill and are associated with many of the same side effects and precautions as oral contraceptives.

Emergency contraceptives contain high doses of estrogen and progestin. They are intended for use only after contraceptive failure or unprotected intercourse. They should never be taken by a pregnant woman.

Contraceptive drugs in any form are associated with risks. These risks are greatest in women over age 35 who smoke and have high blood pressure.

Cautions and Warnings

You should not use contraceptive drugs if you are or might be **pregnant,** have had **blood clots** in veins or arteries, **stroke,** any **blood-coagulation disorder,** known or suspected **cancer** of the breast or sex organs, or liver cancer.

Contraceptive drugs may cause **eye problems.** Call your doctor at once if you develop visual difficulties of any kind.

Women taking the combination product Seasonale will only have their period once every 3 months. It is absolutely essential for you to verify you are not pregnant if you miss that period or think you may be pregnant for any reason.

The risks of contraceptive drugs increase if you are **physically immobile** or have **asthma; cardiac insufficiency; epilepsy; migraine; kidney problems;** a strong family history of **breast cancer; benign breast disease; diabetes; endometriosis; gallbladder disease or gallstones; liver problems,** including jaundice; **high blood cholesterol; high blood pressure; estrogen or progestin intolerance; depression; tuberculosis;** or **varicose veins.**

There is an increased risk of **heart attack** in women who have used contraceptive drugs for more than 10 years, or who are between age 40 and 49 and have other coronary risk factors such as smoking, obesity, high blood pressure, diabetes, and high blood cholesterol. This risk remains even after the medication is stopped. Smokers who use contraceptive drugs are 5 times more likely to have a heart attack than nonsmokers taking contraceptives and 10 to 12 times more likely to have a heart attack than nonsmokers who do not use the pill.

Women with a history of **headaches, high blood pressure,** or **varicose veins** should avoid estrogen-containing products, as should older women and those who have experienced estrogen side effects.

Contraceptive drugs may mask the onset of **menopause.**

Progestin-only products are associated with an increased risk of **blood-clotting problems.**

The progestin in Yasmin raises **blood potassium levels.** Women with **kidney, liver, or adrenal gland disease** should use Yasmin with caution.

Intrauterine inserts have been associated with an increased risk of **pelvic inflammatory disease** (PID). The highest risk usually occurs within the first 20 days after insertion. Do not use intrauterine inserts if you have had an **ectopic pregnancy.**

Possible Side Effects

▼ Common: Common side effects often result from using a product that is poorly suited to your body chemistry. Determining the right amount and type of hormone often minimizes these effects. If you are taking too much estrogen, you may experience nausea, bloating, high blood pressure, migraine, or breast tenderness. Too little estrogen may cause early or mid-cycle breakthrough bleeding, spotting, or reduced periodic flow. Too much progestin is associated with weight gain and increased appetite, tiredness or weakness, low periodic flow, acne, depression, breast regression, and oily scalp. Too little progestin may cause late breakthrough bleeding, excessive periodic bleeding, or missed periods.

▼ Less common: abdominal cramps, infertility after discontinuance of the drug, breast tenderness, weight change, headache, rash, vaginal itching and burning, general vaginal infection, nervousness, dizziness, depression, cataracts, changes in sex drive, hair loss, and increased sensitivity to the sun.

▼ Rare: Women who use contraceptive drugs are more likely to develop several serious conditions, including blood clots in the deep veins, stroke, heart attack, liver cancer, gallbladder disease, and high blood pressure. Women who smoke cigarettes are at much higher risk for some of these adverse effects.

Drug Interactions

• Atorvastatin, rifampin, barbiturates, phenylbutazone, phenytoin, ampicillin, neomycin, penicillin, tetracycline, chloramphenicol, sulfa drugs, griseofulvin, nitrofurantoin, protease inhibitor drugs for AIDS, tranquilizers, and antimigraine drugs make contraceptive drugs less effective. Use backup birth control while taking these medications together.

• Contraceptive drugs may elevate blood levels of benzodiazepine tranquilizers and sleeping pills, caffeine, metoprolol, corticosteroids, theophylline drugs, and tricyclic antidepressants, increasing the risk of side effects.

• Contraceptive drugs may increase the toxic liver effects of acetaminophen and reduce the drug's effectiveness. Contraceptive drugs may increase or decrease the effect of anti-coagulant (blood-thinning) drugs. Discuss the risks of this combination with your doctor.

• Contraceptive drugs may decrease the effects of salicylate pain relievers including aspirin, clofibrate, lorazepam, oxazepam, and temazepam.

• Contraceptive drugs may increase blood-cholesterol levels and interfere with blood tests for thyroid function and blood sugar.

• Since Yasmin raises blood potassium levels, it should not be used if you are taking spironolactone or another potassium-sparing diuretic, potassium supplements, angiotensin-converting enzyme (ACE) inhibitors, angiotensin receptor antagonists, heparin, nonsteroidal anti-inflammatory drugs (NSAIDs), or other medications on a long-term basis that may further increase potassium levels.

Food Interactions

None known.

Usual Dose

Single-Phase, 2-Phase, and 3-Phase Combinations: The first day of bleeding is day 1 of the menstrual cycle. Beginning on the first day of the cycle, take 1 pill a day for 20–21 days according to the number of pills supplied by the manufacturer. If menstrual flow has not begun 7 days after taking the last pill, begin the next month's cycle of pills. Some manufacturers recommend starting the pills on a Sunday to make it easy to remember to take them. In this case, start taking your pills on the first Sunday after your period begins. If menstruation begins on a Sunday, take the first pill that day.

Seasonale: Take 1 pink tablet every day for 84 consecutive days. Do not skip a day. Then, take 1 white pill a day for 7 days. You may be pregnant if you do not have a period while you are taking the white pills. Then, start a new pill cycle.

Progestin-Only Mini-Pill: Take 1 pill every day.

Contraceptive Patch: Apply a new patch to the thigh, abdomen, or arm. Remove the patch after 3 weeks and then reapply a new patch after 1 week. Be sure to always apply a new patch on the same day of the week. If you are switching from birth control pills, apply the first patch on the same day you would start a new cycle of pills.

Vaginal Ring: Keep the vaginal ring in the vaginal canal for 3 weeks. Remove it and put a new one in 1 week later. If you did not use a hormonal contraceptive in the previous month, insert the ring between day 1 and day 5 of your cycle.

If you are switching from a combination birth control pill, insert the ring anytime during the week after you took your last pill but before you would have started your next cycle of pills. No additional contraception is necessary.

If you are switching from a mini-pill, insert the ring on the day after you take your last mini-pill.

If you are switching from a progestin implant or an IUD, insert the ring on the same day your implant or IUD is removed.

If you are switching from a progestin injection, insert the ring on the same day you would have received your next injection.

If you are switching from a progestin-only mini-pill, implant, injection, or IUD, use another form of contraception for the first 7 days after you insert the ring.

Emergency Contraception: Emergency contraceptive kits have only a few pills. Take half the pills (1 or 2 depending on the brand you use) within 72 hours of unprotected sex. Take the rest of the pills 12 hours after the first dose.

Overdosage

An overdose may cause nausea and withdrawal bleeding in adult women. Overdose victims should be taken to a hospital emergency room. ALWAYS bring the prescription package.

Special Information

Use backup birth control to prevent pregnancy in the first 3 weeks after you begin taking contraceptive drugs.

Oral contraceptives do not protect against sexually transmitted diseases.

Take your pill at the same time each day to establish a routine and ensure maximum contraceptive protection.

Call your doctor immediately if you experience severe abdominal pain; severe or sudden headache; pain in the chest, groin, or leg, especially the calf; sudden slurring of speech; changes in vision; weakness, numbness, or pain in the arms or legs; coughing up of blood; loss of coordination; or shortness of breath. These symptoms may require emergency treatment.

Other problems that may require medical attention are bulging eyes; changes in vaginal bleeding; fainting; frequent or painful urination; a gradual increase in blood pressure; breast lumps or secretions; depression; yellowing of the skin or whites of the eyes; rash; redness or irritation; upper abdominal swelling, pain, or tenderness; an unusual or dark-colored mole; thick, white vaginal discharge; or vaginal itching or tenderness.

See your doctor for a check-up every 6 to 12 months.

Some manufacturers include 7 inert or iron pills in their packaging to be taken on days when the drug is not taken. This makes it easier for women to stay on schedule with their pills. The 7 pills bridge the gap between contraceptive cycles and allow women to take 1 pill every day without stopping.

For single- or 2-phase combinations: If you forget to take a pill for 1 day, take 2 pills the following day. If you miss 2 consecutive days, take 2 pills for the next 2 days. Then return to your schedule of 1 pill a day. If you miss 3 consecutive days, do not take any pills for the next 7 days and use another form of contraception; then start a brand new cycle.

Seasonale: The risk of pregnancy increases with each pink tablet you forget. Use another method of non-hormonal back-up contraception any time you miss 2 or more pink tablets until you have taken a pink tablet every day for seven consecutive days. You are protected against pregnancy if you miss 1 or more white tablets, as long as you begin taking the pink tablets again on the proper day.

For 3-phase combinations: If you forget to take a pill for 1 day, take 2 pills the following day. If you miss 2 consecutive days, take 2 pills for the next 2 days. Then return to your schedule of 1 pill a day. If you forget to take a pill for 3 days in a row, stop taking the drug and use an alternate means of contraception until your period starts. ALWAYS use a backup contraceptive method for the remainder of your cycle if you forget even 1 pill of a 3-phase combination.

If you forget to apply the contraceptive patch on the same day of the week once every 4 weeks, you risk a loss of effectiveness on the days after you should have applied it. If the patch comes off or is partially detached in mid-cycle, you must start a new 3-week cycle at once by removing the old patch and applying a new one.

If the vaginal ring is accidentally expelled during the 3 weeks it is normally retained, rinse it off with water and replace it within 3 hours. Do not use hot water. If the ring is not reusable, insert a new ring and continue with your regular schedule. If you do not replace the ring within 3 hours, its effectiveness may be reduced. Use an additional form of contraceptive until the ring has been worn for 7 consecutive days.

Missing a pill reduces your protection. If you keep forgetting to take your pills, you must use another birth control method.

If you take drugs that reduce the effectiveness of contraceptive drugs (see "Drug Interactions"), use a backup contraceptive method during that cycle to prevent accidental pregnancy.

Good dental hygiene is essential while taking contraceptive drugs. See your dentist regularly and brush and floss carefully because contraceptive drugs may increase the risk of an oral infection.

Contraceptive drugs may increase your sensitivity to the sun.

Wearing contact lenses may be uncomfortable while taking contraceptive drugs because the pills can cause minor changes in the shape of your eyes.

All contraceptive prescriptions come with a "patient package insert." It gives detailed information about the drug and is required by federal law.

Special Populations

Pregnancy/Breast-feeding
Contraceptive hormones cause birth defects and may interfere with fetal development. They are not safe for use during pregnancy. If you think you are pregnant, use another form of contraception and stop taking your birth control pills.

Contraceptive hormones pass into breast milk. Combination contraceptive products reduce the amount of milk produced. Nursing mothers who must use any of these drugs should consider bottle-feeding.

Seniors
These products are not intended for women who have completed menopause.

Coreg *see Carvedilol, page 202*

Type of Drug

Corticosteroids, Eye Products

(kor-tih-koe-STER-oids)

Brand Names

Generic Ingredient: Dexamethasone Ⓖ

AK-Dex   Maxidex
Decadron

Generic Ingredient: Fluorometholone Ⓖ

Flarex   FML Forte
Fluor-Op   FML-S
FML

Generic Ingredient: Loteprednol Etabonate

Alrex   Lotemax

Generic Ingredient: Medrysone

HMS

Generic Ingredient: Prednisolone

AK-Pred   Pred Mild
Econopred   Pred Forte
Econopred Plus

Generic Ingredient: Rimexolone

Vexol

Prescribed For

Allergic and inflammatory eye conditions and to speed healing after eye surgery or injury.

General Information

Corticosteroid eye products are prescribed for general relief of inflammation due to allergy and other causes. They are also used after eye surgery or serious eye injury to aid the healing process by reducing the natural inflammatory process. Very severe eye conditions that do not respond to these products may require treatment with corticosteroid drugs taken by mouth. Fluorometholone, medrysone, and prednisolone (up to 0.125%) are preferred for long-term treatment because they are least likely to raise the fluid pressure inside the eye. Corticosteroid eye products have not been widely studied in children, though fluorometholone has been proven safe for use in children age 2 and over.

Cautions and Warnings

Do not use any of these products if you are **allergic** or **sensitive** to corticosteroids. These products should be used with caution if you have a **fungal, herpes, tuberculosis, or viral infection of the eye,** or have **cataracts, glaucoma,** or **diabetes**. Do not use any of these products without your doctor's knowledge.

Long-term use of these products can lead to **eye damage,** including glaucoma, infection, and nerve damage.

Do not use any of these products in **children** without consulting a doctor.

Possible Side Effects

▼   Rare: watery eyes, glaucoma, optic nerve damage, gradual blurring, reduction, or loss of vision, eye pain, nausea, vomiting, eye infections, drooping eyelid, and eye burning, stinging, or redness.

Drug Interactions

• Corticosteroids applied to the eye may interfere with the effect of antiglaucoma drugs.

• The risk of raising fluid pressure inside the eye is increased when corticosteroid eye products are taken with anticholinergic drugs, especially atropine, over a long period of time.

Food Interactions

None known.

Usual Dose

Eyedrops: 1–2 drops several times a day.

Eye Ointment: Place a thin strip of ointment into the affected eye several times a day.

Overdosage

Swallowing a container of corticosteroid eyedrops or ointment usually does not produce serious effects. Call your local poison center or a hospital emergency room for more information.

Special Information

If you forget to administer a dose, do so as soon as you remember. If it is almost time for your next dose, skip the one you forgot and continue with your regular schedule.

To prevent infection, keep the eyedropper from touching your fingers, eyelids, or any surface. Wait at least 5 minutes before using any other eyedrops.

If the brand you are taking contains benzalkonium chloride, wait at least 15 minutes before inserting contact lenses. In some cases, you may be instructed not to wear contact lenses for the duration of treatment.

Special Populations

Pregnancy / Breast-feeding

Using large amounts of corticosteroid eyedrops during pregnancy may affect the adrenal gland of the fetus. When your doctor considers one of these products crucial, its potential benefits must be carefully weighed against its risks.

Oral corticosteroids pass into breast milk, but it is not known if this is also true of corticosteroid eyedrops. Nursing mothers who must use one of these medications should consider bottle-feeding.

Seniors

Seniors may use these products without special precaution.

Type of Drug

Corticosteroids, Inhalers

(kor-tih-koe-STER-oids)

Brand Names

Generic Ingredient: Beclomethasone Dipropionate

Beclovent	Vancenase Pockethaler
QVAR 40	Vanceril
QVAR 80	Vanceril Double Strength

Generic Ingredient: Budesonide
Pulmicort Turbuhaler   Pulmicort Respules

Generic Ingredient: Flunisolide
AeroBid   AeroBid-M

Generic Ingredient: Fluticasone Propionate
Flovent   Flovent Rotadisk
Flovent Diskus

Generic Ingredient: Triamcinolone Acetonide
Azmacort

Prescribed For

Chronic asthma and bronchial disease.

General Information

Corticosteroid inhalers relieve the symptoms associated with asthma and bronchial disease by reducing inflammation of bronchial mucous membranes, making it easier to breathe. Corticosteroid inhalers produce the same treatment effect as oral corticosteroids, with some important differences. Because inhalers deliver the drug directly to the lungs, smaller dosages can be used. They also have fewer side effects because little of the drug reaches the bloodstream. Corticosteroid inhalers can prevent asthma attacks if used regularly but do not relieve them once they start.

Cautions and Warnings

Do not use any of these drugs if you are **allergic** to corticosteroids.

Corticosteroid inhalers should not be used as the primary treatment of severe **asthma**. They are recommended only for people who take prednisone or another oral corticosteroid, or for people who do not respond to other asthma drugs.

In people with asthma, death from **adrenal gland failure** has occurred during and after switching from an oral corticosteroid to an inhaler. Adrenal function is impaired for several months after the switch.

Combining an oral corticosteroid with a corticosteroid inhaler may cause **pituitary gland suppression**.

During a period of severe **stress,** you may have to switch to an oral corticosteroid if the inhaler does not control your asthma. During periods of stress or a severe asthmatic attack, people who have stopped using an inhaler should ask their doctors about taking an oral corticosteroid.

Corticosteroid inhalers may be associated with immediate or delayed **drug reactions,** including breathing difficulties, rash, and bronchospasm.

Corticosteroid inhalers are not recommended for **children under age 6**.

Possible Side Effects

▼ Most common: dry mouth, hoarseness, rash, and bronchospasm.

▼ Rare: cough, wheezing, infection, and facial swelling. Cough and wheezing are probably caused by an ingredient in the inhaler other than the corticosteroid itself.

Drug Interactions

• Ketoconazole may increase blood levels of budesonide and fluticasone.

• Using an inhaled corticosteroid and an oral corticosteroid together may increase the effect of both drugs. Use with caution.

Food Interactions

None known.

Usual Dose

Beclomethasone

Adult and Child (age 13 and over): 2 inhalations (84 mcg) 3–4 times a day, or 4 inhalations twice a day. People with severe asthma may take up to 16 inhalations a day.

Child (age 6–12): 1–2 inhalations 3–4 times a day.

Budesonide

Adult: starting dose—200–400 mcg (1 to 2 inhalations) twice a day. Do not exceed 800 mcg twice a day.

Child (age 6 and over): 200 mcg (1 inhalation) twice a day. Do not exceed 400 mcg twice a day.

Budesonide Respules

Child (age 1–8): 1–2 ml once or twice a day via jet nebulizer connected to an air compressor.

Flunisolide
   Adult and Child (age 16 and over): 2 inhalations (500 mcg) morning and evening. Do not exceed 8 inhalations a day.
   Child (age 6–15): 2 inhalations (500 mcg) morning and evening. Do not exceed 4 inhalations a day.

Fluticasone Inhalation
   Adult and Child (age 12 and over): 88–880 mcg twice a day.
   Child (6–12): 88–440 mcg twice a day.

Fluticasone Rotadisk and Diskus
   Adult and Child (age 12 and over): 100–1000 mcg twice a day.
   Child (age 4–11): 50–100 mcg twice a day.

Triamcinolone
   Adult and Child (age 13 and over): 2 inhalations (200 mcg) 3–4 times a day. Do not exceed 16 inhalations a day without your doctor's knowledge.
   Child (age 6–12): 1–2 inhalations (100–200 mcg) 3–4 times a day. Do not exceed 12 inhalations a day.

Overdosage

Serious adverse effects are unlikely. Excessive use of large amounts of an inhaled corticosteroid may cause overdose symptoms and require gradually stopping the drug. Call your local poison control center or a hospital emergency room for more information.

Special Information

People using both a corticosteroid inhaler and a bronchodilator, such as albuterol, should use the bronchodilator first, wait a few minutes, and then use the corticosteroid inhaler. This allows more corticosteroid to be absorbed.

These drugs are for preventive therapy only and will not affect an asthma attack. Inhaled corticosteroids must be taken regularly, as directed. Wait at least 1 minute between inhalations.

To properly take this medication, thoroughly shake the inhaler if it is one that must be shaken. Take a drink of water to moisten your throat. Place the inhaler 2 finger-widths away from your mouth and tilt your head back slightly. While activating the inhaler, take a slow, deep breath for 3 to 5 seconds, then hold your breath for about 10 seconds, and finally breathe out slowly. Allow at least 1 minute between puffs. Rinse your mouth after each use to reduce dry mouth and hoarseness.

If you forget to administer a dose, do so as soon as you remember. If it is almost time for your next dose, skip the dose you forgot and continue with your regular schedule. Do not take a double dose.

Special Populations

Pregnancy/Breast-feeding

Corticosteroids may cause birth defects or interfere with fetal development. When any of these drugs is considered crucial by your doctor, its potential benefits must be carefully weighed against its risks.

It is not known if inhaled corticosteroids pass into breast milk, though oral corticosteroids do. Nursing mothers who must take an inhaled corticosteroid should consider bottle-feeding.

Seniors

Seniors may use corticosteroid inhalers without special restriction. Tell your doctor if you have bone or bowel disease, colitis, diabetes, glaucoma, fungal or herpes infections, high blood pressure, high blood cholesterol, an underactive thyroid, or heart, kidney, or liver disease.

Type of Drug

Corticosteroids, Nasal (kor-tih-koe-STER-oids)

Brand Names

Generic Ingredient: Beclomethasone Dipropionate
Beconase AQ   Vancenase Pockethaler
Vancenase AQ

Generic Ingredient: Budesonide
Rhinocort Aqua

Generic Ingredient: Flunisolide Ⓖ
Nasalide   Nasarel

Generic Ingredient: Fluticasone Propionate
Flonase

Generic Ingredient: Mometasone Furoate Monohydrate
Nasonex

Generic Ingredient: Triamcinolone Acetonide
Nasacort AQ

Prescribed For

Rhinitis (nasal inflammation) associated with seasonal or chronic allergy and other causes; also used to prevent recurrence of nasal polyps.

General Information

Nasal corticosteroids are used to treat severe symptoms of seasonal allergy that have not responded to other drugs such as decongestants. They work by reducing inflammation of the mucous membranes that line the nasal passages, making it easier to breathe. These drugs may take several days to produce an effect. Some nasal corticosteroids are approved for both allergic and non-allergic rhinitis.

Cautions and Warnings

Do not use a nasal corticosteroid if you are **allergic** to any of its ingredients. Rarely, serious and life-threatening drug-sensitivity reactions have occurred.

Combining prednisone or another oral corticosteroid with a nasal corticosteroid may cause **pituitary gland suppression,** although nasal corticosteroids alone rarely cause this problem.

Use nasal corticosteroids with caution if you have **tuberculosis** or a serious **fungal, bacterial, or viral infection.**

Rarely, *Candida* **(yeast) infections** of the nose and throat develop.

During a period of severe **stress,** you may have to switch to an oral corticosteroid drug if the nasal form does not control your symptoms.

Possible Side Effects

▼ Most common: mild irritation of the nose, nasal passages, and throat; burning; stinging; dryness; and headache.

▼ Less common: light-headedness, nausea, nosebleed or bloody mucus, unusual nasal congestion,

---

Possible Side Effects *(continued)*

bronchial asthma, sneezing attacks, runny nose, throat discomfort, and loss of the sense of taste.

▼ Rare: ulcers of the nasal passages, watery eyes, sore throat, vomiting, hypersensitivity reactions (symptoms include itching, rash, swelling, bronchospasms, and breathing difficulties), nasal infection, wheezing, perforation of the wall between the nostrils, and increased eye pressure.

Very rarely, deaths caused by failure of the adrenal gland have occurred in people taking adrenal corticosteroid tablets or syrup who were switched to a nasal corticosteroid. This is a rare complication and usually results from stopping the liquid or tablets suddenly instead of gradually.

Drug Interactions

• Ephedrine, phenobarbital, and rifampin may decrease the effect of nasal corticosteroids.

• Use caution when combining ketoconazole with nasal corticosteroids.

Usual Dose

Beclomethasone
   Adult and Child (age 13 and over): 1 spray (42 mcg) in each nostril 2–4 times a day.
   Child (age 6–12): 1 spray (42 mcg) in each nostril 3 times a day.

Budesonide
   Adult and Child (age 6 and over): 2 sprays (64 mcg) in each nostril morning and evening, or 4 sprays in the morning.
   Child (under age 6): not recommended.

Flunisolide
   Adult and Child (age 15 and over): 2 sprays (50 mcg) in each nostril 2 times a day to start; may be increased up to 8 sprays a day in each nostril.
   Child (age 6–14): 1 spray (25 mcg) in each nostril 3 times a day, or 2 sprays in each nostril 2 times a day.

Fluticasone

Adult: 2 sprays (100 mcg) in each nostril once a day or divided in 2 doses, to start. Dosage may be reduced in half in a few days, if tolerated.

Child (age 4 and over): 1 spray (50 mcg) in each nostril once a day; may be increased to 2 sprays a day in each nostril, if needed.

Child (under age 4): not recommended.

Mometasone

Adult and Child (age 12 and over): 2 sprays (100 mcg) in each nostril once a day; may be increased to 4 sprays a day in each nostril.

Triamcinolone

Adult and Child (age 13 and over): 2 sprays (220 mcg) in each nostril once a day; may be increased to 4 sprays a day in each nostril.

Child (age 6–12): 1 (Nasacort AQ) or 2 (Nasacort) sprays in each nostril once a day; may be increased to 2 sprays a day in each nostril, if needed.

Child (under age 6): not recommended.

Overdosage

Serious adverse effects are unlikely after accidental ingestion. Excessive use of large amounts of nasal corticosteroids may cause overdose symptoms and require gradual discontinuation of the drug. Call your local poison control center or a hospital emergency room for more information.

Special Information

It may be necessary to clear your nasal passages with a nasal decongestant before using a nasal corticosteroid to allow it to reach the mucous membranes.

Some of these drugs take 10 to 14 days to start working. Beclomethasone, budesonide, and triamcinolone work faster, in 3 to 7 days; in some cases, triamcinolone and budesonide provide relief in 12 hours. Flunisolide may take up to 2 weeks. Do not use any of these drugs continuously for more than 3 weeks unless you have experienced a definite benefit.

If you are using more than one spray at a time, wait at least 1 minute between sprays.

Nasal corticosteroids may cause irritation and drying of mucous membranes in the nose. Call your doctor if this effect persists or if symptoms get worse.

Rarely, nasal *Candida* infections develop in people using a nasal corticosteroid. These infections may require treatment with an antifungal drug, as well as the discontinuance of the nasal corticosteroid.

People using a nasal corticosteroid to prevent the return of nasal polyps after surgery may experience nosebleeds because the drug can slow healing of the wound.

If you forget to administer a dose, do so as soon as you remember. If it is almost time for your next dose, skip the dose you forgot and continue with your regular schedule. Do not take a double dose.

Special Populations

Pregnancy/Breast-feeding

Taking large amounts of corticosteroids during pregnancy may slow fetal growth. While the small amount of drug absorbed into the blood after nasal application is unlikely to have any effect, consult your doctor before taking any corticosteroid if you are or might be pregnant.

Dexamethasone passes into breast milk. Nursing mothers who must use this drug should bottle-feed. It is not known if other nasal corticosteroids pass into breast milk, though oral corticosteroids do. Nursing mothers should be cautious about using any of these drugs.

Seniors

Seniors may use nasal corticosteroids without special restriction. Tell your doctor if you have bone or bowel disease, colitis, diabetes, glaucoma, fungal or herpes infections, high blood pressure, high blood cholesterol, an underactive thyroid, or heart, kidney, or liver disease.

Type of Drug

Corticosteroids, Oral (kor-tih-koe-STER-oids)

Brand Names

Generic Ingredient: Betamethasone
Celestone

Generic Ingredient: Budesonide
Entocort EC

Generic Ingredient: Cortisone Acetate Ⓖ
Cortone

Generic Ingredient: Dexamethasone Ⓖ

Decadron   Hexadrol
Dexameth   Mymethasone
Dexone

Generic Ingredient: Hydrocortisone Ⓖ

Colocort   Cortifoam
Cortef   Hydrocortone
Cortenema

Generic Ingredient: Methylprednisolone Ⓖ
Medrol

Generic Ingredient: Prednisolone Ⓖ

Orapred   Prelone
Pediapred Ⓢ Ⓐ

Generic Ingredient: Prednisone Ⓖ

Deltasone   Prednicen-M
Liquid Pred   Prednisone Intensol
Meticorten   Sterapred
Orasone   Sterapred DS
Panasol-S

Generic Ingredient: Triamcinolone Ⓖ

Aristocort   Kenacort
Atolone

Prescribed For

A wide variety of disorders from rash to cancer, including adrenal disease, adrenal hormone replacement, bursitis, arthritis, severe skin reactions including psoriasis and other rashes, severe or disabling allergies, asthma, drug or serum sickness, severe respiratory diseases including pneumonitis, blood disorders, gastrointestinal (GI) disease including ulcerative colitis and Crohn's disease, and inflammation of the nerves, heart, or other organs. Dexamethasone is also used to treat mountain sickness, vomiting, bronchial disease in premature babies, excessive hairiness, and hearing loss associated with bacterial meningitis. Prednisone is used to improve strength and function of some muscular dystrophy patients. Methylprednisolone is used to decrease mortality in some patients suffering from severe alcoholism and chronic active hepatitis.

General Information

Produced by the adrenal gland, natural corticosteroids are hormones that affect almost every body system. The major differences among corticosteroid drugs are potency and variation in secondary effects. Doctor preference and past experience with a corticosteroid usually determine which drug to prescribe for a specific disease.

Cautions and Warnings

If you are **allergic** to one corticosteroid, you are probably allergic to all corticosteroids and should avoid using them.

Corticosteroids may mask symptoms of an **infection**. Because these drugs compromise the immune system, new infections may occur during corticosteroid treatment; when this happens, a relatively minor infection that would respond to ordinary treatment can turn serious. Corticosteroids may impair immune response to **hepatitis B**, prolonging recovery. They may reactivate dormant **amebiasis** (an amoebic infection usually acquired in the tropics). Corticosteroids should not be taken if you have a **fungal blood infection,** because they can allow the infection to spread more easily. They should be used with caution by people with **tuberculosis**.

Long-term use of any corticosteroid may increase the risk of developing **cataracts, glaucoma,** or **eye infections,** especially viral or fungal.

When stopping a corticosteroid, dosage must be reduced gradually under a doctor's supervision—otherwise you may experience **adrenal gland failure**.

If you are taking large corticosteroid doses, you should not receive any **live virus vaccine** because corticosteroids interfere with the body's reaction to the vaccine.

Hydrocortisone and cortisone may lead to **high blood pressure**. Other corticosteroids are less likely to affect blood pressure.

Corticosteroids should be used with caution if you have severe **kidney disease**.

High-dose or long-term corticosteroid therapy may aggravate or worsen **stomach ulcers**. This may occur when total dosage reaches 1000 mg of prednisone, 150 mg of betamethasone or dexamethasone, 5000 mg of cortisone, 4000 mg of hydrocortisone, 1000 mg of prednisolone, or 800 mg of triamcinolone or methylprednisolone.

People who have recently stopped taking a corticosteroid and are going through a period of **stress** may need small doses of a rapid-acting corticosteroid, such as hydrocortisone to get them through this period. Call your doctor if you think you might be experiencing this kind of stress reaction.

Use corticosteroids with caution if you have had a recent **heart attack** or have **ulcerative colitis, heart failure, high blood pressure, blood-clotting tendencies, thrombophlebitis, osteoporosis, antibiotic-resistant infections, Cushing's disease, myasthenia gravis, metastatic cancer, diabetes, underactive thyroid disease, cirrhosis of the liver,** or **seizure disorders**.

Corticosteroid psychosis (symptoms include euphoria or feeling "high," delirium, sleeplessness, mood swings, personality changes, and severe depression) may develop in people taking dosages greater than 40 mg a day of prednisone. These symptoms may also develop with other corticosteroids taken in equivalent doses (see "Usual Dose" for relative equivalencies). Symptoms of corticosteroid psychosis usually develop within 15 to 30 days of beginning treatment. These symptoms may also be linked to other factors—women and those with a family history of psychosis are more at risk.

Corticosteroids can cause **loss of calcium,** which may result in bone fractures and aseptic necrosis of the femoral and humoral heads (a condition in which the large bones in the hip degenerate from loss of calcium).

Prednisone may aggravate **emotional instability**.

Corticosteroids do not cure multiple sclerosis (MS) or slow its progression, though they may speed recovery from attacks of the disease.

Corticosteroid products often contain **tartrazine dyes** and **sulfite preservatives**. Many people are allergic to these chemicals.

Possible Side Effects

▼ Most common: upset stomach, possibly leading to stomach or duodenal ulcer.

▼ Common: water retention, heart failure, potassium loss, muscle weakness, loss of muscle mass, slowed

---

Possible Side Effects *(continued)*

healing of wounds, black-and-blue marks, increased sweating, allergic rash, itching, convulsions, dizziness, and headache.

▼ Less common: irregular menstruation; slowed growth in children, particularly after lengthy periods of corticosteroid treatment; adrenal or pituitary gland suppression; diabetes; drug sensitivity or allergic reactions; blood clots; insomnia; weight gain; increased appetite; nausea; feeling unwell; euphoria; mood swings; personality changes; and severe depression.

Drug Interactions

- Tell your doctor if you are taking any oral anticoagulant (blood-thinning) drug. If you begin taking a corticosteroid, your anticoagulant dosage may have to be adjusted.
- Combining a corticosteroid and a diuretic such as hydrochlorothiazide may cause loss of blood potassium. Low blood potassium may increase the side effects of digitalis drugs.
- Oral contraceptives (the "pill"), estrogen, erythromycin, azithromycin, clarithromycin, and ketoconazole may increase the risk of corticosteroid side effects.
- Barbiturates, aminoglutethimide, phenytoin and other hydantoin anticonvulsants, rifampin, ephedrine, colestipol, and cholestyramine may reduce the effectiveness of corticosteroids.
- Corticosteroids may decrease the effects of aspirin and other salicylates, growth hormones, and isoniazid.
- Combining a corticosteroid and a theophylline drug may require a dosage adjustment of either or both drugs.
- Corticosteroids may interfere with laboratory tests. Tell your doctor if you are taking any of these drugs so that tests are properly analyzed.

Food Interactions

Take corticosteroids with food or a small amount of antacid to avoid stomach upset. If stomach upset continues, notify your doctor.

Usual Dose

Once-daily doses should be taken in the morning.

Betamethasone: starting dosage—0.6–7.2 mg a day. Maintenance dosage—0.6–7.2 mg a day.

Budesonide: 9 mg a day.

Cortisone: starting dosage—25–300 mg a day. Maintenance dosage—25–300 mg a day.

Dexamethasone: 0.75–9 mg a day. Daily dosage sometimes exceeds 9 mg. A temporary dosage increase may be necessary if you are experiencing emotional stress. In alternate-day therapy, twice the usual daily dose is taken every other day.

Hydrocortisone: 20–240 mg a day.

Methylprednisolone: starting dosage—4–48 mg or more a day. Maintenance dosage varies. A temporary dosage increase may be necessary if you are experiencing emotional stress. In alternate-day therapy, twice the usual daily dose is taken every other day.

Prednisone and Prednisolone: 5–60 mg a day. Daily dosage sometimes exceeds 60 mg. A temporary dosage increase may be necessary if you are experiencing emotional stress. In alternate-day therapy, twice the usual daily dose is taken every other day.

Equivalent doses: Using 5 mg of prednisone as the basis for comparison, equivalent doses of other corticosteroids are 0.6 mg–0.75 mg of betamethasone, 25 mg of cortisone, 0.75 mg of dexamethasone, 20 mg of hydrocortisone, 4 mg of methylprednisolone, 5 mg of prednisolone, and 4 mg of triamcinolone.

Overdosage

Symptoms of overdose are anxiety, depression or stimulation, stomach bleeding, increased blood sugar, high blood pressure, and water retention. The victim should be taken to a hospital emergency room immediately. ALWAYS bring the prescription bottle or container.

Special Information

Do not stop taking this medication without your doctor's knowledge. Suddenly stopping any corticosteroid drug may have severe consequences; the dosage must be gradually reduced by your doctor.

Call your doctor if you develop unusual weight gain, black or tarry stools, swelling of the feet or legs, muscle weakness, vomiting of blood, menstrual irregularity, prolonged sore throat, fever, cold or infection, appetite loss, nausea and vomiting, diarrhea, weight loss, weakness, dizziness, or low blood sugar.

If you take several doses a day and forget a dose, take the dose you forgot as soon as possible. If it is almost time for your next dose, skip the one you forgot and double the next dose. If you take 1 dose a day and forget a dose, skip the dose you forgot and continue with your regular schedule. Do not take a double dose.

If you take a corticosteroid every other day and forget a dose, take it immediately if you remember it in the morning of your regularly scheduled day. If it is much later in the day, skip the dose you forgot and take it the following morning, then go back to your regular schedule. Do not take a double dose.

Special Populations

Pregnancy/Breast-feeding

Studies have shown that long-term corticosteroid therapy at high dosages may cause birth defects, as may chronic corticosteroid use during the first 3 months of pregnancy. When this drug is considered crucial by your doctor, its potential benefits must be carefully weighed against its risks.

Corticosteroids taken by mouth may pass into breast milk. Most nursing mothers who must take a corticosteroid should bottle-feed, though low dosages of some of these drugs may be taken for short periods while breast-feeding. Consult your doctor.

Seniors

Seniors are more likely to develop high blood pressure while taking an oral corticosteroid. Older women are more susceptible to osteoporosis (a condition characterized by loss of bone mass due to depletion of minerals, especially calcium) associated with high dosages of oral corticosteriods. Lower dosages are just as effective in seniors and cause fewer side effects.

Type of Drug

Corticosteroids, Topical

(kor-tih-koe-STER-oids)

Brand Names

Generic Ingredient: Alclometasone Dipropionate
Aclovate

Generic Ingredient: Amcinonide G
Cyclocort

Generic Ingredient: Augmented Betamethasone Dipropionate G
Diprolene   Diprolene AF

Generic Ingredient: Betamethasone G

Alphatrex	Maxivate
Betaderm	Psorion Cream
Betatrex	Teladar
Beta-Val	Valisone
Dermabet	Valisone Reduced Strength
Diprosone	Valnac
Luxiq	

Generic Ingredient: Clobetasol Propionate G

Clobex	Olux
Cormax	Temovate
Embeline	Temovate E
Embeline E	

Generic Ingredient: Clocortolone Pivalate
Cloderm

Generic Ingredient: Desonide G
DesOwen   Tridesilon

Generic Ingredient: Desoximetasone G
Topicort   Topicort LP

Generic Ingredient: Dexamethasone G
Aeroseb-Dex   Decaspray
Decadron

Generic Ingredient: Diflorasone Diacetate G
Florone   Maxiflor
Florone E   Psorcon E

Generic Ingredient: Fluocinolone Acetonide G
Derma-Smoothe/FS   FS Shampoo
Fluonid   Synalar
Flurosyn   Synalar-HP

Generic Ingredient: Fluocinonide G
Fluonex   Lidex-E
Lidex

Generic Ingredient: Flurandrenolide
Cordran   Cordran Tape
Cordran SP

Generic Ingredient: Fluticasone Propionate
Cutivate

Generic Ingredient: Halcinonide
Halog   Halog-E

Generic Ingredient: Halobetasol Propionate
Ultravate

Generic Ingredient: Hydrocortisone G
1% HC   Delcort
Acticort 100   Dermacort
Ala-Cort   Dermol HC
Ala-Scalp   Dermolate
Analpram-HC   Dermtex HC with Aloe
Anucort-HC   Eldecort
Anumed HC   Epicort
Anusol-HC   Gynecort
Bactine Hydrocortisone   Hemril HC Uniserts
Cetacort   Hi-Cor 1.0
CortaGel   Hi-Cor 2.5
Cortaid with Aloe   Hycort
Cortaid Intensive Therapy   Hydrocort
Cort-Dome   HydroTex
Cortenema   Hytone
Cortifoam   LactiCare-HC
Cortizone-5   Lanacort-5
Cortizone-10   Lanacort-10
Cortril   Locoid

Generic Ingredient: Hydrocortisone [G]

Maximum Strength Cortaid
Maximum Strength Cortaid-
Faststick
Maximum Strength KeriCort-
10
NutracortPandel
Penecort
Pramoxine HC
Procort
Proctocort

Proctocream-HC
Proctofoam-HC
Scalpicin
S-T Cort
Stie-Cort
Synacort
Tegrin-HC
Texacort
T Scalp
Westcort

Generic Ingredient: Mometasone Furoate [G]

Elocon

Generic Ingredient: Prednicarbate

Dermatop

Dermatop E Emollient

Generic Ingredient: Triamcinolone Acetonide [G]

Aristocort
Aristocort A
Delta-Tritex
Flutex
Kenalog

Kenalog-H
Kenonel
Triacet
Triderm
Trymex

Prescribed For

Inflammation, itching, eczema, dermatitis, or other local skin problems; may also be used to treat psoriasis and severe diaper rash.

General Information

Topical corticosteroids do not cure the underlying cause of skin problems, but they can relieve symptoms of rash, itching, or inflammation by interfering with the body mechanisms that produce them. You should never use a topical corticosteroid without your doctor's knowledge because it could mask a symptom important in diagnosing your condition. Some generic versions of topical corticosteroids vary in potency from related brand-name forms. Ask your doctor or pharmacist which products are interchangeable.

Cautions and Warnings

Do not use a topical corticosteroid as the sole treatment for **bacterial and viral skin diseases** such as herpes, **fungal skin infections** such as athlete's foot, or **tuberculosis** of the skin. These drugs should not be used in the **ear** if the eardrum is perforated. Do not use these drugs if you are **allergic** to any component of the aerosol, cream, gel, lotion, ointment, or solution.

Rectal corticosteroid products should not be used if you have any serious **bowel condition,** including bowel perforation, obstruction, abscess, and systemic fungal infection.

The **rectal foam** is not expelled after it has been applied and may result in higher drug blood levels than those associated with rectal enema products. The risk of systemic (whole-body) side effects is greater when more of the drug enters the blood. If there is no improvement after 2 or 3 weeks of using a rectal corticosteroid, contact your doctor.

Using a topical corticosteroid around the eyes for prolonged periods may cause **cataracts** or **glaucoma.**

Children may be more susceptible to serious side effects from topical corticosteroids, especially if they are applied to large areas over long periods. Augmented betamethasone propionate, clobetasol, desoximetasone, fluticasone, and halobetasol are not recommended for use on children's skin.

Possible Side Effects

▼ Most common: burning, itching, irritation, acne, dry and cracking skin, skin tightening, secondary infection, and skin discoloration. These effects are more likely when the treated area is covered with an occlusive bandage (one that prevents contact with water and air).

Significant quantities of corticosteroids may be absorbed into the bloodstream if large amounts are used for long periods. This can result in systemic effects and may cause serious problems, particularly in people with liver disease.

Drug Interactions

None known.

Usual Dose

Cream, Ointment, Solution, and Aerosol: Apply a thin film to the skin 2–4 times a day.

Rectal Enema: 100 mg nightly for 21 days.

Rectal Foam: 1 applicator's worth, 1–2 times a day for 2–3 weeks.

Overdosage

Serious adverse effects are unlikely after accidental ingestion. Excessive use of large amounts of topical corticosteroids may cause overdose symptoms and require gradual discontinuation of the drug. Call your local poison control center or a hospital emergency room for more information.

Special Information

To prevent secondary infection, clean the skin before applying the drug. Apply a very thin film and rub in gently—effectiveness depends on contact area, not the thickness of the layer applied.

Do not wash, rub, or put clothing on the area until the medication has dried.

Topical corticosteroids have an additive effect: with continuous use, 1 or 2 applications a day may be as effective as 3 or more. Once the drug begins to take effect, your doctor may recommend reducing the dose to the minimum level needed to control the condition.

Flurandrenolide tape comes with specific directions for use; follow them carefully.

If your doctor instructs you to apply plastic wrap or any other occlusive dressing, follow directions carefully. These dressings can increase the penetration of the drug into your skin by as much as 10 times, which may be a crucial element in the medication's effectiveness. Occlusive dressings should not be used with augmented betamethasone, betamethasone propionate, clobetasol, halobetasol, or mometasone.

If you are using one of these products for diaper rash, do not use tight-fitting diapers or plastic pants, which can cause too much drug to be absorbed into the blood.

Your doctor may prescribe a specific form of the product with good reason. Do not change forms without your doctor's knowledge; a different form may not be as effective.

If you forget to administer a dose, do so as soon as you remember. If it is almost time for your next dose, skip the one you forgot and continue with your regular schedule. Do not administer a double dose.

Special Populations

Pregnancy/Breast-feeding

Corticosteroids applied to the skin in large amounts or for long periods of time may cause birth defects. When any of these drugs is considered crucial by your doctor, its potential benefits must be carefully weighed against its risks. Over-the-counter hydrocortisone products should not be used for more than a few days without your doctor's knowledge.

It is not known if topical corticosteroids pass into breast milk, though oral corticosteroids do. Nursing mothers who must use a topical corticosteroid should consider bottle-feeding. If you apply a corticosteroid to the nipple area, be sure to completely clean the area prior to nursing. Nursing mothers should never use clobetasol.

Seniors

Seniors are more susceptible to high blood pressure and osteoporosis (a condition characterized by loss of bone mass due to depletion of minerals, especially calcium) associated with large dosages. These effects are unlikely with topical corticosteroids unless a high-potency medication is used over a large area for an extended period.

Brand Name

Cortisporin Otic

Generic Ingredients

Hydrocortisone + Neomycin Sulfate + Polymyxin B Sulfate Ⓖ

Other Brand Names

AK-Spore H.C. Otic
AntibiOtic
Cortatrigen Ear Drops
Drotic
Ear-Eze

LazerSporin-C
Octicair
Otic-Care
Otic-Care
Otocort

Other Brand Names
Otomycin-HPN Otic   UAD
Pediotic

Type of Drug

Antibiotic-corticosteroid combination.

Prescribed For

Superficial ear infection, ear inflammation or itching, and other outer ear problems.

General Information

Cortisporin Otic contains a corticosteroid to reduce inflammation and 2 antibiotics to treat local ear infections. This combination can be quite useful for local ear problems because of its dual method of action and its relatively broad applicability.

Cautions and Warnings

Do not use this product if you are **sensitive** or **allergic** to any of its ingredients.

Cortisporin Otic is designed for use in the ear. It can be **very damaging if placed into the eye**.

Cortisporin Otic should not be used if you have a **perforated eardrum**.

Possible Side Effects

▼ Local irritation, such as itching or burning, may occur as a drug sensitivity or allergic reaction.

Drug Interactions

None known.

Usual Dose

3–4 drops in the affected ear 3–4 times a day. Treatment should not last beyond 10 days.

Overdosage

The amount of drug contained in each bottle is too small to cause serious problems. Call a hospital emergency room or your local poison control center for more information. If you seek treatment, ALWAYS bring the prescription bottle or container.

Special Information

Use only when prescribed by a physician. Overuse of this or similar products can result in the growth of new organisms, such as fungi. If new infections or problems appear, stop using the drug and contact your doctor.

Wash your hands, then hold the closed bottle in your hand for a few minutes to warm it to body temperature. Shake well for 10 seconds. For best results, drops should not be self-administered, but given by another person. The person receiving the drops should lie on his or her side with the affected ear facing upward. Fill the dropper and instill the required number of drops directly in the ear canal.

If the drops are being given to an infant, hold the earlobe down and back to allow the drops to run in. If the drops are being given to an older child or adult, hold the earlobe up and back to allow them to run in. Do not put the dropper into the ear or allow it to touch any part of the ear or bottle. Keep the ear tilted for about 2 minutes after the drops have been put in or insert a soft cotton plug, whichever is recommended by your doctor.

If you forget to administer a dose of Cortisporin Otic, do so as soon as you remember. If it is almost time for your next dose, skip the dose you forgot and continue with your regular schedule. Do not apply a double dose.

Special Populations

Pregnancy/Breast-feeding
Pregnant and breast-feeding women may use this product.

Seniors
Seniors may use this product without special restriction.

Brand Name
Cosopt

Generic Ingredients
Dorzolamide + Timolol

Type of Drug

Carbonic-anhydrase inhibitor and beta blocker combination.

Prescribed For

Open-angle glaucoma and ocular hypertension.

General Information

Cosopt contains 2 glaucoma drugs that work in different ways. It is intended for people whose glaucoma does not respond to either drug used alone. Small amounts of dorzolamide and timolol—the active ingredients in Cosopt—enter the bloodstream.

Cautions and Warnings

Do not use Cosopt if you are **sensitive** or **allergic** to either of its ingredients or cannot take sulfa drugs or beta blockers. Cosopt should not be used by people with bronchial **asthma**, severe **chronic obstructive pulmonary disease, slow heart rate** or **heart block, heart failure,** or who are in **shock**.

People with **diabetes** or an **overactive thyroid** should use Cosopt with caution since beta blockers can mask the signs of low blood sugar or hyperthyroidism.

Small amounts of both ingredients enter the bloodstream and can produce the same kinds of **systemic (whole-body) reactions** associated with larger dosages of either a sulfa drug or beta blocker. Stop using the drug at once and call your doctor if a serious reaction develops.

Beta blockers may have to be discontinued prior to **major surgery** because they can affect the heart's ability to respond normally. Some people taking a beta blocker experience severe reductions while undergoing general anesthesia.

Dorzolamide should not be used by people with **kidney disease** and has not been studied in people with **liver disease**.

People with a history of **severe allergic reactions** who take a beta blocker may be at increased risk of experiencing a reaction because the drug blocks part of the body's natural allergic response.

Timolol can worsen the muscle weakness that accompanies **myasthenia gravis.**

Possible Side Effects

▼ Most common: changes in sense of taste, especially bitterness or sourness; increased sensitivity to light; and a burning or stinging sensation in the eye.

▼ Common: eye redness, blurred vision, and eye irritation or itching.

▼ Less common: abdominal pain, back pain, eyelid inflammation, bronchitis, cloudy vision, eye discharge or swelling, conjunctivitis (pinkeye), corneal erosion, corneal staining, lens cloudiness, cough, dizziness, dry eye, upset stomach, drug particles in the eye, eye pain, tearing, eyelid scaling, eyelid pain or discomfort, sensation of something in the eye, headache, high blood pressure, influenza, lens discoloration, nausea, sore throat, cataracts, sinus irritation, respiratory infection, urinary infection, visual problems, and retinal detachment.

▼ Rare: slow heartbeat, heart failure, chest pain, stroke, depression, diarrhea, dry mouth, breathing difficulties, low blood pressure, heart attack, stuffy nose, rash, tingling in the hands or feet, kidney stones, and vomiting. Other rare side effects associated with oral dorzolamide or timolol may occur.

Drug Interactions

• If you use more than 1 eyedrop medication, separate doses of these drugs by at least 10 minutes.

• Cosopt can increase the effect of other carbonic-anhydrase inhibitors.

• Combining Cosopt with an oral beta blocker or another calcium antagonist may increase the risk of side effects, especially changes in heart rhythm and low blood pressure.

• Do not combine Cosopt and another beta-blocking eyedrop.

• Combining Cosopt and reserpine can lead to low blood pressure, slowing of heartbeat, and dizziness or fainting.

• Combining Cosopt with digitalis and a calcium antagonist, or with quinidine, can slow heartbeat.

Usual Dose

Adult: 1 drop in the affected eye 2 times daily.

Overdosage

Little is known about the effects of Cosopt overdose or accidental ingestion. Possible overdose symptoms include dizziness, headache, shortness of breath, slow heartbeat, breathing difficulties, heart attack, and nervous system effects. Call your local poison control center or a hospital emergency room for more information. If you seek treatment, ALWAYS bring the prescription bottle or container.

Special Information

Conjunctivitis and eyelid reactions can occur due to an allergic reaction or as the result of local irritation. If you experience either of these problems, stop using the drug and call your doctor so that your condition can be evaluated.

To prevent infection, do not allow the eyedropper to touch your fingers, eyelids, or any surface. Wait at least 10 minutes before using any other eyedrops.

Cosopt contains benzalkonium chloride (a preservative), which may be absorbed by soft contact lenses. Remove your soft contact lenses before using the eyedrops; you may put them back in 15 minutes after a dose.

If you forget a dose of Cosopt, take it as soon as you remember. If it is almost time for your next dose, skip the forgotten dose and continue with your regular schedule.

Store Cosopt away from sunlight.

Special Populations

Pregnancy/Breast-feeding

The safety of using Cosopt is not known. When this drug is considered crucial by your doctor, its potential benefits must be carefully weighed against its risks.

It is not known if dorzolamide passes into breast milk, though timolol does. Nursing mothers who must use Cosopt should bottle-feed.

Seniors

Seniors may use Cosopt without precaution.

Coumadin   see *Warfarin, page 1150*

Cozaar *see Angiotensin II Blockers, page 84*

Generic Name

Cromolyn (KROE-muh-lin) Ⓖ

Brand Names

Crolom	Intal
Cromoptic	Nasalcrom
Gastrocrom	Opticrom

The information in this profile also applies to the following drug:

Generic Ingredient: Nedocromil

Alocril	Tilade

Type of Drug

Allergy preventive and antiasthmatic.

Prescribed For

Prevention of severe allergy reactions, including asthma, runny nose, and mastocytosis; also prescribed for food allergies, eczema, dermatitis, chronic itching, and hay fever. It may be used to treat and prevent chronic inflammatory bowel disease. The eyedrops are used to treat conjunctivitis (pinkeye) and other eye irritations.

General Information

Unlike antihistamines, which work against histamine that has been released into the system, cromolyn sodium prevents allergy, asthma, and other conditions by stabilizing mast cells, a key component in any allergic reaction because they release histamine. Cromolyn prevents the release of histamine and other chemicals from mast cells. The drug works only in the areas to which it is applied; only 7% to 8% of an inhaled dose and 1% of a swallowed capsule is absorbed into the blood. Even the oral capsules, which one would normally expect to be absorbed into the blood, treat only gastrointestinal-tract allergies. Cromolyn products must be used on a regular basis to be effective in reducing the frequency and intensity of allergic reactions.

Cautions and Warnings

Cromolyn should never be used to treat an acute allergy attack. It is intended only to prevent or reduce the number of allergic attacks and their intensity. Once the proper dosage level has been established for you, reducing that level may result in a recurrence of attacks.

Rarely, people have experienced **severe allergic attacks** after taking cromolyn. People allergic to cromolyn should not take any product containing it.

People with **kidney or liver disease** require reduced dosage.

Cough or **bronchial spasm** may occasionally occur after the inhalation of a cromolyn dose. Severe bronchospasm is rare.

Cromolyn aerosol should be used with caution in people with **abnormal heart rhythm** or **diseased coronary blood vessels** because of a possible reaction to the propellants used in the product.

Possible Side Effects

▼ Most common: rash and itching. Capsules— headache and diarrhea. Most capsule side effects are minor and may be attributable to the underlying condition; a variety have been reported but cannot be tied conclusively to the drug.

▼ Less common: local irritation, including nasal stinging, sneezing, tearing, cough, and stuffy nose; urinary difficulty or frequency; dizziness; headache; joint swelling; muscle pain; a bad taste in the mouth; nosebleeds; abdominal pain; and nausea.

▼ Rare: severe drug reactions, consisting of coughing, difficulty in swallowing, hives, itching, breathing difficulties, or swelling of the eyelids, lips, or face.

Drug Interactions

None known.

Food Interactions

Inhaled or swallowed cromolyn products should not be mixed with any food, juice, or milk. The nasal and eye products may be taken without regard to food or meals.

Usual Dose

Inhaled Capsules or Solution

Adult and Child (age 2 and over): starting dose—20 mg 4 times a day. Children under age 5 may inhale cromolyn powder if their allergies are severe. The solution must be given with a power-operated nebulizer and face mask. Handheld nebulizers are not adequate. To prevent exercise asthma, 20 mg may be inhaled up to 1 hour before exercise.

Aerosol

Adult and Child (age 5 and over): up to 2 sprays 4 times a day, spaced equally throughout the day. To prevent exercise asthma, 2 puffs may be inhaled up to 1 hour before exercise.

Nasal Solution

Adult and Child (age 6 and over): 1 spray in each nostril 3–6 times a day at regular intervals. First blow your nose, and then inhale the spray.

Oral Capsules

Adult: 2 dissolved capsules a half hour before meals and at bedtime.

Child (age 2–12): 1 dissolved capsule (100 mg) 4 times a day a half hour before meals and at bedtime. Dosage may be increased to about 13–18 mg per lb. of body weight in 4 equal doses.

Child (under age 2): about 10 mg per lb. of body weight a day divided into 4 equal doses. This product is recommended in infants and young children only if absolutely necessary.

Eyedrops

Adult and Child (age 4 and over): 1–2 drops in each eye 4–6 times a day at regular intervals.

Overdosage

No action is necessary other than medical observation. Call your local poison control center or a hospital emergency room for more information.

Special Information

Cromolyn is taken to prevent or minimize severe allergic reactions. It is imperative that you take cromolyn products on a regular basis to provide equal protection throughout the day.

If you are taking cromolyn to prevent seasonal allergies, it is essential that you start taking the medication before you come into contact with the cause of the allergy and that you continue treatment while you are exposed to it.

Cromolyn oral capsules should be opened and their contents mixed with about 4 oz. of hot water. Stir until the powder completely dissolves and the solution is completely clear; then fill the rest of the glass with cold water. Drink the entire contents of the glass. Do not mix the solution with food, juice, or milk.

Do not wear soft contact lenses while using cromolyn eyedrops. The lenses may be replaced a few hours after you stop taking the drug. To prevent contamination, do not touch the applicator tip to any surface including the eyes.

Call your doctor if you develop wheezing, coughing, a severe drug reaction (see "Possible Side Effects"), rash, or any bothersome or persistent side effect.

Call your doctor if your symptoms do not improve or if they worsen.

If you forget to administer a dose, do so as soon as you remember and space the remaining daily dosage evenly throughout the day. Do not take a double dose.

Special Populations

Pregnancy/Breast-feeding
In animal studies, very large dosages of cromolyn administered by vein have affected the fetus, though no birth defects were reported. When this drug is considered crucial by your doctor, its potential benefits must be carefully weighed against its risks.

It is not known if cromolyn passes into breast milk. Nursing mothers who must use cromolyn should consider bottle-feeding.

Seniors
Older adults with reduced kidney or liver function may require lower dosages.

Generic Name

Cyclobenzaprine (sye-cloe-BEN-zuh-prene) Ⓖ

Brand Name

Flexeril

Type of Drug

Skeletal muscle relaxant.

Prescribed For

Serious muscle spasm and acute muscle pain; also used to treat fibrositis (muscular rheumatism).

General Information

Cyclobenzoprine hydrochloride is used to treat severe muscle spasms; it is prescribed as part of a coordinated program of rest, physical therapy, and other measures.

Cautions and Warnings

Do not take cyclobenzaprine if you are **allergic** to it. This drug should not be taken for several weeks following a **heart attack** or by people with **abnormal heart rhythms, heart failure, heart block** (disruption of the electrical impulses that control heart rate), or **hyperthyroidism** (overactive thyroid gland).

Cyclobenzaprine should be avoided by people with **urinary retention, glaucoma,** or **increased eye pressure.** This drug may increase the chances of **cavities** or **gum disease.**

Cyclobenzaprine is intended only for **short-term use** of 2 to 3 weeks.

Cyclobenzaprine is chemically similar to tricyclic antidepressants and may produce some of the more serious side effects associated with those drugs. Abruptly stopping cyclobenzaprine may cause **nausea, headache,** and **feelings of ill health;** this is not a sign of addiction.

Possible Side Effects

▼ Most common: dry mouth, drowsiness, and dizziness.

▼ Less common: muscle weakness, fatigue, nausea,

Possible Side Effects *(continued)*

---

constipation, upset stomach, unpleasant taste, blurred vision, headache, nervousness, and confusion.

▼ Rare: Rare side effects can occur in almost any part of the body. Contact your doctor if you experience any side effect not listed above.

Many other side effects have been reported by people taking cyclobenzaprine, but their relationship to the drug has not been established.

Drug Interactions

• The effects of alcohol, sedatives, or other nervous system depressants may be increased by cyclobenzaprine.

• Cyclobenzaprine may increase some side effects of atropine, ipratropium, and other anticholinergic drugs. These include blurred vision, constipation, urinary difficulties, dry mouth, confusion, and drowsiness.

• The combination of cyclobenzaprine and a monoamine oxidase inhibitor (MAOI) antidepressant may produce very high fever, convulsions, and possibly death. Do not take these drugs within 14 days of each other.

• Cyclobenzaprine may increase the effects of haloperidol, loxapine, molindone, pimozide, anticoagulant (blood-thinning) drugs, anticonvulsants, thyroid hormones, antithyroid drugs, phenothiazines, thioxanthenes, and nasal decongestants such as naphazoline, oxymetazoline, phenylephrine, and xylometazoline.

• Barbiturates and carbamazepine may counteract the effects of cyclobenzaprine.

• Fluoxetine, ranitidine, cimetidine, methylphenidate, estramustine, estrogens, and oral contraceptives may increase the effects and side effects of cyclobenzaprine.

• Cyclobenzaprine may counteract the effects of clonidine, guanadrel, and guanethidine.

Food Interactions

None known.

Usual Dose

Adult and Child (age 15 and over): 10 mg 3 times a day; may be increased up to 60 mg a day.

Child (under age 15): not recommended.

Overdosage

Cyclobenzaprine overdose may cause confusion, loss of concentration, hallucinations, agitation, overactive reflexes, fever or vomiting, rigid muscles, and other side effects of the drug. It may also cause drowsiness, low body temperature, rapid or irregular heartbeat and other kinds of abnormal heart rhythms, heart failure, dilated pupils, convulsions, very low blood pressure, stupor, coma, and sweating. Overdose victims must be taken to a hospital emergency room. ALWAYS bring the prescription bottle or container.

Special Information

Cyclobenzaprine causes drowsiness, dizziness, or blurred vision in more than 40% of people who take it, which may interfere with the ability to perform complex tasks like driving or operating equipment. Avoid alcohol, sedatives, and other nervous system depressants because they can enhance sedative effects of cyclobenzaprine.

Call your doctor if you develop rash; hives; itching; urinary difficulties; clumsiness; confusion; depression; convulsions; difficulty breathing; irregular heart rate; chest pain; fever; yellowing of the skin or whites of the eyes; swelling of the face, lips, or tongue; or any other persistent or bothersome side effect.

If you forget a dose of cyclobenzaprine, take it as soon as you remember. If you take cyclobenzaprine once a day and it is almost time for your next dose, skip the one you forgot and continue with your regular schedule. If you take cyclobenzaprine twice a day and it is almost time for your next dose, take 1 dose as soon as you remember, another in 5 or 6 hours, and then go back to your regular schedule. If you take cyclobenzaprine 3 times a day and it is almost time for your next dose, take 1 dose as soon as you remember, another in 3 or 4 hours, and then go back to your regular schedule. Never take a double dose.

Special Populations

Pregnancy/Breast-feeding

As with all drugs, cyclobenzaprine should be avoided by pregnant women unless the potential benefits clearly outweigh the risks.

It is not known if cyclobenzaprine passes into breast milk, but antidepressants with a similar chemical structure do pass into breast milk. Nursing mothers who must take this drug should consider bottle-feeding.

Seniors

Seniors are more likely to be sensitive to the effects of cyclobenzaprine.

Generic Name

Cyclosporine (sye-kloe-SPOR-in) [G]

Brand Names

Gengraf   Sandimmune
Neoral

Type of Drug

Immunosuppressant.

Prescribed For

Kidney, heart, or liver transplantation; also used for bone-marrow, heart-lung, and pancreas transplants; also prescribed for patchy hair loss, rheumatoid arthritis, aplastic anemia, atopic dermatitis, Behçet's disease, cirrhosis of the liver, ulcerative colitis, dermatomyositis, eye symptoms of Graves' disease, insulin-dependent diabetes, kidney inflammation, multiple sclerosis (MS), severe psoriasis and psoriasis-related arthritis, myasthenia gravis, pemphigus, sarcoidosis of the lung, and pyoderma gangrenosum.

General Information

Cyclosporine is used to prevent rejection of transplanted organs. It works by blocking the activity of T-cells, which protect the body against invading microorganisms or foreign substances. Cyclosporine also prevents the production of a substance known as interleukin-II that activates T-cells. In 1995, a new form of cyclosporine called Neoral, a microemulsion, was introduced by its manufacturer. This form is as safe and effective as the original product but is better absorbed into the bloodstream and requires less medication to achieve the same effect.

Cautions and Warnings

Cyclosporine should be prescribed only by doctors experienced in immunosuppressive therapy and the care of organ-transplant patients. Sandimmune is always used with corticosteroid drugs like prednisone. Neoral has been used with a corticosteroid and azathioprine, an immune suppressant. When combined with other immune suppressants, cyclosporine must be used with great care because oversuppression of the immune system may lead to **lymphoma** or extreme susceptibility to **infection**.

Sandimmune, the original oral form of cyclosporine, is poorly absorbed into the bloodstream; it must be taken in a dosage that is 3 times greater than the injectable dosage. People taking this drug by mouth for a long period of time should have their blood checked for **cyclosporine levels** so that the dosage may be adjusted if necessary. Since more Neoral is absorbed into the blood you will probably need less of it. Do not substitute Neoral for Sandimmune; they are not equivalent to each other.

Cyclosporine causes **kidney toxicosis** (kidney poisoning)—different from transplant rejection—in 25% to 35% of people taking it to prevent organ rejection. Mild symptoms usually start after about 2 or 3 months of treatment. Reducing drug dosage may control this effect. In one study, clonidine skin patches used before and after surgery decreased toxic risks to the kidney.

Liver toxicosis is seen in about 5% of transplant patients taking cyclosporine. It usually appears in the first month and may be controlled by reducing dosage.

Convulsions may develop, especially in people also taking high dosages of corticosteroids. Other nervous system side effects are listed below (see "Possible Side Effects").

Cyclosporine may cause **high blood-potassium or uric-acid levels**.

In one study, cyclosporine increased **cholesterol** and other blood-fat levels. It is not known how this affects people who take the drug on a long-term basis.

There is conflicting information on how cyclosporine affects blood sugar. Kidney-transplant patients taking the drug have developed **insulin-dependent diabetes,** which is related to the dosage of cyclosporine and reverses itself when you stop taking the drug. On the other hand, cyclosporine preserves the function of insulin-producing cells in the pancreas and has allowed many insulin-dependent diabetics to live without taking insulin.

Possible Side Effects

▼ Most common: Cyclosporine is known to be toxic to the kidneys. Your doctor will carefully monitor your kidney function while you are taking it. Other side effects are high blood pressure, increased hair growth, and enlargement of the gums. Lymphoma may develop in people whose immune systems are excessively suppressed. Almost 85% of people treated with cyclosporine develop an infection, compared with 94% of people on other immune-system suppressants.

▼ Less common: tremors, cramps, acne, brittle hair or fingernails, convulsions, headache, confusion, diarrhea, nausea or vomiting, tingling in the hands or feet, facial flushing, reduced white-blood-cell and platelet counts, sinus inflammation, swollen and painful male breasts, drug allergy (symptoms include rash, itching, hives, and breathing difficulties), conjunctivitis (pinkeye), fluid retention and swelling, ringing or buzzing in the ears, hearing loss, high blood sugar, and muscle pain.
retention and swelling, ringing or buzzing in the ears, hearing loss, high blood sugar, and muscle pain.

▼ Rare: blood in the urine, heart attack, itching, anxiety, depression, lethargy, weakness, mouth sores, difficulty swallowing, intestinal bleeding, constipation, pancreas inflammation, night sweats, chest pain, joint pain, visual disturbances, and weight loss.

Drug Interactions

• Cyclosporine should be used carefully with other kidney-toxic drugs including nonsteroidal anti-inflammatory drugs (NSAIDs) such as ibuprofen, naproxen, and others; gentamicin; tobramycin; vancomycin; trimethoprim-sulfamethoxazole; melphalan; amphotericin B; ketoconazole; azapropazon; diclofenac; cimetidine; ranitidine; and tacrolimus.

• Drugs that may increase blood levels of cyclosporine include calcium channel blockers, oral contraceptives, corticosteroids, foscarnet; amiodarone; diltiazem; nicardipine;

verapamil; fluconazole; itraconazole; clarithromycin; danazol; erythromycin; methyltestosterone; methylprednisolone—this combination also causes convulsions; allopurinol; bromocriptine; danazol; and metoclopramide. With ketoconazole, your doctor may use this drug interaction to reduce your cyclosporine dosage.

• Drugs that decrease cyclosporine levels and may lead to organ rejection include terbinafine, nafcillin, rifabutin, rifampin, carbamazepine, probucol, phenobarbital, and phenytoin.

• Cyclosporine interferes with the body's ability to clear digoxin, etoposide, prednisolone, and lovastatin. People taking any of these drugs who start on cyclosporine must have their drug dosage reduced.

• Combining colchicine and cyclosporine may lead to liver, kidney, stomach, and other side effects. Avoid this combination.

• Combining cyclosporine and nifedipine may lead to gum overgrowth.

• Cyclosporine increases blood potassium. Excessive blood-potassium levels may be reached if cyclosporine is taken with enalapril, lisinopril, a potassium-sparing diuretic such as spironolactone, salt substitutes, potassium supplements, or high potassium—low sodium—food.

• Cyclosporine prevents the normal body response to live vaccines. People taking cyclosporine should be vaccinated only after specific discussions with their doctors. You must wait for a period of several months to several years after stopping the medication before vaccination may be considered again.

Food Interactions

Cyclosporine may be taken with food if it upsets your stomach. For optimal effectiveness, avoid eating a fatty meal within half an hour of taking Neoral.

You may mix Neoral in a glass—not a paper or plastic cup—with room-temperature orange or apple juice or chocolate milk to make it taste better. DO NOT DRINK GRAPEFRUIT JUICE BECAUSE IT SPEEDS THE BREAKDOWN OF CYCLOSPORINE. Drink immediately after mixing, then put more juice or chocolate milk in the glass and drink it to be sure that the entire dose has been taken. Neoral should not be taken with unflavored milk because it may be unpalatable.

Usual Dose

In general, the usual dosage of Neoral is lower than Sandimmune, but dosage must be individualized for you by your doctor. Do not substitute one brand for the other.

Sandimmune

   Adult: The usual oral dosage of cyclosporine is 6–8 mg per lb. of body weight a day. The first dose is given 4–12 hours before the transplant operation or immediately after surgery. This dosage is continued after the operation for 1–2 weeks and then slowly reduced to 2.25–4.5 mg per lb. of body weight.

   Child: Similar dosages are usually prescribed, but because children tend to release the drug from their bodies faster than adults, larger and more frequent doses may be needed.

Neoral

   Adult: The usual oral dosage of Neoral is 3–4 mg per lb. of body weight a day divided into 2 doses. The first dose is given 4–12 hours before the transplant operation or immediately after surgery. This dosage is continued after the operation for 1–2 weeks and then slowly reduced to maintain a target amount of cyclosporine in the body. Dosage may vary according to the organ transplanted.

   Child: Similar dosages are usually prescribed but, because children tend to release the drug from their bodies faster than adults, larger and more frequent doses may be needed.

Overdosage

Overdose victims may be expected to develop side effects and symptoms of extreme immunosuppression. Induce vomiting with ipecac syrup—available at any pharmacy—which is recommended up to 2 hours after the overdose was taken. Call your doctor or local poison control center before inducing vomiting. If you must go to a hospital emergency room, ALWAYS bring the prescription bottle or container.

Special Information

Call your doctor at the first sign of fever; sore throat; tiredness; weakness; nervousness; unusual bleeding or bruising; tender or swollen gums; convulsions; irregular heartbeat; confusion; numbness or tingling of your hands, feet, or lips; breathing difficulties; severe stomach pain with nausea; or blood in the urine. Other side effects such as shaking or trembling of the hands, increased hair growth, acne, headache, leg cramps, nausea, or vomiting are less serious but should be brought to your doctor's attention, particularly if they are bothersome or persistent.

Maintain good dental hygiene while taking cyclosporine and use extra care when brushing and flossing because the drug increases your risk of oral infection. Cyclosporine may also cause swollen gums. See your dentist regularly.

Continue taking your medication as long as your doctor prescribes it. Do not stop taking it without your doctor's knowledge. If you cannot take one of the oral forms, cyclosporine can be given by injection.

Do not keep either brand of the oral liquid in the refrigerator. After the bottle is opened, use the medication within 2 months. At temperatures below 68°F, Neoral can form a gel and a light sediment can form in Sandimmune. These do not affect the potency of either product. They can still be used and are effective.

If you forget a dose, take it as soon as you remember if it is within 12 hours of your regular dose. If not, skip the dose you forgot and continue with your regular schedule. Do not take a double dose.

Special Populations

Pregnancy/Breast-feeding
In animal studies cyclosporine damages the fetus. Though a small number of pregnant women have taken cyclosporine without major problems, it is recommended that pregnant women avoid cyclosporine. When this drug is considered crucial by your doctor, its potential benefits must be carefully weighed against its risks.

Cyclosporine passes into breast milk. Nursing mothers who must take cyclosporine should bottle-feed.

Seniors
Due to decreased kidney function, seniors are more susceptible to kidney toxicosis.

Generic Name

Delavirdine (deh-LAV-er-dene)

Brand Name

Rescriptor

Type of Drug

Antiviral.

Prescribed For

Human immunodeficiency virus (HIV) infection, in combination with other antiviral drugs.

General Information

Delavirdine mesylate is a non-nucleoside reverse transcriptase inhibitor (NNRTI). Delavirdine inhibits the reverse transcriptase (RT) enzyme, necessary for reproduction of HIV in body cells, by binding directly to RT. If delavirdine is not taken with other antivirals, resistance to the drug may develop as soon as 8 weeks after treatment begins. For this reason, delavirdine is recommended only in combination with other anti-HIV drugs.

Delavirdine is broken down in the liver. Delavirdine inhibits the enzymes that break it down, so it actually stays in the body longer as treatment continues. Women reach 30% higher delavirdine blood levels than men.

Cautions and Warnings

Delavirdine **drug interactions may be serious or life threatening** (see "Drug Interactions").

Delavirdine is primarily broken down in the liver; people with **liver disease** should use it with caution. People taking delavirdine should have their liver enzymes measured periodically.

The chances of developing a drug **rash** while taking delavirdine are almost 1 in 5.

Anyone who develops a severe rash, rash with fever, blisters, mouth sores, eye irritation, swelling, or muscle or joint ache should stop taking delavirdine and call their doctor.

Possible Side Effects

▼ Most common: nausea and rash.

▼ Common: headache and tiredness.

▼ Less common: diarrhea, vomiting, liver irritation, and itching. Other less common side effects can occur in almost any part of the body. Contact your doctor if you experience any side effect not listed above.

Drug Interactions

Some delavirdine drug interactions, which occur because of delavirdine's effect on liver enzymes, are potentially life threatening.

• Anticonvulsants, rifabutin, and rifampin may reduce the amount of delavirdine in the blood.

• Antacids and didanosine may reduce the amount of delavirdine in the blood by interfering with its absorption in the blood; take these drugs and delavirdine at least 1 hour apart.

• When delavirdine and clarithromycin are combined, the amount of either drug in the blood may be doubled.

• Delavirdine interferes with the breakdown of protease inhibitors. A protease inhibitor dosage reduction may be needed.

• Fluoxetine and ketoconazole increase the amount of delavirdine in the blood by about 50%.

• Cimetidine, ranitidine, and similar drugs may reduce the amount of delavirdine absorbed. Do not combine these drugs with delavirdine for any length of time.

• Delavirdine may increase the amount of certain calcium channel blockers or sildenafil in the blood. Do not take more than a single 25 mg dose of sildenafil in a 48-hour period when taking delavirdine.

• Do not take delavirdine with certain antimicrobials, including dapsone and rifabutin; benzodiazepine tranquilizers and sleeping medication; ergot drugs; quinidine; and warfarin.

Food Interactions

This drug may be taken with or without food.

Usual Dose

Adult: 400 mg 3 times a day.

Overdosage

Little is known about the effects of delavirdine overdose. Overdose victims should be taken to a hospital emergency room for treatment. ALWAYS bring the prescription bottle or container.

Special Information

Delavirdine solution is somewhat better absorbed than the tablets. The amount of drug absorbed from delavirdine tablets can be increased by allowing the 100 mg tablet to disintegrate in water and then swallowing the mixture. 200 mg tablets do not dissolve in water.

People with achlorhydria (absence of stomach acid) should take delavirdine with an acidic drink, such as orange or cranberry juice.

Delavirdine does not cure HIV. It will not prevent you from transmitting the HIV virus to another person; you must still practice safe sex. People taking delavirdine for HIV can still develop HIV-related conditions. The long-term effects of delavirdine are not known. People taking this drug should be under a doctor's care at all times.

If you develop a severe rash, or rash with fever, blisters, mouth sores, eye irritation, swelling, or muscle or joint ache, stop taking delavirdine and see your doctor.

Take the medication every day exactly as prescribed. It is important to follow your doctor's directions and not miss doses. If you forget to take a dose of delavirdine, take it as soon as you remember. If it is almost time for your next dose, skip the dose you forgot and continue with your regular schedule. Do not take a double dose.

Special Populations

Pregnancy/Breast-feeding

Delavirdine causes birth defects in laboratory animals. Of 7 unplanned pregnancies reported in delavirdine studies, 3 women had ectopic pregnancies, 3 had normal, healthy babies, and one baby was born prematurely with a heart valve defect. However, there are no specific studies of delavirdine in pregnant women. This drug should not be taken unless you have discussed the possible benefits and risks with your doctor.

Delavirdine passes into breast milk in concentrations that are 3 to 5 times the concentrations found in the mother's blood and should not be taken by nursing mothers. In any case, mothers who are HIV positive should bottle-feed their babies to avoid transmitting the virus through their milk.

Seniors
Seniors may take delavirdine without special precaution.

Depakote   see Valproic Acid, page 1139

Generic Name

Desmopressin (dez-moe-PRES-in) Ⓖ

Brand Names

Concentraid	Minirin
DDAVP	Stimate

Type of Drug

Pituitary hormone replacement.

Prescribed For

Nighttime bed-wetting and diabetes insipidus (central or cranial diabetes); also used to control bleeding in certain forms of hemophilia A and von Willebrand's disease.

General Information

Desmopressin is a synthetic version of antidiuretic hormone (ADH). When ADH is lacking, the body has difficulty retaining fluid. People lacking ADH experience excessive thirst, increased urination, and dehydration; desmopressin controls these symptoms. When used for nighttime bed-wetting, desmopressin should be used in conjunction with behavioral or other non-drug therapies.

Cautions and Warnings

People **allergic** to desmopressin should not take this drug.

People, especially children and seniors and people with **cystic fibrosis** and **electrolyte imbalances,** should only drink enough fluid to satisfy their thirst while taking desmopressin because of the risk of water intoxication, which can result in seizures. People with **coronary artery disease, heart disease,** or **high blood pressure** should use this drug with caution.

Heart attacks and **strokes** after treatment with desmopressin have been reported in people at risk for them, but there is no definite link to desmopressin use.

People using desmopressin should have their urine checked regularly by their doctor. Your doctor should also check for nasal swelling, congestion, and scarring.

Possible Side Effects

▼ Rare: slight increases in blood pressure, loss of sodium, water intoxication (symptoms include coma, confusion, drowsiness, continuing headache, decreased urination, rapid weight gain, and seizures), edema, stomach or abdominal cramps, nausea, redness or flushing of the skin, passing headaches, vulvar pain, and stuffy or runny nose.

Drug Interactions

• Desmopressin may increase the effects of other drugs that raise blood pressure. This only happens with large dosages.

• Chlorpropamide and carbamazepine may increase the effects of desmopressin.

Food Interactions

None known.

Usual Dose

Nasal Solution—Nighttime Bed-Wetting
   Adult and Child (age 6 and over): 20 mcg (0.2 ml) at bedtime.

Nasal Solution—Diabetes Insipidus
   Adult: 0.1–0.4 ml a day in 1–3 doses.

Child (age 3 months–12 years): 0.05–0.3 ml a day in 1–2 doses.

Tablets—Diabetes Insipidus
   Adult: Begin with 0.05 mg 2 times a day. Daily dosage should be increased according to individual need, up to 1.2 mg a day divided into 2–3 doses.
   Child: Begin with 0.05 mg and adjust according to individual need.

Overdosage

Symptoms include headache, difficulty breathing, abdominal cramps, nausea, and facial flushing. Call your doctor or a hospital emergency room if you suspect an overdose. Because there is no known antidote to desmopressin, your dosage may be temporarily reduced until overdose symptoms subside. If you seek treatment, ALWAYS bring the prescription bottle or container.

Special Information

Call your doctor if you develop headache, breathing difficulties, heartburn, nausea, abdominal or stomach cramps, or vulvar pain.

   The Stimate Nasal Solution spray pump and Minirin spray must be primed before its first use. To prime the pump, press down 4 times. Stimate delivers 25 doses per bottle. Throw away the bottle after 25 doses have been used, because anything remaining after the 25th dose is likely to deliver less drug than is needed.

   If you forget a dose of desmopressin, take it as soon as you remember. If you don't remember until your next dose, skip the forgotten dose and continue with your regular schedule.

Special Populations

Pregnancy/Breast-feeding
The safety of using desmopressin during pregnancy is not known, though it has been used to treat diabetes insipidus in pregnant women without apparent harm to the fetus. When this drug is considered crucial by your doctor, its potential benefits must be carefully weighed against its risks.

   Desmopressin may pass into breast milk. Nursing mothers who must use this drug should consider bottle-feeding.

Seniors

Seniors should avoid drinking too much fluid while taking desmopressin.

Detrol LA *see Tolterodine, page 1082*

Generic Name

Diazepam (dye-AZ-uh-pam) Ⓖ

Brand Names

Diastat	Valium
Diazepam Intensol	Valrelease

The information in this profile also applies to the following drugs:

Generic Ingredient: Halazepam
Paxipam

Generic Ingredient: Lorazepam Ⓖ

Ativan	Lorazepam Intensol

Generic Ingredient: Oxazepam Ⓖ
Serax

Generic Ingredient: Prazepam Ⓖ
Centrax

Type of Drug

Benzodiazepine tranquilizer.

Prescribed For

Anxiety, tension, fatigue, agitation (particularly due to alcohol withdrawal), muscle spasm, and seizures; also prescribed for irritable bowel syndrome and panic attacks.

General Information

Diazepam and other benzodiazepines directly affect the brain. They can relax you and make you more tranquil or sleepy, or they can slow nervous system transmissions in such a way as to act as an anticonvulsant.

Cautions and Warnings

Do not take diazepam if you know you are **sensitive** or **allergic** to it or to another benzodiazepine drug, including clonazepam.

Diazepam can aggravate narrow-angle **glaucoma,** but you may take it if you have open-angle glaucoma.

Other conditions in which diazepam should be avoided are severe **depression,** severe **lung disease, sleep apnea** (intermittent cessation of breathing during sleep), **liver disease, drunkenness,** and **kidney disease**. In all of these conditions, the depressive effects of diazepam may be enhanced or could be detrimental to your overall condition.

Diazepam should not be taken by **psychotic patients**. It is not effective for them and can trigger unusual excitement, stimulation, and rage.

Diazepam is not intended for more than 3 to 4 months of continuous use. Your condition should be reassessed before continuing your medication beyond that time.

Diazepam may be **addictive**. Drug withdrawal may develop if you stop taking it after only 4 weeks of regular use but is more likely after longer use. It may start with anxiety and progress to tingling in the hands or feet, sensitivity to bright light, sleep disturbances, cramps, tremors, muscle tension or twitching, poor concentration, flu symptoms, fatigue, appetite loss, sweating, and changes in mental state.

Possible Side Effects

▼ Most common: mild drowsiness during the first few days of therapy. Weakness and confusion may occur, especially in seniors and in those who are sickly. If these effects persist, contact your doctor.

▼ Less common: depression, lethargy, disorientation, headache, inactivity, slurred speech, stupor, dizziness, tremors, constipation, dry mouth, nausea, inability to control urination, sexual difficulties, irregular menstrual cycle, changes in heart rhythm, low blood pressure, fluid retention, blurred or double vision, itching, rash, hiccups, nervousness, hysteria, psychosis, inability to fall asleep, and occasional liver dysfunction. If you have any

---

Possible Side Effects *(continued)*

of these symptoms, stop taking the drug and contact your doctor at once.

▼ Rare: Rare side effects can affect your heart, stomach and intestines, urinary tract, blood, muscles, and joints. Contact your doctor if you experience any side effect not listed above.

Drug Interactions

• Diazepam is a central-nervous-system depressant. Avoid alcohol, other tranquilizers, narcotics, barbiturates, monoamine oxidase inhibitors (MAOIs), antihistamines, and antidepressants. Taking diazepam with these drugs may lead to excessive depression, drowsiness, or difficulty breathing.

• Smoking may reduce diazepam's effectiveness by increasing the rate at which it is broken down by the body.

• Effects of diazepam may be prolonged when taken with cimetidine, oral contraceptives, disulfiram, fluoxetine, isoniazid, ketoconazole, rifampin, metoprolol, probenecid, propoxyphene, propranolol, and valproic acid.

• Theophylline may reduce the sedative effects of diazepam.

• If you take antacids, separate them from your diazepam dose by at least 1 hour to prevent them from interfering with the passage of diazepam into the bloodstream.

• Diazepam may increase blood levels of digoxin and the chances for digoxin toxicity.

• Levodopa's effects may be decreased if it is taken with diazepam.

• Combining diazepam and phenytoin may increase phenytoin blood concentrations and the risk of phenytoin toxicity.

Food Interactions

Diazepam is best taken on an empty stomach, but it may be taken with food if it upsets your stomach.

Usual Dose

Solution or Tablets

Adult: 4–40 mg a day. Dosage must be adjusted to individual response for maximum effect. In seniors, less of the drug is usually required to control tension and anxiety.

Child (6 months and over): 1–2.5 mg 3 or 4 times a day; more may be needed to control anxiety and tension.

Child (under 6 months): not recommended.

Rectal Gel

Adult and Child (age 12 and over): 0.09 mg per lb. of body weight. Approximate dosage: 5 mg if 31–60 lbs., 10 mg if 61–110 lbs., 15 mg if 111–165 lbs., or 20 mg if 166–244 lbs.

Child (age 6–11): 0.14 mg per lb. of body weight. Approximate dosage: 5 mg if 22–40 lbs., 10 mg if 41–82 lbs., 15 mg if 83–121 lbs., or 20 mg if 122–163 lbs.

Child (age 2–5): 0.23 mg per lb. of body weight. Approximate dosage: 5 mg if 13–24 lbs., 10 mg if 25–49 lbs., 15 mg if 50–73 lbs., or 20 mg if 74–97 lbs.

An extra 2.5 mg of the rectal gel may be given if a more precise dosage is needed or as a partial replacement for people who do not retain the full dosage after it is first inserted rectally.

Overdosage

Symptoms of overdose include confusion, sleepiness, poor coordination, lack of response to pain, loss of reflexes, shallow breathing, low blood pressure, and coma. The victim should be taken to a hospital emergency room. ALWAYS bring the prescription bottle or container.

Special Information

Diazepam can cause tiredness, drowsiness, inability to concentrate, or similar symptoms. Be careful if you are driving, operating machinery, or performing other activities that require concentration.

People taking diazepam for more than 3 or 4 months at a time may develop drug withdrawal reactions if the medication is stopped suddenly (see "Cautions and Warnings").

If you forget a dose of diazepam, take it as soon as you remember. If it is almost time for your next dose, skip the one you forgot and continue with your regular schedule. Do not take a double dose.

Special Populations

Pregnancy/Breast-feeding

Diazepam may cause birth defects if taken during the first 3 months of pregnancy. Avoid taking any benzodiazepine if you are or might be pregnant.

Diazepam may pass into breast milk. Nursing mothers who must take this drug should bottle-feed.

Seniors

Seniors, especially those with liver or kidney disease, are more sensitive to the effects of diazepam and generally require smaller doses to achieve the same effect.

Generic Name

Dicyclomine (dih-SYE-kloe-meen) Ⓖ

Brand Names

Bemote	Byclomine
Bentyl	Di-Spaz

Type of Drug

Antispasmodic and anticholinergic.

Prescribed For

Irritable bowel, spastic colon, and similar digestive problems.

General Information

Dicyclomine hydrochloride has been used for many years to calm "nervous stomach." It and other anticholinergics work by blocking the effects of the neurohormone acetylcholine in the gastrointestinal (GI) tract. This reduces the mobility of the GI tract and slows the production of enzymes and other secretions.

Cautions and Warnings

Do not take dicyclomine if you are **allergic** to it.

This drug should be used with caution if you have **heart disease, Down's syndrome, spastic paralysis, reduced mobility of the stomach and lower esophagus, fever, stomach obstruction, glaucoma, urinary difficulties, acute bleeding, hiatal hernia, intestinal paralysis, myasthenia gravis, kidney or liver disease, rapid heartbeat, hyperthyroidism (overactive thyroid gland), high blood pressure,** or **ulcerative colitis.**

Dicyclomine reduces your ability to sweat and may lead to **heat exhaustion** and **heatstroke,** which can be life-threatening.

Avoid extended heavy exercise and limit your exposure to high temperatures.

Anticholinergenic **psychosis** has been reported by those taking anticholinergics, but it usually resolves after discontinuation of the drug.

Possible Side Effects

▼ Common: constipation, decreased sweating, and dry mouth, throat, or skin.

▼ Less common: reduced breast-milk flow, difficulty swallowing, blurred vision, and sensitivity to bright light.

▼ Rare: drug allergy (symptoms include rash, itching, hives, and breathing difficulties), confusion, eye pain, dizziness when rising quickly from a sitting or lying position, a bloated feeling, difficult or painful urination, drowsiness, unusual tiredness or weakness, headache, memory loss, and nausea or vomiting.

Drug Interactions

• Antacids containing calcium or magnesium, citrates, sodium bicarbonate, and carbonic-anhydrase inhibitor drugs may increase dicyclomine's therapeutic effect and side effects.

• Combining dicyclomine with other anticholinergic drugs including atropine, belladonna, clidinium, glycopyrrolate, hyoscyamine, isopropamide, propantheline, and scopolamine may intensify side effects.

• Dicyclomine may reduce stomach acidity and blood levels of oral ketoconazole (an antifungal).

• Dicyclomine may counteract the effect of metoclopramide in reducing nausea and vomiting.

• Taking dicyclomine with a narcotic pain reliever may cause severe constipation.

• Taking this or any drug that slows the movement of stomach and intestinal muscles with a potassium chloride supplement—especially one in wax-matrix tablet form—may lead to excessive irritation of the stomach.

• Combining dicyclomine and the antiviral amantadine may increase dicyclomine side effects.

• Dicyclomine may increase the effects of atenolol and digoxin.

• Phenothiazine drugs and tricyclic antidepressants may increase side effects of dicyclomine. The effectiveness of phenothiazines to control psychotic symptoms may be decreased.

Food Interactions

Take dicyclomine on an empty stomach, a half hour before or 2 hours after a meal.

Usual Dose

Adult: 80–160 mg a day. Seniors should receive the lowest possible dosage and increase only as needed.

Child (age 2 and over): 5–10 mg 3–4 times a day.

Child (age 6 months–2 years): 5–10 mg of syrup 3–4 times a day.

Child (under 6 months): not recommended.

Overdosage

Symptoms include blurred vision; clumsiness; confusion; breathing difficulties; dizziness; drowsiness; dry mouth, nose, or throat; rapid heartbeat; fever; hallucinations; weakness; slurred speech; excitement, restlessness, or irritability; warmth; and dry or flushed skin. Take the victim to a hospital emergency room at once. ALWAYS bring the prescription bottle or container.

Special Information

Children taking dicyclomine may be more likely to develop high body temperature in hot weather and other side effects and should be carefully watched for side effects.

Call your doctor if you develop diarrhea, rash, flushing, eye pain, dry mouth, urinary difficulties, constipation, increased sensitivity to light, or any bothersome or persistent side effect.

Brush and floss your teeth regularly while taking this drug. Because dicyclomine may cause dry mouth, you may be more likely to develop cavities or other dental problems. Ice or hard candy may relieve dry mouth.

Constipation may be treated by using a laxative.

Dicyclomine may make you drowsy or tired and cause blurred vision. Be careful when driving or doing any task that requires concentration.

If you forget a dose, take it as soon as you remember. If it is almost time for your next dose, skip the dose you forgot and continue with your regular schedule. Do not take a double dose.

Special Populations

Pregnancy/Breast-feeding

A few cases of human malformation were linked to dicyclomine, but studies have shown that the drug has no effect on the fetus. When this drug is considered crucial by your doctor, its potential benefits must be carefully weighed against its risks.

Dicyclomine can reduce the amount of milk produced. Infants given dicyclomine may faint, go limp, and develop breathing problems and seizures. Nursing mothers who must take this drug should bottle-feed.

Seniors

Seniors may be more susceptible to side effects, especially memory loss, changes in mental state, and glaucoma. Seniors may obtain maximum benefit with smaller dosages.

Generic Name

Didanosine (dye-DAN-oe-zene)

Brand Name

Videx   Videx EC

Type of Drug

Antiviral.

Prescribed For

Acquired immunodeficiency syndrome (AIDS).

General Information

Didanosine interferes with the human immunodeficiency virus (HIV) that causes AIDS by interrupting the internal DNA manufacturing process essential to the reproduction of HIV. Didanosine is an important part of the multi-drug cocktail approach to treating HIV/AIDS. It is usually one of the first drugs prescribed for people with HIV/AIDS.

Cautions and Warnings

Do not take didanosine if you are **allergic** to it or any ingredient in the didanosine tablet.

The most serious—and potentially fatal—side effects of didanosine are nervous system inflammation and inflammation of the pancreas.

Up to 50% of patients who take didanosine experience symptoms of **nervous system inflammation** and about 33% need to reduce their dosage to control these symptoms. Symptoms generally manifest as numbness, tingling, and pain in the hands and feet. People who already have these signs of nerve damage should not take didanosine.

Potentially fatal **inflammation of the pancreas** has occurred in up to 3% of people taking didanosine. Of people with a history of pancreatic inflammation who take didanosine, 33% are likely to develop this problem again. Symptoms of inflammation of the pancreas include major changes in blood-sugar levels, increased triglyceride blood levels, a drop in blood calcium, nausea, vomiting, and abdominal pain. People who develop pancreatic inflammation must stop taking didanosine.

Lactic acidosis and **enlargement of the liver** have been reported with didanosine.

Liver failure may develop in people taking this drug; 15% to 20% will begin to test abnormally for liver function. A small number of these patients may develop fatal liver disease.

Four children taking didanosine developed **severe eye disease,** resulting in some loss of sight. The progress of the eye disease slowed or stopped when dosage was reduced. Children taking this drug should have an eye examination every 6 months or if vision starts to worsen.

Kidney and liver disease may interfere with the elimination of didanosine from the body. Reduced doses may be required to accommodate these conditions.

Possible Side Effects

▼ Most common: diarrhea, nervous system inflammation, fever, chills, itching, rash, abdominal pain, weakness, headache, nausea, vomiting, infection, pneumonia, and pancreatic inflammation.

Possible Side Effects (continued)

▼ Less common: tumors, muscle pain, appetite loss, dry mouth, convulsions, abnormal thought patterns, breathing difficulties, drug allergy, anxiety, nervousness, twitching, confusion, depression, and blood component abnormalities.

▼ Rare: Rare side effects can occur in almost any part of the body. Contact your doctor if you experience any side effect not listed above.

Almost all children who take didanosine experience side effects. They are likely to experience many of the same reactions as adults, most commonly chills, fever, weakness, appetite loss, nausea and vomiting, diarrhea, liver dysfunction, headache, nervousness, sleeplessness, cough, runny nose, asthma or breathing difficulties, rash, and skin problems.

Drug Interactions

• Other drugs that may cause inflammation of the nervous system such as chloramphenicol, cisplatin, dapsone, disulfiram, ethionamide, glutethimide, gold, hydralazine, isoniazid, metronidazole, nitrofurantoin, ribavirin, and vincristine should be avoided while you are taking didanosine.

• Use extreme caution when combining didanosine with stavudine in pregnant women, as fatal lactic acidosis has been reported with this combination.

• Didanosine should not be taken with zalcitabine.

• Drugs that may cause inflammation of the pancreas, including intravenous pentamidine, should not be taken with didanosine.

• The use of allopurinol with didanosine is not recommended.

• Quinolone anti-infectives, tetracycline antibiotics, and other drugs whose absorption into the bloodstream may be affected by antacids should not be taken within 2 hours of taking didanosine because of its high magnesium and aluminum content.

Food Interactions

Food may prevent the absorption of a dose of didanosine by up to 50%. Take didanosine on an empty stomach.

Usual Dose

Adult: 250–400 mg a day (tablets); 167–250 mg every 12 hours (powder).
Child: 50–250 mg a day, based on weight and height.

Dosage should be adjusted to the level of kidney and liver function.

Overdosage

Didanosine overdose will cause many of the drug's usual side effects, especially inflammation of the nervous system or pancreas, diarrhea, and liver failure. Overdose victims should be taken to a hospital emergency room for testing and monitoring. ALWAYS remember to bring the prescription bottle or container.

Special Information

Didanosine does not cure AIDS. It will not prevent you from transmitting the HIV virus to another person; you must still practice safe sex. People may still develop AIDS-related opportunistic infections while taking this drug.

Didanosine may affect components of the blood system. Your doctor should perform blood tests to check for any changes.

People taking didanosine should take good care of their teeth and gums to minimize the possibility of oral infections.

Call your doctor if you develop any of the following symptoms of didanosine toxicity: numbness and pain in the hands and feet, nausea, vomiting, or abdominal pain.

If you are taking didanosine in chewable tablets, be sure to thoroughly chew each tablet. You may also completely dissolve the tablets in about ¼ cup of water and drink the entire mixture immediately. Do not mix didanosine tablets with juice or any other acidic drink.

If you are using the powdered form of didanosine, make a solution by pouring the entire contents of a packet into ½ cup of water. Stir until dissolved and drink immediately. Do not mix didanosine powder with juice or any other acidic drink. For children, your pharmacist will prepare a mixture of 10 mg per ml of didanosine and an equal amount of Mylanta Double Strength Antacid or Maalox TC Antacid. This mixture must be stored in a refrigerator and can be kept for 30 days. Shake well before using. Spilled didanosine should be cleaned immediately to prevent accidental poisoning.

If you forget to take a dose of didanosine, take it as soon as you remember. If it is almost time for your next dose, allow 4 to 8 hours to pass between the dose you took late and your next dose, and then continue with your regular schedule. Call your doctor for more specific advice if you forget to take several doses.

Special Populations

Pregnancy/Breast-feeding

Didanosine was slightly toxic to pregnant animals receiving doses 12 times human levels. There are no studies of pregnant women taking this drug; however, women who are or might become pregnant should only take didanosine if absolutely necessary and should use effective contraception to avoid passing on the virus.

It is not known if didanosine passes into breast milk. In any case, mothers who are HIV positive should bottle-feed their babies to avoid transmitting the virus through their milk.

Seniors

People with reduced kidney or liver function—common in seniors—should receive smaller dosages of didanosine than those with normal function.

Diflucan see *Triazole Antifungals,* page 1107

Generic Name

Digoxin (dih-JOX-in) Ⓖ

Brand Names

Digitek   Lanoxin
Lanoxicaps

Type of Drug

Cardiac glycoside.

Prescribed For

Congestive heart failure (CHF) and other heart conditions involving a very rapid heartbeat.

General Information

Digoxin works directly on heart muscle. It improves the heart's pumping ability or helps to control its beating rhythm. People with heart failure often develop swelling of the lower legs, feet, and ankles; digoxin improves these symptoms by improving blood circulation. Digoxin is generally used as part of the lifelong treatment of CHF.

Cautions and Warnings

Do not use digoxin if you are **allergic** or **sensitive** to it. Digoxin allergies are rare.

Digoxin should not be used in people with **ventricular fibrillation**.

Digoxin has been used to treat obesity. The risk of fatal heart rhythms associated with such treatment makes it extremely **dangerous as weight-loss medication**. Many **heart disease symptoms** may be associated with digoxin. Report any unusual side effects to your doctor at once. **Kidney disease** may increase blood levels of digoxin. Your dosage may need adjustment.

Long-term use of a digoxin may cause the body to lose **potassium**, especially since it is generally used in combination with diuretics (agents that increase urination). For this reason, be sure to eat a balanced diet and high-potassium foods—bananas, citrus fruits, melons, and tomatoes.

Digoxin should be used with caution in people with **electrolyte disorders**.

Digoxin requirements vary with **thyroid status**. If you are taking digoxin and your thyroid status changes, your doctor will have to alter your digoxin dosage.

Possible Side Effects

Adults and Seniors

▼ Most common: appetite loss, nausea, vomiting, diarrhea, and blurred or disturbed vision. If you experience any of these problems, call your doctor immediately.

▼ Less common: headache, weakness, apathy, drowsiness, dizziness, blurred or yellow-tinted vision, seeing halos around bright lights, depression, psychoses, confusion or disorientation, restlessness,

---

Possible Side Effects *(continued)*

---

hallucinations, delirium, seizure, nerve pain, abnormal heart rhythms, and slow pulse.

▼ Rare: Enlargement of the breasts has been reported after long-term use of digoxin.

Children

▼ Children are more likely to develop abnormal heart rhythms before they see yellow or green halos or spots and before they develop nausea, vomiting, diarrhea, or stomach pain. Any abnormal heart rhythms that develop while a child is taking digoxin should be assumed to be a side effect.

Drug Interactions

• Drugs that may increase the effect of digoxin are amiloride aminoglycoside antibiotics, amiodarone, anticholinergic drugs, benzodiazepines, bepredil, captopril, cyclosporine, diltiazem, dipyridamole, erythromycin, esmolol, felodipine, flecainide, hydroxychloroquine, ibuprofen, indomethacin, itraconazole, nifedipine, omeprazole, propafenone, propantheline, quinidine, quinine, tetracycline, tolbutamide, triamterene, and verapamil.

• Drugs that may decrease blood levels of digoxin include aminoglutethimide, aminoglycosides, aminosalicylic acid, antacids, anti-cancer combinations, antidiabetes medication, antihistamines, barbiturates, cholestyramine, colestipol, kaolin-pectin mixtures, metoclopramide, oral kanamycin, oral neomycin, oral sulfonylureas, phenylbutazone, phenytoin and related anti-seizure drugs, rifampin, St. John's wort, sucralfate, and sulfasalazine.

• Disopyramide may alter the effects of digoxin, although the exact interaction is not well understood.

• Thiazide diuretics, furosemide, ethacrynic acid, and bumetanide increase digoxin's effect and increase the risk of side effects.

• Spironolactone may increase or decrease the side effects of digoxin; amiloride may reduce the effect of digoxin on the force of heart contraction.

• The effects of digoxin on the heart may be additive to those of ephedrine, epinephrine and other stimulants, beta-blockers, calcium salts, procainamide, and rauwolfia drugs.

• Digoxin dosage must be adjusted when it is combined with a thyroid drug.

Food Interactions

These drugs may generally be taken without regard to meals. Taking your medication after a high-fiber meal reduces the amount of drug absorbed into your blood.

Usual Dose

Adult and Child (age 11 and over): Starting dosage—known as the digitalizing or loading dose—is about 4–7 mcg per lb. of body weight. Digitalization may also be accomplished with a lower dosage over 7 days. Maintenance dosage—0.125–0.5 mg; it must be corrected for kidney function. For seniors, a lower dosage is required.

Child (under age 11): Starting dosage—5–30 mcg per lb. of body weight. Maintenance dosage—20%–35% of the starting dosage. Careful measurement of your child's digoxin dosage is crucial to safe and effective treatment.

Overdosage

Adult: Symptoms include appetite loss, nausea, vomiting, diarrhea, headache, weakness, apathy, blurred vision, yellow or green spots or halos before the eyes, yellowing of the skin or whites of the eyes, and changes in heartbeat.

Senior: Vomiting, diarrhea, and eye trouble are frequently seen.

Child: An early sign is a change in heart rhythms.

Call your doctor immediately if any of these symptoms appear. Take the victim to a hospital emergency room. ALWAYS bring the prescription bottle or container.

Special Information

Take each day's dose at the same time of day.

Do not stop taking digoxin without your doctor's knowledge.

Lanoxicaps are better absorbed than tablet forms of digoxin. For this reason, each dose of Lanoxicaps is slightly lower than the corresponding digoxin tablet.

Avoid over-the-counter diet and cold medications containing stimulants.

Call your doctor at once if you develop side effects.

There may by some variation between digoxin tablets from different manufacturers. Do not change drug brands without telling your doctor.

Check your pulse every day—your doctor will teach you how—and call your doctor if it drops below 60 beats per minute.

If you forget a dose and remember at least 12 hours before your next dose, take it right away. If you do not remember until it is less than 12 hours before your next dose, skip the one you forgot and continue with your regular schedule. Do not take a double dose. Call your doctor if you miss a dose for 2 or more days.

Special Populations

Pregnancy/Breast-feeding

Digoxin crosses into the fetal circulation. While digoxin is sometimes used during pregnancy to treat fetal heart disease, women who are or might be pregnant should not take digoxin without their doctor's approval. When your doctor considers this drug crucial, its potential benefits must be carefully weighed against its risks.

Small amounts of digoxin pass into breast milk. Nursing mothers who take digoxin should consider bottle-feeding their babies.

Seniors

Seniors are more sensitive to digoxin's effects, especially appetite loss. Seniors with impaired renal function may need lower dosages.

Dilantin see *Phenytoin*, *page 854*

Generic Name

Diltiazem (dil-TYE-uh-zem) Ⓖ

Brand Names

Cardizem	Cardizem LA
Cardizem CD	Cardizem SR

Cartia XT
Dilacor XR
Diltia XT

Taztia XT
Tiamate
Tiazac

Type of Drug

Calcium channel blocker.

Prescribed For

Angina pectoris, chronic stable angina, Raynaud's disease, prevention of second heart attacks, tardive dyskinesia (severe side effects associated with antipsychotic and other drugs), and hypertension (high blood pressure).

General Information

Diltiazem hydrochloride is one of many calcium channel blockers available in the U.S. These drugs block the passage of calcium, an essential factor in muscle contraction, into the heart and smooth muscles. Such blockage of calcium interferes with the contraction of these muscles, which in turn dilates (widens) the veins and vessels that supply blood to them. This dilating effect reduces blood pressure, the amount of oxygen used by the heart muscles, and the risk of blood vessel spasm. Diltiazem is therefore useful in treating not only hypertension but also angina pectoris (a condition characterized by brief attacks of chest pain), a condition related to poor oxygen supply to the heart muscles.

Diltiazem affects the movement of calcium only into muscle cells; it has no effect on calcium in the blood.

Cautions and Warnings

Diltiazem can slow your heart and interfere with normal electrical conduction. For people with a condition called **sick sinus syndrome,** this can result in temporary heart stoppage.

Diltiazem should not be taken if you are having a **heart attack** or if you have **lung congestion**. Diltiazem should be taken with caution by people with **heart failure** because it can worsen that condition.

Low blood pressure may occur, especially in people also taking a beta blocker.

Diltiazem can cause severe **liver damage** and should be taken with caution if you have had hepatitis or any other liver condition.

Caution should also be exercised if you have a history of **kidney problems,** although no clear tendency toward causing kidney damage is seen with this drug.

Possible Side Effects

▼ Common: dizziness, light-headedness, weakness, headache, and fluid accumulation in the hands, legs, or feet.

▼ Less common: low blood pressure, fainting, increase or decrease in heart rate, abnormal heart rhythm, heart failure, nervousness, fatigue, nausea, rash, tingling in the hands or feet, hallucinations, temporary memory loss, difficulty sleeping, diarrhea, vomiting, constipation, upset stomach, itching, unusual sensitivity to sunlight, painful or stiff joints, liver inflammation, and increased urination, especially at night.

Drug Interactions

• Diltiazem taken with a beta-blocking drug for hypertension is usually well tolerated, but may lead to heart failure in people with already weakened hearts.

• Calcium channel blockers, including diltiazem, may add to the effects of digoxin. This effect is not observed with any consistency, however, and only affects people with a large amount of digoxin already in their systems.

• Cimetidine and ranitidine increase the amount of diltiazem in the bloodstream and may account for a slight increase in the drug's effect.

• Diltiazem may increase blood levels of cyclosporine, carbamazepine, encainide, and theophylline, and thus increase the chance of side effects from these drugs.

• Diltiazem may cause a decrease in blood lithium levels, possibly undermining lithium's antimanic effect.

Food Interactions

Diltiazem is best taken on an empty stomach, at least 1 hour before or 2 hours after meals.

Usual Dose

Immediate-Release Products
30–60 mg 4 times a day.

Sustained-Release/Extended-Release Products
Cardizem SR: 60–180 mg twice a day.
Cardizem CD: 120–480 mg once a day.
Cardizem LA: 120–150 mg once a day.
Dilacor XR: 180–480 mg once a day.
Diltia XT: 180–480 mg once a day.
Taztia XT: 120–150 mg once a day.
Tiamate: 120–240 mg once a day.
Tiazac: 180–360 mg once a day.

Overdosage

Symptoms of diltiazem overdose are very low blood pressure and reduced heart rate. Overdose victims must be made to vomit with ipecac syrup—available at any pharmacy—within 30 minutes of taking the overdose. DO NOT INDUCE VOMITING IF THE VICTIM HAS FAINTED OR IS CONVULSING. If overdose symptoms have developed or more than 30 minutes have passed, vomiting is of little value. Take the victim to a hospital emergency room immediately. ALWAYS bring the prescription bottle or container.

Special Information

Call your doctor if you develop any of the following symptoms: swelling of the hands, legs, or feet; severe dizziness; constipation or nausea; or very low blood pressure.

Do not open, chew, or crush sustained-release capsules of Dilacor XR.

If you take your diltiazem 3 or 4 times a day and forget a dose, take it as soon as you remember. Space the remaining doses throughout the rest of the day. If you take diltiazem 1 or 2 times a day and forget to take a dose, take it as soon as you remember. If it is almost time for your next dose, skip the one you forgot and continue with your regular schedule. Never take a double dose.

Special Populations

Pregnancy / Breast-feeding

In animal studies, high doses of diltiazem interfered with the development of the fetus. Diltiazem should not be taken by women who are or might be pregnant. When your doctor considers this drug crucial, its potential benefits must be carefully weighed against its risks.

Because diltiazem passes into breast milk, nursing mothers taking this drug should bottle-feed.

Seniors

Seniors may be more sensitive to the effects of this drug because it takes longer to pass out of their bodies.

Generic Name

Dimenhydrinate (dye-men-HYE-drih-nate) G

Brand Names

Calm-X   Dramamine
Dimetabs   Triptone

The information in this profile also applies to the following drug:

Generic Ingredient: Meclizine G

Antivert   Bonine
Antivert 25   Meni-D
Antrizine   Ru-Vert-M

Type of Drug

Antihistamine and antiemetic (an agent that prevents or relieves nausea and vomiting).

Prescribed For

Nausea, vomiting, vertigo, and dizziness associated with motion sickness.

General Information

Dimenhydrinate, which depresses middle ear function, is a mixture of diphenhydramine—an antihistamine believed to be the active ingredient—and another ingredient. Meclizine is an antihistamine. It takes a little longer to start working than dimenhydrinate, but its effects last much longer. Meclizine does a better job of preventing motion sickness than treating its symptoms. It takes 30 minutes to 1 hour to work and lasts for 12 to 24 hours.

Cautions and Warnings

People with a **prostate condition, stomach ulcer, intestinal obstruction, bladder problems, difficulty urinating, glau-**

coma, asthma, or abnormal heart rhythms should use dimenhydrinate only while under a doctor's care. Newborn babies and people who are allergic or sensitive to dimenhydrinate should not be given this drug.

Because it controls nausea and vomiting, dimenhydrinate may hide the symptoms of appendicitis or overdoses of other drugs.

Possible Side Effects

▼ Most common: drowsiness.

▼ Less common: confusion; nervousness; excitation; restlessness; headache; sleeplessness, especially in children; tingling; heavy or weak hands; fainting; dizziness; tiredness; rapid heartbeat; low blood pressure; heart palpitations; blurred or double vision; difficult or painful urination; increased sensitivity to the sun; appetite loss; nausea; vomiting; diarrhea; upset stomach; constipation; nightmares; rash; drug reaction (symptoms include rash, itching, hives, and breathing difficulties); ringing or buzzing in the ears; dry mouth, nose, or throat; stuffy nose; wheezing; and increased chest phlegm or chest tightness.

Drug Interactions

• This drug should not be taken with a monoamine oxidase inhibitor (MAOI) antidepressant.

• Taking dimenhydrinate with an alcoholic beverage, other antihistamine, tranquilizer, or other central nervous system (CNS) depressant may cause excessive dizziness, drowsiness, or other signs of depression.

• Combining dimenhydrinate and certain antibiotics that cause dizziness or other ear-related side effects may mask early signs of these side effects, especially in infants and children.

Food Interactions

Take dimenhydrinate with food or milk if it upsets your stomach.

Usual Dose

Dimenhydrinate
   Adult and Child (age 13 and over): 50–100 mg—1 or 2 tablets or 4–8 tsp.—every 4–6 hours; do not take more than 400 mg a day.

Child (age 6-12): 25–50 mg—½ or 1 tablet or 2–4 tsp.—every 6–8 hours; do not take more than 150 mg a day.

Child (age 2–5): up to 25 mg—½ or 1 tablet or 2 tsp.—every 6–8 hours; do not take more than 75 mg a day.

Child (under age 2): Consult your doctor.

Meclizine

Adult and Child (age 13 and over): 25–50 mg 1 hour before travel; repeat every 24 hours for duration of journey. Up to 100 mg a day in divided doses may be needed to control dizziness from other causes.

Child: not recommended.

Overdosage

Symptoms of overdose include drowsiness, clumsiness, unsteadiness, feeling faint, facial flushing, and dry mouth, nose, or throat. Convulsions, coma, and breathing difficulties may also develop. Overdose victims should be taken to a hospital emergency room for treatment. ALWAYS bring the prescription bottle or container.

Special Information

For maximum effectiveness against motion sickness, take dimenhydrinate 1 to 2 hours before traveling; it may still be effective if taken 30 minutes before traveling.

This drug may cause drowsiness: Be extremely cautious when driving, operating hazardous machinery, or doing anything that requires concentration.

Dimenhydrinate may cause dry mouth, nose, or throat. Sugarless candy, gum, or ice chips can usually relieve these symptoms. Constant dry mouth may increase the likelihood of developing tooth decay or gum disease. Pay special attention to oral hygiene while you are taking dimenhydrinate, and contact your doctor if dry mouth lasts more than 2 weeks.

If you forget to take a dose of dimenhydrinate, take it as soon as you remember. If it is almost time for your next dose, skip the one you forgot and continue with your regular schedule. Do not take a double dose.

Special Populations

Pregnancy/Breast-feeding

Animal studies suggest that meclizine may cause birth defects. Do not take any antihistamine without your doctor's knowledge if you are or might be pregnant—especially during the last 3 months of pregnancy, because newborns may have severe reactions to antihistamines.

Small amounts of dimenhydrinate may pass into breast milk. Dimenhydrinate may also slow milk production. Nursing mothers who must take dimenhydrinate should bottle-feed.

Seniors
Seniors are more sensitive to antihistamine side effects and should take the lowest effective dose.

Diovan   see *Angiotensin II Blockers, page 85*

Diovan HCT   see *Angiotensin II Blockers, page 85*

Generic Name

Diphenhydramine Hydrochloride
(dye-fen-HYE-druh-mene hye-droe-KLOR-ide) Ⓖ

Brand Names

AllerMax	Dytuss
Banophen	Genahist
Benadryl Allergy	Siladryl
Diphen AF	Tusstat
Diphenhist	

Type of Drug
Antihistamine.

Prescribed For
Stuffy and runny nose, itchy eyes, and scratchy throat caused by seasonal allergy and for other symptoms of allergy such as itching, rash, and hives; also prescribed for motion sickness, insomnia, and Parkinson's disease.

General Information

Antihistamines generally work by blocking the release of histamine (a chemical released by body tissue during an allergic reaction), drying the nose, throat, and eye secretions. Diphenhydramine is the most common active ingredient found in nonprescription sleep-aids.

Cautions and Warnings

This drug should not be used if you are **allergic** to it. It should be avoided or used with extreme care if you have narrow-angle **glaucoma, stomach ulcer, intestinal obstruction, other stomach problems, difficulty urinating,** or **enlarged prostate**. It should not be used by people who have **sleep apnea** or **deep-breathing problems** such as **asthma**. Use with care if you have a history of **thyroid disease, heart disease, emphysema, chronic bronchitis,** or **high blood pressure**.

Possible Side Effects

▼ Common: drowsiness and weakness.

▼ Less common: itching, rash, sensitivity to bright light, perspiration, chills, lowering of blood pressure, headache, rapid heartbeat, sleeplessness, dizziness, disturbed coordination, confusion, restlessness, nervousness, irritability, euphoria (feeling "high"), tingling and weakness of the hands or feet, blurred or double vision, ringing in the ears, upset stomach, appetite loss, nausea, vomiting, constipation, diarrhea, urinary difficulties, thickening of lung secretions, tightness of the chest, wheezing, nasal stuffiness, and dry mouth, nose, or throat.

Drug Interactions

• This drug should not be taken with a monoamine oxidase inhibitor (MAOI) antidepressant.

• The effects of tranquilizers, sedatives, sleeping medications, and other central nervous system (CNS) depressants will be intensified when combined with diphenhydramine hydrochloride; it is extremely important that doses of these drugs are properly adjusted.

• This drug increases the intoxicating and sedating effects of alcohol.

Food Interactions

Take this drug with food if it upsets your stomach.

Usual Dose

Allergy
  Adult: 25–50 mg 3–4 times a day.
  Child (over 20 lbs.): 12.5–25 mg 3–4 times a day.

Nighttime Sedation
  Adult and Child (age 12 and over): 25–50 mg at bedtime.

Cough Syrup
  Adult and Child (age 13 and over): 25 mg every 4 hours.
  Child (age 6–12): 12.5 mg every 4 hours.
  Child (age 2–6): 6.25 mg every 4 hours.

Overdosage

Symptoms of overdose include depression or stimulation—especially in children; dry mouth; fixed or dilated pupils; flushing; and upset stomach. Overdose victims should be made to vomit with ipecac syrup—available at any pharmacy. Take the overdose victim to a hospital emergency room immediately if you cannot induce vomiting. ALWAYS bring the prescription bottle or container.

Special Information

This drug may cause drowsiness. Be extremely cautious when driving or operating hazardous equipment.

If you are taking this medication for motion sickness, take the first dose at least 30 minutes prior to exposure.

If you forget to take a dose of diphenhydramine hydrochloride, take it as soon as you remember. If it is almost time for your next dose, skip the one you forgot and continue with your regular schedule. Do not take a double dose.

Special Populations

Pregnancy/Breast-feeding

Animal studies have shown that some antihistamines may cause birth defects. Do not take any antihistamine without your doctor's knowledge if you are or might be pregnant—especially during the last 3 months of pregnancy—because newborns may have severe reactions to antihistamines.

Small amounts of antihistamine pass into breast milk. Nursing mothers who must take this drug should bottle-feed.

Seniors

Seniors are more sensitive to antihistamine side effects and may require lower dosages.

Generic Name

Dirithromycin (dye-rith-roe-MYE-sin)

Brand Name

Dynabac

Type of Drug

Macrolide antibiotic.

Prescribed For

Respiratory tract infections, skin infections, tonsillitis, and pharyngitis caused by streptococcus, staphylococcus, and other bacteria against which penicillin or tetracycline antibiotics cannot be used.

General information

Dirithromycin and other macrolide antibiotics are either bactericidal (bacteria-killing) or bacteriostatic (inhibiting bacterial growth), depending on the organism in question and amount of antibiotic present. The drug is not broken down by the liver and passes out of the body through the stool.

Cautions and Warnings

Do not take dirithromycin if you are **allergic** to it or any macrolide.

Dirithromycin should not be used for **serious blood infections** or *Haemophilus influenzae* infection, a very contagious infection that often affects children in daycare centers and their families.

Dosage changes are not needed for people with mild liver disease or with kidney disease. This drug has not been studied in people with **severe liver disease** but should be used with caution.

Colitis (bowel inflammation) has been associated with all antibiotics (see "Possible Side Effects").

Possible Side Effects

▼ Most common: abdominal pain, headache, nausea, and diarrhea. Colitis (symptoms include severe abdominal cramps and severe, persistent, and possibly bloody diarrhea) may develop.

▼ Less common: increased blood-platelet count, vomiting, upset stomach, increased blood potassium, dizziness, pain, weakness, stomach disorders, increasing cough, gas, rash, breathing difficulties, itching, and sleeplessness. Blood tests can also be affected.

▼ Rare: serious abnormal heart rhythms. Rare side effects can occur in almost any part of the body. Contact your doctor if you experience any side effect not listed above.

Drug Interactions

• The amount of dirithromycin absorbed into the blood increases slightly when it is taken immediately after an antacid containing aluminum or magnesium, or an H_2 antagonist such as cimetidine, famotidine, nizatidine, or ranitidine. This effect is not considered important.

• Pimozide should not be taken with dirithromycin. Two people died after combining a macrolide and pimozide.

Food Interactions

For optimum effectiveness, take with food or within 1 hour of having eaten.

Usual Dose

Adult and Child (age 12 and over): 500 mg a day for 5–14 days.

Child (under age 12): not recommended.

Overdosage

Overdose may result in nausea, vomiting, stomach cramps, and diarrhea. Call your local poison control center or a hospital emergency room for more information. If you seek treatment, ALWAYS bring prescription bottle or container.

Special Information

Call your doctor if you develop nausea, vomiting, diarrhea, stomach cramps, severe abdominal pain, or any severe or persistent side effect. Stop taking this medication and immediately call your doctor if you experience breathing difficulties, chest pain, hives, rash, itching, mouth sores, or unusual sensitivity to light.

Dirithromycin is not the antibiotic of choice for severe infections.

Do not crush, cut, or chew dirithromycin tablets.

If you forget a dose, take it as soon as you remember. If you do not remember until the next day, skip the dose you forgot and go back to your regular schedule. Call your doctor if you forget more than 1 dose.

Remember to take the full course of dirithromycin exactly as prescribed, even if you feel well sooner.

Special Populations

Pregnancy/Breast-feeding

Dirithromycin affected the fetus in animal studies. When this drug is considered crucial by your doctor, its potential benefits must be carefully weighed against its risks.

It is not known if dirithromycin passes into breast milk, but other macrolides do. Nursing mothers who take this drug should bottle-feed.

Seniors

Seniors may use dirithromycin without special restriction.

Generic Name

Disopyramide (die-soe-PIE-rah-mide) G

Brand Names

Norpace   Norpace CR

Type of Drug

Antiarrhythmic.

Prescribed For

Abnormal heart rhythms.

General Information

Disopyramide phosphate slows the rate at which nerve impulses are carried through heart muscle, reducing the response of heart muscle to those impulses. It acts on the heart similarly to the more widely used antiarrhythmic medications procainamide hydrochloride and quinidine sulfate. Disopyramide is often prescribed for people who do not respond to other antiarrhythmic drugs.

Cautions and Warnings

Do not take disopyramide if you are **allergic** to it.

This drug can worsen **heart failure** or trigger severely **low blood pressure**. It should be used in combination with another antiarrhythmic agent or beta blocker, only with caution.

In rare instances, disopyramide has caused a **reduction in blood-sugar levels**. Therefore, the drug should be used with caution by diabetics, older adults—who are more susceptible to this effect—and people with poor kidney or liver function. Ask your doctor if you should have your blood-sugar levels checked while taking this drug.

Because of its anticholinergic effects, men with a severe **prostate condition** and people who have **glaucoma, myasthenia gravis,** or severe **difficulty urinating** should use disopyramide with caution.

People with **liver or kidney disease** must take a reduced dose of disopyramide.

Possible Side Effects

▼ Most common: heart failure, low blood pressure, and urinary difficulty.

▼ Common: dry mouth, throat, or nose; constipation; and blurred vision.

▼ Less common: urination, dizziness, fatigue, headache, nervousness, breathing difficulties, chest pain, nausea, stomach pain or bloating, gas, appetite loss, diarrhea, vomiting, itching, rashes, muscle weakness, generalized aches and pains, not feeling well, low blood-potassium levels, increases in blood-cholesterol and triglyceride levels, and dry eyes.

▼ Rare: Rare side effects can occur in almost any part of the body. Contact your doctor if you experience any side effect not listed above.

Drug Interactions

• Phenytoin and rifampin may increase the rate at which the body removes disopyramide from the blood. Your disopyramide dose may need alteration if this combination is used. Other drugs known to increase drug breakdown by the liver, such as barbiturates and primidone, may also have this effect.

• Other antiarrhythmic drugs, such as procainamide and quinidine, may increase the effect of disopyramide, making dosage reduction necessary. At the same time, disopyramide may reduce the effectiveness of quinidine.

• When disopyramide is combined with a beta-blocking drug, increased disopyramide effects, additive effects, or depression of heart function may result.

• Erythromycin may increase the amount of disopyramide in your blood, causing abnormal heart rhythms or other cardiac effects.

• Disopyramide may reduce the effectiveness of oral anticoagulant (blood-thinning) drugs. Your doctor should check your anticoagulant dosage to be sure you are getting the right amount.

• Hydantoins may cause a decrease in the effectiveness of disopyramide.

• Disopyramide may increase the amount of digoxin in your blood, though the amount of the increase is not likely to affect your heart.

Food Interactions

Disopyramide should be taken on an empty stomach at least 1 hour before or 2 hours after meals.

Usual Dose

Adult: 400–800 mg a day (divided into 2 or 4 doses for the immediate-release form). In severe cases, 400 mg every 6 hours may be required. This level of dosage should be monitored in the hospital. The sustained-release preparation is taken every 12 hours. People with reduced kidney function should receive a lower dosage, depending on the degree of kidney function present. People with liver failure should take 400 mg a day.

Child (age 13–18): 2.5–7 mg a day per lb. of body weight.

Child (age 5–12): 4.5–7 mg a day per lb. of body weight.

Child (age 1–4): 4.5–9 mg a day per lb. of body weight.

Child (under age 1): 4.5–13.5 mg a day per lb. of body weight.

Overdosage

Overdose symptoms are breathing difficulties, abnormal heart rhythms, and unconsciousness. In severe cases, overdosage can lead to death. Overdose victims should be made to vomit with ipecac syrup—available at any pharmacy—to remove any remaining drug from the stomach. Call your doctor or poison control center before doing this. If you must go to a hospital emergency room, ALWAYS bring the prescription bottle or container. Prompt and vigorous treatment can mean the difference between life and death in severe overdosage.

Special Information

Disopyramide may cause symptoms of low blood sugar: anxiety, chills, cold sweats, drowsiness, excessive hunger, nausea, nervousness, rapid pulse, shakiness, unusual weakness, tiredness, or cool, pale skin. If this happens to you, eat some chocolate, candy, or other high-sugar food, and call your doctor at once.

Disopyramide can cause dry mouth, urinary difficulty, constipation, or blurred vision. Call your doctor if these symptoms become severe or intolerable, but do not stop taking the medication without your doctor's approval.

If disopyramide is required for a child and capsules are not appropriate, your pharmacist can make a liquid product. Do not do this at home: This medication requires special preparation. The liquid should be refrigerated and protected from light and should be thrown away after 30 days.

If you forget to take a dose of disopyramide, take it as soon as possible. However, if it is within 4 hours of your next dose, skip the dose you forgot and go back to your regular schedule. Do not take a double dose.

Special Populations

Pregnancy/Breast-feeding

Do not take this drug if you are pregnant or planning to become pregnant while using it, because it will pass into the fetus and may affect its development. When disopyramide is considered crucial by your doctor, its potential benefits must carefully be weighed against its risks.

Disopyramide passes into breast milk. Nursing mothers who must take this drug should bottle-feed.

Seniors

Seniors, especially those with liver or kidney disease, are more sensitive to the effects of this drug.

Ditropan XL *see Oxybutynin, page 812*

Generic Name

Dofetilide (DOH-fet-a-lyed)

Brand Name

Tikosyn

Type of Drug

Antiarrhythmic.

Prescribed For

Specific abnormal heart rhythms.

General Information

Dofetilide is used to establish and maintain normal sinus rhythm in the heart. Dofetilide is available only to hospitals and doctors who receive specific training and education on how to use this drug because of the risks associated with using it.

Cautions and Warnings

Dofetilide is reserved for people whose abnormal heart rhythms have not responded to other drugs. People taking dofetilide must be in a **hospital** or other facility for at least three days where appropriate **blood tests** can be performed to monitor kidney and heart function.

This drug is cleared through the kidneys. **Poor kidney function** increases the amount of dofetilide in the body. Liver disease has no effect on dofetilide blood levels.

Dofetilide, like other antiarrhythmic drugs, can cause severe and sometimes **fatal abnormal rhythms** of its own.

Women may be at a greater risk for some **arrhythmias** caused by dofetilide.

Possible Side Effects

Serious heart arrhythmias can develop in up to 3½ percent of patients taking up to 1000 mcg a day of dofetilide. People taking daily doses above 1000 mcg a day are at up to 5 times greater risk for arrhythmias.

▼ Most common: headache, chest pain, and respiratory infection.

▼ Common: difficulty breathing, nausea, and dizziness.

▼ Less common: flu, sleeplessness, accidental injury, back pain, diarrhea, abdominal pain, angina, anxiety, joint pain, weakness, atrial and ventricular arrhythmia, high blood pressure, pain, heart palpitations, swollen legs, ankles or arms, sweating, and urinary infections.

▼ Rare: some arrhythmias, heart attack, hives, slow heartbeat, stroke, facial or other paralysis, tingling in the hands or feet, cough, liver damage, migraine, fainting, and sudden death.

Drug Interactions

Dofetilide should not be given with drugs that are known to interact with it. Dofetilide must be stopped at least 2 days before any potentially interacting drug is taken.

• Do not mix dofetilide with any product containing verapamil, a calcium channel blocker, or trimethoprim, used for urinary infections. These combinations can substantially raise the amount of dofetilide into the blood.

• Some drugs may increase the amount of dofetilide in the blood by inhibiting enzymes that break it down in the liver. They include delavirdine, indinavir, ritonavir, saquinavir, amiodarone, cimetidine, ciprofloxacin, clarithromycin, cannabis, diltiazem, erythromycin, fluconazole, fluvoxamine, itraconazole, ketoconazole, mifepristone, nefazodone, norfloxacin, mibefradil, troleandomycin and zafirlukast.

• Some drugs may reduce the amount of dofetilide in the blood by stimulating enzymes that break it down in the liver, including efavirenz, nevirapine, carbamazepine, corticosteroids, modafinil, phenobarbital and other barbiturates, phenytoin, pioglitazone, and rifampin. Amiloride, metformin, megestrol, and triamterene can interfere with the elimination of dofetilide via the kidney, raising blood levels of the drug.

• Other drugs that can increase the effects of dofetilide are other antiarrhythmic drugs, bepridil, phenothiazines, and tricyclic antidepressants.

• Mixing dofetilide with digoxin may lead to a ventricular arrhythmia called torsade de pointes. Thiazides, furosemide, and other potassium-depleting diuretics can also increase the risk of this arrhythmia.

Food Interactions

Grapefruit juice may increase dofetilide blood levels.

Usual Dose

125–500 mcg twice a day.

Overdosage

Dofetilide overdose is likely to cause significant heart rhythm problems. Overdose victims must be treated symptomatically by their cardiologist.

Special Information

Read all information supplied to you before you begin taking this medication and read it again if anything in your treatment program changes.

Tell your doctor about any changes in your prescription or non-prescription drug use or in your use of vitamins, minerals, and other dietary supplement products.

Be sure that any other doctor or hospital that treats you and might prescribe another drug knows you are taking dofetilide.

Call your doctor at once if you develop any signs of altered electrolyte balance including excessive or prolonged diarrhea, sweating, vomiting, appetite changes or excessive thirst.

If you forget to take a dose, take it as soon as you remember. If it is almost time for your next dose, skip the dose you forgot and continue with your regular schedule. Do not take a double dose.

Special Populations

Pregnancy/Breast-feeding

Dofetilide causes birth defects in animal studies. Pregnant women should take this drug only after discussing with their doctors its potential benefits and risks.

It is unknown whether dofetilide passes into breast milk. Nursing mothers who take it should bottle-feed.

Seniors

Older adults may take this drug without special restriction.

Brand Name

Donnatal

Generic Ingredients

Atropine Sulfate + Hyoscyamine Sulfate + Phenobarbital + Scopolamine Hydrobromide Ⓖ

Other Brand Names

Barbidonna   Hyosophen
Bellatal   Spasmolin
Donnatel Extencaps   Susano
Hyonatal

The information in this profile also applies to the following drugs:

Generic Ingredient: Hyoscyamine Sulfate Ⓖ

Anaspaz   Levsin
A-Spas S/L   Levsinex Timecaps
Cytospaz   Medispaz
Donnamar   NuLev
Hyosol   Spasdel
Hyosyne   Symax
Levbid

Generic Ingredients: Belladonna Alkaloids + Phenobarbital Ⓖ
Donnapine

Generic Ingredient: Propantheline Ⓖ
Pro-Banthine

Type of Drug

Anticholinergic combination.

Prescribed For

Stomach spasm and gastrointestinal (GI) cramps; also used to treat motion sickness.

General Information

Donnatal is a mild antispasmodic sedative. Its principal action is to counteract the effect of acetylcholine, an important neurohormone. Donnatal is used only to relieve symptoms, not to treat the underlying condition, and there is considerable doubt among medical experts that this drug lives up to its claims. In addition to the brand names listed above, there are about 50 other anticholinergic combinations with similar properties. All are used to relieve cramps and all are about equally effective. Some have additional ingredients to reduce or absorb excess gas in the stomach, to coat the stomach, or to control diarrhea. Donnatal and products like it should not be used for more than the temporary relief of symptoms.

Cautions and Warnings

Donnatal should not be used by people with **glaucoma, rapid heartbeat,** severe **intestinal disease** such as **ulcerative colitis, intestinal obstruction, urinary difficulties, asthma, myasthenia gravis, acute intermittent porphyria,** or a history of **allergy** to any of the ingredients of this drug.

Donnatal can reduce your ability to sweat and may lead to **heat exhaustion**. Avoid extended heavy exercise and limit your exposure to high temperatures.

Donnatal should be used with caution in children and in people with **brain damage, spastic paralysis, Down's syndrome,** a history of **drug addiction, heart disease, high blood pressure, hyperthyroidism** (overactive thyroid gland), **kidney or liver disease, autonomic neuropathy, gastric ulcer,** or **hiatal hernia.**

Possible Side Effects

▼ Most common: blurred vision, dry mouth, urinary difficulties, flushing, and dry skin.

▼ Less common: rapid or unusual heartbeat, increased sensitivity to bright light, loss of the sense of taste, headache, nervousness, tiredness, weakness, dizziness, sleeplessness, nausea, vomiting, fever, stuffy nose, heartburn, loss of sex drive, decreased sweating, constipation, feeling bloated, and allergic reactions such as fever and rash.

Drug Interactions

• Although Donnatal contains only a small amount of phenobarbital, it is wise to avoid alcohol or other sedative drugs. Although unlikely, phenobarbital interactions are possible with anticoagulants, adrenal corticosteroids, tranquilizers, narcotics, sleeping pills, digitalis or other cardiac glycosides, and antihistamines.

• Some phenothiazine drugs, tranquilizers, tricyclic antidepressants, and narcotics may increase the side effects of the atropine sulfate ingredient in Donnatal, causing dry mouth, urinary difficulties, and constipation. The effectiveness of phenothiazines to control psychotic symptoms may be decreased.

• Combining Donnatal and the antiviral amantadine may increase the side effects of Donnatal.

• Donnatal may increase the side effects of atenolol and digoxin.

• Antacids may decrease Donnatal's effectiveness; do not take antacids within one hour of taking Donnatal.

Food Interactions

Take Donnatal 30 to 60 minutes before meals.

Usual Dose

Donnatal
    Adult (age 13 and over): 1–2 tablets, capsules, or tsp. 3–4 times a day.
    Child (age 2–12): ½ the adult dosage.
    Child (under age 2): not recommended.

Propantheline
    Adult: 7.5–15 mg 3 times a day, and 30 mg at bedtime.
    Senior: 7.5 mg 3 times a day.
    Child (under age 12): not recommended.

Overdosage

Symptoms of overdose include dry mouth; difficulty swallowing; thirst; blurred vision; sensitivity to bright light; flushed, hot, or dry skin; rash; fever; abnormal heart rate; high blood pressure; urinary difficulties; restlessness; confusion; delirium; and breathing difficulties. The victim should be taken to a hospital emergency room immediately. ALWAYS bring the prescription bottle or container.

Special Information

Call your doctor if you experience persistent diarrhea, bloating, fever, heart palpitations, rash, flushing or eye pain.

Do not crush or chew Donnatal tablets.

Dry mouth usually can be relieved by chewing gum or sucking hard candy or ice chips. Constipation can be treated with a stool-softening laxative.

Donnatal may reduce the amount of saliva in your mouth, making it easier for bacteria to grow there. Pay special attention to dental hygiene while taking this medication to prevent cavities and gum disease.

Donnatal may cause drowsiness and blurred vision. Be careful when driving or operating hazardous equipment.

If you forget to take a dose of Donnatal, take it as soon as you remember. If it is almost time for your next dose, skip the one you forgot and continue with your regular schedule. Do not take a double dose.

Special Populations

Pregnancy/Breast-feeding

Donnatal may cause drug dependency or breathing problems in newborns and may interfere with labor and delivery. When this drug is considered crucial by your doctor, its potential must be carefully weighed against its risks.

Donnatal passes into breast milk and may reduce the amount of milk produced. It may cause tiredness, shortness of breath, and a slower-than-normal heartbeat in infants. Nursing mothers who must take this medication should consider bottle-feeding.

Seniors

Seniors are often more sensitive to the side effects of Donnatal, such as excitement, confusion, drowsiness, agitation, constipation, dry mouth, and urinary difficulties. Memory may be impaired and glaucoma worsened.

Generic Name

Doxazosin (dok-SAY-zoe-sin) G

Brand Name

Cardura

Type of Drug

Antihypertensive.

Prescribed For

High blood pressure and benign prostatic hyperplasia (BPH); also used with digoxin and diuretic drugs to treat congestive heart failure.

General Information

Doxazosin mesylate and other alpha-adrenergic blocking agents, or alpha blockers, reduce blood pressure by dilating (widening) blood vessels. They achieve this effect by blocking nerve endings known as alpha$_1$ receptors. The maximum blood-pressure-lowering effect of doxazosin is seen between 2 and 6 hours after taking a dose. In BPH, doxazosin works by relaxing smooth muscles in the prostate and neck of the bladder. Doxazosin helps the symptoms of BPH, and taking it for several years may eliminate the need for surgery or allow the use of a less invasive type of surgery. Doxazosin's effect lasts for 24 hours. It is mostly broken down in the liver; little passes out of the body via the kidneys.

Cautions and Warnings

Doxazosin may cause **dizziness** and **fainting,** especially the first few doses. This is known as a first-dose effect, which can be minimized by limiting the first dose to 1 mg at bedtime. First-dose effects occur in about 1% of people taking an alpha blocker and may recur if the drug is stopped for a few days and then started again.

Doxazosin should be taken with caution if you have **liver disease**.

People **allergic** or **sensitive** to any alpha blocker should avoid doxazosin.

Doxazosin may slightly reduce cholesterol levels and improve the ratio of high-density lipoprotein (HDL)—"good" cholesterol—and low-density lipoprotein (LDL), a positive step for people with a blood-cholesterol problem.

White-blood-cell counts may be slightly decreased in people taking doxazosin.

Possible Side Effects

▼ Most common: headache, dizziness, and weakness.

▼ Less common: heart palpitations, abnormal heart rhythms, chest pain, nausea, diarrhea, constipation, abdominal pain or discomfort, gas, breathing difficulties, nosebleed, sore throat, runny nose, muscle or joint pain, visual disturbances, conjunctivitis (pinkeye), ringing in the ears, fainting, depression, decreased sex drive or sexual function, tingling in the hands or feet, nervousness, tiredness, anxiety, sleeplessness, poor muscle coordination, muscle stiffness, poor bladder control, frequent urination, itching, rash, sweating, fluid retention, facial swelling and flushing, and back, neck, shoulder, arm, or leg pain.

▼ Rare: vomiting, dry mouth, sinus irritation, bronchitis, cold or flu symptoms, worsening of asthma, coughing, hair loss, weight gain, and fever.

Drug Interactions

• Doxazosin may interact with beta blockers to increase the risk of dizziness or fainting after the first dose of doxazosin.

• The blood-pressure-lowering effect of doxazosin may be reduced by indomethacin.

• When taken with other blood-pressure-lowering drugs, doxazosin produces a severe reduction of blood pressure.

• The blood-pressure-lowering effect of clonidine may be reduced by doxazosin.

Food Interactions

None known.

Usual Dose

1 mg at bedtime to start; may be increased to a total of 16 mg, taken once a day.

Overdosage

Overdose may produce drowsiness, poor reflexes, and very low blood pressure. Overdose victims should be taken to a hospital emergency room at once. ALWAYS bring the prescription bottle or container.

Special Information

Take doxazosin exactly as prescribed. Do not stop taking it unless directed to do so by your doctor. Avoid over-the-counter drugs that contain stimulants because they may increase your blood pressure.

Doxazosin may cause dizziness, headache, and drowsiness, especially 2 to 6 hours after you take your first dose, although these effects can persist after the first few doses. Use caution when getting up from a sitting or lying position.

Call your doctor if you develop severe dizziness, heart palpitations, or any bothersome or persistent side effect.

Wait 12 to 24 hours after taking your first dose of doxazosin before driving or doing anything that requires concentration. Take your dose at bedtime to minimize this problem.

If you forget a dose, take it as soon as you remember. If it is almost time for your next dose, skip the dose you forgot and continue with your regular schedule. Do not take a double dose.

Special Populations

Pregnancy/Breast-feeding

The safety of using doxazosin during pregnancy is not known, although animal studies have shown that alpha blockers may affect fetal development. When this drug is considered crucial by your doctor, its potential benefits must be carefully weighed against its risks.

Small amounts of doxazosin pass into breast milk. Nursing mothers who must take this drug should bottle-feed.

Seniors

Seniors, especially those with liver disease, may be more sensitive to the effects and side effects of doxazosin.

Generic Name

Doxercalciferol Ⓖ (docks-er-kal-SIH-fer-ahl)

Brand Name

Drisdol Liquid   Hectorol Capsules

Type of Drug

Vitamin D supplement.

Prescribed For

Elevated parathyroid hormone levels in patients undergoing kidney dialysis.

General Inforamation

Doxercalciferol is a synthetic form of vitamin D that is processed in the body to form active vitamin D. Vitamin D, along with parathyroid hormone, are key elements of the calcium-regulating system in the body. Normally, your body releases parathyroid hormone if blood calcium levels are too low. Parathyroid hormones move calcium from the place where it is found in greatest quantity—your bones—into the bloodstream. This can have disastrous effects for a wide variety of body functions where calcium is crucial including muscle contraction, nervous system function, bone fragility, and blood clotting. Doxercalciferol helps to stabilize the system and normalize parathyroid hormone levels that can be artificially elevated in dialysis patients.

Cautions and Warnings

Do not use doxercalciferol if you are **sensitive** or **allergic** to it.

People with a tendency toward **high calcium** or **vitamin D levels** should not take doxercalciferol.

Possible Side Effects

▼ Common: swelling, headache, general discomfort, nausea, vomiting, dizziness, difficulty breathing, itching, loss of appetite, indigestion, weight gain, joint pain, constipation, and sleepiness.

Drug Interactions

• Do not take antacids that contain magnesium while you are taking doxercalciferol.

• Cholestyramine may reduce the absorption of doxercalciferol.

• Prolonged use of mineral oil may reduce the absorption of doxercalciferol.

• Do not combine any other over-the-counter or prescription medicines and doxercalciferol without first talking with your doctor.

Food Interactions

You may need to limit your consumption of vitamin D. Consult your doctor.

Usual Dose

Starting dose—10 mcg 3 times a week during kidney dialysis treatment. Dosage may be adjusted to 2.5 mcg at 8-week intervals if necessary.

Overdosage

Symptoms include weakness, headache, drowsiness, nausea, vomiting, dry mouth, metallic taste in mouth, constipation, muscle pain, and bone pain. Call your local poison control center or a hospital emergency room for more information. If you seek treatment, ALWAYS bring the prescription bottle or container.

Special Information

Compliance with dosage instruction, diet, and calcium supplementation is important while taking doxercalciferol.

Lab tests are required to monitor therapy while taking doxercalciferol.

Doxercalciferol may cause dizziness. Use caution while driving or performing other tasks requiring alertness, coordination, or physical dexterity.

Special Populations

Tell your doctor or pharmacist if you are pregnant, planning on becoming pregnant, or breastfeeding.

The safety of using doxercalciferol during pregnancy is not known. When this drug is considered crucial by your doctor, its potential benefits must be carefully weighed against its risks.

It is not known if doxercalciferol passes into breast milk. Nursing mothers who must use this drug should consider bottle-feeding.

Seniors

Seniors may use this drug without special precaution.

Generic Name

Dronabinol (droe-NAB-ih-nol)

Brand Name

Marinol

Type of Drug

Antinauseant.

Prescribed For

Nausea and vomiting associated with cancer chemotherapy, and appetite stimulation and weight-loss prevention in people with acquired immunodeficiency syndrome (AIDS).

General Information

Dronabinol is a legal form of marijuana. The psychoactive chemical in marijuana is delta-9-THC. Dronabinol has all of the psychological effects of marijuana and is therefore considered to be a highly abusable drug. It can cause personality changes, feelings of detachment, hallucinations, and euphoria (feeling "high"). Younger adults have reported a greater success rate with dronabinol, probably because they are better able to tolerate these effects.

Most people start taking dronabinol while in the hospital so their response to the drug and its possible adverse effects can be monitored. Dronabinol has also been studied as a glaucoma treatment.

Cautions and Warnings

Dronabinol should not be used to treat **nausea** and **vomiting** caused by anything other than cancer chemotherapy. It should not be used by people who are **allergic** to it, to marijuana, or to sesame oil.

Dronabinol has a profound effect on **mental states**; it will impair your ability to operate complex equipment or engage in any activity that requires intense concentration, sound judgment, or coordination—such as driving a car.

Dronabinol produces **withdrawal symptoms** when the drug is stopped. These may develop within 12 hours of the drug's discontinuation and include restlessness, sleeplessness, and irritability. Within a day after the drug has been stopped, stuffy nose, hot flashes, sweating, loose stools, hiccups, or appetite loss may occur. The symptoms usually subside within a few days.

Dronabinol should be used with caution by people with **heart disease** or **high blood pressure**. Dronabinol should be used with caution by people with a **manic-depressive or schizophrenic history** because it may aggravate the underlying disease.

Possible Side Effects

▼ Most common: drowsiness, euphoria, dizziness, anxiety, muddled thinking, perceptual difficulties, poor coordination, irritability, a separation in time and space, depression, weakness, sluggishness, headache, hallucinations, memory lapses, loss of muscle coordination, unsteadiness, paranoia, depersonalization, disorientation, confusion, rapid heartbeat, and dizziness when rising from a sitting or lying position.

▼ Less common: difficulty talking or slurred speech, facial flushing, excessive perspiration, nightmares, ringing or buzzing in the ears, fainting, diarrhea, loss of bowel control, and muscle pain.

Drug Interactions

• Dronabinol increases the effects of alcohol, tranquilizers, sleeping pills, sedatives, and other depressants. It also enhances the effects of psychoactive drugs including tricyclic antidepressants, amphetamines, cocaine, and other stimulants.

• Dronabinol may increase the effects of fluoxetine and disulfiram.

• The effects of theophylline drugs are reduced by dronabinol.

• Combining dronabinol and antihistamines or anticholinergic drugs may cause either rapid heartbeat or excessive drowsiness.

Food Interactions

This drug may be taken without regard to food or meals; as an appetite stimulant, it is often taken before meals.

Usual Dose

Antiemetic: 5 mg 1–3 hours before starting chemotherapy treatment and repeated every 2–4 hours after treatment, for a total of 4–6 doses a day. Dosage may be increased up to 15 mg per dose if needed; psychiatric side effects increase greatly at higher dosages.

Appetite Stimulant: 2.5 mg before lunch or dinner, or 2.5 mg at bedtime. Dosage may be increased to 20 mg a day.

Overdosage

Overdose symptoms may occur at usual dosages or at higher dosages if the drug is being abused. The primary symptoms of overdose are the psychological symptoms listed above (see "Possible Side Effects"). In some cases, overdose may lead to panic reactions or seizure. Contact a hospital or local poison center for more information. If you seek treatment, ALWAYS bring the prescription bottle or container.

Special Information

Be careful when driving or performing any task that requires concentration. Avoid alcohol and other central nervous system (CNS) depressants.

Dronabinol may cause acute psychiatric or psychological side effects. Call your doctor if any develop.

The capsules must be stored in the refrigerator.

If you forget a dose, take it as soon as you remember. If it is almost time for your next dose, skip the one you forgot and continue with your regular schedule. Do not take a double dose.

Special Populations

Pregnancy/Breast-feeding

Animal studies have shown adverse effects on the fetus. When this drug is considered crucial by your doctor, its benefits must be carefully weighed against its risks.

Dronabinol passes into breast milk. Nursing mothers who must take this drug should bottle-feed.

Seniors

Seniors may be more sensitive to this drug, especially its psychological effects.

Duragesic *see Codeine, page 282*

Brand Name

Dyazide

Generic Ingredients

Hydrochlorothiazide + Triamterene G

Other Brand Names
Maxide   Maxzide-25

The information in this profile also applies to the following drugs:

Generic Ingredients: Amiloride + Hydrochlorothiazide G
Moduretic

Generic Ingredients: Spironolactone + Hydrochlorothiazide G
Aldactazide   Spirozide
Spironazide

Type of Drug

Diuretic (an agent that increases urination).

Prescribed For

Hypertension (high blood pressure) or any condition where it is desirable to eliminate excess water from the body.

General Information

Dyazide combines a thiazide diuretic and a potassium-sparing diuretic. The latter, triamterene, helps the body retain potassium while producing a diuretic effect. This balances the other ingredient, hydrochlorothiazide, which normally causes a loss of potassium. Different products contain differing concentrations of these 2 drugs. Dyazide should be used only when you need its exact proportion of ingredients.

Cautions and Warnings

Do not use Dyazide if you have **nonfunctioning kidneys,** are **allergic** to this drug or any sulfa drug, or have a history of **allergy** or **bronchial asthma**.

Do not combine any **potassium supplement** and Dyazide without your doctor's knowledge.

Possible Side Effects

▼ Most common: appetite loss, drowsiness, lethargy, headache, gastrointestinal upset, cramping, and diarrhea.

▼ Less common: rash, mental confusion, fever, feeling unwell, impotence, bright red tongue, burning sensation in the tongue, tingling in the toes and fingers, restlessness, anemia or other effects on blood components, increased sensitivity to sunlight, and dizziness when rising quickly from a sitting position. Dyazide may also produce muscle spasms, gout, weakness, and blurred vision.

Drug Interactions

• Dyazide increases the effect of other blood-pressure-lowering drugs. This is why other blood–pressure drugs are often prescribed with Dyazide, but dosage adjustments may be required.

• Combining Dyazide and digitalis drugs, amphotericin B, or adrenal corticosteroids increases the risk of body-fluid imbalance. If you are taking insulin or an oral antidiabetic drug and begin taking Dyazide, the insulin or antidiabetic dosage may have to be modified.

• Dyazide may increase the risk of allopurinol side effects.

• Dyazide may decrease the effects of oral anticoagulant (blood-thinning) drugs.

• Antigout drug dosage may have to be modified since Dyazide raises uric-acid levels.

• Dyazide may prolong the effects of chemotherapy drugs on reducing white-blood-cell counts.

• Dyazide may increase the effects of diazoxide, which may lead to symptoms of diabetes.

• Dyazide should not be taken with loop diuretics because the combination can lead to an extreme diuretic effect and an extreme effect on blood-sodium levels.

• Dyazide may increase the effect of vitamin D, which may cause high blood-calcium levels.

• Propantheline and other anticholinergics may increase the diuretic effect of Dyazide.

• Lithium carbonate taken with Dyazide should be monitored carefully by a doctor due to an increased risk of lithium side effects.

• Cholestyramine and colestipol prevent Dyazide from being absorbed. Dyazide should be taken at least 2 hours before cholestyramine or colestipol.

• Methenamine and other urinary agents may reduce the effect of Dyazide.

• Some nonsteroidal anti-inflammatory drugs (NSAIDs), particularly indomethacin, may reduce the effect of Dyazide. Sulindac, another NSAID, may increase its effect.

Food Interactions

Take this drug with food if it upsets your stomach.

Usual Dose

Amilioride combination: 1–2 tablets daily with meals.
Spironolactone combination: 1–8 tablets daily.
Triamterene combination: 1–2 capsules or tablets a day.

Overdosage

Symptoms may include tingling in the arms or legs, weakness, fatigue, changes in heartbeat, a sickly feeling, dry mouth, restlessness, muscle pain or cramps, urinary difficulties, nausea, and vomiting. In some cases, low blood pressure and decreased respiration may occur. Take the victim to a hospital emergency room immediately. ALWAYS bring the prescription bottle or container.

Special Information

Dyazide causes excess urination at first, but this subsides after several weeks of use. Diuretics are usually taken early in the day to prevent excessive nighttime urination that may interfere with sleep.

Dyazide may make you drowsy. Be careful when driving or performing any task that requires concentration.

Call your doctor if you develop muscle pain, sudden joint pain, weakness, cramps, nausea, vomiting, restlessness, excessive thirst, tiredness, drowsiness, increased heart or pulse rate, diarrhea, dizziness, headache, or rash.

People with diabetes may experience an increased blood-sugar level and require dosage adjustments of their antidiabetic medications.

Avoid other drugs while taking Dyazide unless otherwise directed by your doctor. Avoid alcohol.

If you are taking Dyazide for the treatment of hypertension or congestive heart failure (CHF), avoid over-the-counter cough, cold, or allergy medications, which may contain stimulants.

Take Dyazide exactly as prescribed. Be aware that all triamterene-hydrochlorothiazide products are not equal to each other and should not be freely substituted. Check with your doctor and pharmacist before switching brands.

If you forget a dose, take it as soon as you remember. If it is almost time for your next dose, skip the dose you forgot and continue with your regular schedule. Do not take a double dose.

Special Populations

Pregnancy/Breast-feeding

Dyazide may enter the fetal circulation, though it is sometimes used to treat specific conditions in pregnant women. When this drug is considered crucial by your doctor, its potential benefits must be carefully weighed against its risks.

The thiazide diuretic in Dyazide passes into breast milk. Nursing mothers who must take Dyazide should consider bottle-feeding.

Seniors

Seniors are more sensitive to the effects of Dyazide.

Generic Name

Econazole (ee-KON-uh-zole)

Brand Name

Spectazole

Type of Drug

Antifungal.

Prescribed For

Fungal infections of the skin, including athlete's foot, jock itch, and ringworm.

General Information

Econazole nitrate can kill fungal organisms that may have penetrated to deep layers of the skin. Very small amounts of econazole are absorbed into the bloodstream.

Cautions and Warnings

Do not use econazole if you have had an **allergic reaction** to it or any other ingredient in this product. Do not apply econazole cream in or near your **eyes**.

Long-term application of this product to large areas of skin may cause **liver damage**.

Possible Side Effects

▼ Most common: burning, itching, stinging, and redness in the areas to which the cream has been applied.

Drug Interactions

None known.

Usual Dose

Apply enough of the cream to cover affected areas with a thin layer 1–2 times a day.

Overdosage

Accidental ingestion may cause nausea, upset stomach, drowsiness, and liver inflammation or damage. Call your local poison control center for more information.

Special Information

Clean the affected areas before applying econazole cream unless otherwise directed by your doctor. Dry the infected area thoroughly, and wear loose-fitting clothes to keep the area cool and dry.

Call your doctor if the treated area burns, stings, or becomes red.

This product can be expected to relieve symptoms within 1 or 2 days after you begin using it. Follow your doctor's directions for the complete 2- to 4-week course of treatment to gain maximum benefit. Stopping the drug too soon can lead to a relapse.

If you forget a dose of econazole, apply it as soon as you remember. If it is almost time for your next dose, skip the one you forgot and continue with your regular schedule. Do not apply a double dose.

Special Populations

Pregnancy/Breast-feeding

When given by mouth to pregnant animals in high doses, econazole was toxic to the fetus. It should be strictly avoided during the first 3 months of pregnancy. During the last 6 months of pregnancy, it should be used only if absolutely necessary.

Econazole may pass into breast milk. Nursing mothers who must take this drug should consider bottle-feeding.

Seniors

Seniors may take this drug without special restriction.

Generic Name

Efalizumab (ef-ah-LIZ-u-mab)

Brand Name

Raptiva

Type of Drug

Immune system suppressant.

Prescribed For

Chronic to severe plaque psoriasis.

General Information

Efalizumab is a manmade antibody that works by binding to specific areas of certain white blood cells called *leukocytes*. This prevents the leukocytes from interacting with other cells and interrupts inflammation that is involved in the development of patches of psoriatic skin. The molecule that efaluzimab interacts with is found on many other key cells found in the immune system, and this is the source of many of the drug's more serious side effects.

Cautions and Warnings

Do not use this drug if you are **sensitive** or **allergic** to it.

People taking efalizumab are at a greater risk of **infection** because it suppresses the immune system. Contact your doctor if you develop any kind of infection, including a common cold. Serious infections may require hospitalization.

The chances of **malignancy** may be increased by efalizumab because it suppresses the immune system. People with any type of cancer should not use this drug.

Efalizumab may lead to **bleeding** because it can cause a drastic reduction in blood platelet counts. People with a history of **low blood platelet counts** should be extremely cautious about using efalizumab.

Psoriasis can get worse or recur during or after efalizumab treatment in a small number of people. Call your doctor immediately if your condition worsens while you are taking efalizumab.

Possible Side Effects

Headache, fever, nausea, and vomiting are common after taking the very first dose of efalizumab. A "conditioning" dose of about 0.3 mg per pound of body weight is often given to minimize these reactions.

▼ Most common: headache, infections, chills, nausea, and pain.

▼ Common: muscle aches, flu-like symptoms, itching, and fever.

▼ Less common: back pain, arthritis, lung inflammation, and acne.

▼ Rare: psoriasis, arthritis, joint pain, malignancy, low blood platelet count, and drug allergy or sensitivity. Other rare side effects can occur in almost any part of the body. Contact your doctor if you experience any side effect not listed above.

Drug Interactions

• Efalizumab is an immune system suppressant and should not be combined with other immune suppressant drugs because of the increased risk of infection and malignancy.

• Combining vaccines (live and acellular) with efalizumab may exaggerate the body's response to the vaccine and increase the risk of developing the disease against which the vaccination is being administered. People taking efalizumab should not receive vaccines.

Food Interactions

None known.

Usual Dose

Adult: 0.3 mg per lb. of body weight to start. Then about $1/2$ mg per lb. of body weight once a week on the same day. The maximum dose is 200 mg by subcutaneous injection. Mix your dose immediately before it is to be injected and throw away any unused medicine.

Child: not recommended.

Overdosage

Doses up to 4 times the recommended dose have been taken for 10 weeks without additional side effects. However, overdose victims should be taken to a hospital emergency room for observation. ALWAYS bring the prescription bottle or container.

Special Information

See your doctor regularly while you are taking efaluzimab. Regular blood tests are required to make sure your blood platelets are not unusually low.

Tell your doctor if you gain or lose weight, since doses of efaluzimab are based on how much you weigh.

Tell your doctor about all medicines you are taking including other medicines for psoriasis, non-prescription drugs, vitamins, and herbal supplements.

Store unused medicine in the refrigerator. Throw away medicine that has been mixed but not used.

Call your doctor immediately if you develop bleeding gums, black and blue marks, any kind of infection, begin to bruise easily, or if you are told by another doctor that you have any kind of cancer.

This drug is given by injection under the skin. For more information on how to properly administer this drug, see page 1188.

Special Populations

Pregnancy/Breast-feeding

It is not known how efaluzimab will affect a growing fetus. Animal studies using doses equal to 30 times the human dose showed no adverse effects. While animal studies of efaluzimab reveal no damage to the fetus, this drug should be used only during pregnancy after carefully weighing its potential benefits against its risks.

It is not known if efaluzimab passes into breast milk, although it might affect the nursing infant's developing immune system. Nursing mothers who must take this drug should bottle-feed.

Seniors

Seniors should be cautious about using efaluzimab because of the increased risk of infection.

Generic Name

Efavirenz (ef-ah-VIE-renz)

Brand Name

Sustiva

Type of Drug

Antiviral.

Prescribed For

Human immunodeficiency virus (HIV).

General Information

Efavirenz is a non-nucleoside reverse transcriptase inhibitor (NNRTI). It inhibits the reverse transcriptase (RT) enzyme, necessary for reproduction of HIV in body cells, by binding directly to it. The duration of any benefit from taking this drug may be limited because liver enzymes that break down efavirenz grow more potent as you continue to take it, removing it from your blood faster as time passes. The HIV virus can become resistant to efavirenz. For this reason, efavirenz is prescribed as part of a multi-drug anti-HIV "cocktail." Drug combinations containing efavirenz are just as effective in children as in adults.

Cautions and Warnings

Do not take this drug if you are **allergic** or s**ensitive** to it.

HIV becomes **resistant** to efavirenz if it is used alone. Treatment must always include at least 1 other anti-HIV drug.

Efavirenz can be toxic to the **liver**. People with a history of hepatitis should have their liver function evaluated periodically and probably should use an alternate therapy. Efavirenz can raise blood **cholesterol** by 10%–20%.

Efavirenz has been associated with serious psychiatric side effects including delusional and psychotic behavior. People with a history of **psychiatric disorders** may be at greater risk for these events. Contact your doctor immediately if you begin to experience psychiatric symptoms while taking this medication.

This drug has not been studied in **children** under age 3 or those who weigh less than 22 lbs.

Possible Side Effects

More than half of people who take efavirenz experience some nervous system and psychiatric side effects and rash. About 2% have to stop treatment because of them. Children are more likely than adults to develop rash.

▼ Most common: nausea, dizziness, sleeplessness, headache, and temporary rash.

▼ Common: abnormal dreaming, poor concentration, tiredness, and diarrhea.

▼ Less common: itching, sweating, stomach pain or gas, upset stomach, reduced sensitivity to stimulation, depression, appetite loss, hallucinations, and nervousness.

▼ Rare: blisters, wet ulcers, peeling skin, blood in the urine, delusions, inappropriate behavior, and severe depression. Blood cholesterol can rise 10% to 20%. Other rare side effects can occur in almost any part of the body. Contact your doctor if you experience any side effect not listed above.

Drug Interactions

• Combining efavirenz and astemizole; midazolam, triazolam, or other benzodiazepine drugs; or ergot-containing products can lead to life-threatening abnormal heart rhythms, excessive sedation, or severe breathing difficulties. DO NOT COMBINE these drugs.

• Efavirenz increases the nervous-system effects of alcohol, tranquilizers, antidepressants, and other psychoactive drugs.

• Combining efavirenz with ritonavir increases blood levels of both drugs. This interaction increases the effectiveness of anti-HIV therapy as well as the risk of side effects.

• Efavirenz reduces indinavir and amprenavir blood levels. Your indinavir or amprenavir dosage may need to be increased.

• Efavirenz significantly reduces saquinavir blood levels.

• Combining efavirenz with clarithromycin, ethinyl estradiol, nelfinavir, or rifampin can alter blood levels of either drug. The importance of this interaction is unclear and dosage adjustments are unnecessary.

• Rifambutin decreases blood levels of efavirenz. Dosage adjustments may be necessary.

• Nevirapine decreases blood levels of efavirenz.

• Efavirenz decreases blood levels of methadone.

• Combining efavirenz and warfarin may increase the risk of excessive bleeding.

• The effect of efavirenz on oral contraceptives ("the pill") is not known. People combining these drugs should use an additional contraceptive method.

Food Interactions

This drug may be taken with or without food, but do not take efavirenz with a high-fat meal because it will increase the amount of efavirenz absorbed by about 50%, raising the risk of adverse events.

Usual Dose

Adult: 600 mg once a day, preferably at bedtime at first.
Child (88 lbs. and over): 600 mg a day.
Child (71.5–87 lbs.): 400 mg a day.
Child (55–71.5 lbs.): 350 mg a day.
Child (44–54 lbs.): 300 mg a day.
Child (33–43 lbs.): 250 mg a day.
Child (22–32 lbs.): 200 mg a day.
Child (under age 3 or less than 22 lbs.): not recommended.

Overdosage

Symptoms may include dizziness, nausea, loss of concentration, and other nervous system effects. Take the victim to a hospital emergency room. ALWAYS bring the prescription bottle or container.

Special Information

It is imperative for you to take your HIV medication exactly as prescribed. Missing or skipping doses of efavirenz increases your risk of becoming resistant to the drug and losing the benefits of efavirenz therapy.

Efavirenz does not cure acquired immunodeficiency syndrome (AIDS). It does not prevent you from transmitting the HIV virus to another person; you must still practice safe sex.

About half of people taking efavirenz develop dizziness, loss of concentration, depression, delusions, or drowsiness. Call your doctor if this occurs or if strange behavior develops. Do not combine efavirenz with alcohol, tranquilizers, or other psychoactive drugs.

Be careful when driving or performing any task that requires concentration. Take your medication at bedtime to better tolerate the depressant effects of efavirenz.

If you forget a dose, take it as soon as you remember. Contact your doctor if you forget your medication for 1 day.

Special Populations

Pregnancy/Breast-feeding

Animal studies of efavirenz showed that it can cause birth defects. Before starting on efavirenz, women should be tested to ensure they are not pregnant. When this drug is considered crucial by your doctor, its potential benefits must be carefully weighed against its risks.

Efavirenz passes into breast milk. Nursing mothers with HIV should always bottle-feed, regardless of whether they take this drug, to avoid transmitting the virus.

Seniors

Seniors may take this drug without special precaution.

Effexor XR   *see Venlafaxine, page 1143*

Generic Name

Eflornithine   (eh-FLOOR-nih-thene)

Brand Name

Vaniqa

Type of Drug

Hair growth retardant.

Prescribed For

Removal of unwanted facial hair by women.

General Information

This drug has only been studied for its ability to prevent hair growth on the face and chin and should not be used on other body areas. It works by interfering with enzymes in the skin necessary for hair growth, slowing the rate at which hair will grow. Improvement may be seen as soon as 4 to 8 weeks after you start using eflornithine, but the condition will return within 8 weeks after you stop using it.

Cautions and Warnings

Do not use eflornithine if you are **sensitive** or **allergic** to it.

Possible Side Effects

Eflornithine side effects are similar to those of a placebo (sugar pill).
▼ Most common: acne, bumps, or small pustules on the skin.
▼ Common: stinging.
▼ Less common: headache, dizziness, burning, itching, redness, tingling, irritation, rash, hair loss, upset stomach, and appetite loss.
▼ Rare: fainting, ingrown hairs, inflamed hair follicles, facial swelling, nausea, bleeding, contact dermatitis, inflammation of one or both lips, herpes breakout, numbness, and dilated blood vessels and pores on the nose and cheeks.

Food and Drug Interactions

None known.

Usual Dose

Adult and Child (age 12 and over): Apply a thin layer of cream to affected areas and rub in thoroughly 2 times a day at least 8 hours apart. Do not wash your face until at least 4 hours after you have applied eflornithine cream. Wait at least 5 minutes after hair removal to apply eflornithine.

   Child (under age 12): not recommended.

Overdosage

Little is known about the effects of eflornithine overdose or accidental ingestion. Call your local poison control center for more information.

Special Information

If you forget to apply a dose of eflornithine, apply it as soon as you remember. Bear in mind that at least 8 hours must elapse between doses and you cannot wash the area for another four hours after application. If it is almost time for your next dose, skip the dose you forgot and continue with your regular schedule.

   This product slows hair growth. It is not a depilatory. You will have to continue shaving, tweezing, or using another hair removal technique.

   Call your doctor if your skin becomes irritated or if you develop other side effects. If skin irritation continues, you may have to stop using eflornithine.

Special Populations

Pregnancy/Breast-feeding

Eflornithine cream may cause birth defects. When this drug is considered crucial by your doctor, its potential benefits must be carefully weighed against its risks.

   It is not known if this drug passes into breast milk. Nursing mothers should consider bottle-feeding.

Seniors

Seniors may use this product without special restriction.

Brand Name

EMLA

Generic Ingredients

Lidocaine + Prilocaine

Type of Drug

Topical anesthetic.

Prescribed For

Skin pain.

General Information

EMLA—which stands for Eutectic Mixture of Local Anesthetics—is a mixture of anesthetics that turns to liquid on contact with the skin. EMLA penetrates all layers of skin, dulling nerve endings and providing a local anesthetic effect comparable with that produced by injectable drugs. EMLA can prevent virtually any kind of skin pain and may be used by people of almost any age. The cream must be applied under an occlusive bandage (one that prevents contact with air or water), which intensifies the contact between skin and anesthetic. It works after being on the skin for at least 1 hour but may be more effective if left on for 2 or 3 hours. The anesthetic effect remains for 2 hours after the cream has been removed. EMLA is also available in patch form.

EMLA cream has been used to relieve the pain of intravenous catheter placement, minor plastic and skin surgery, shingles, and injections such as those used during vaccinations and blood donation.

Cautions and Warnings

Do not use EMLA cream if you are **allergic** to either of its anesthetics. People with **methemoglobinemia** (a rare blood condition) should not use EMLA.

Do not apply EMLA cream beyond the area prescribed by your doctor—otherwise, too much anesthetic may enter your blood and cause side effects. Do not apply EMLA to **open wounds, burns,** or **broken or inflamed skin.** Do not put EMLA in your **eyes, ears,** or **mouth.**

People with severe **liver disease** should use EMLA with caution because they may have difficulty removing the absorbed anesthetics from the blood.

Possible Side Effects

▼ Most common: irritation, redness, and swelling of the area to which it is applied.

▼ Common: skin pallor, patches of white skin, itching, rash, and changes in how you sense skin temperature.

▼ Rare: severe allergic reaction (symptoms include breathing difficulties, rash, intense itching, and elevated

Possible Side Effects *(continued)*

pulse). In rare cases when EMLA is applied in excess, is used too often, or too much anesthetic is absorbed, the following reactions may occur: nervous system excitation; nervousness; apprehension; light-headedness; euphoria (feeling "high"); confusion; dizziness; drowsiness; ringing or buzzing in the ears; blurred or double vision; vomiting; feelings of warmth, coldness, or numbness; twitching; tremors; convulsions; unconsciousness; or a very slow breathing rate or cessation of breathing.

Drug Interactions

• Drugs associated with causing methemoglobinemia should not be taken with EMLA. This interaction is generally limited to children under age 1. Some of these drugs are acetaminophen, sulfa drugs, oral antidiabetes drugs, thiazide diuretics, phenacetin, phenobarbital, phenytoin, primaquine, and quinine.

• Combining EMLA and antiarrhythmic drugs such as tocainide and mexiletine may increase the risk of serious side effects.

Usual Dose

Cream

Adult and Child (age 1 month and over): Apply a thick layer—2.5 g or ½ tsp.—and cover with the dressing provided in the package or some other occlusive bandage. Leave in place for at least 1–2 hours. The cream should be wiped away immediately before any surgical procedure or injection.

Patch

Apply to designated area and leave in place for at least 1–2 hours before removing.

Overdosage

Accidental ingestion of EMLA may affect the heart by making it less efficient. Call your local poison control center or a hospital emergency room for more information. If you seek treatment, ALWAYS bring the prescription bottle or container.

Special Information

EMLA numbs the skin. Be careful not to accidentally scratch or burn yourself after the product has been applied.

When you apply the cream, place the entire dose in the center of the designated area. Then cover it with the occlusive dressing and allow the pressure of the dressing to spread the cream.

Call your doctor if you develop severe, persistent, or bothersome side effects.

If you forget to apply EMLA, do so as soon as you can.

Special Populations

Pregnancy/Breast-feeding

The safety of using EMLA cream during pregnancy is not known, though there is no evidence that it interferes with fetal development. When this drug is considered crucial by your doctor, its potential benefits must be carefully weighed against its risks.

The anesthetics in EMLA cream pass into breast milk. Nursing mothers who must use this drug should consider bottle-feeding.

Seniors

Seniors may be more sensitive to side effects, especially after repeated applications.

Generic Name

Emtricitabine (em-trih-SIT-ah-bean)

Brand Name

Emtriva

Type of Drug

Antiviral.

Prescribed For

Human immunodeficiency virus (HIV) infection, in combination with other anti-HIV drugs.

General Information

Emtricitabine, is a nucleoside-type antiviral that works on the HIV virus in the same way as zalcitabine (ddC), zidovidudine (AZT), stavudine, and other drugs of this type. It is generally given in combination with AZT and a protease inhibitor. Emtricitabine is rapidly absorbed into the blood. Most of it passes out of the body in the urine.

Cautions and Warnings

Do not take emtricitabine if you are **sensitive** or **allergic** to it.

People with **kidney disease** require lower dosages of emtricitabine than people with normal kidney function.

The HIV virus can become **resistant** to emtricitabine. HIV strains that are resistant to emtricitabine were also resistant to lamivudine and zalcitabine but remained sensitive to many other antiviral drugs including abacavir, delavirdine, didanosine, efavirenz, nevirapine, stavudine, tenofovir, and zidovudine.

Emtricitabine and other antiretrovirals can cause **liver enlargement** and **lactic acidosis** (a potentially fatal metabolic imbalance). This frequently occurs in women but obesity and long-term treatment with emtricitabine may also be risk factors. However, people with no known risk factors have also developed these problems. Symptoms of lactic acidosis include **heart problems, bluish discoloration of the skin, cold hands or feet, rapid heartbeat, low blood pressure, dehydration, rapid breathing or difficulty breathing, lethargy, stupor or coma, vomiting, and/or abdominal pain**. Call your doctor immediately if you develop any of these or other unusual symptoms.

People taking emtricitabine or other anti-HIV drugs may experience unusual fat accumulation or redistribution leading to **buffalo hump, breast enlargement, abnormal thinness,** or a **round, moon-shaped face**. The reasons for this are not known.

Possible Side Effects

Because this drug is always taken with other antiviral drugs, the listed side effects are those of the drugs in combination. The risk of developing specific side effects can be different depending on the exact drug combination you are taking. The long-term effects of emtricitabine are not known.

▼ Most common: rash, itching, allergic reactions, cough, runny nose, nausea, weakness, diarrhea, abdominal pain, depression, and headache.

Possible Side Effects *(continued)*

▼ Common: discoloration of the soles of the feet or palms of the hands, upset stomach, vomiting, joint or muscle pain, unusual dreams, dizziness, sleeplessness, and tingling or pain in the hands or feet.

▼ Rare: Rare side effects can occur in almost any part of the body. Contact your doctor if you experience any side effect not listed above.

Drug Interactions

None known.

Food Interactions

This drug may be taken with or without food.

Usual Dose

Adult (age 18 and over): 200 mg once a day. People with reduced kidney function may take as little as 200 mg once every 4 days. Dialysis patients take one dose after dialysis is complete.

Child: not recommended.

Overdosage

Individual doses up to 1,200 mg a day have been studied, but little is known about the effects of emtricitabine overdose. Call your local poison control center or a hospital emergency room for more information. If you seek treatment, ALWAYS bring the prescription bottle or container.

Special Information

Emtricitabine does not cure AIDS. It will not prevent you from transmitting the HIV virus to another person; you must still practice safe sex. People taking this drug may still develop opportunistic infections and other complications of AIDS.

It is very important to take emtricitabine exactly as prescribed. If you forget a dose, take it as soon as you remember. If it is almost time for your next dose, skip the dose you forgot and continue with your regular schedule. Call your doctor if you forget 2 or more doses in a row.

Call your doctor immediately if your child develops signs of pancreas inflammation while taking emtricitabine. Symptoms include severe abdominal pain, tense abdominal muscles, sweating, feeling very ill, shallow and rapid breathing, fever, and possible fainting.

Special Populations

Pregnancy/Breast-feeding

Emtricitabine enters the fetal circulation. When this drug is considered crucial by your doctor, its potential benefits must be carefully weighed against its risks.

It is not known if emtricitabine passes into breast milk. Nursing mothers who must take emtricitabine should bottle-feed. In any case, nursing mothers who are HIV positive should bottle-feed to avoid transmitting the virus to their child.

Seniors

Seniors generally require lower doses of emtricitabine because of possible reductions in liver, renal, or cardiac function.

Generic Name

Enalapril (uh-NAL-uh-pril) G

Brand Name

Vasotec

Combination Products

Generic Ingredients: Enalapril + Hydrochlorothiazide G
Vaseretic

Generic Ingredients: Enalapril + Felodipine
Lexxel

Type of Drug

Angiotensin-converting enzyme (ACE) inhibitor.

Prescribed For

Hypertension (high blood pressure) and heart failure; also prescribed for diabetic kidney disease and heart attack treatment when the function of the left ventricle has been affected.

General Information

Enalapril maleate and other ACE inhibitors work by preventing the conversion of a hormone called angiotensin I to another hormone called angiotensin II, a potent blood-vessel constrictor. Preventing this conversion relaxes blood vessels, thus reducing blood pressure and relieving symptoms of heart failure. Enalapril also affects the production of other hormones and enzymes that participate in the regulation of blood-vessel dilation. Enalapril begins working about 1 hour after you take it and continues to work for 24 hours.

Some people who start taking enalapril after they are already on a diuretic (an agent that increases urination) experience a rapid drop in blood pressure after their first doses or when their dosage is increased. To prevent this from happening, your doctor may tell you to stop taking your diuretic 2 or 3 days before starting enalapril or to increase your salt intake during that time. The diuretic may then be restarted gradually.

Cautions and Warnings

Do not take enalapril if you are **allergic** to it.

Enalapril occasionally causes **very low blood pressure**.

Enalapril may affect your **kidney function,** especially if you have congestive **heart failure**. Your doctor should check your urine for protein content during the first few months of treatment. Dosage adjustment of enalapril is necessary if you have reduced kidney function.

Enalapril can affect white-blood-cell counts, possibly increasing your susceptibility to **infection**. Your doctor should monitor your blood counts periodically.

Enalapril may cause serious injury or death to the fetus if taken during pregnancy. Pregnant women should not take enalapril.

Possible Side Effects

▼ Most common: dizziness, fatigue, headache, nausea, and chronic cough. The cough usually goes away a few days after you stop taking the medication.

▼ Less common: chest tightness or pain, dizziness when rising from a sitting or lying position, fainting,

Possible Side Effects *(continued)*

abdominal pain, nausea, vomiting, diarrhea, bronchitis, urinary tract infection, breathing difficulties, weakness, and rash.

▼ Rare: Rare side effects can occur in almost any part of the body. Contact your doctor if you experience any side effect not listed above.

Drug Interactions

• The blood-pressure-lowering effect of enalapril is additive with diuretic drugs and beta blockers. Any other drug that causes a rapid drop in blood pressure should be used with caution if you are taking enalapril.

• Enalapril may increase blood-potassium levels, especially when taken with Dyazide or other potassium-sparing diuretics.

• Enalapril may increase the effects of lithium; this combination should be used with caution.

• Antacids and enalapril should be taken at least 2 hours apart.

• Capsaicin may trigger or aggravate the cough associated with enalapril therapy.

• Indomethacin may reduce the blood-pressure-lowering effects of enalapril.

• Phenothiazine tranquilizers and antiemetics may increase the effects of enalapril.

• Rifampin may reduce the effects of enalapril.

• The combination of allopurinol and enalapril increases the chance of side effects. Avoid this combination.

• Enalapril increases blood levels of digoxin, which may increase the chance of digoxin-related side effects.

Food Interactions

You may take enalapril with food if it upsets your stomach.

Usual Dose

5–40 mg a day in 1 or 2 doses. People with poor kidney function need less medication.

Overdosage

The principal effect of enalapril overdose is a rapid drop in blood pressure, as evidenced by dizziness or fainting. Take the overdose victim to a hospital emergency room immediately. ALWAYS bring the prescription bottle or container.

Special Information

Enalapril can cause swelling of the face, lips, hands, or feet. This swelling can also affect the larynx (throat) or tongue and interfere with breathing. If this happens, go to a hospital emergency room at once. Call your doctor if you develop a sore throat, mouth sores, abnormal heartbeat, chest pain, persistent rash, or loss of taste perception.

You may get dizzy if you rise to your feet too quickly from a sitting or lying position.

Avoid strenuous exercise or very hot weather because heavy sweating or dehydration can cause a rapid drop in blood pressure.

While taking enalapril, avoid over-the-counter diet pills, decongestants, and other stimulants that can raise blood pressure.

If you take enalapril once a day and forget to take a dose, take it as soon as you remember. If it is within 8 hours of your next dose, skip the one you forgot and continue with your regular schedule. If you take enalapril twice a day and miss a dose, take it right away. If it is within 4 hours of your next dose, take 1 dose immediately and another in 5 or 6 hours, then go back to your regular schedule. Never take a double dose.

Special Populations

Pregnancy/Breast-feeding

ACE inhibitors can cause fetal injury or death. Women who are or might become pregnant should not take ACE inhibitors. Sexually active women of childbearing age who must take enalapril must use an effective contraceptive method to prevent pregnancy. If you become pregnant, stop taking the medication and call your doctor immediately.

Small amounts of enalapril pass into breast milk. Nursing mothers who must take this drug should consider bottle-feeding.

Seniors

Seniors may be more sensitive to the effects of this drug due to age-related losses in kidney or liver function.

Generic Name

Enfuvirtide (en-FUV-jr-tide)

Brand Name

Fuzeon

Type of Drug

Antiviral fusion inhibitor.

Prescribed For

Human immunodeficiency virus (HIV) infection and acquired immunodeficiency syndrome (AIDS).

General Information

Enfuvirtide is the first of a new class of anti-HIV drugs. Unlike all other anti-HIV medicines, it works by preventing the HIV virus from fusing to healthy CD4 cells, a key part of the human immune system. This helps fight AIDS by having fewer HIV-infected cells as well as a healthier immune system to fight off the HIV virus. Enfuvirtide is always prescribed in combination with other antiviral medicines. It is possible for the HIV virus to become resistant to enfuvirtide, but this drug can work against types of the virus that have become resistant to other anti-HIV therapies.

Cautions and Warnings

Do not take enfuvirtide if you are **sensitive** or **allergic** to it. Symptoms of drug allergy can include generalized itching, rash, severe chills, and low blood pressure.

People taking enfuvirtide may be more likely to develop **bacterial pneumonia**. See your doctor regularly and report any difficulty breathing or unusual respiratory reactions.

Enfuvirtide may **raise blood sugar levels,** worsen **diabetes,** or trigger latent diabetes. People with diabetes who take this drug may need to have the dosage of their anti-diabetes medication adjusted.

Possible Side Effects

▼ Most common: allergic skin reaction at the site of injection (symptoms include itching, rash, and swelling

---

Possible Side Effects *(continued)*

of tissue under the skin), diarrhea, nausea, fatigue, and sleeplessness.

▼ Common: tingling in the hands or feet, depression, anxiety, cough, sinusitis, herpes infection, weight loss, appetite loss, weakness, itching, and muscle ache.

▼ Less common: taste changes, small skin tumors, flu infection, constipation, abdominal pain, pancreas inflammation, conjunctivitis, and lymph gland inflammation.

▼ Rare: Rare side effects can affect the blood, immune system, kidneys, urinary tract, and central nervous system.

Drug Interactions

Enfuvirtide is not broken down in the liver and does not affect liver enzyme systems, so it is not likely to be involved in common drug interactions.

Food Interactions

None known.

Usual Dose

Adult and Child (age 17 and over): 90 mg injected under the skin into the upper arm, thigh, or abdomen 2 times a day.

Child (age 6–16): 0.91 mg per lb. of body weight 2 times a day, up to 90 mg per injection. Be sure to increase enfuvirtide dosage as your child's weight increases.

Child (under age 6): not recommended.

Overdosage

Little is known about the effects of enfuvirtide overdose. Take the victim to a hospital emergency room. ALWAYS bring the prescription bottle or container.

Special Information

Enfuvirtide does not cure the HIV infection or AIDS. It will not prevent you from transmitting the HIV virus to another person; you must still practice safe sex. You may still develop opportunistic infections or other illnesses associated with advanced HIV disease.

This drug is given by injection under the skin. For information on how to properly administer this drug, see page 1188.

Do not use a vial of enfuvirtide if the final solution has particles floating in it. It should be completely clear, colorless, and have no bubbles in the vial.

You may keep enfuvirtide in the refrigerator and use it for up to 24 hours after it has been mixed. After that, it must be thrown away.

Tell your doctor if you are pregnant, become pregnant or plan to become pregnant.

Do not stop taking this, or any other anti-HIV medicine, without first consulting your doctor.

Special Populations

Pregnancy/Breast-feeding
While animal studies of enfuvirtide reveal no damage to the fetus, this drug should only be used during pregnancy after carefully weighing its potential benefits against its risks. A national registry has been established to gather information on pregnant women who take this drug.

It is not known if enfuvirtide passes into breast milk. Nursing mothers with HIV should always bottle-feed, regardless of whether they take this drug, to avoid transmitting the virus to their child.

Seniors
The effects of enfuvirtide in seniors is unknown.

Generic Name

Entacapone (in-TACK-a-pohn)

Brand Name

Comtan

Type of Drug

Anti-parkinsonian.

Prescribed For

Parkinson's disease patients for whom levodopa and carbidopa are losing their effectiveness.

General Information

Entacapone is always used in combination with levodopa and carbidopa. Some patients experience signs and symptoms of an end-of-dose "wearing-off" effect despite taking levodopa and carbidopa. Entacapone enhances the effect of levodopa and carbidopa by reversing the action of an enzyme known as catechol-O-methyltransferase (COMT), which is primarily responsible for breaking down levodopa in the body.

Cautions and Warnings

Do not take this drug if you are **sensitive** or **allergic** to any of its ingredients.

People with **liver disease** may accumulate twice as much of this drug in their blood as people with normal liver function.

Entacapone has been rarely associated with the formation of **fibrous tissues** in unusual places such as the urinary tract and lungs. It has also caused **fluid in the lungs**.

Entacapone may cause **kidney toxicity**.

Possible Side Effects

▼ Most common: difficulty performing voluntary muscle functions, excessive muscle activity, nausea, diarrhea, urine discoloration, and diarrhea.

▼ Common: reduced muscle activity, dizziness, fatigue, constipation, and abdominal pain.

▼ Less common: low blood pressure and fainting when rising from a sitting or lying position, severe diarrhea, hallucinations, anxiety, agitation, gastritis or other stomach disorders, stomach gas, upset stomach, dry mouth, vomiting, increased sweating, back pain, taste changes, shortness of breath, easy bruising, weakness, and bacterial infection.

▼ Rare: muscle damage or death, high fever, and confusion.

Drug Interactions

• Do not mix entacapone with the monamine oxidase inhibitor (MAOI) drugs phenelzine or tranylcypromine. Entacapone may be taken with the MAOI selegiline.

• Other drugs broken down by COMT will also be affected by entacapone. Isoproterenol, epinephrine, ephedrine, norepinephrine, isoetharine, and others will interact with entacapone, even when taken by inhalation. The result may be increased heart rate, arrythmias, and excessive changes in blood pressure.

• Cholestyramine, probenecid, erythromycin, rifampicin, ampicillin, and chloramphenicol may interfere with the elimination of entacapone from the body.

• Entacapone may enhance the effects of sedatives, tranquilizers, and other nervous system depressants.

Food Interactions

This drug may be taken with or without food.

Usual Dose

200 mg with each levodopa and carbidopa dose, up to 8 tablets a day.

Overdosage

Theoretically, a massive entacapone overdose could prove lethal by completely inhibiting COMT throughout the body. There have been no reports of significant entacapone overdose but theoretically, a massive dose could be fatal. Doses up to 800 mg have been taken and side effects were mainly abdominal pain and loose stools. Other effects that might be expected include difficulty breathing, loss of muscle coordination, reduced level of activity, and convulsions. Overdose victims should be taken to a hospital emergency room as soon as possible. ALWAYS bring the prescription bottle or container.

Special Information

Always take your entacapone dose together with your levodopa and carbidopa dose. If you forget a dose, take it as soon as you remember. If it is within 2 hours of your next dose, skip the dose you forgot and continue with your regular schedule.

This drug can cause dizziness, nausea, sweating, or fainting when rising quickly from a sitting or lying position, especially at the beginning of treatment.

Increased body movements and twitching, twisting, or uncontrolled tongue, lip, face, arm, or leg movement may occur. If this happens, your doctor may need to adjust your dose of levodopa and carbidopa.

Exercise caution when performing tasks, such as driving, that require coordination and concentration until your body has become accustomed to the effects of entacapone.

Gradually reducing the dose of entacapone decreases some drug side effects.

Entacapone can cause your urine to turn a brownish-orange color. This change is harmless.

Special Populations

Pregnancy/Breast-feeding
Entacapone causes birth defects, miscarriage and abortion in pregnant animals. When this drug is considered crucial by your doctor, its potential benefits must be weighed against its risks.

Entacapone passes into the breast milk of animals but no information on humans is available. Nursing mothers should consider bottle-feeding.

Seniors
Seniors may take this drug without special precaution.

Brand Name

Entex PSE

Generic Ingredients

Guaifenesin + Pseudoephedrine [G]

Other Brand Names

Anatuss LA	Dynex
Aquatab	Endal-SR
Coldmist	Fedahist Expectorant
Congess	GFN/PSE
Congestac	GP-500
Contuss	Guaifed
Deconsal II	Guaifed-PD
Defen LA	Guaifenex GP
Durasal II	Guaifenex PSE
Duratuss	Guaifenex RX

Guaimax-D
Guaimax-S
Guaipax PSE
Guaitab
Guaitex PSE
Guaituss PE
Guai-Vent PSE
H 9600 SR
Histalet X
Iosal II
Maxifed
Maxifed G
Med-RX
Miraphen PSE
Nasabid
Nasabid-SR
Nasatab LA
Nesstab LA
PanMist LA
PanMist-Jr.
PanMist Syrup

Profen II
Pseudovent
Pseudovent-PED
Refenesen Plus
Respa-1st
Respaire
Respaire-120 SR
Robitussin PE
Ru-Tuss DE
Rymed
Sinufed Timecelles
Stamoist E
Sudal
Syn-RX
Touro LA
Tuss-LA
V-Dec-M
Versacaps
Zephrex
Zephrex LA

The information in this profile also applies to the following drugs:

Generic Ingredients: Guaifenesin + Ephedrine G
Broncholate
Bronkaid Dual Action
Dynafed Asthma Relief
MiniThin Asthma Relief
Primatine

Generic Ingredients: Guaifenesin + Phenylephrine G
Deconsal Sprinkle
Endal
Entex LA
Liquibid
PhenaVent
Sinupan
Sinuvent PE Tablets

Type of Drug

Decongestant and expectorant combination.

Prescribed For

Cold or allergy and for nasal congestion, stuffy nose, and runny nose associated with other upper respiratory conditions.

General Information

The decongestant ingredient in Entex PSE, pseudoephedrine, dramatically reduces congestion and stuffiness. The decongestant ingredients ephedrine and phenylephrine act similarly. The expectorant, guaifenesin, is used to help loosen thick mucus that may contribute to chest congestion; the effectiveness of guaifenesin and other expectorants has not been established. There are other drugs on the market using this same general formula—an expectorant plus a decongestant—but they use different decongestant ingredients or a combination of decongestants plus guaifenesin. Nothing cures a cold or allergy, but Entex PSE may provide relief from symptoms.

Cautions and Warnings

Entex PSE may cause **anxiety** or **nervousness** or interfere with **sleep**.

Do not use Entex PSE if you have **diabetes, heart disease, hypertension** (high blood pressure), **thyroid disease, glaucoma, stomach ulcer, urinary blockage,** or a **prostate condition**.

Entex PSE should not be used over extended periods of time to treat **persistent or chronic cough** especially one that may be caused by cigarette smoking, asthma, or emphysema.

Possible Side Effects

▼ Most common: fear, anxiety, restlessness, sleeplessness, tension, excitation, nervousness, dizziness, drowsiness, hallucinations, headache, psychological disturbances, tremor, and convulsions.

▼ Less common: nausea, vomiting, upset stomach, low blood pressure, heart palpitations, chest pain, rapid heartbeat, abnormal heart rhythms, irritability, euphoria (feeling "high"), eye irritation and tearing, hysterical reaction, appetite loss, urinary difficulties in men with a prostate condition, weakness, loss of facial color, and breathing difficulties.

Drug Interactions

• Entex PSE should be avoided if you are taking a monoamine oxidase inhibitor (MAOI) antidepressant for depression or hypertension because the MAOI may cause a very rapid rise in blood pressure or increase side effects such as dry mouth or nose, blurred vision, and abnormal heart rhythms.

• The decongestant in Entex PSE may interfere with blood-pressure-lowering medication.

Food Interactions

Take Entex PSE with food if it upsets your stomach.

Usual Dose

Capsules: 1 twice a day.

Liquid: 2 tsp. 4 times a day.

Overdosage

Most cases of overdose are not severe. Symptoms include sedation, sleepiness, increased sweating, and increased blood pressure. Hallucinations, convulsions, nervous-system depression, and breathing difficulties are more prominent in older adults. Most cases of overdose are not severe. Induce vomiting with ipecac syrup—available at any pharmacy. Call you local poison control center or a hospital emergency room before doing this. If you seek treatment, ALWAYS bring the prescription bottle or container.

Special Information

Call your doctor if your side effects are severe or gradually become intolerable.

If you forget a dose, take it as soon as you remember. If it is almost time for your next dose, skip the one you forgot and continue with your regular schedule. Do not take a double dose.

Special Populations

Pregnancy/Breast-feeding
Women who are or might be pregnant should avoid Entex PSE. When your doctor considers this drug crucial, its potential benefits must be carefully weighed against its risks.

The decongestant in Entex PSE may pass into breast milk. Nursing mothers who must take Entex PSE should consider bottle-feeding.

Seniors
Seniors are more sensitive to the effects of Entex PSE.

Generic Name

Epoetin (Ee-poh-eh-tin)

Brand Name

Epogen   Procrit

Type of Drug

Red blood cell growth stimulator.

Prescribed For

Anemia; may also be used for reducing the need for blood or red blood cell transfusions.

General Information

Epoetin is a natural hormone that stimulates the bone marrow to produce red blood cells. It is used for anemia that does not respond to iron supplements. In most cases of anemia, there are plenty of red blood cells circulating, but they lack iron—a necessary element in the manufacture of hemoglobin—which carries oxygen to body tissues. Hemoglobin is contained in red blood cells. People who need epoetin do not have enough red blood cells. Epoetin stimulates the production of new red blood cells to carry needed oxygen.

Cautions and Warnings

Do not use epoetin if you are **sensitive** or **allergic** to albumin or products manufactured from animal cells.

People with **uncontrolled high blood pressure** should not use epoetin.

Some people with **chronic kidney failure** and **severe anemia** should not take epoetin. Epoetin is not a replacement for emergency blood transfusion.

Epoetin is not intended for **anemia caused by folate or iron deficiency, hemodialysis, or GI bleeding.**

People using epoetin may require anticoagulant medicine to prevent **blood clotting** during treatment.

In rare cases, people taking epoetin may have **seizures.** Avoid driving or any other activities where a sudden seizure could be dangerous.

Epoetin should be avoided in patients with **blood cancers** such as lymphoma, because it can act as a growth factor for the tumor.

Possible Side Effects

Side effects reported in studies of epoetin were similar to those reported with an inactive placebo.

▼ Most common: high blood pressure, headache, constipation, diarrhea, nausea, joint pain, fever, fatigue, itching, rash, and difficulty breathing.

▼ Common: swelling, vomiting, chest pain, skin reactions at the site of injection, weakness, dizziness, urinary infections, diarrhea, upset stomach, blood clots, anxiety, tingling in the hands or feet, and trunk pain.

▼ Rare: stroke and heart attack.

Food and Drug Interactions

None known.

Usual Dose

Adult: Starting dose—23 to 69 units per lb. of body weight 3 times a week by intravenous or subcutaneous injection. Final dose is based on response and need. Surgery patients take 138 units per lb. for 10 days before surgery or 276 units once a week for 3 weeks before surgery and another dose on the day of surgery.

Child (under age 12): 23 units per lb. of body weight 3 times a week by intravenous or subcutaneous injection. Final dose is based on response and need.

Dialysis patients take epoetin once a week.

Overdosage

Little is known about the effects of epoetin overdose. Call your local poison control center or a hospital emergency room for information. If you seek treatment, ALWAYS bring the prescription bottle or container.

Special Information

People taking epoetin should have regular blood tests to assure the drug is working well. Your doctor may want to take blood samples 2 times a week for several weeks and then test your blood regularly.

Epoetin has been used by athletes to enhance physical performance. This is called blood doping and has resulted in several deaths because the hematocrit (percentage of red blood cells in a blood sample) could rise to very high levels.

Epoetin must be stored in a refrigerator.

This drug is given by infection under the skin. To give a subcutaneous (under the skin) injection, slowly draw the exact amount prescribed into the syringe being careful to avoid air bubbles in the solution. Insert the needle at a 45⁰ angle to the skin, pinch up your skin to prevent injecting the drug into a muscle, and pull back slightly on the plunger to be sure you have not entered a vein. If blood enters the syringe remove it and throw it away. If not, you may slowly depress the syringe plunger until the contents have been completely injected. Your doctor will teach you about this procedure.

Special Populations

Pregnancy/Breast-feeding
Animal studies suggest that epoetin may enter fetal circulation. When this drug is considered crucial by your doctor its potential benefits must be carefully weighed against its risks.

It is not known if epoetin passes into breast milk. Nursing mothers who must take it should bottle-feed.

Seniors
Seniors may use this product without special precaution.

Brand Name

Equagesic

Generic Ingredients

Aspirin + Meprobamate

Other Brand Names
Epromate-M   Meprogesic Q
Heptogesic   Micrainin
Meprogesic

Type of Drug

Analgesic combination.

Prescribed For

Pain from muscle spasms, sprains, strains, or bad backs.

General Information

Equagesic is one of several combination products containing a tranquilizer and an analgesic; it is used to relieve pain associated with muscle spasms.

Cautions and Warnings

Do not take this medication if you are **allergic** to any of its ingredients or carisoprodol, or if you have **acute intermittent porphyria**.

Meprobamate should be used with caution in people with **liver** or **kidney disease,** people with **epilepsy,** or people at **risk for suicide**.

Equagesic should be used with caution by people with a history of drug or alcohol dependence. The meprobamate in this product can become **habit-forming** and possibly **addictive,** especially when taken with other tranquilizers or depressant drugs. Avoid using this product for more than a few weeks at a time. Abruptly stopping this medication may lead to drug withdrawal (symptoms include anxiety, appetite loss, insomnia, vomiting, tremors, muscle weakness or twitching, confusion, and hallucinations) or recurrence of symptoms. The dose should be gradually reduced over a period of 1 to 2 weeks.

For additional information see "Cautions and Warnings" in Aspirin (p. 111).

Possible Side Effects

▼ Most common: clumsiness, unsteadiness, and drowsiness.

▼ Common: nausea, vomiting, dizziness, diarrhea, headache, changes in vision, euphoria (feeling "high"), weakness and tiredness.

▼ Less common: allergy, itching, rash, swelling in the arms or legs, and fainting spells.

▼ Rare: confusion, irregular heartbeat, sore throat and fever, unusual bleeding or bruising, breathing difficulties, and changes in blood components.

For additional information see "Possible Side Effects" in Aspirin (p. 111).

Drug Interactions

• In high doses, meprobamate can cause sleepiness, drowsiness, or difficulty breathing. Avoid taking this medication with other central nervous system (CNS) depressants, including alcohol, barbituates, narcotics, sleeping pills, tranquilizers, and some antihistamines.

For additional information see "Drug Interactions" in Aspirin (p. 111).

Food Interactions

This medication may be taken with food if it upsets your stomach.

Usual Dose

Adult and Child (age 17 and over): 1–2 tablets 3–4 times a day.

Child (under age 17): not recommended.

Overdosage

Overdoses are serious. Symptoms are drowsiness, lightheadedness, sleepiness, nausea, and vomiting. Victims should be taken to a hospital emergency room immediately. ALWAYS bring the prescription bottle or container.

Special Information

Equagesic may cause drowsiness, dizziness, or blurred vision. Be careful when driving or performing complex tasks while taking this medication.

Call your doctor immediately if you experience fever, sore throat, rash, or any other sign of an allergic reaction, or if side effects become bothersome or persistent.

If you forget a dose, take it as soon as you remember. If it is almost time for your next dose, skip the one you forgot and continue with your regular schedule. Do not take a double dose.

For additional information see "Special Information" in Aspirin (p. 111).

Special Populations

Pregnancy/Breast-feeding

These drugs cross into the fetal blood circulation.

Meprobamate has been known to increase the risk of birth defects if taken during the first 3 months of pregnancy and taking too much aspirin late in the pregnancy may decrease a newborn's weight and cause other problems. When this medication is considered essential by your doctor, its potential benefits must be carefully weighed against its risks.

These drugs pass into breast milk. Nursing mothers taking this medication should speak to their doctors before using Equagesic.

Seniors

Seniors are more sensitive to the effects of this medication, especially drowsiness or sleepiness, and should take the lowest effective dose.

Type of Drug

Erectile Dysfunction Drugs

Generic Ingredient: Sildenafil Citrate
Viagra

Generic Ingredient: Tadalafil
Cialis

Generic Ingredient: Vardenafil
Levitra

Prescribed For

Erectile dysfunction (ED).

General Information

The chemical nitric oxide is released in the penis during sexual stimulation. Nitric oxide causes the release of enzyme called cyclic guanosine monophosphate (cGMP), which increases blood flow into the penis, producing an erection. cGMP is broken down by the enzyme phosphodiesterase type 5 (PDE5). In men with low levels of cGMP, these medicines help achieve and maintain an erection by inhibiting PDE5, thus causing higher levels of cGMP. ED can be the result of nerve, blood vessel, or psychological problems. These drugs, which are effective in about 70% of men, only help when poor blood flow is the cause of the dysfunction. Women have reported some benefit from sildenafil, though it has been widely studied only in men. Vardenafil and tadalafil are intended only for men. These medicines start working in 30 to 60 minutes and their effects usually last from 2 to 4 hours, though some have noted an effect as long as 24 hours or more. Tadalafil begins working in 30 to 60 minutes and can last for up to 36 hours. The drug remains in the body for more than 2 days, much longer than the other medicines in this group. Some drug interactions and kidney or liver diseases extend this time even more.

Cautions and Warnings

These medicines **lower blood pressure** and should be avoided if you have high (greater than 170/100) or low (less than 90/50) blood pressure. Several people have died from a sudden blood pressure drop after combining erectile dysfunction medications with other medications that can reduce blood pressure.

People with **heart disease** may experience heart problems with sildenafil or vardenafil, including a heart attack. These reactions can occur during or shortly after sexual activity.

These medicines should never be taken by those taking heart medications called **nitrates,** as fatal reactions have occurred.

Avoid these medicines if you have had a **heart attack, stroke,** or life-threatening **abnormal heart rhythms** in the past 6 months, or if you have **heart failure,** unstable **angina pectoris, damage to the penis,** or a progressive eye disease called **retinitis pigmentosa.**

People taking sildenafil or vardenafil have experienced difficulties seeing blue or green colors and may see things with a blue tinge surrounding them. This happens because they affect an enzyme in the eye. The effect clears up after the drug passes out of your body.

People with **kidney or liver damage** retain these medicines in their bodies longer than people whose kidneys and liver function normally. People with kidney or liver problems should always begin with the lowest possible dosage.

People with **priapsm** (painful erection lasting more than 6 hours) or a condition that predisposes them to priapism—such as **leukemia** or **multiple myeloma**—should be cautious about taking these medicines.

Vardenafil should be avoided by people with **stomach or bleeding ulcers** because its effect on these conditions is not known.

Possible Side Effects

Sildenafil

▼ Most common: headache and flushing.

▼ Less common: upset stomach, stuffy nose, urinary infection, diarrhea, rash, dizziness, seizure, anxiety, prolonged and possibly painful erection, double vision, visual changes, blood-shot eyes, burning eyes, swelling in the eye, and blood vessel diseases in the retina.

▼ Rare: Rare side effects can occur in almost any part of the body. Call your doctor if you experience any side effect not listed above.

Tadalafil

▼ Most common: headache.

▼ Common: upset stomach. Back pain and muscle aches can develop 12 to 24 hours after taking tadalafil and go away on their own after 2 days.

▼ Less common: flushing, nasal congestion, and arm or leg pain.

▼ Rare: prolonged or painful erections. Other rare side effects can occur in almost any part of the body. Call your doctor if you experience any side effect not listed above.

Vardenafil

▼ Most common: headache and flushing.

▼ Less common: upset stomach, sinus infection, flu-like symptoms, dizziness, and nausea.

▼ Rare: Rare side effects can occur in almost any part of the body. Call your doctor if you experience any side effect not listed above.

Drug Interactions

• Combining cimetidine and sildenafil leads to a substantial (more than 50%) increase in the amount of sildenafil in the blood. Vardenafil is not affected by cimetidine.

• Erythromycin, itraconazole, ketoconazole, and protease inhibitors—used to combat HIV—drugs can cause sildenafil blood levels to almost double. Vardenafil levels can increase by 400% to 1,000% when combined with these medicines. If you are taking one of these medicines, do not take more than the lowest possible dose of your erectile dysfunction drug. Do not take tadalafil more than once every 3 days if you are also taking one of these medicines.

• Rifampin can be expected to reduce the effect of erectile dysfunction medicines by reducing the amount of drug in the blood. Other drugs that may reduce the effects of these drugs are carbamazepine, phenobarbital, and phenytoin.

• Dihydrocodeine—a widely used prescription pain reliever—may increase the effects of sildenafil, yielding substantially prolonged erections, sometimes lasting for hours.

• Do not combine sildenafil, tadalafil, and vardenafil. The effects of combining these drugs are not known.

• Do not combine either sildenafil or vardenafil with nitrates (such as nitroglycerin) and other drugs that lower blood pressure. The combination can cause a sudden, rapid drop in blood pressure.

• Do not take vardenafil if you are taking an alpha blocker (such as alfuzosin, doxazosin, prazosin, tamsulosin, or terazosin). Tadalafil may be taken only with tamsulosin. You may take sildenafil with an alpha blocker, but you must separate them by at least 4 hours.

• Do not take vardenafil if you are taking any medicine to treat an abnormal heartbeat, including amiodarone, procainamide, quinidine, and sotalol.

• Alcohol adds to the blood pressure-lowering effects of these medicines.

Food Interactions

Grapefruit juice may increase the amount these drugs in the blood. Taking sildenafil with a high-fat meal reduces the amount of drug absorbed. Tadalafil and vardenafil may be taken without regard to food or meals.

Usual Dose

Sildenafil

Adult: 50 mg taken about 1 hour before sexual activity. Individual doses can range from 25–100 mg. The maximum dosing frequency is once a day.

Senior: begin with 25 mg and gradually increase dosage as needed.

Tadalafil

Adult: 10 mg taken about 1 hour before sexual activity. Individual doses can range from 5–20 mg. Do not take more than 1 dose of tadalafil a day.

Senior: begin with 5 mg and gradually increase dosage as needed.

Vardenafil

Adult: 10 mg taken about 1 hour before sexual activity. Individual doses can range from 5–20 mg.

Senior: begin with 5 mg and gradually increase dosage as needed.

Overdosage

Sildenafil and tadalafil overdose are likely to produce exaggerated drug side effects. Vardenafil overdose may cause neck pain, muscle aches, or vision changes. Call your local poison control center or hospital emergency room for more information. If you seek treatment, ALWAYS bring the prescription bottle or container.

Special Information

Call your doctor and do not engage in sexual activity if the erection produced by sildenafil is painful or lasts 4 or more hours, or if you experience dizziness, nausea, or chest pain after taking sildenafil.

People who use organic nitrates for gardening or other purposes can experience a severe and dangerous blood pressure drop if they take sildenafil or vardenafil. It is not known how long you have to wait to resume nitrate use.

These drugs do not protect against sexually transmitted diseases.

Special Populations

Pregnancy/Breast-feeding
There is no evidence that sildenafil or vardenafil harm the fetus; however, they are not intended for pregnant women or nursing mothers.

Seniors
Men age 65 and over eliminate these drugs more slowly than younger men and should begin with the lowest possible dosage.

Generic Name

Ergoloid Mesylates

(ER-goe-loid MES-il-ates) Ⓖ

Brand Names

Gerimal   Hydergine LC
Hydergine

Type of Drug

Psychotherapeutic agent.

Prescribed For

Age-related decline in mental capacity.

General Information

Ergoloid mesylates is used to treat decreased mental capacity of unknown cause in people over age 60. This drug should not be used for any condition that is treatable with another drug or that may be reversible. People who respond to ergoloid mesylates are likely to have Alzheimer's disease or some other cause of dementia. Nobody knows exactly how ergoloid mesylates produce their effect, but they improve the supply of blood to the brain in test animals, reduce their heart rate, and improve muscle tone in blood vessels. Some studies show the drug to be very effective in relieving mild symptoms of mental impairment, while others find it to be only moderately effective. It is most beneficial in people whose symptoms are due to the effects of high blood pressure in the brain.

Cautions and Warnings

Ergoloid mesylates should not be taken if you are **allergic** or **sensitive** to them or have **psychotic symptoms** or **psychosis**.

Ergoloid mesylates should be used with caution in people with **liver disease, low blood pressure,** or **slow heartbeat.**

Possible Side Effects

▼ Common: Ergoloid mesylates does not produce serious side effects. When taken under the tongue, this drug may cause irritation, nausea, or upset stomach. Other side effects are drowsiness, slow heartbeat, and rash.

Drug Interactions

None known.

Food Interactions

Do not eat, drink, or smoke while you have an ergoloid mesylates pill under your tongue.

Usual Dose

1–2 mg 3 times a day. Do not exceed 12 mg a day.

Overdosage

Symptoms include blurred vision, dizziness, fainting, flushing, headache, appetite loss, nausea, vomiting, stomach cramps, and stuffy nose. Take the victim to a hospital emergency room. ALWAYS bring the prescription bottle or container.

Special Information

The effects of ergoloid mesylates are gradual and frequently not seen for up to 6 months. A 6-month period of treatment with ergoloid mesylates is recommended before your doctor can fully evaluate your response to the drug. Your doctor should periodically reevaluate your condition to determine if ergoloid mesylates is still needed and that it is working for you.

Dissolve sublingual tablets under the tongue. Do not chew or crush them; they are not effective if swallowed whole.

If you forget a dose, skip it and go back to your regular schedule. Do not take a double dose. Call your doctor if you miss 2 or more consecutive doses.

Special Populations

Pregnancy/Breast-feeding

Ergoloid mesylates may interfere with fetal development. When this drug is considered crucial by your doctor, its potential benefits must be carefully weighed against its risks.

Ergoloid mesylates pass into breast milk. Nursing mothers who must take this drug should bottle-feed.

Seniors

Seniors are more likely to develop side effects, especially hypothermia (low body temperature).

Generic Name

Erythromycin (eh-rith-roe-MYE-sin) Ⓖ

Brand Names

A/T/S	Erymax
Akne-mycin	EryPads
Benzamycin	Ery-Tab
Del-Mycin	Erythra-Derm
E-Base	Erythromycin DR
Emgel	Erythromycin Filmtabs
E-Mycin	Ilotycin
Eryc	PCE Dispertab
Erycette	Staticin
Eryderm	Theramycin Z
Erygel	T-Stat

The information in this profile also applies to all forms of erythromycin:

Generic Ingredient: Erythromycin Estolate Ⓖ

Ilosone	Ilosone Pulvules

Generic Ingredient: Erythromycin Ethylsuccinate Ⓖ

E.E.S. 200	EryPed 400
E.E.S. 400	EryPed Drops
EryPed	Erythromycin ES
EryPed 200	Pediamycin

Generic Ingredients: Erythromycin Ethylsuccinate + Sulfisoxasole

Eryzole	Pediazole

Generic Ingredient: Erythromycin Stearate Ⓖ

Erythrocin Stearate

Type of Drug

Macrolide antibiotic.

Prescribed For

Infections of virtually any part of the body: upper and lower respiratory tract infections; sexually transmitted diseases; urinary tract infections; infections of the mouth, gums, or teeth; and infections of the nose, ears, or sinuses. It is prescribed for acne and may be used for mild to moderate skin infections. Erythromycin is effective against diphtheria and dysentery. It is also prescribed for legionnaires' disease, rheumatic fever, whooping cough, and bacterial endocarditis. It is prescribed to patients with pelvic inflammatory disease as an alternative to penicillin. The eye ointment is used to prevent newborn gonococcal or chlamydial eye infections.

General Information

Erythromycin and other macrolide antibiotics are either bactericidal (bacteria-killing) or bacteriostatic (inhibiting bacterial growth) depending on the organism in question and amount of antibiotic present. Erythromycin is deactivated by stomach acid, so the tablet form is made to bypass the stomach and dissolve in the intestine.

Since the action of this antibiotic depends on its concentration in the invading bacteria, it is crucial that you follow your doctor's directions regarding the spacing of doses as well as the number of days you must take the medication—otherwise this antibiotic may be much less effective.

Cautions and Warnings

Do not take erythromycin if you are **allergic** to it or any macrolide.

Erythromycin is excreted primarily through the liver. People with **liver disease or damage** should consult their doctors. Those on long-term therapy with erythromycin should have periodic blood tests. If you restart erythromycin after having experienced liver damage, it is likely that symptoms will recur within 48 hours.

Erythromycin estolate has occasionally produced **liver problems** (symptoms include fatigue, nausea, vomiting, abdominal cramps, and fever). If you are susceptible to stomach problems, erythromycin may cause mild to moderate **stomach upset**; discontinuing the drug will reverse this condition.

Colitis (bowel inflammation) has been associated with all antibiotics (see "Possible Side Effects").

Possible Side Effects

▼ Most common: nausea, vomiting, stomach cramps, and diarrhea. Colitis (symptoms include severe abdominal cramps and severe, persistent, and possibly bloody diarrhea) may develop. Side effects of the topical erythromycin include peeling, dryness, itching, and oiliness.

▼ Less common: hairy tongue, itching, irritation of the anal or vaginal region, eye irritation, and skin tenderness. If any of these symptoms appear, call your physician immediately.

▼ Rare: hearing loss—which reverses itself after the drug is stopped and occurs most often in people with liver and kidney problems—and abnormal heart rhythms.

Drug Interactions

• Antacids may slightly affect the release of erythromycin from your body. This effect is not considered important.

• Do not combine erythromycin with astemizole or terfenadine.

• Erythromycin may slow the breakdown of carbamazepine (an anticonvulsant prescribed for seizures). Avoid this combination.

• Mixing erythromycin with rifabutin or rifampin can interfere with the antibiotic's effect and increase the risk of intestinal side effects.

• Do not mix erythromycin with sparfloxacin (a fluoroquinolone antibiotic). This mixture can lead to severe, possibly fatal, abnormal heart rhythms. Grepafloxacin (another fluoroquinolone) should only be mixed with erythromycin in hospitalized patients whose hearts can be monitored during treatment.

• Do not combine erythromycin and pimozide. Two people died after combining pimozide and a macrolide.

• Erythromycin may neutralize penicillin. It may also neutralize the antibiotics lincomycin and clindamycin.

• Erythromycin interferes with the elimination of theophylline from the body, possibly leading to theophylline overdose. It may also increase the effects of caffeine.

• Mixing erythromycin with a statin cholesterol-lowering drug increases the risk of developing a potentially fatal condition involving severe muscle pain and destruction.

• Combining erythromycin and alfentanil (an injectable pain reliever), bromocriptine, buspirone, digoxin, disopyramide, ergotamine, cyclosporine, methylprednisolone (a corticosteroid), tacrolimus, vinblastine, or benzodiazepines (such as alprazolam, diazepam, midazolam, and triazolam), increases the risk of drug side effects.

• Erythromycin estolate may increase the liver side effects of other drugs that affect the liver.

• Erythromycin may increase the anticoagulant (blood-thinning) effects of warfarin in people who take it regularly, especially older adults. People taking this combination should be tested regularly.

Food Interactions

Grapefruit juice slows the breakdown of erythromycin, increasing the amount of drug in the blood. For optimum effectiveness, take erythromycin base and erythromycin stearate on an empty stomach with a 6 to 8 oz. glass of water. 1 hour before or 2 hours after meals. Other forms of erythromycin can be taken without regard to food or meals.

Usual Dose

Tablet and Suspension
  Adult: 250–400 mg every 6 hours, taken 1 hour before meals. Maximum dose is 4 g a day.
  Child: 15–25 mg per lb. of body weight a day in divided doses depending on age, weight, and severity of infection.

Eye Ointment
½ in. 2–6 times a day.

Topical Solution
Apply morning and night.

  Doses of erythromycin ethylsuccinate are 60% higher due to differences in chemical composition.

Overdosage

Overdose may cause severe side effects, especially nausea, vomiting, stomach cramps, and diarrhea. Mild hearing loss, ringing or buzzing in the ears, or fainting may also occur. Call your local poison control center or a hospital emergency room for more information.

Special Information

Erythromycin is used instead of penicillin for mild to moderate infections in people who are allergic to penicillin. Erythromycin is not the antibiotic of choice for severe infections.

Erythromycin products should be stored at room temperature, except for oral and topical liquids, which should be kept in the refrigerator.

Call your doctor if you develop nausea; vomiting; diarrhea; stomach cramps; severe abdominal pain; rash, itching, or redness; dark or amber-colored urine; yellowing of the skin or whites of the eyes; or any severe or persistent side effect.

If you forget a dose of oral erythromycin, take it as soon as you remember. If it is almost time for your next dose, space the next 2 doses over 4 to 6 hours, then continue with your regular schedule. Do not take a double dose.

Remember to complete the full course of therapy prescribed even if you feel well before you finish the medication.

Special Populations

Pregnancy/Breast-feeding

Erythromycin passes into the fetal circulation. Erythromycin estolate has caused mild liver inflammation in about 10% of pregnant women who took it and should not be used if you are or might be pregnant. Other forms of erythromycin have been used safely without difficulty.

Erythromycin passes into breast milk. Nursing mothers who must take erythromycin should bottle-feed.

Seniors

Seniors with liver disease should use caution. Seniors taking high doses of erythromycin may be at an increased risk of hearing loss.

Generic Name

Estazolam (es-TAZ-oe-lam) G

Brand Name

ProSom

Type of Drug

Benzodiazepine sedative.

Prescribed For

Insomnia and sleep disturbances.

General Information

Estazolam is a member of the group of drugs known as benzodiazepines. They work by a direct effect on the brain. Benzodiazepines make it easier to go to sleep and decrease the
number of times you wake up during the night. Estazolam is
considered an intermediate-acting sedative and generally
remains in your body long enough to give you a good night's
sleep with minimal "hangover."

Cautions and Warnings

People with **respiratory disease** taking estazolam may experience **sleep apnea** (intermittent cessation of breathing during
sleep).

People with **kidney or liver disease** should be carefully
monitored while taking estazolam. Take the lowest possible
dose to help you sleep.

Clinical **depression** may be increased by estazolam, which
can depress the nervous system. Intentional overdose is
more common among depressed people who take sleeping
pills than among those who do not.

All benzodiazepines can be **addictive** if taken for long periods of time and can cause drug withdrawal symptoms if discontinued suddenly. Withdrawal symptoms include tremors,
muscle cramps, insomnia, agitation, diarrhea, vomiting,
sweating, and convulsions.

Possible Side Effects

▼ Common: drowsiness, headache, dizziness, talkativeness, nervousness, apprehension, poor muscle coordination, light-headedness, daytime tiredness, muscle
weakness, slowness of movement, hangover, and euphoria (feeling high).

▼ Less common: nausea, vomiting, rapid heartbeat,
confusion, temporary memory loss, upset stomach, stomach cramps and pain, depression, blurred or double vision
and other visual disturbances, constipation, changes in

Possible Side Effects (continued)

sense of taste, appetite changes, stuffy nose, nosebleeds, common cold symptoms, asthma, sore throat, cough, breathing difficulties, diarrhea, dry mouth, allergic reaction, fainting, abnormal heart rhythm, itching, acne, dry skin, sensitivity to bright light or to the sun, rash, nightmares or strange dreams, sleeplessness, tingling in the hands or feet, ringing or buzzing in the ears, ear or eye pain, menstrual cramps, frequent urination and other urinary difficulties, blood in the urine, discharge from the penis or vagina, lower back and joint pain, muscle spasms and pain, fever, swollen breasts, and weight changes.

▼ Rare: Rare side effects can affect your heart, stomach and intestines, urinary tract, blood, muscles, and joints. Contact your doctor if you experience any side effect not listed.

Drug Interactions

• As with all benzodiazepines, the effects of estazolam are enhanced if it is taken with an alcoholic beverage, antihistamine, tranquilizer, barbiturate, anticonvulsant medication, antidepressant, or monoamine oxidase inhibitor drug (MAOI).

• Oral contraceptives, cimetidine, disulfiram, and isoniazid may increase the effect of estazolam by interfering with the drug's breakdown in the liver. Probenecid also increases estazolam's effects.

• Cigarette smoking, rifampin, and theophylline may reduce the effect of estazolam.

• Levodopa's effectiveness may be decreased by estazolam.

• Estazolam may increase the amount of zidovudine (an AIDS drug—also known as AZT), phenytoin, or digoxin in your bloodstream, increasing the chances of side effects.

• The combination of clozapine and benzodiazepines has led to respiratory collapse in a few people. Estazolam should be stopped at least 1 week before starting clozapine treatment.

Food Interactions

Estazolam may be taken with food if it upsets your stomach.

Usual Dose

Adult (age 18 and over): 1–2 mg about 60 minutes at bedtime.

Senior: starting dose—0.5–1 mg. Dosage should be increased cautiously.

Child (under age 18): not recommended.

Overdosage

The most common overdose symptoms are confusion, sleepiness, depression, loss of muscle coordination, and slurred speech. Coma and death may also occur. People who take an estazolam overdose must be made to vomit with ipecac syrup—available at any pharmacy—to remove any remaining drug from the stomach: Call your doctor or a poison control center before doing this. The victim must be taken to a hospital emergency room for treatment if 30 minutes have passed since the overdose was taken or if symptoms have begun to develop. ALWAYS bring the prescription bottle or container.

Special Information

Never take more estazolam than your doctor has prescribed.

Avoid alcoholic beverages and other nervous system depressants while taking estazolam.

Exercise caution while performing tasks that require concentration and coordination; estazolam may make you tired, dizzy, or light-headed.

If you take estazolam daily for 3 or more weeks, you may experience some withdrawal symptoms when you stop taking the drug.

If you forget to take a dose of estazolam and remember within about 1 hour of your regular time, take it right away. If you do not remember until later, skip the dose you forgot and go back to your regular schedule. Do not take a double dose.

Special Populations

Pregnancy/Breast-feeding

Estazolam absolutely should not be used by pregnant women or by women who may become pregnant.

Estazolam passes into breast milk. The drug should not be taken by nursing mothers.

Seniors

Seniors are more susceptible to the effects of estazolam.

Type of Drug

Estrogens (ES-troe-jens)

Brand Names

Generic Ingredient: Chlorotrianisene
TACE

Generic Ingredient: Conjugated Estrogens
Premarin

Generic Ingredient: Conjugated Estrogens (Synthetic)
Cenestin

Generic Ingredients: Conjugated Estrogens +
Medroxyprogesterone
Prempro   Premphase

Generic Ingredient: Dienestrol
Ortho Dienestrol

Generic Ingredient: Esterified Estrogens
Estratab   Menest

Generic Ingredients: Esterified Estrogens + Methyltestosterone
Estratest   Syntest HS
Estratest HS   Syntest DS

Generic Ingredient: Estradiol G
Alora Transdermal System   Femring
Climara   Gynodiol
Esclim   Innofem
Estrace   NuvaRing
Estraderm   Vagifem
Estrasorb   Vivelle
Estring   Vivelle-Dot
FemPatch

Generic Ingredients: Estradiol + Norethindrone Acetate
Activella   CombiPatch

Generic Ingredients: Estradiol + Levonorgestrel
Climara Pro Transdermal System

Generic Ingredients: Estradiol + Norgestimate
Ortho-Prefest

Generic Ingredient: Estropipate G

Ogen   Ortho-Est

Generic Ingredient: Ethinyl Estradiol

Estinyl

Generic Ingredients: Ethinyl Estradiol + Norethindrone Acetate

femhrt

Prescribed For

Moderate to severe menopausal symptoms including hot flashes, night sweats and sleep problems, and vaginal dryness and irritation; also prescribed for ovarian failure, osteoporosis prevention, male breast cancer, advanced prostate cancer, abnormal bleeding of the uterus, vaginal irritation, female castration, Turner's syndrome, and birth control.

General information

Six estrogens have been identified in women but only 3 are present in large amounts: estradiol, estrone, and estriol. Estradiol is the most potent and important. Other estrogens are produced by chemical conversions in the body. Estradiol, for example, is transformed into estrone, which in turn becomes estriol. Estrogens all have the same actions and side effects; only potency varies. More potent types require smaller dosages to produce the same effect.

Estrogens are largely responsible for the growth and maintenance of the female reproductive system and sex characteristics. They affect the release of hormones from the pituitary gland (controller of hormone production and regulator of basic bodily functions). These hormones control the functioning of capillaries (smallest blood vessels), may cause fluid retention, affect protein breakdown in the body, prevent ovulation and breast engorgement after childbirth, and influence the shaping and maintenance of the skeleton through an effect on calcium.

Estrogen products differ in their hormone content and dosage. Some may affect one part of the body more than another. Generally, though, estrogens are interchangeable as long as dosage differences are taken into account.

Many women have taken hormone replacement therapy to manage menopausal symptoms, but there are risks associated with this form of treatment.

Cautions and Warnings

Women with an intact uterus who choose hormone replacement therapy for menopausal symptoms should take the lowest effective dose for the shortest possible time to minimize their risk of **heart disease, cancer, blood clots,** and **strokes.** The results of a very large study called the Women's Health Initiative were published in 2002 and have drastically changed the face of estrogen replacement therapy. The study found that women taking long-term estrogen replacement therapy have a small but important increase in the risk of **nonfatal heart attacks.** The risk for **invasive breast cancer** is 26% higher and tumors are harder to detect when taking estrogen therapy. The risk of a **stroke** was increased by 41% and the risk of **blood clots** forming in the body was doubled in women taking hormone therapy. This study did show some benefits of the effects of long-term hormone replacement in colon cancer and osteoporosis but these benefits do not necessarily outweigh the risks.

Women with **blood clotting problems** and those who are **allergic** to estrogens should not take them.

Estrogens may increase the risk of **endometrial cancer** by 4.5 to 14 times in postmenopausal women taking them without progestin for prolonged periods of time; the risk depends on duration of treatment and dosage.

Women with **breast cancer** should not take estrogens, except some being treated for breast cancer that has spread, nor should those with an estrogen-dependent cancer or **abnormal vaginal bleeding** whose cause is unknown. Women who have a strong family **history of breast cancer** or who have **breast nodules or cysts** or an **abnormal mammogram** should be cautious about using estrogens. Women taking an estrogen for breast cancer that has spread to their bones can develop large increases in blood **calcium.**

Oral contraceptives ("the pill") containing norgestrel and ethinyl estradiol have been used as emergency **"morning-after" contraception.** The drug must be taken no more than 72 hours after intercourse to be effective and can harm the fetus if pregnancy is not prevented.

Postmenopausal women taking estrogen are more likely to develop **gallbladder disease** or **dementia.**

Estrogens can raise **blood pressure.** Pressure usually returns to normal when the drug is stopped.

There is an increased risk of **thrombosis** in men taking estrogens for prostate cancer.

People with **thrombophlebitis** should avoid these drugs. The risk is greatest with very high dosages. Low dosages may not be a problem.

Estrogens should not be used to treat painful **breast enlargement** that sometimes develops after giving birth.

Estrogens can cause significant increases in blood **triglycerides** and **pancreas inflammation** in women with inherited **blood-fat disorders**.

Oral contraceptives may be associated with an increase in depression; patients with a history of depression should be watched carefully.

Vaginal estrogen cream may stimulate **bleeding of the uterus**. It may also cause **breast tenderness, vaginal discharge,** and **withdrawal bleeding** if the product is suddenly stopped. Women with **endometriosis** may experience heavy vaginal bleeding.

Possible Side Effects

▼ Most common: breast enlargement or tenderness, ankle and leg swelling, appetite loss, weight changes, water retention, nausea, vomiting, abdominal cramps, and a feeling of abdominal bloating. The estrogen patch may cause rash, irritation, and redness where it is applied.

▼ Less common: bleeding gums, breakthrough vaginal bleeding, vaginal spotting, changes in menstrual flow, painful menstruation, premenstrual syndrome (PMS), absence of menstrual periods during and after estrogen use, uterine fibroid enlargement, vaginal *Candida* infection, a cystitis-like condition, mild diarrhea, yellowing of the skin or whites of the eyes, eye lesions, contact-lens intolerance, rash, hair loss, development of new hairy patches, migraine, mild dizziness, depression, increased sex drive (women), and decreased sex drive (men).

▼ Rare: stroke, blood-clot formation, dribbling or sudden passage of urine, loss of coordination, chest pain, leg pain, breathing difficulties, slurred speech, and changes in vision. Men who take large estrogen dosages for prostate cancer have a greater risk of heart attack, phlebitis, and blood clots in the lungs.

Drug Interactions

• Phenytoin, ethotoin, and mephenytoin may interfere with estrogen's effects.

• Estrogens may reduce the effect of oral anticoagulant (blood-thinning) drugs. Your anticoagulant dosage may need an adjustment.

• Estrogens increase the amount of calcium absorbed from the stomach. This interaction is used to help women with osteoporosis increase their calcium level.

• Estrogens may increase the side effects of antidepressants and phenothiazine tranquilizers.

• Low estrogen dosages may increase phenothiazine's effectiveness.

• Estrogens may increase cyclosporine and corticosteroid blood levels. Dosage adjustments of the non-estrogen drugs may be needed.

• Rifampin, barbiturates, and other drugs that stimulate the liver to break down drugs may reduce estrogen blood levels.

• Estrogens may interfere with tamoxifen and bromocriptine.

• Women, especially those over age 35, who smoke cigarettes and take estrogen have a much greater risk of developing stroke, hardening of the arteries, and blood clots in the lungs. The risk increases with age and tobacco use.

• Estrogens interfere with many diagnostic tests. Make sure your doctor knows you are taking estrogen before conducting any blood tests or other diagnostic procedures.

Food Interactions

Estrogens may be taken with food to reduce nausea and upset stomach. Avoid drinking grapefruit juice if you are taking this drug.

Usual Dose

Dosage varies. All of these products, including the transdermal skin patch, may be taken continuously or on a cyclic schedule of 3 weeks on, 1 week off.

Tablets
Chlorotrianisene: 12–200 mg.
   Conjugated estrogens: 0.3–30 mg.
   Conjugated estrogens, synthetic: 0.625–1.25 mg.
   Esterified estrogens: 0.3–30 mg.
   Estradiol: 0.5–30 mg.

Estropipate: 0.625–7.5 mg.
Ethinyl estradiol: 0.02–3.0 mg.

Estradiol Lotion
Apply 3 grams (about ¹/₂ teaspoon) to the legs, thighs, or calves once a day.

Estradiol Transdermal Patch (0.025, 0.0375, 0.05, 0.075, or 0.1 mg)
Alora, Estraderm, and Esclim: 1 patch twice a week; or use 1 patch twice a week for 3 weeks, stop for 1 week, then start again.

Climara and Fempatch: 1 patch every week; or use 1 patch once a week for 3 weeks, stop for 1 week, then start again.

Vaginal Cream
Conjugated estrogens: 0.5–2.0 g a day for 3 weeks; stop for 1 week, then start again.

Dienestrol: 1 applicatorful 1–2 times a day for 1–2 weeks, half the original dosage for another 1–2 weeks, then 1 applicatorful 1–3 times a week.

Estradiol: 2–4 g a day for 2 weeks, half the starting dosage for another 2 weeks, then 1 g 1–3 times a week.

Estropipate: 2–4 g a day for 3 weeks; stop for 1 week, then start again.

Estradiol Ring
Insert once every 3 months.

Overdosage

Symptoms may include nausea and vaginal bleeding in adult women. Call your local poison control center or a hospital emergency room for information. If you seek treatment, ALWAYS bring the prescription bottle or container.

Special Information

Many experts note that the risk of serious health complications for an individual woman taking hormone replacement therapy is small. Be sure your decision to take hormones is based on a complete discussion of the facts and your individual situation with your doctor.

Call your doctor if you develop breast pain or tenderness, swelling of the feet and lower legs, rapid weight gain, chest pain, breathing difficulties, pain in the groin or calves, unusual or persistent vaginal bleeding, missed menstrual period, lumps in the breast, sudden severe headache, dizziness or fainting, disturbances in speech or vision, weakness or numbness in the arms or legs, abdominal pain, depression, yellowing of the skin or whites of the eyes, or jerky or involuntary muscle movement.

Women taking estrogens or combined estrogen and progestin therapy should have yearly breast exams, perform monthly breast self-examinations, and have regular mammograms.

Talk to your doctor about ways to reduce risk factors for heart disease (such as blood pressure control, healthy diet, and stopping tobacco use) and osteoporosis (such as vitamin D and calcium supplements, healthy diet, and weight-bearing exercise).

Your doctor should reevaluate your need for estrogen vaginal cream every 3–6 months. Do not stop using the drug suddenly because this may increase your risk of developing unpredicted or breakthrough vaginal bleeding.

Women using the cream who develop breast tenderness, start to bleed, or have other vaginal discharge should contact their doctors at once.

Women who smoke cigarettes and take estrogen have a greater risk of cardiovascular side effects including stroke and blood clotting.

Estrogen skin patches should be applied to a clean, dry, non-oily, hairless area of intact skin, preferably on the abdomen. Do not apply them to your breasts or waist, or to any area where tight-fitting clothes may loosen the patch from your skin. The application site should be rotated to prevent irritation and each site should have a patch-free period for 7 days.

Good dental hygiene is important while taking estrogen because estrogen may increase your risk of oral infection. Dental work should be completed prior to starting estrogen, if possible.

Vaginal estrogen cream should be inserted high into the vagina, about ⅔ of the length of the applicator.

Press the vaginal ring into an oval and insert as deeply as possible in the upper ⅓ of the vagina.

Some of these products contain tartrazine (a commonly used orange dye and food-coloring). If you are allergic to tartrazine or have asthma, check with your pharmacist to find out if your estrogen product contains this coloring agent.

If you forget a dose, take it as soon as you remember. If it is almost time for your next dose, skip the one you forgot and continue with your regular schedule. Do not take a double dose.

Special Populations

Pregnancy/Breast-feeding

Estrogens harm the fetus and should never be used during pregnancy for any reason.

Estrogens pass into breast milk and reduce its flow. Nursing mothers who must take them should bottle-feed.

Seniors

The risk of side effects increases with age, especially if you smoke. Women age 65 or over taking estrogens may be more likely to develop dementia.

Generic Name

Etanercept (eh-TAN-er-sept)

Brand Name

Enbrel

Type of Drug

Immune system modulator.

Prescribed For

Rheumatoid arthritis, juvenile rheumatoid arthritis, psoriatic arthritis, ankylosing spondylitis, and psoriasis.

General Information

Etanercept binds to a specific protein in the body known as tumor necrosis factor (TNF) and blocks it from interacting with cell surfaces. TNF is involved in normal inflammatory and immune responses and the inflammatory processes of rheumatoid arthritis, juvenile rheumatoid arthritis, and other conditions. Etanercept can also interfere with biological actions that are either caused or regulated by TNF.

Cautions and Warnings

Do not use this drug if you are **sensitive** or **allergic** to it.

Serious infections and **malignancies** are possible in people using etanercept because of its ability to suppress the immune response. This may be more common in people with other conditions that predispose them to infections such as advanced or uncontrolled **diabetes**.

Levels of blood platelets and some white blood cells may be reduced in rare cases, leading to **persistent fever, bruising, bleeding,** and **pale skin.** Contact your doctor if any of these symptoms develop.

Etanercept may increase the risk of some **nervous system disorders** including multiple sclerosis.

Etanercept may cause or worsen **congestive heart failure.**

People taking etanercept should not receive any **live vaccines,** because the body may not be able to respond as expected to the vaccine.

Possible Side Effects

Reactions may develop at the site where etanercept is injected. Injection sites should be rotated among the thigh, abdomen, and upper arm to avoid excessive bruising or other skin damage.

▼ Most common: infection, injection site reactions, upper respiratory infection, headache, and runny nose.

▼ Common: nausea, dizziness, sore throat, cough, weakness, abdominal pain, rash, and respiratory problems.

▼ Less common: upset stomach, sinus irritation, vomiting, swelling in the legs or feet, mouth sores, and hair loss.

▼ Rare: malignancy, stroke, seizure, tingling in the hands or feet, nervous system irritation similar to multiple sclerosis, eye inflammation, joint pain, generalized pain, appetite loss, blood vessel inflammation in the skin, dry eyes, lumps under the skin, fever, flu symptoms, weight gain, chest pain, flushing, diarrhea, taste changes, difficulty breathing, worsening of existing lung conditions, itching, and skin reactions.

Drug Interactions

• Do not mix etanercept in the same syringe as another drug.

Food Interactions

None known.

Usual Dose

Adult: 25 mg twice a week injected under the skin 3–4 days apart.

Child (age 4–17): 0.2 mg per lb. of body weight, up to 25 mg twice a week, injected under the skin 3–4 days apart.

Child (under age 4): not recommended.

Overdosage

In one study, a patient accidentally self-administered 62 mg of etanercept 2 times a week for 3 weeks with no problems. Call your local poison control center or a hospital emergency room for more information. If you seek treatment, ALWAYS bring the prescription bottle or container.

Special Information

Etanercept is taken by injection under the skin. Be sure you understand how to measure the proper dose of etanercept and how to self-inject it.

To mix and inject etanercept: Withdraw all the water supplied with the medicine into a syringe and slowly inject it into the vial containing etanercept. Swirl the mixture gently to avoid excess foaming in the vial. *Do not shake the vial.*

Do not combine etanercept with any other injectable drug.

Etanercept should be mixed just before you inject it, but may be stored in a refrigerator for up to 6 hours after it is mixed. The mixed vial must be discarded if not used in 6 hours.

If you forget to administer a dose, do so as soon as you remember. Remember that etanercept doses must be administered at least 3 days apart. Call your doctor or pharmacist if you have any questions about how to time your etanercept doses.

Special Populations

Pregnancy/Breast-feeding

The safety of using etanercept during pregnancy is not known. When this drug is considered crucial by your doctor, its potential benefits must be carefully weighed against its risks.

It is not known if this drug passes into breast milk. Nursing mothers who must take it should bottle-feed.

Seniors

Seniors are more likely to develop infections while using etanercept.

Generic Name

Etodolac (ee-TOE-doe-lak) G

Brand Names

Lodine   Lodine XL

Type of Drug

Nonsteroidal anti-inflammatory drug (NSAID).

Prescribed For

Osteoarthritis; may also be used to treat rheumatoid arthritis, ankylosing spondylitis, mild to moderate pain, tendinitis, bursitis, painful shoulder, and gout.

General Information

Etodolac and other NSAIDs are used to relieve pain and inflammation. We do not know exactly how NSAIDs work, but they may achieve their effects by blocking the body's production of a hormone called prostaglandin and the action of other body chemicals. Etodolac starts relieving pain in about 30 minutes and its effects last for 4 to 12 hours. Etodolac is broken down in the liver and eliminated through the kidneys.

Cautions and Warnings

People who are **allergic** to etodolac or any other NSAID and those with a history of **asthma** attacks brought on by an NSAID, iodides, or aspirin should not take etodolac.

Etodolac may cause **gastrointestinal (GI) bleeding, ulcers,** and **stomach perforation**. This can occur at any time, with or without warning, in people who take etodolac regularly. People with a history of active GI bleeding should be cautious about taking any NSAID. People who develop bleeding or ulcers and continue NSAID treatment should be aware of the possibility of developing more serious side effects.

Etodolac may affect platelets and **blood clotting** at high doses, and should be avoided by people with clotting problems and those taking warfarin.

People with **heart problems** who use etodolac may experience swelling in their arms, legs, or feet.

Etodolac may cause severe toxic effects to the **kidney**. Report any unusual side effects to your doctor, who may need to periodically test your kidney function.

People with **impaired kidney or liver function** may need lower dosages of etodolac.

Etodolac may make you **unusually sensitive to the effects of the sun**.

Possible Side Effects

▼ Most common: dizziness, weakness, diarrhea, nausea, vomiting, constipation, gas, stomach upset or irritation, and appetite loss, especially during the first few days of treatment.

▼ Less common: stomach ulcers, GI bleeding, depression, hepatitis, gallbladder attacks, painful urination, poor kidney function, kidney inflammation, blood and protein in the urine, fainting, nervousness, depression, hallucinations, confusion, disorientation, tingling in the hands or feet, light-headedness, itching, increased sweating, dry nose and mouth, heart palpitations, chest pain, breathing difficulties, and muscle cramps.

▼ Rare: severe allergic reactions including closing of the throat, fever and chills, changes in liver function, jaundice (yellowing of the skin or whites of the eyes), and kidney failure. People who experience such effects must be promptly treated in a hospital emergency room or doctor's office. NSAIDs have caused severe skin reactions; if this happens to you, see your doctor immediately.

Drug Interactions

• Etodolac may increase the effects of oral anticoagulant (blood-thinning) drugs such as warfarin. Your anticoagulant dose may need to be reduced.

• Taking etodolac with cyclosporine may increase the kidney-related side effects of both drugs. Methotrexate side effects may be increased in people also taking etodolac.

• Etodolac may increase phenytoin side effects. Lithium blood levels may be increased by etodolac.

• Etodolac blood levels may be affected by cimetidine.

• Probenecid may increase the risk of etodolac side effects.

• Aspirin and other salicylates should never be combined with etodolac.

• Combining etodolac and bisphosphonates may increase the risk of gastric ulceration.

• Colestipol may decrease the effectiveness of etodolac.

• Etodolac may decrease the effectiveness of ACE inhibitors and diuretics.

• Etodolac may increase lithium levels.

Food Interactions

Take etodolac with food or a magnesium-aluminum antacid if it upsets your stomach.

Usual Dose

200–400 mg every 6–12 hours, not to exceed 1200 mg a day. People weighing 132 lbs. or less should not take more than 20 mg for every 2.2 lbs. of body weight.

Overdosage

People have died from NSAID overdoses. Common signs of overdose are drowsiness, nausea, vomiting, diarrhea, abdominal pain, rapid breathing, rapid heartbeat, increased sweating, ringing or buzzing in the ears, confusion, disorientation, stupor, and coma. Take the victim to a hospital emergency room at once. ALWAYS bring the prescription bottle or container.

Special Information

Take each dose with a full glass of water and do not lie down for 15 to 30 minutes afterward.

Etodolac can make you drowsy or tired: Be careful when driving or operating hazardous equipment. Do not take any over-the-counter products containing acetaminophen or aspirin while taking etodolac. Avoid alcoholic beverages.

Contact your doctor if you develop rash or itching, visual disturbances, weight gain, breathing difficulties, fluid retention, hallucinations, black or tarry stools, persistent headache, or any unusual or intolerable side effect.

If you forget a dose of etodolac, take it as soon as you remember. If you take etodolac once a day and it is within 8 hours of your next dose, or if you take several doses a day and it is within 4 hours of your next dose, skip the dose you forgot and continue with your regular schedule. Never take a double dose.

Special Populations

Pregnancy/Breast-feeding

NSAIDs may affect the fetal heart during the second half of pregnancy. Pregnant women should not take etodolac without their doctor's approval. When the drug is considered crucial by your doctor, its potential benefits must be carefully weighed against its risks.

NSAIDs may pass into breast milk. There is a possibility that a nursing mother taking etodolac might affect her baby's heart or cardiovascular system. Nursing mothers who must take this drug should bottle-feed.

Seniors

Seniors may be more susceptible to side effects, especially ulcer disease.

Evista *see Raloxifene, page 919*

Generic Name

Exemestane (ex-eh-MES-tane)

Brand Name

Aromasin

Type of Drug

Aromatase inhibitor.

Prescribed For

Breast cancer. Also prescribed for prostate cancer prevention.

General Information

Some breast cancers depend on the presence of the hormone estrogen to stimulate their growth. Depriving these cancers of estrogen is an effective way of treating the condition. Exemestane significantly reduces the amount of estrogen in the blood by binding permanently to an enzyme called aromatase, an essential element in the conversion of androgen (male hormones) to estrogen in premenopausal and postmenopausal women. Exemestane does not affect other hormones in the body. Exemestane is broken down in the liver.

Cautions and Warnings

Do not take this drug if you are **sensitive** or **allergic** to it.

Exemestane may be prescribed only for postmenopausal women.

Possible Side Effects

▼ Most common: fatigue, hot flashes, pain, depression, sleeplessness, anxiety, nausea, and breathing difficulties.

▼ Common: flu-like symptoms, leg swelling, high blood pressure, dizziness, headache, vomiting, abdominal pain, leg swelling or other fluid retention, sweating, appetite loss, constipation, and coughing.

▼ Less common: increased appetite, diarrhea, fever, weakness, tingling in the hands or feet, broken bones, bronchitis, sinusitis, rash, itching, urinary infection, and swollen lymph glands.

▼ Rare: chest pain, confusion, reduced sensitivity to stimulation, upset stomach, joint, back, or other bone pain, respiratory infection, sore throat, runny nose, and hair loss.

Drug Interactions

• Estrogen-containing drugs reduce the effectiveness of exemestane. Do not combine these drugs.

Food Interactions

Take this drug with a meal. The amount of exemestane absorbed into the blood is increased by 40% when taken with a high-fat meal.

Usual Dose

Adult: 25 mg once a day with or just after a meal. Dose adjustment is not needed in people with kidney or liver disease.

Child: not recommended.

Overdosage

Doses as large as 600 mg have been well tolerated by women with advanced breast cancer. Overdose victims should be taken to a hospital emergency room for evaluation and treatment. ALWAYS bring the prescription bottle or container.

Special Information

If you forget a dose, skip the forgotten dose and continue with your regular schedule. Contact your doctor if you skip more than one dose.

Contact your doctor if you develop a cough or hoarseness; difficulty breathing; fever or chills; high blood pressure; lower back or side pain; depression; hand, ankle, foot, or lower leg swelling; chest tightness or pain; difficulty urinating; burning or painful urination; the urge to urinate frequently; headache; sore throat; unexplained broken bones; or wheezing.

Special Populations

Pregnancy/Breast-feeding

Exemestane is intended only for postmenopausal women. It can cause birth defects and miscarriage and should not be used by pregnant women or women who may become pregnant.

Exemestane may pass into breast milk. Nursing mothers who must take it should bottle-feed.

Seniors

Seniors may take this drug without special precaution.

Generic Name

Ezetimibe (eh-ZEH-tim-ibe)

Brand Name

Zetia

Type of Drug

Cholesterol-lowering agent.

Prescribed For

High cholesterol, high LDL ("bad") cholesterol, high triglycerides, and low HDL ("good") cholesterol; also prescribed for two rare genetic disorders called homozygous familial hypercholesterolemia and homozygous sitosterolemia.

General Information

Ezetimibe was the first of a new class of medicines used to treat blood lipid problems. Unlike the widely used statin drugs, ezetimibe interferes with the absorption of cholesterol through the intestine and into the bloodstream. Another group of cholesterol-lowering drugs called bile acid sequestrants (such as cholestyramine, colestipol, and colsevelam) prevents cholesterol absorption by binding to bile acids in the intestine. Ezetimibe may be taken by itself or together with a statin drug. Ezetimibe may be helpful for people whose LDL ("bad") cholesterol remains high despite treatment with a statin drug. Cholesterol-lowering medicines should always be used together with appropriate diet and exercise.

Cautions and Warnings

Do not take this drug if you are **sensitive** or **allergic** to it.

People with **liver disease** or **elevated liver enzyme** measurements should not take ezetimibe because its effects on the liver are not known.

Possible Side Effects

Ezetimibe side effects are similar to those reported by people taking a placebo.

▼ Most common: headache, back pain, joint pain, and abdominal pain.

▼ Common: muscle ache and respiratory infection.

▼ Less common: fatigue, chest pain, diarrhea, sore throat, and cough.

Drug Interactions

• Cholestyramine reduces the amount of ezetimibe absorbed in the blood. Separate these drugs by 2 hours or more.

• Cyclosporine (to prevent organ transplant rejection) may substantially reduce the amount of ezetimibe in the blood. This combination must be monitored closely by your doctor.

• Gemfibrozil (another blood fat-reducer) can increase the amount of ezetimibe in the blood.

Food Interactions

This drug can be taken without regard to food or meals.

Usual Dose

Adult and Child (age 10 and over): 10 mg once a day.
Child (age 9 and under): not recommended.

Overdosage

Little is known about the effects of ezetimibe overdose. Call your local poison control center or a hospital emergency room for information. If you seek treatment, ALWAYS bring the prescription bottle or container.

Special Information

If you are taking more than one drug to lower cholesterol or another blood fat, consider the side effects of all of those drugs combined.

Special Populations

Pregnancy/Breast-feeding

Little is known about the effects of ezetimibe during pregnancy. When this drug is considered crucial by your doctor, its potential benefits must be carefully weighed against its risks. Statin drugs should never be taken by a pregnant woman or nursing mother.

It is not known if ezetimibe passes into breast milk. Nursing mothers who must take it should bottle-feed.

Seniors

Seniors may use this drug without special precaution.

Generic Name

Famciclovir (fam-SYE-kloe-vere)

Brand Name

Famvir

Type of Drug

Antiviral.

Prescribed For

Herpes zoster (shingles), genital herpes, and herpes simplex in HIV-infected people.

General Information

Famciclovir is absorbed into the body and converted to the antiviral penciclovir, the drug that actually works against shingles by interfering with the reproduction of DNA in the herpes virus. Penciclovir does not affect DNA in uninfected body cells. Penciclovir is broken down by the liver and eliminated from the body through the kidneys.

Cautions and Warnings

People **sensitive** or **allergic** to famciclovir should not take this drug. Those with **reduced kidney function** should have their dosage adjusted accordingly. **Severe liver disease** reduces the maximum possible concentration of penciclovir in the blood and increases the time it takes to reach this maximum level; however, dosage adjustment is not normally required.

Possible Side Effects

▼ Most common: headache, nausea, and diarrhea.

▼ Less common: fever, fatigue, pain, vomiting, constipation, appetite loss, dizziness, tingling in the hands or feet, sleepiness, sore throat, sinus irritation, itching, and signs of shingles.

▼ Rare: chills, abdominal pain, back or joint pain, and upset stomach.

Drug Interactions

• Probenecid, cimetidine, and theophylline interfere with the elimination of penciclovir from the body, possibly leading to higher levels of penciclovir in the blood.

• People who took famciclovir and digoxin together experienced increased digoxin in their blood.

Food Interactions

None known.

Usual Dose

Shingles
   Adult (age 18 and over): 500 mg every 8 hours for 1 week. People with reduced kidney function may require a reduced dose taken as infrequently as once a day.

Genital Herpes
   Adult (age 18 and over): 125 mg twice a day for 5 days; or 250 mg twice a day for up to 1 year for suppression; or 250 mg 3 times a day for 7 days for initial episode. People with reduced kidney function take the same dose but less often, as infrequently as once every 2 days. HIV-infected people should take 500 mg twice a day for 7 days.

Overdosage

Little is known about the effects of famciclovir overdose. Overdose victims should be taken to a hospital emergency room for treatment. ALWAYS bring the prescription bottle or container.

Special Information

Famciclovir treatment should be started as soon as shingles is diagnosed. For maximum benefit, be sure to complete the full week of treatment.

Famciclovir is not a cure for genital herpes and it is not known if it will prevent the transmission of the herpes virus to another person. Avoid sexual intercourse when herpes lesions are present even while taking famciclovir for genital herpes.

Begin taking famciclovir at the first sign of a herpes attack (symptoms include pain, tenderness, burning, itching, tingling, ulcers, or scabs). The effectiveness of starting famciclovir 6 hours or more after symptoms or lesions appear has not been established.

Call your doctor if you experience any unusual or intolerable side effects.

If you forget a dose of famciclovir, take it as soon as you remember. If it is almost time for your next dose, skip the dose you forgot. Do not take a double dose. Call your doctor if you forget more than 2 doses in a row.

Special Populations

Pregnancy/Breast-feeding

Famciclovir should only be taken by a pregnant woman if it is absolutely necessary and the possible benefits outweigh the risks to the fetus.

In animal studies, penciclovir (the active form of famciclovir) passed into breast milk in high concentrations but it is not known if this holds true for humans. Nursing mothers who must take this drug should bottle-feed.

Seniors

Seniors clear penciclovir from the bloodstream more slowly than younger people and should have their dosage adjusted according to their level of kidney function.

Generic Name

Famotidine (fam-OE-tih-dine) G

Brand Names

Pepcid   Pepcid Complete
Pepcid AC   Pepcid RPD

Type of Drug

Histamine H$_2$ antagonist.

Prescribed For

Ulcers of the stomach and duodenum (upper intestine). This drug is also used to treat gastroesophageal reflux disease (GERD), stress ulcer, and other conditions characterized by the production of large amounts of gastric fluids; to prevent stress ulcer and stomach and upper intestinal bleeding; and to stop the production of stomach acid during surgery. Pepcid AC is approved for heartburn.

General Information

Histamine H_2 antagonists work by turning off the system that produces stomach acid and other secretions. Famotidine is effective in treating the symptoms of ulcer and preventing complications of the disease, although an ulcer that does not respond to another histamine H_2 antagonist will probably not respond to famotidine. Histamine H_2 antagonists differ only in their potency. Cimetidine is the least potent; 1000 mg are roughly equal to 300 mg of either nizatidine or ranitidine, or 40 mg of famotidine. All these drugs have roughly equivalent success rates in treating ulcer disease and comparable risk of side effects.

Cautions and Warnings

Do not take famotidine if you have had an **allergic reaction** to it or any histamine H_2 antagonist.

People with **kidney or liver disease** should take famotidine with caution because ⅓ of each dose is broken down in the liver and the rest passes out of the body through the kidneys.

Possible Side Effects

▼ Most common: headache.

▼ Less common: dizziness, mild diarrhea, and constipation.

▼ Rare: Rare side effects can occur in almost any part of the body. Contact your doctor if you experience any side effect not listed above.

Drug Interactions

• Enteric-coated tablets should not be taken with famotidine. The change in stomach acidity that famotidine produces causes the tablets to disintegrate prematurely in the stomach.

• Antacids, anticholinergics, and metoclopramide may slightly reduce the amount of famotidine absorbed into the blood. No special precaution is needed.

Food Interactions

Famotidine may be taken without regard to food or meals.

Usual Dose

Adult: 20–40 mg at bedtime, or 20 mg twice a day for 4–8 weeks. Dosage should be reduced in people with severe kidney disease.

Child (age 1–16): 0.23–0.45 mg per lb. of body weight, at bedtime or in 2 divided doses, up to 40 mg a day.

Overdosage

Little is known about the effects of famotidine overdose, but victims may experience exaggerated side effects. Your local poison control center may advise giving ipecac syrup—available at any pharmacy—to induce vomiting and remove any remaining drug from the stomach. Victims who have definite symptoms should be taken to a hospital emergency room. ALWAYS bring the prescription bottle or container.

Special Information

Take famotidine exactly as directed and follow your doctor's instructions regarding diet and other treatment in order to get the maximum benefit from the drug. Antacids may be taken together with famotidine if needed.

Cigarettes worsen stomach ulcers and may reduce famotidine's effectiveness.

Call your doctor at once if you develop any unusual side effects such as bleeding or bruising, tiredness, diarrhea, dizziness, or rash. Black, tarry stools or vomiting material that resembles coffee grounds may indicate your ulcer is bleeding.

If you forget a dose of famotidine, take it as soon as you remember. If it is almost time for your next dose, skip the one you forgot and continue with your regular schedule. Do not take a double dose.

Special Populations

Pregnancy/Breast-feeding

Although animal studies revealed no damage to the fetus, famotidine should be avoided by women who are or might be pregnant. When this drug is considered crucial by your doctor, its possible benefits must be carefully weighed against its risks.

Famotidine may pass into breast milk. Nursing mothers who must take this drug should consider bottle-feeding.

Seniors

Seniors may need lower doses due to loss of kidney function and may be more susceptible to side effects.

Generic Name

Felbamate (FEL-bam-ate)

Brand Name

Felbatol

Type of Drug

Anticonvulsant.

Prescribed For

Partial seizure and Lennox-Gastaut syndrome in children.

General Information

Felbamate is related to the older tranquilizer-sedative meprobamate (Miltown). Exactly how felbamate works is not known, but it raises the seizure threshold and prevents the seizure impulse from spreading in the brain, as do other anticonvulsants. Felbamate should only be used when other seizure drugs have failed because of the risks associated with it. About half of each dose passes out of the body through the kidneys; the other half is broken down and eliminated by the liver.

Cautions and Warnings

Felbamate is associated with an increase in the risk of **aplastic anemia,** a potentially fatal condition.

Possibly fatal **liver failure** occurs in people taking felbamate much more often than normal. Regular liver function tests are recommended.

Felbamate should never be **suddenly stopped** or seizures may become more frequent. Dosage should be gradually reduced or replaced by another anticonvulsant.

People who are **allergic** to felbamate or related drugs should not take it.

Felbamate may cause **increased sensitivity to the sun.** Wear protective clothing and use sunscreen while taking this drug.

People with **kidney disease** may require lower doses.

Possible Side Effects

Adults

▼ Most common: sleeplessness, sleepiness, fatigue, headache, dizziness, nervousness, upset stomach, vomiting, constipation, nausea, appetite loss.

▼ Common: anxiety, tremors, walking unusually, depression, tingling in the hands or feet, diarrhea, liver inflammation, abdominal pains, respiratory infections, abnormal vision, taste changes.

▼ Less common: weakness, dry mouth, stupor, abnormal thinking, rash, sinus irritation, sore throat, muscle aches, fever, chest pain.

▼ Rare: Rare side effects can occur in almost any part of the body. Contact your doctor if you experience any side effect not listed above.

Children

▼ Most common: abdominal pain, fever, respiratory infections, sleeplessness, sleepiness, nervousness, vomiting, constipation, black and blue marks.

▼ Common: headache, appetite loss, hiccups, sore throat, coughing, middle ear infections, fatigue, weight loss, temporary loss of urine control, pain, walking unusually, weakness, abnormal thinking, emotional instability, pinpoint pupils, rash, upset stomach, low white blood cell count.

▼ Rare: Rare side effects can occur in almost any part of the body. Contact your doctor if your child experiences any side effect not listed above.

Drug Interactions

• Combining felbamate and other antiseizure drugs usually requires dosage adjustments due to the risk of drug interaction.

• Combining felbamate and carbamazepine reduces blood levels of both drugs by roughly half. Dosage adjustments are necessary.

• Combining phenobarbital and felbamate increases the amount of phenobarbital in the blood and decreases felbamate levels. Dosage adjustments are necessary.

• If you combine felbamate and phenytoin, your phenytoin dosage may have to be reduced by as much as 40%. This combination also decreases felbamate blood levels by almost 50%.

• Felbamate increases blood levels of valproic acid and methsuximide.

Food Interactions

Felbamate is best taken on an empty stomach but may be taken with food if it causes upset stomach.

Usual Dose

Adult and Child (age 14 and over): 1200–3600 mg a day, divided into 3–4 doses.

Child (age 2–13): 6.8–20.5 mg per lb. a day, divided into 3–4 doses.

Overdosage

Overdose symptoms may include upset stomach, increased heart rate, and felbamate side effects. Call your local poison control center or a hospital emergency room for more information. If you seek treatment, ALWAYS bring the prescription bottle or container.

Special Information

Do not take more felbamate than your doctor has prescribed.

Felbamate can cause drowsiness; be careful when driving or performing tasks that require concentration.

Avoid prolonged exposure to the sun while taking felbamate.

Call your doctor if you develop any bothersome or persistent side effect.

Maintain good dental hygiene while taking felbamate and use extra care when brushing or flossing because this drug can cause swollen gums. See your dentist regularly.

If you forget a dose, take it as soon as you remember. If it is almost time for your next dose, take 1 dose right away and another in 3 or 4 hours, then go back to your regular schedule. Do not take a double dose.

Special Populations

Pregnancy/Breast-feeding

This drug may cross into fetal circulation. When the drug is considered crucial by your doctor, its potential benefits must be carefully weighed against its risks.

Felbamate passes into breast milk. Nursing mothers who must take this drug should consider bottle-feeding.

Seniors

Seniors, especially those with liver, kidney, or heart disease, may be more sensitive to the effects of this drug and should receive lower doses.

Generic Name

Felodipine (feh-LOE-dih-pene)

Brand Name

Plendil

Type of Drug

Calcium channel blocker.

Prescribed For

High blood pressure.

General Information

Felodipine is one of many calcium channel blockers available in the U.S. Its once-daily dosage schedule makes it particularly suited to treating high blood pressure. Felodipine blocks the passage of calcium, an essential factor in muscle contraction, into the heart and smooth muscles. Such blockage interferes with the contraction of these muscles, which in turn dilates (widens) the veins and vessels that supply blood to them. This dilating effect reduces blood pressure, the amount of oxygen used by the heart muscle, and the risk of blood vessel spasm. Felodipine is therefore useful in treating not only high blood pressure but also angina pectoris (brief attacks of chest pain), a condition related to poor oxygen supply to the heart muscles.

Felodipine only affects the movement of calcium into muscle cells; it has no effect on calcium in the blood.

Cautions and Warnings

Felodipine should not be taken if you have had an **allergic reaction** to it in the past.

On rare occasions, felodipine may cause very **low blood pressure** that may lead to stimulation of the heart and rapid heartbeat and can worsen angina. This reaction may happen when treatment is first started, when dosage is increased, or if the drug is rapidly withdrawn; it may be avoided by reducing dosage gradually.

Studies have shown that people taking calcium channel blockers—usually those taken several times a day, not those taken only once daily—have a greater chance of having a **heart attack** than do people taking beta blockers or other medications for the same purpose. Discuss this with your doctor to be sure you are receiving the best possible treatment.

Patients taking a beta-blocking drug who begin taking felodipine may develop **heart failure** or increased **angina**.

People with severe **liver disease** may require dosage adjustments.

People taking felodipine who have had a **heart attack** and have **lung congestion** may experience worsened heart failure, since this drug can actually reduce the force of each heartbeat.

Possible Side Effects

Side effects produced by calcium channel blockers are generally mild and rarely cause people to stop taking them. Side effects are more common with higher doses and in older patients.

▼ Most common: swelling in the ankles, feet, or legs; dizziness; light-headedness; muscle weakness or cramps; facial flushing; and headache.

▼ Less common: respiratory infections, cough, tingling in the hands or feet, upset stomach, abdominal pains, chest pains, nausea, constipation, diarrhea, heart palpitations, sore throat, runny nose, back pain, and rash.

▼ Rare: Rare side effects can affect the heart, stomach, blood and joints. It can affect your mood, sex drive, and urinary tract. Contact your doctor if you experience any side effect not listed above.

Drug Interactions

• Felodipine may increase the amount of beta-blocking drugs in the bloodstream. This can lead to heart failure, very low blood pressure, or an increased incidence of angina.

However, in many cases these drugs have been taken together with no problem.

• Felodipine increases the effects of other blood-pressure-lowering drugs. Such drug combinations are often used to treat hypertension.

• Cimetidine, ranitidine, and azole antifungals increase the amount of felodipine in the blood and may account for a slight increase in the drug's effect.

• Phenytoin and other hydantoin antiseizure medicines, carbamazepine, and barbiturate sleeping pills and sedatives may decrease the amount of felodipine in the blood, reducing its effect on the body.

• Erythromycin and cyclosporine may increase the side effects of felodipine.

• Felodipine may increase the effects of digoxin, theophylline (prescribed for asthma and other respiratory problems), and oral anticoagulant (blood-thinning) drugs.

• Felodipine may also interact with quinidine (prescribed for abnormal heart rhythm) to produce low blood pressure, very slow heart rate, abnormal heart rhythms, and swelling in the arms or legs.

Food Interactions

You may take felodipine with food if it upsets your stomach. Avoid taking felodipine with concentrated grapefruit juice—it doubles the amount of drug absorbed.

Usual Dose

2.5–10 mg a day. No patient should take more than 20 mg a day. Do not stop taking felodipine abruptly. The dosage should be reduced gradually over a period of time.

Overdosage

Felodipine overdose can cause low blood pressure. If you think you have taken an overdose of felodipine, call your doctor or go to a hospital emergency room. ALWAYS bring the prescription bottle or container.

Special Information

Call your doctor if you develop constipation, nausea, very low blood pressure, breathing difficulties, increased heart pain, dizziness, or light-headedness, or if other side effects are bothersome or persistent.

Swelling of the hands or feet may develop within 2 or 3 weeks of starting felodipine. The chances of this happening depend on age and dosage. It occurs in less than 10% of people under age 50 taking 5 mg a day and in more than 30% of those over age 60 taking 20 mg a day.

Be sure to continue taking your medication even if you feel well, and follow any instructions for diet restriction or other treatments to help maintain lower blood pressure.

Do not break or crush felodipine tablets.

It is important to maintain good dental hygiene while taking felodipine and to use extra care when using your toothbrush or dental floss because of the chance that the drug will make you more susceptible to certain infections.

If you forget to take a dose of felodipine, take it as soon as you remember. If it is almost time for your next dose, skip the dose you forgot and continue with your regular schedule. Do not take a double dose.

Special Populations

Pregnancy/Breast-feeding

Animal studies of felodipine have shown that it crosses into the fetal circulation and causes birth defects. Women who are or who might become pregnant while taking this drug should not take it without their doctor's approval. The potential benefit of taking felodipine must be carefully weighed against its risks.

It is not known if felodipine passes into breast milk. Before breast-feeding, you must consider the drug's potential effect on the nursing infant.

Seniors

Seniors, especially those with liver disease, are more sensitive to the effects of this drug.

Generic Name

Fenofibrate (fen-oe-FIH-brate)

Brand Name

Lofibra   Tricor

Type of Drug

Anti-hyperlipidemic (blood-fat reducer).

Prescribed For

High blood cholesterol and/or triglycerides; also prescribed for syndrome X, a condition which increases the risk of type 2 diabetes.

General Information

Fenofibrate works by interfering with the body's ability to make triglyceride. It also reduces uric acid levels. This drug should only be used in people with very high triglyceride levels who are at risk for pancreatitis (inflammation of the pancreas) and have not responded to other treatments.

Cautions and Warnings

People taking fenofibrate and other triglyceride-lowering drugs are more likely to die from causes unrelated to triglyceride levels. It has not been established whether fenofibrate helps people live longer. For both these reasons, fenofibrate should **only be used if absolutely necessary**.

People taking fenofibrate, gemfibrozil, and clofibrate may develop **pancreatitis** (inflammation of the pancreas).

People with **liver or severe kidney disease** should avoid fenofibrate. People with less severe kidney disease require reduced dosage.

People taking fenofibrate are more likely to develop **gallstones**.

Fenofibrate can destroy muscle cells, leading to **kidney failure,** especially when combined with a statin cholesterol-lowering drug (see "Drug Interactions").

Possible Side Effects

▼ Most common: abnormal liver function, abdominal pain, and respiratory disorders.

▼ Common: rash, headache, upset stomach, pain, weakness, tiredness, and flu-like symptoms.

▼ Less common: joint pain, abnormal heart rhythms, reduced sex drive, dizziness, increased appetite, sleeplessness, tingling in the hands or feet, nausea, vomiting, diarrhea, abdominal pain, constipation, stomach noise or gas, frequent urination, vaginal irritation, runny nose, cough, sinus irritation, eye irritation, blurred vision, conjunctivitis (pinkeye), earache, and tiny particles inside the eye ("floaters").

Possible Side Effects *(continued)*

▼ Rare: allergic reactions including severe rash, itching, liver inflammation or enlargement, gallstones, gallbladder disease, muscle aches, and increased sensitivity to the sun.

Drug Interactions

• Combining fenofibrate and a statin cholesterol-lowering drug (atorvastatin, cerivastatin, fluvastatin, lovastatin, pravastatin, or simvastatin) can lead to severe muscle pain, muscle cell destruction, and kidney failure. If you have extremely high blood-fat levels, the potential benefits of this combination may outweigh the risks. In people taking this combination, the health of muscles and kidneys must be monitored regularly via blood tests.

• Fenofibrate increases the effects of anticoagulant (blood-thinning) drugs. Your anticoagulant dosage may need an adjustment.

• Combining fenofibrate and cyclosporine can increase the risk of kidney toxicity. This combination should only be used if it is absolutely necessary and the lowest possible dosage is taken.

• If you are taking cholestyramine or colestipol (both are used to reduce blood-fat levels) as well as fenofibrate, take the fenofibrate at least 1 hour before or 4 to 6 hours after these drugs.

• If you take a bile acid sequestrant, take fenofibrate at least 1 hour beforehand, or 4 to 6 hours afterward.

Food Interactions

Take fenofibrate with food to get the best effect from it.

Usual Dose

Adult: 54–160 mg a day.

Senior: Begin with 54 mg a day. This dosage also applies to people with kidney disease.

Child: not recommended.

Overdosage

Little is known about the effects of fenofibrate overdose. Victims should be taken to a hospital emergency room. ALWAYS bring the prescription bottle or container.

Special Information

People should take fenofibrate only after a triglyceride-lowering diet and other medications have failed. While taking fenofibrate, follow the diet recommended by your doctor.

If you forget a dose, take it as soon as you remember. If it is almost time for your next dose, skip the forgotten dose and continue with your regular schedule.

Special Populations

Pregnancy/Breast-feeding

Fenofibrate causes fetal injury and death in animal studies. When this drug is considered crucial by your doctor, its potential benefits must be carefully weighed against its risks.

This drug should not be taken by nursing mothers because of its potential to affect the nursing infant.

Seniors

Seniors are more likely to experience side effects and should never start with more than 1 capsule (67 mg) a day.

Generic Name

Finasteride (fin-ASS-ter-ide)

Brand Names

Proscar   Propecia

The information in this profile also applies to the following drug:

Generic Ingredient: Dutasteride
Avodart   Duagen

Type of Drug

Alpha-reductase inhibitor.

Prescribed For

Benign prostatic hyperplasia (BPH) and male pattern baldness. May also play a role in preventing prostate cancer.

General Information

Finasteride works by interfering with the action of the enzyme alpha-reductase, which converts testosterone into 5-

dihydrotestosterone (DHT). By suppressing DHT levels, finasteride reduces the size of the prostate in most men who take the drug for BPH. You may need to take finasteride for 6 to 12 months before its effects can be assessed.

Urine flow improves in about 60% of men taking finasteride for BPH and symptoms improve in about 30%. In one study, men experienced a significant regression in prostate size after 3 months and the reduction was maintained through the 12-month study period; these men experienced a significant improvement in urine flow that could be maintained up to 36 months.

Studies of finasteride for hair loss on the top and back-middle of the scalp show new hair growth in 65% to 80% of men taking the drug continuously for 2 years. The drug must be taken for 3 months or more before it begins to have an effect and must be taken continuously to maintain hair growth. Once you stop taking this drug, any new hair you have grown is likely to fall out in the next 12 months. Between 14 to 17% of men taking the drug continued to lose hair throughout the study period.

Finasteride has been studied as therapy following radical prostatectomy surgery and in the prevention of first-stage prostate cancer, acne in women, and unusual hairiness.

Cautions and Warnings

Do not take finasteride if you are **allergic** to any of its ingredients. This drug must not be used in **women** or **children**.

People who do not respond to finasteride may have a condition that causes BPH-like symptoms, such as prostate cancer, bladder or nerve disorders, or physical obstruction of the urinary tubes. Finasteride cannot be used to treat these conditions.

Because it is broken down in the liver, finasteride must be used with caution by people with **liver disease**.

Finasteride may mask symptoms of **prostate cancer** by causing a reduction in the level of prostate-specific antigen (PSA), an increasingly acknowledged indicator of prostate cancer.

Possible Side Effects

Side effects are generally mild and often subside with continued use of the drug.

Possible Side Effects *(continued)*

▼ Common: impotence, loss of sex drive, decreased amount of semen, breast tenderness and enlargement, testicular pain, and drug sensitivity reaction including lip swelling and rash.

Drug Interactions

• Finasteride may reduce the effectiveness of theophylline and aminophylline, though dosage adjustments usually are not required.

• Finasteride affects the PSA blood test used for prostate cancer screening. Be sure your doctor knows you are taking this drug if you have a PSA test done or are being tested for prostate cancer.

• Dustasteride blood levels may increase when mixed with ritonavir, ketoconazole, cimetidine, and ciprofloxacin, all of which are inhibitors of a liver enzyme called CYP3A4. Blood levels of dutasteride also increase with verapamil and diltiazem, however, no change in concentration is seen when dutasteride is mixed with amlodipine.

• There is no interaction between dutasteride and tamsulosin, terazosin, warfarin, digoxin, or cholestyramine.

Food Interactions

You may take finasteride with food if it upsets your stomach.

Usual Dose

Dutasteride
   Adult: 0.5 mg (1 capsule) once a day.
   Child: not recommended.

Finasteride
   Adult: BPH—5 mg once a day. Male pattern baldness—1 mg once a day.
   Child: not recommended.

Women should not take finasteride.

Overdosage

Side effects are unlikely. Doses of dutasteride as high as 40 mg a day have been taken with no adverse side effects. Call your local poison control center or a hospital emergency room for more information. If you seek treatment, ALWAYS bring the prescription bottle or container.

Special Information

Women who are or might be pregnant should not handle crushed finasteride tablets because small amounts of the drug may be absorbed into the blood, possibly affecting the fetus.

If your sexual partner is or might be pregnant and you start taking finasteride, you must wear a condom during sex to avoid directly exposing her to finasteride in the semen.

Semen volume may decrease while on finasteride. Impotence or reduced sex drive is also a risk.

If you forget a dose, take it as soon as you remember. If it is almost time for your next dose, skip the one you forgot and continue with your regular schedule. Do not take a double dose. Call your doctor if you miss a dose for 2 or more days.

Special Populations

Pregnancy/Breast-feeding

This drug is not intended for women. Finasteride will harm the fetus if taken during pregnancy. It is not known if finasteride passes into breast milk.

Seniors

Seniors with liver disease should use this drug with caution.

Brand Name

Fioricet

Generic Ingredients

Acetaminophen + Butalbital + Caffeine ⒢

Other Brand Names

Esgic	Fiorpap
Esgic-Plus	Isocet
Femcet	Repan

Type of Drug

Barbiturate and analgesic (pain reliever) combination.

Prescribed For

Migraine and other pain.

General Information

Fioricet is one of many combination products containing a barbiturate—butalbital—and an analgesic—acetaminophen. Products of this kind also often contain a tranquilizer or a narcotic. Other analgesic combinations, such as Fiorinal, substitute aspirin for acetaminophen.

Cautions and Warnings

Do not take Fioricet if you are **allergic** or **sensitive** to it. Use this drug with extreme caution if you suffer from **asthma or other breathing problems,** have **kidney or liver disease,** or a **viral infection of the liver.** This medication should also be used with caution if you have **diabetes, hyperthyroidism** (overactive thyroid gland), severe **heart disease**, or a history of **porphyria.** Chronic (long-term) use of Fioricet may lead to drug dependence or **addiction.**

Butalbital is a respiratory depressant and affects the central nervous system (CNS), producing **drowsiness, tiredness,** and an **inability to concentrate**. Alcohol increases the CNS depression caused by this drug.

For additional information see "Caution and Warnings" in Acetaminophen (p.13).

Possible Side Effects

▼ Most common: light-headedness, dizziness, sedation, nausea, vomiting, sweating, appetite loss, and mild stimulation.

▼ Less common: weakness, headache, upset stomach, sleeplessness, agitation, tremor, uncoordinated muscle movement, mild hallucinations, disorientation, visual disturbances, euphoria (feeling "high"), dry mouth, constipation, facial flushing, changes in heart rate, palpitations, feeling faint, urinary difficulties, rash, itching, confusion, rapid breathing, and diarrhea.

For additional information see "Possible Side Effects" in Acetaminophen (p.13).

Drug Interactions

• Combining Fioricet with alcohol, tranquilizers, barbiturates, sleeping pills, antihistamines, or other CNS depressants may cause tiredness, drowsiness, and trouble concentrating.

• The barbiturate ingredient in this medication may reduce the effectiveness of corticosteroids and contraceptives ("the pill") containing estrogen.

For additional information see "Drug Interactions" in Acetaminophen (p.13).

Food Interactions

Fioricet is best taken on an empty stomach but may be taken with food if it upsets your stomach.

Usual Dose

1–2 tablets or capsules every 4 hours or as needed; do not exceed 6 doses a day.

Overdosage

Symptoms include breathing difficulties, nervousness progressing to stupor or coma, pinpointed pupils, cold and clammy skin and lowered heart rate or blood pressure, nausea, vomiting, dizziness, ringing in the ears, facial flushing, sweating, and thirst. Take the victim to a hospital emergency room immediately. ALWAYS bring the prescription bottle or container.

Special Information

Fioricet may cause drowsiness. Be careful when driving or performing any task that requires concentration.

If you have been taking this medication for more than a few weeks, do not stop taking it without your doctor's instructions. Suddenly stopping Fioricet may lead to withdrawal symptoms.

Call your doctor if your headache or pain persists or gets worse, or if you develop side effects that are bothersome or persistent.

If you forget a dose, take it as soon as you remember. If it is almost time for your next dose, skip the one you forgot and continue with your regular schedule. Do not take a double dose.

For additional information see "Special Information" in Acetaminophen (p. 13).

Special Populations

Pregnancy/Breast-feeding

Fioricet should not be taken during pregnancy. It is associated with birth defects, prolonged labor and delayed delivery, and breathing problems in newborns. Regular use of Fioricet during the last 3 months of pregnancy may also cause drug dependency in the newborn.

Fioricet passes into breast milk. Breast-feeding while using Fioricet may cause babies to become tired, short of breath, or have a slow heartbeat. Nursing mothers who must take this drug should consider bottle-feeding.

Seniors

Fioricet may have a greater depressant effect on seniors. Seniors are also more likely to experience stimulation and disorientation.

Brand Name

Fiorinal

Generic Ingredients

Aspirin + Butalbital + Caffeine [G]

Other Brand Names

Amaphen	Fiorital
Anoquan	Lanorinal
Butal Compound	Margesic
Butalbital Compound	Medigesic
Endolor	Triad
Femcet	

Type of Drug

Barbiturate and analgesic (pain reliever) combination.

Prescribed For

Migraine and other pain.

General Information

Pain relief products often combine an analgesic with a sedative. The analgesic ingredient in Fiorinal is aspirin; other brand-name products, such as Esgic and Fioricet, contain acetaminophen. The sedative ingredient in pain-relief combinations may be a barbiturate, narcotic, or other tranquilizer. Fiorinal contains the barbiturate butalbital. Fiorinal also contains caffeine, which is often used in analgesic combinations that treat headache because it enhances the pain-relieving effect of aspirin.

Cautions and Warnings

Do not take Fiorinal if you are **allergic** or **sensitive** to any of its ingredients. Use Fiorinal with extreme caution if you suffer from **asthma or other breathing problems**. This drug should be used with caution if you have **kidney or liver disease, diabetes, hyperthyroidism** (overactive thyroid gland), severe **heart disease** or a history of **porphyria**.

Long-term use of this drug may cause drug dependence and **addiction**.

Butalbital is a respiratory depressant and affects the central nervous system (CNS), producing **drowsiness, tiredness,** and an **inability to concentrate**. Alcohol increases the CNS depression caused by butalbital.

For additional information see "Cautions and Warnings" in Aspirin (p. 111).

Possible Side Effects

▼ Most common: light-headedness, dizziness, sedation, nausea, vomiting, sweating, upset stomach, appetite loss, and mild stimulation.

▼ Less common: weakness, headache, sleeplessness, agitation, tremor, uncoordinated muscle movements, mild hallucinations, disorientation, visual disturbances, euphoria (feeling "high"), dry mouth, constipation, facial flushing, changes in heart rate, palpitations, faintness, urinary difficulties, rash, itching, confusion, rapid breathing, and diarrhea.

For additional information see "Possible Side Effects " in Aspirin (p. 111).

Drug Interactions

• Combining Fiorinal with alcohol, tranquilizers, barbiturates, sleeping pills, antihistamines, or other CNS depressants may cause tiredness, drowsiness, and trouble concentrating.

• The barbiturate ingredient in this medication may reduce the effectiveness of corticosteroids and oral contraceptives ("the pill") containing estrogen.

For additional information see "Drug Interactions" in Aspirin (p. 111).

Food Interactions

Fiorinal is best taken on an empty stomach but may be taken with food if it upsets your stomach.

Usual Dose

1–2 tablets or capsules every 4 hours or as needed. Do not exceed 6 doses a day.

Overdosage

Symptoms include breathing difficulties, nervousness progressing to stupor or coma, pinpointed pupils, cold and clammy skin, lowered heart rate or blood pressure, nausea, vomiting, dizziness, ringing in the ears, flushing, sweating, and thirst. Symptoms of mild overdose are rapid and deep breathing, nausea, vomiting, dizziness, ringing or buzzing in the ears, flushing, sweating, thirst, headache, drowsiness, diarrhea, and rapid heartbeat. Severe overdose may cause fever, excitement, confusion, convulsions, liver or kidney failure, coma, and bleeding. Take the victim to a hospital emergency room immediately. ALWAYS bring the prescription bottle or container.

Special Information

Fiorinal may cause drowsiness. Be careful when driving or performing any task that requires concentration.

If you have been taking this medication for more than a few weeks, do not stop taking it without your doctor's instructions. Suddenly stopping this drug may lead to withdrawal symptoms.

Call your doctor if your headache pain persists or gets worse, or if you develop any bothersome or persistent side effect.

If you forget a dose, take it as soon as you remember. If it is almost time for your next dose, skip the dose you forgot and continue with your regular schedule. Do not take a double dose.

For additional information see "Special Information" in Aspirin (p. 111).

Special Populations

Pregnancy/Breast-feeding

Fiorinal should not be taken during pregnancy. Pregnant women taking it may experience prolonged labor, delayed delivery, and bleeding problems. Fiorinal increases the risk of birth defects and may cause breathing or bleeding problems in newborns. Regular use of Fiorinal during the last 3 months of pregnancy may also cause drug dependency in the newborn.

Fiorinal passes into breast milk. Breast-feeding while using Fiorinal may cause tiredness, shortness of breath, or slowed heartbeat in the baby. Nursing mothers who must take Fiorinal should consider bottle-feeding.

Seniors

Fiorinal may have a greater depressant effect on seniors. Seniors are also more likely to experience stimulation and disorientation.

Brand Name

Fiorinal with Codeine

Generic Ingredients

Aspirin + Butalbital + Caffeine + Codeine Phosphate Ⓖ

Type of Drug

Barbiturate, narcotic, and analgesic (pain reliever) combination.

Prescribed For

Migraine or other pain.

General Information

Fiorinal with Codeine is one of many combination products containing a barbiturate, an analgesic, and a narcotic. In Fiorinal with Codeine, butalbital is the barbiturate, aspirin is the analgesic, and codeine is the narcotic. These products often also contain a tranquilizer, and acetaminophen may be substituted for aspirin.

Cautions and Warnings

Do not take Fiorinal with Codeine if you are **allergic** or **sensitive** to any of its ingredients.

Use this drug with extreme caution if you suffer from **asthma or other breathing problems**. This medication should be used with caution if you have **kidney or liver disease, head injuries, brain disease,** a history of **seizures, inflammatory bowel disease, gallstones or gallbladder disease, enlarged prostate, urinary difficulties, diabetes, hyperthyroidism** (overactive thyroid), severe **heart disease,** or a history of **porphyria**.

Fiorinal with Codeine may cause postural **low blood pressure** (symptoms include dizziness or fainting when rising from a sitting or lying position).

Long-term use of this drug may cause drug dependence or **addiction**.

Fiorinal with Codeine is a respiratory depressant and affects the central nervous system (CNS), producing **sleepiness, tiredness,** or **inability to concentrate**. Alcohol increases the depression caused by codeine and butalbital.

For additional information see "Cautions and Warnings" in Aspirin (p. 111).

Possible Side Effects

▼ Most common: light-headedness, dizziness, sleepiness, nausea, vomiting, appetite loss, and sweating. If these occur, ask your doctor to consider lowering the dosage. Usually the side effects disappear if you lie down.

▼ Less common: euphoria (feeling "high"), breathing difficulties, weakness, sleepiness, headache, agitation, uncoordinated muscle movement, minor hallucinations, disorientation and visual disturbances, dry mouth, constipation, facial flushing, rapid heartbeat, palpitations, feeling faint, urinary difficulties or hesitancy, reduced sex drive or potency, itching, rash, anemia, lowered blood sugar, and yellowing of the skin or whites of the eyes. Narcotic analgesics may aggravate convulsions in those who have had them.

For additional information see "Possible Side Effects" in Aspirin (p. 111).

Drug Interactions

• Interaction with alcohol, tranquilizers, barbiturates, sleeping pills, antihistamines, or other drugs that produce sedation may cause tiredness, drowsiness, and trouble concentrating.

• The barbiturate ingredient in this medication may reduce the effectiveness of corticosteroids and oral contraceptives ("the pill") containing estrogen.

For additional information see "Drug Interactions" in Aspirin (p. 111).

Food Interactions

Fiorinal with Codeine is best taken on an empty stomach but may be taken with food if it upsets your stomach.

Usual Dose

1–2 tablets or capsules every 4 hours or as needed; do not exceed 6 doses a day.

Overdosage

Usual overdose symptoms include breathing difficulties, nervousness progressing to stupor or coma, pinpointed pupils, cold clammy skin and lowered heart rate or blood pressure, nausea, vomiting, dizziness, ringing in the ears, flushing, sweating, and thirst. Symptoms of mild overdose include rapid and deep breathing, nausea, vomiting, dizziness, ringing or buzzing in the ears, flushing, sweating, thirst, headache, drowsiness, diarrhea, and rapid heartbeat. Severe overdose may cause fever, excitement, confusion, convulsions, liver or kidney failure, coma, or bleeding. Take the victim to a hospital emergency room immediately. ALWAYS bring the prescription bottle or container.

Special Information

This drug may cause drowsiness. Be careful when driving or performing any task that requires concentration.

If you have been taking this medication for more than a few weeks, do not stop taking it without your doctor's instruction. Suddenly stopping this drug may lead to withdrawal symptoms.

Call your doctor if you experience breathing difficulties, or persistent nausea, vomiting, or constipation.

If you forget a dose, take it as soon as you remember. If it is almost time for your next dose, skip the one you forgot and continue with your regular schedule. Do not take a double dose.

For additional information see "Special Information" in Aspirin (p. 111).

Special Populations

Pregnancy/Breast-feeding

Fiorinal with Codeine should not be used during pregnancy. Pregnant women taking it may experience prolonged labor, delayed delivery, and bleeding problems. This drug increases the risk of birth defects and may cause breathing or bleeding problems in newborns. Regular use of Fiorinal with Codeine during the last 3 months of pregnancy may also cause drug dependency in the newborn.

Fiorinal with Codeine passes into breast milk. Breast-feeding while using this drug may cause tiredness, shortness of breath, or a slow heartbeat in the baby. Nursing mothers who must take this drug should consider bottle-feeding.

Seniors

This drug may have a greater depressant effect on seniors. Other effects that may be more prominent are stimulation, disorientation, light-headedness and dizziness or fainting when rising suddenly from a sitting or lying position.

Generic Name

Flecainide (FLEH-kan-ide) G

Brand Name

Tambocor

Type of Drug

Antiarrhythmic.

Prescribed For

Abnormal heart rhythm.

General Information

Flecainide is prescribed in situations where the abnormal rhythm is so severe as to be life-threatening and does not respond to other drug treatments. Like other antiarrhythmic drugs, flecainide works by affecting the movement of nervous impulses within the heart. Flecainide's effects may not become apparent for 3 to 4 days after you start taking it.

Cautions and Warnings

As with other antiarrhythmic drugs, there is no proof that flecainide helps people live longer or avoid sudden death. Do not take flecainide if you are **allergic** or **sensitive** to it or if you have **heart block,** unless you have a cardiac pacemaker.

Flecainide causes **new arrhythmias** or worsens already existing ones in 7% of people who take it; this risk increases with certain kinds of underlying heart disease and higher doses of the drug. Flecainide causes or worsens **heart failure** in about 5% of people taking it because it tends to reduce the force and rate of each heartbeat.

Flecainide is extensively broken down in the liver. People with **poor liver function** should not take flecainide unless the benefits clearly outweigh the risks.

Changes in the **pH of urine** may affect the effectiveness of flecainide.

Possible Side Effects

▼ Most common: dizziness, fainting, light-headedness, unsteadiness, visual disturbances including blurred vision and seeing spots before the eyes, breathing difficulties, headache, nausea, fatigue, heart palpitations, chest pain, tremors, weakness, constipation, bloating, and abdominal pain.

▼ Less common: new or worsened heart arrhythmias or heart failure, heart block, slowed heart rate, vomiting, diarrhea, upset stomach, loss of appetite, stomach gas, a bad taste in your mouth, dry mouth, tingling in the hands or feet, partial or temporary paralysis, loss of muscle control, flushing, sweating, ringing or buzzing in the ears, anxiety, sleeplessness, depression, not feeling well, twitching, weakness, convulsions, speech disorders, stupor, memory loss, personality loss, nightmares, apathy, eye pain, unusual sensitivity to bright light, sagging eye-

---

Possible Side Effects *(continued)*

lids, reduced white-blood-cell or blood-platelet counts, impotence, reduced sex drive, frequent urination, urinary difficulty, itching, rash, fever, muscle ache, closing of the throat, and swollen lips, tongue, or mouth.

Drug Interactions

• The combination of propranolol and flecainide may cause an exaggerated lowering in heart rate. Other drugs that slow the heart may also interact with flecainide to produce an excessive slowing of heart rate.

• Avoid megadoses of vitamin C while taking this drug.

• The amount of flecainide in your blood and its effect on your heart may be increased if it is taken together with amiodarone, cimetidine, disopyramide, or verapamil.

• Smokers may need a larger dose of flecainide than nonsmokers.

• Flecainide may increase the amount of digoxin in the bloodstream, increasing the chance of side effects.

Food Interactions

A vegetarian diet may affect the effectiveness of flecainide.

Usual Dose

Starting dose—50–100 mg every 12 hours. Maximum dosage is 400 mg a day.

Overdosage

Flecainide overdose affects heart function, causing slower heart rate, low blood pressure, and possible death from respiratory failure. Victims of flecainide overdose should be taken to a hospital emergency room for treatment. ALWAYS bring the prescription bottle or container.

Special Information

Flecainide can make you dizzy, light-headed, or disoriented. Take care while driving or performing complex tasks.

Call your doctor if you develop chest pains, an abnormal heartbeat, breathing difficulties, bloating in your feet or legs, tremors, fever, chills, sore throat, unusual bleeding or bruising, yellowing of the whites of your eyes, or any other intolerable side effect.

If you forget to take a dose of flecainide and remember within 6 hours, take it as soon as possible. If you do not remember until later, skip the dose you forgot and continue with your regular schedule. Do not take a double dose.

Special Populations

Pregnancy/Breast-feeding

At high doses, flecainide damages an animal fetus. When this drug is considered crucial by your doctor, its potential benefits must be weighed against its risks.

Flecainide passes into breast milk. Nursing mothers who must take this drug should bottle-feed.

Seniors

Seniors with reduced kidney or liver function are more likely to develop side effects and require a lower dosage.

Flomax   *see Tamsulosin, page 1016*

Flonase   *see Corticosteroids, Nasal, page 306*

Flovent   *see Corticosteroids, Inhalers, page 303*

Generic Name

Flucytosine   (floo-SYE-toe-sene)

Brand Name

Ancobon

Type of Drug

Antifungal.

Prescribed For

Serious blood-borne fungal infections.

General Information

Flucytosine is meant for fungal infections—*Candida, chromomycoses,* and *cryptococcus*—carried in the blood that affect the urinary tract, respiratory tract, central nervous system, heart, and other organs. It is not meant for fungal infections of the skin, such as common athlete's foot.

Cautions and Warnings

Do not take this drug if you are **allergic** to it. Flucytosine can worsen **bone-marrow depression** in people whose immune systems are already compromised. Liver and kidney function and blood composition should be monitored while you are taking this drug.

People with **kidney disease** must be closely monitored by their doctors and should take this medication with extreme caution; daily dosage must be reduced.

Possible Side Effects

▼ Most common: unusual tiredness or weakness, liver inflammation, yellowing of the eyes or skin, abdominal pain, diarrhea, loss of appetite, nausea, vomiting, rash, redness, itching, sore throat, fever, and unusual bleeding or bruising.

▼ Less common: chest pains, breathing difficulties, sensitivity to the sun or bright light, dry mouth, duodenal ulcers, severe bowel irritation, stomach bleeding, interference with kidney function, kidney failure, reduced red- and white-blood-cell counts or other changes in blood composition, headache, hearing loss, confusion, dizziness, weakness, shaking, sedation or tiredness, psychosis, hallucinations, heart attack, and low blood-sugar and potassium levels.

Drug Interactions

• Amphotericin B increases flucytosine's effectiveness; this combination is generally used to produce better results.
• Flucytosine may interfere with some routine blood tests.
• Cytosine may inactivate the antifungal activity of flucytosine.

Food Interactions

Take flucytosine with food if it upsets your stomach.

Usual Dose

22–66 mg per lb. a day, in divided doses.

Overdosage

Little is known about the effects of flucytosine overdose, but it may cause exaggerated drug side effects.

Special Information

Take the capsules a few at a time over 15 minutes to avoid nausea and vomiting.

Call your doctor if you develop unusual tiredness or weakness; yellowing of the skin or whites of the eyes; rash, redness, or itching; sore throat or fever; unusual bleeding or bruising; or any persistent or intolerable side effect.

Maintain good dental hygiene while taking flucytosine. Use extra care when using your toothbrush or dental floss because of the risk that flucytosine will make you more susceptible to infection. Dental work should be completed prior to starting on this drug.

Exposure to sunlight may cause rash, itching, redness, discoloration of the skin, or severe sunburn. Stay out of direct sunlight when taking flucytosine.

If you forget a dose, take it as soon as you remember. If it is almost time for your next dose, take 1 dose right away and another in 3 or 4 hours, then go back to your regular schedule. Do not take a double dose.

Special Populations

Pregnancy/Breast-feeding

Flucytosine causes birth defects in animals and crosses the placenta. Flucytosine should be used by pregnant women only when its potential benefits clearly outweigh its risks.

It is not known if flucytosine passes into breast milk. Nursing mothers who must take this drug should bottle-feed.

Seniors

Dosage adjustment may be required due to loss of kidney function.

Type of Drug

Fluoroquinolone Anti-Infectives

(flor-oe-QUIN-oe-lone)

Brand Names

Generic Ingredient: Ciprofloxacin
Ciloxan   Cipro XR
Cipro

Generic Ingredient: Enoxacin
Penetrex

Generic Ingredient: Gatifloxacin
Tequin

Generic Ingredient: Gemifloxacin
Factive

Generic Ingredient: Levofloxacin
Levaquin   Quixin Eyedrops

Generic Ingredient: Lomefloxacin
Maxaquin

Generic Ingredient: Moxifloxacin
Avelox   Vigamox Eyedrops

Generic Ingredient: Norfloxacin
Chibroxin   Noroxin

Generic Ingredient: Ofloxacin
Floxin   Ocuflox Eyedrops
Floxin Otic

Generic Ingredient: Sparfloxacin
Zagam

Generic Ingredients: Trovafloxacin
Trovan

Prescribed For

Infections of the lower respiratory system, sinuses, urinary tract, skin, bone and joints, lungs, and prostate; also prescribed for sexually transmitted diseases, prostatitis, infectious diarrhea, bronchitis, pneumonia, typhoid fever, anthrax, and traveler's diarrhea. The eyedrops are used to treat ocular infections; the eardrops for for ear infections.

General Information

Fluoroquinolone anti-infectives work against many organisms that traditional antibiotics have trouble killing. They do not work against the common cold, flu, or other viral infections. These medications are chemically related to an older antibacterial called nalidixic acid but work better than that drug against urinary infections. Some fluoroquinolone drugs such as ciprofloxacin are used to treat a variety of infections all over the body. Others are used for more specific purposes.

Cautions and Warnings

Do not take a fluoroquinolone if you are **allergic** to any drug in this group or have had a reaction to related medications like nalidixic acid. Severe, possibly fatal, allergic reactions can occur even after the very first dose. These reactions include cardiovascular collapse, loss of consciousness, tingling, swelling of the face or throat, breathing difficulties, itching, and rash. Stop taking the drug if this happens and seek medical help at once.

Fluoroquinolones may cause increased pressure on parts of the brain, leading to **convulsions** and **psychotic reactions**. Other possible effects include **tremors, restlessness, light-headedness, confusion,** and **hallucinations**. Fluoroquinolones should be used with caution in people with **head trauma, seizure disorders,** or other nervous system conditions.

Moxifloxacin should not be used by people with **liver disease**. It and gatifloxacin should be avoided by people with **heart rhythm problems** or those taking drugs that can affect heart rhythm. Dosage of trovafloxacin must be reduced in people with **chronic liver disease**. People taking trovafloxacin have developed **severe liver damage or liver failure leading to death**. Trovafloxacin should be reserved for treating severe infections when other drugs have failed.

People with **kidney disease** require reduced dosage of these drugs, except in the case of trovafloxacin and moxifloxacin.

People taking fluoroquinolones may be unusually **sensitive to the sun**. Avoid the sun while taking this drug and for several days following therapy, EVEN IF YOU ARE USING SUNSCREEN.

People taking a fluoroquinolone may develop **colitis** that could range from mild to very serious. Contact your doctor if you develop diarrhea or cramps.

Prolonged fluoroquinolone use can lead to **fungal overgrowth**. Follow your doctor's directions exactly.

Possible Side Effects

Side effects are rarely serious.

▼ Most common: nausea (most likely with ciprofloxacin and moxifoxacin), vomiting (most likely with enoxacin), and diarrhea (may be most likely with moxifloxacin, gatifloxacin, and ofloxacin).

▼ Less common: dizziness, vomiting, abdominal pain, headache, and liver inflammation. Taking trovafloxacin-alatrofloxacin for more than 2 weeks increases the risk of serious liver injury.

▼ Rare: Rare side effects can occur in almost any part of the body. Contact your doctor if you experience any side effect not listed above.

Drug Interactions

• Separate your fluoroquinolone dose from that of antacids, didanosine, iron supplements, or zinc by 2 to 6 hours. These drugs decrease the amount of fluoroquinolone absorbed. Moxifloxacin must be taken 4 hours before or 8 hours after antacids, iron, or zinc.

• Sucralfate reduces the amount of fluoroquinolone absorbed in the blood. Take sucralfate at least 6 hours after taking a fluoroquinolone.

• Probenecid may increase the risk of some fluoroquinolone side effects. Cimetidine may also increase fluoroquinolone blood levels.

• Fluoroquinolones (excepting moxifloxacin and gatifloxacin) may increase the effect of oral anticoagulant drugs such as warfarin. Your anticoagulant dosage may have to be reduced.

• Fluoroquinolones may increase the toxic effects of cyclosporine (used for organ transplants) on your kidneys.

• Fluoroquinolones (excepting moxifloxacin and gatifloxacin) may increase theophylline blood levels and the risk of side effects.

• Azlocillin may increase the risk of ciprofloxacin side effects.

• Ciprofloxacin, enoxacin, and norfloxacin may increase caffeine's effects.

• Nitrofurantoin may antagonize norfloxacin's antibacterial effects. Do not take these drugs together.

• Sparfloxacin, moxifloxacin, and gatifloxacin can increase the risk of abnormal heart rhythms. Combining these drugs with astemizole, bepridil, erythromycin, tricyclic antidepressants, and phenothiazine antipsychotics increases the risk of abnormal heart rhythms associated with those drugs.

• People taking drugs to correct abnormal heart rhythms should avoid fluoroquinolones, especially sparfloxacin, which has the greatest effect on the heart.

• Enoxacin increases blood levels of digoxin. Dosage adjustment may be needed.

• NSAIDs and anti-inflammatory drugs should not be combined with fluoroquinolones because of the increased risk of stimulation and seizures.

• Bismuth subsalicylate (Pepto-Bismol) reduces the amount of enoxacin absorbed in the blood. Take these drugs at least 1 hour apart.

• People receiving intravenous morphine accumulate less trovafloxacin in the blood, possibly reducing its effectiveness.

Food Interactions

Gatifloxacin, levofloxacin, lomefloxacin, moxifloxacin, and sparfloxacin may be taken with or without food. Take enoxacin, ofloxacin, norfloxacin, and trovafloxacin at least 2 hours before or 2 hours after meals or antacids. Ciprofloxacin is best taken 1 hour before or 2 hours after meals, but may be taken with food. Dairy products and calcium-fortified orange juice interfere with the absorption of ciprofloxacin and should be avoided.

Usual Dose

Tablets (Adults, age 18 and over; not recommended for use in children)

Ciprofloxacin: 100–750 mg twice a day.

Ciprofloxacin XR: 1,000 mg once a day.

Enoxacin: 200–400 mg every 12 hours; a single dose of 400 mg may be taken for gonorrhea.

Gatifloxacin: 200–400 mg a day.

Gemifloxacin: 320 mg once a day.

Levofloxacin: 250–750 mg once a day.

Lomefloxacin: 400 mg a day.

Moxifloxacin: 400 mg a day.

Norfloxacin: 400 mg every 12 hours; a single dose of 800 mg may be taken for gonorrhea.

Ofloxacin: 200–400 mg every 12 hours.

Sparfloxacin: two 200-mg tablets on the first day, then one 200-mg tablet a day.

Trovafloxacin and alatrofloxacin: 100–200 mg once a day for up to 28 days.

Dosage of most fluoroquinolones must be reduced in the presence of kidney failure. In the case of trovafloxacin and alatrofloxacin, dosage adjustment is unnecessary.

Eyedrops

Ciprofloxacin or norfloxacin: 1–2 drops in the affected eye several times a day.

Levofloxacin: days 1–2—1–2 drops in the affected eye every 2 hours while awake, up to 8 times a day. Days 3–7— 1–2 drops in the affected eye every 4 hours while awake, up to 4 times a day.

Ofloxacin: bacterial conjunctivitis—days 1–2, place 1–2 drops in the affected eye every 2–4 hours while awake; days 3–7, place 1–2 drops in the affected eye every 4–6 hours while awake. Bacterial corneal ulcer— days 1–2, place 1–2 drops in the affected eye every 30 minutes while awake; awaken 4–6 hours after you go to sleep for one more dose; days 3–7 or 9, place 1–2 drops in the affected eye every hour while awake; days 7–9, or through the end of treatment, place 1–2 drops in the affected eye 4 times a day.

Moxifloxacin: 1 drop in the affected eye 3 times a day for 1 week.

Eardrops

Ofloxacin: 5–10 drops in the affected ear twice a day.

Overdosage

Symptoms generally include drug side effects. Overdose may cause kidney failure and, in the case of moxifloxacin, abnormal heart rhythms. Call your local poison control center or a hospital emergency room for more information. You may be told to induce vomiting with ipecac syrup—available at any pharmacy—before taking the victim to an emergency room. If you seek treatment, ALWAYS bring the prescription bottle or container.

Special Information

Take each dose with a full glass of water. Be sure to drink at least 8 glasses of water a day while taking this drug to help avoid side effects.

If you are taking an antacid, didanosine, sucralfate, or an iron or zinc supplement while taking a fluoroquinolone, separate the doses by at least 4 hours to avoid a drug interaction. Moxifloxacin must be taken 4 hours before or 8 hours after antacids, iron, or zinc.

Drug sensitivity reactions can develop even after only 1 dose. Stop taking the drug and get immediate medical attention if you feel faint or develop itching, rash, facial swelling, breathing difficulties, convulsions, depression, visual disturbances, dizziness, headache, light-headedness, or any sign of a drug reaction.

Colitis can be caused by any anti-infective medication. If diarrhea develops, call your doctor at once.

Avoid excessive sunlight. Call your doctor if you become sensitive to the sun.

Follow your doctor's directions exactly. Complete the full course of drug therapy, even if you feel well.

Eyedrops

To avoid infection, do not let the eyedropper tip touch your finger, eyelid, or any surface. Wait 5 minutes before using another eyedrop or eye ointment.

Call your doctor at once if your vision declines or if eye stinging, itching or burning, redness, irritation, swelling, or pain worsens.

Fluoroquinolones can cause changes in vision, dizziness, drowsiness, and light-headedness. Be careful when driving or performing any task that requires concentration.

If you forget to administer a dose, do so as soon as you remember. If it is almost time for your next dose, skip the missed dose and continue with your regular schedule. Do not take a double dose.

Special Populations

Pregnancy/Breast-feeding

Animal studies have shown that fluoroquinolones may damage the fetus or reduce the likelihood of a successful pregnancy. When a fluoroquinolone is considered crucial by your doctor, its potential benefits must be carefully weighed against its risks.

Fluoroquinolones pass into breast milk. Nursing mothers who must take them should bottle-feed.

Seniors

With the exception of moxifloxacin and gatifloxacin, seniors may require reduced dosage due to decreases in kidney function. In the case of eyedrops, seniors may also need less medication.

Generic Name

Fluoxymesterone (flue-OX-ee-MES-ter-one) G

Brand Name

Halotestin

Type of Drug

Androgen (male hormone).

Prescribed For

Men: hormone replacement or augmentation and male menopause; also prescribed as male contraception for up to 12 months, and for delayed puberty.

Women: breast pain and fullness in women who have given birth, and inoperable breast cancer.

General Information

Fluoxymesterone is an androgen. Androgens are responsible for the normal growth and development of male sex organs and for maintaining secondary sex characteristics including hair distribution, vocal cord thickening, muscle development, and fat distribution.

Cautions and Warnings

Androgens do not improve athletic performance and may cause serious side effects.

Women taking any androgen may develop **deepening of the voice, oily skin, acne, hairiness, increased sex drive,** and

menstrual irregularities. Androgens should be avoided if possible by young boys who have not gone through puberty.

Fluoxymesterone worsens **gynecomastia** (a condition characterized by swollen male breast tissue).

Men with unusually **high blood levels of calcium,** known or suspected **prostate cancer** or **prostate destruction,** or **breast cancer** should not use fluoxymesterone, nor should anyone with severe **liver, heart, or kidney disease**.

Long-term, high-dose androgen therapy may cause severe **liver disease,** including hepatitis and cancer, **reduced sperm count,** and water retention. **Blood cholesterol** may be raised by androgens. This can be a problem for people who have heart disease.

Androgens may cause or worsen **sleep apnea**.

For patients with **diabetes mellitus,** this drug may affect blood sugar levels.

Possible Side Effects

Men

▼ Most common: inhibition of testicle function, impotence, chronic erection, and painful enlargement of breast tissue.

Women

▼ Most common: unusual hairiness, male pattern baldness, deepening of the voice, and enlargement of the clitoris. These changes are usually IRREVERSIBLE once they occur. Increased blood calcium and menstrual irregularities may also develop.

Men and Women

▼ Most common: changes in sex drive, headache, anxiety, depression, a tingling feeling, sleep apnea (condition characterized by intermittent cessation of breathing during sleep), flushing, rash, acne, habituation (the drug may be habit forming), excitation, chills, sleeplessness, water retention, nausea, vomiting, diarrhea, hepatitis (symptoms include yellowing of the skin or whites of the eyes), liver inflammation, and liver cancer. Symptoms resembling those of a stomach ulcer may also develop.

Drug Interactions

• Fluoxymesterone may increase the effect of an oral anti-coagulant (blood thinner); dosage of the anticoagulant may have to be reduced. It may also have an effect on the glucose-tolerance test, a blood test used to screen for diabetes. Androgens may interfere with tests of thyroid function.

• Combining an androgen and imipramine or another tricyclic antidepressant may result in a severe paranoid reaction.

• Androgens may decrease insulin requirements.

Food Interactions

Take fluoxymesterone with meals if it upsets your stomach.

Usual Dose

2.5–40 mg a day.

Overdosage

Symptoms include nausea, vomiting, and diarrhea. Call your local poison control center or a hospital emergency room for more information. If you seek treatment, ALWAYS bring the prescription bottle or container.

Special Information

Androgens must be taken only under the close supervision of your doctor. The dosage and clinical effects of fluoxymesterone vary widely and require constant monitoring.

Call your doctor if you develop nausea or vomiting, swelling of the legs or feet, yellowing of the skin or whites of the eyes, or a painful or persistent erection. Women should call their doctors immediately if they develop a deep or hoarse voice, acne, hairiness, male pattern baldness, or menstrual irregularities.

If you forget a dose, take it as soon as you remember. If it is almost time for your next dose, skip the one you forgot and continue with your regular schedule. Do not take a double dose.

Special Populations

Pregnancy/Breast-feeding

Fluoxymesterone should never be taken by pregnant or nursing women because it can affect the developing fetus and nursing infant.

Seniors

Seniors are more likely to develop prostate enlargement or prostate cancer. A marked increase in sex drive may also occur.

Generic Name

Flurazepam (fluh-RAZ-uh-pam) Ⓖ

Brand Name

Dalmane

Type of Drug

Benzodiazepine sedative.

Prescribed For

Insomnia and sleep disturbances.

General Information

Flurazepam is a member of the group of drugs known as benzodiazepines. Benzodiazepines work by a direct effect on the brain. They make it easier to go to sleep and decrease the number of times you wake up during the night. Flurazepam and quazepam remain in your bloodstream longer than other drugs in this class, thus resulting in the greatest incidence of morning "hangover."

Cautions and Warnings

People with **kidney or liver disease** should be carefully monitored while taking flurazepam. Take the lowest possible dose to help you sleep.

People with **respiratory disease** may experience **sleep apnea** (intermittent cessation of breathing during sleep) while taking flurazepam.

Clinical **depression** may be increased by flurazepam, which can depress the nervous system. Intentional overdose is more common among depressed people who take sleeping pills than among those who do not.

Some people have experienced **amnesia** while taking flurazepam.

All benzodiazepines can be **addictive** if taken for long periods of time and can cause drug withdrawal symptoms if discontinued suddenly. Withdrawal symptoms include tremors, muscle cramps, insomnia, agitation, diarrhea, vomiting, sweating, and convulsions.

Possible Side Effects

▼ Common: drowsiness, headache, dizziness, talkativeness, nervousness, apprehension, poor muscle coordination, light-headedness, daytime tiredness, muscle weakness, slowness of movement, hangover, and euphoria (feeling high).

▼ Less common: nausea, vomiting, rapid heartbeat, confusion, temporary memory loss, upset stomach, stomach cramps and pain, depression, blurred or double vision and other visual disturbances, constipation, changes in sense of taste, appetite changes, stuffy nose, nosebleeds, common cold symptoms, asthma, sore throat, cough, breathing difficulties, diarrhea, dry mouth, allergic reaction, fainting, abnormal heart rhythm, itching, rash, acne, dry skin, sensitivity to the sun, nightmares or strange dreams, sleeplessness, tingling in the hands or feet, ringing or buzzing in the ears, ear or eye pain, menstrual cramps, frequent urination and other urinary difficulties, blood in the urine, discharge from the penis or vagina, lower back and other pain, muscle spasms and pain, fever, swollen breasts, and weight changes.

▼ Rare: Rare side effects can affect your heart, stomach and intestines, urinary tract, blood, muscles and joints. Contact your doctor if you experience any side effect not listed above.

Drug Interactions

• As with all benzodiazepines, the effects of flurazepam are enhanced if it is taken with an alcoholic beverage, antihistamine, tranquilizer, barbiturate, anticonvulsant medication, antidepressant, or monoamine oxidase inhibitor (MAOI).

• Oral contraceptives, cimetidine, disulfiram, and isoniazid may increase the effect of flurazepam by reducing the drug's breakdown in the liver. Probenecid also increases flurazepam's effects.

• Cigarette smoking, rifampin, and theophylline may reduce the effect of flurazepam on your body by increasing the rate at which it is broken down by the liver.

• Levodopa's effectiveness may be decreased by flurazepam.

• Flurazepam may increase the amount of zidovudine (an AIDS drug—also known as AZT), phenytoin, or digoxin in your bloodstream, increasing the chances of side effects.

• Mixing clozapine with a benzodiazepine has led to respiratory collapse in a few people. Flurazepam should be stopped at least 1 week before starting clozapine treatment.

Food Interactions

Flurazepam may be taken with food if it upsets your stomach.

Usual Dose

Adult and Child (age 15 and over): 15–30 mg at bedtime. Dosage must be individualized for maximum benefit.

Senior: starting dose—15 mg at bedtime.

Child (under age 15): not recommended.

Overdosage

The most common overdose symptoms are confusion, sleepiness, depression, loss of muscle coordination, and slurred speech. Coma may also occur. Patients who overdose on this drug must be made to vomit with ipecac syrup—available at any pharmacy—to remove any remaining drug from the stomach: Call your doctor or a poison control center before doing this. If 30 minutes have passed since the overdose was taken or if symptoms have begun to develop, take the victim immediately to a hospital emergency room for treatment. ALWAYS bring the prescription bottle or container.

Special Information

Never take more flurazepam than your doctor has prescribed.

Avoid alcoholic beverages and other nervous system depressants while taking flurazepam.

Exercise caution while performing tasks that require concentration and coordination. Flurazepam may make you tired, dizzy, or light-headed.

If you take flurazepam daily for 3 or more weeks, you may experience some withdrawal symptoms when you stop taking the drug.

If you forget a dose and remember within 1 hour, take it as soon as you remember. If you do not remember until later, skip the dose you forgot and go back to your regular schedule. Do not take a double dose.

Special Populations

Pregnancy/Breast-feeding
Flurazepam absolutely should not be used by pregnant women or by women who may become pregnant.

Flurazepam passes into breast milk. The drug should not be taken by nursing mothers.

Seniors
Seniors are more susceptible to the effects of flurazepam.

Generic Name

Flutamide (FLUE-tuh-mide) Ⓖ

Brand Name

Eulexin

Type of Drug

Antiandrogen.

Prescribed For

Prostate cancer.

General Information

Prostatic cancer is sensitive to anything that removes the source of androgen (male hormone). Flutamide works by slowing the uptake of androgen or by interfering with the binding of androgen to body tissues. It is always prescribed together with a luteinizing hormone-releasing hormone (LHRH) drug.

Cautions and Warnings

Do not take flutamide if you are **allergic** to it.

This drug may cause **jaundice** and severe blood conditions including **hemolytic anemia**. People with certain **blood disorders** and people who **smoke** are at greater risk for these side effects. Severe **liver injury** may also occur; your doctor should monitor your liver function. People with severe **liver disease** are at greater risk for serious side effects.

Two men taking this drug have developed **breast cancer**. Flutamide may **reduce sperm counts**.

Possible Side Effects

▼ Most common: diarrhea, cystitis, and bleeding from the rectum.

▼ Common: rectal irritation, blood in the urine, hot flashes, loss of libido, impotence, nausea, rash, and swollen breasts.

▼ Less common: drowsiness, confusion, depression, anxiety, nervousness, appetite loss, stomach problems, anemia, low white-blood-cell and blood-platelet counts, arm or leg swelling, urinary and muscle problems, and high blood pressure.

▼ Rare: hepatitis, jaundice, and breathing difficulties.

Drug Interactions

• Flutamide may increase the effects of blood-thinning drugs such as warfarin. Dosage adjustment may be necessary.

Food Interactions

None known.

Usual Dose

Adult: 250 mg (2 capsules) every 8 hours, 3 times a day.

Overdosage

Overdose symptoms may include tiredness or low activity levels, slow breathing, weakness, tearing, appetite loss, vomiting, swollen and tender breasts, and liver inflammation. Overdose victims should be taken to a hospital emergency room. ALWAYS bring the prescription bottle or container.

Special Information

Report anything unusual to your doctor, especially pain or tenderness in the upper right abdomen, yellowing of the skin or whites of the eyes, severe itching, dark urine, persistent appetite loss, and unexplained flu symptoms. These may be signs of severe liver toxicity.

Flutamide can turn your urine amber or yellow-green and cause unusual sun sensitivity. Use sunscreen and wear long-sleeved protective clothing while you are taking flutamide.

Flutamide must be taken exactly as prescribed. Call your doctor if you miss a dose of this drug.

Special Populations

Pregnancy/Breast-feeding
This drug is not intended for use by women.

Seniors
Seniors may take this drug without special precaution.

Fosamax see Bisphosphonates, page 158

Generic Name

Fosfomycin (fos-foe-MYE-sin)

Brand Name

Monurol

Type of Drug

Urinary anti-infective.

Prescribed For

Uncomplicated urinary infections.

General Information

Fosfomycin kills a variety of bacteria. It works by preventing bacteria from sticking to the wall of the urinary tract and by interfering with bacterial cell division. In the body, it is converted to its active form—free fosfomycin. Generally, bacteria that are resistant to other antibiotics are not resistant to fosfomycin, so this drug may work where others have failed.

Cautions and Warnings

Do not take fosfomycin if you are **allergic** to it. Fosfomycin is meant to be taken once, in a single dose. Taking more than 1 packet of fosfomycin only **increases side effects;** it does not improve the drug's effectiveness.

Possible Side Effects

▼ Less common: diarrhea, vaginal irritation, runny nose, nausea, and headache.

▼ Rare: Rare side effects can occur in almost any part of the body. Contact your doctor if you experience any side effect not listed above.

Drug Interactions

• Metoclopramide reduces fosfomycin blood levels.

Food Interactions

You may take fosfomycin with or without food.

Usual Dose

Adult: 1 packet.
Child (under age 12): not recommended.

Overdosage

Little is known about the effects of fosfomycin overdose. Call your local poison control center or a hospital emergency room for more information. If you seek treatment, ALWAYS bring the prescription bottle or container.

Special Information

Do not take fosfomycin powder in its dry form. Mix the contents of the packet with 3 to 4 oz. of cool or cold water until it dissolves. Then drink the solution immediately.

Call your doctor if your infection does not improve within 2 or 3 days.

Special Populations

Pregnancy/Breast-feeding

The safety of using fosfomycin during pregnancy is not known. When this drug is considered crucial by your doctor, its potential benefits must be carefully weighed against its risks.

It is not known if fosfomycin passes into breast milk. Nursing mothers who must take this drug should bottle-feed.

Seniors

Seniors may take fosfomycin without special restriction.

Generic Name

Fosinopril (fos-IN-oe-pril)

Brand Name

Monopril

Combination Products

Generic Ingredients: Fosinopril + Hydrochlorothiazide
Monopril HCT

Type of Drug

Angiotensin-converting enzyme (ACE) inhibitor.

Prescribed For

High blood pressure.

General Information

Fosinopril sodium and other ACE inhibitors work by preventing the conversion of a hormone called angiotensin I to another hormone called angiotensin II, a potent blood-vessel constrictor. Preventing this conversion relaxes blood vessels, thus reducing blood pressure and relieving the symptoms of heart failure. Fosinopril also affects the production of other hormones and enzymes that participate in the regulation of blood vessel dilation. Fosinopril begins working 2 to 6 hours after you take it.

Some people who start taking an ACE inhibitor after they are already on a diuretic (agent that increases urination) experience a rapid drop in blood pressure after their first doses or when the dosage is increased. To prevent this from happening, you may be told to stop taking the diuretic 2 or 3 days before starting the ACE inhibitor or to increase your salt intake during that time. The diuretic may then be restarted gradually.

Cautions and Warnings

Do not take fosinopril if you have had an **allergic reaction** to it.

Fosinopril occasionally causes **very low blood pressure** or affects your **kidneys**. Your doctor should check your urine for changes during the first few months of treatment.

ACE inhibitors can affect your white-blood-cell count, possibly increasing your susceptibility to **infection**. Blood counts should be checked periodically.

Possible Side Effects

▼ Most common: headache and chronic cough. The cough usually goes away a few days after you stop taking the medicine.

▼ Less common: chest pain; low blood pressure; dizziness, especially when rising from a sitting or lying position; fatigue; diarrhea; vomiting; and nausea.

▼ Rare: Rare side effects can affect your heart, sleeping, stomach and intestines, skin, sex drive, and joints. Contact your doctor if you experience any side effect not listed above.

Drug Interactions

• The blood-pressure-lowering effect of fosinopril is additive with diuretic drugs and beta blockers. Any other drug that causes a rapid drop in blood pressure should be used with caution if you are taking an ACE inhibitor.

• Mixing 325 mg a day or more of aspirin with fosinopril carries a higher risk of death than taking lower doses (less than 60 mg a day). People taking aspirin to prevent a heart attack should use lower doses of this drug.

• Fosinopril may increase potassium levels in your blood, especially when taken with Dyazide or other potassium-sparing diuretics.

• Fosinopril may increase the effects of lithium; this combination should be used with caution.

• Antacids and fosinopril should be taken at least 2 hours apart.

• Capsaicin may trigger or aggravate the cough associated with fosinopril therapy.

• Indomethacin may reduce the blood-pressure-lowering effects of fosinopril.

• Phenothiazine tranquilizers and antivomiting drugs may increase the effects of fosinopril.

• The combination of allopurinol and fosinopril increases the chance of side effects.

• ACE inhibitors increase blood levels of digoxin, possibly increasing the chance of digoxin-related side effects.

Food Interactions

You may take fosinopril with food if it upsets your stomach.

Usual Dose

10–80 mg once a day. People with liver disease may require lower dosages.

Overdosage

The principal effect of ACE inhibitor overdose is a rapid drop in blood pressure, as evidenced by dizziness or fainting. Take the overdose victim to a hospital emergency room immediately. ALWAYS bring the prescription bottle or container.

Special Information

Call your doctor if you develop swelling of the face or throat, if you have sudden difficulty in breathing, or if you develop a sore throat, mouth sores, abnormal heartbeat, chest pain, persistent rash, or loss of taste perception. Unexplained swelling of the face, lips, hands, and feet can also affect the larynx (throat) and tongue and interfere with breathing. If this happens, the victim should be taken to a hospital emergency room at once.

You may get dizzy if you rise to your feet quickly from a sitting or lying position.

Avoid strenuous exercise or very hot weather, because heavy sweating or dehydration can cause a rapid decrease in blood pressure.

Avoid over-the-counter diet pills, decongestants, and other stimulants that can raise blood pressure.

If you forget to take a dose of fosinopril, take it as soon as you remember. If it is within 8 hours of your next dose, skip the one you forgot and continue with your regular schedule. Do not take a double dose.

Special Populations

Pregnancy/Breast-feeding

ACE inhibitors can cause fetal injury or death. Women who are or might be pregnant should not take ACE inhibitors.

Stop taking the drug and contact your doctor if you become pregnant.

Large amounts of fosinopril pass into breast milk. Nursing mothers who must take this drug should bottle-feed.

Seniors

Seniors may be more sensitive to the effects of fosinopril.

Generic Name

Ganciclovir (gan-SYE-kloe-vere)

Brand Names

Cytovene   Vitrasert
Valcyte

Type of Drug

Antiviral.

Prescribed For

Cytomegalovirus (CMV) infections of the eye and CMV infections in other parts of the body, in people with compromised immune systems.

General Information

Ganciclovir works by preventing reproduction of the virus CMV. Unlike other antiviral drugs, it works only against this virus and no others. Because viral resistance develops more quickly to the capsules, the capsule form of ganciclovir is restricted to follow-up treatment in people who have received intravenous treatment for CMV infections. The drug is eliminated through the kidneys.

Though most often used for CMV retinitis (eye infection), ganciclovir has also been used for CMV infections of the urine, blood, throat, and semen. It is also used to prevent CMV infection. Ganciclovir is helpful in controlling CMV infection in heart or bone marrow transplant patients.

Cautions and Warnings

Ganciclovir causes **anemia, reduced white-blood-cell count,** and **blood platelet loss**. Regular monitoring of blood and platelet counts is recommended while taking this drug.

Oral ganciclovir is linked to a faster progression of CMV eye infection than the intravenous form of the drug. The **risk of rapid progression of eye infection** should be balanced against the benefits of taking oral CMV.

People **allergic** to acyclovir or ganciclovir should not take ganciclovir.

Ganciclovir is intended only for people who are immuno-compromised. It is not intended to treat or prevent CMV infections in **newborns**.

Detachment of the retina has been noted in people taking ganciclovir, as well as in people with CMV who have not taken the drug. The relationship between ganciclovir and this effect is not well known.

Ganciclovir causes increased **sensitivity to the sun;** use a sunscreen or wear protective clothes when you go outside.

People with **kidney disease** should use ganciclovir with caution, and may require treatment at a lower dosage.

Studies of ganciclovir in African Americans, Hispanics, and Caucasians showed a trend toward higher blood levels among Caucasians than other groups.

Intravenous ganciclovir has been given to a small number of children under age 12 with mixed results. Side effects were similar to those experienced by adults taking the drug.

Possible Side Effects

▼ Most common: fever, diarrhea, abdominal pain, reduced white-blood-cell counts, anemia, rash, sweating, nausea, vomiting, and appetite loss.

▼ Common: infection; chills; stomach gas; low platelet counts (symptoms include bleeding or oozing blood); tingling; burning; numbness or pain in the hands, arms, legs, or feet; itching; pneumonia; weakness; and headache.

▼ Less common: Less common side effects can occur in almost any part of the body. Contact your doctor if you experience any side effect not listed above.

Drug Interactions

• Dapsone, pentamidine, flucytosine, vincristine, vinblastine, adriamycin, amphotericin B, trimethoprim-sulfamethoxazole, and other cytotoxic drugs may increase the side effects of ganciclovir and should be used together only if absolutely necessary, and only if the potential benefits outweigh the risks.

• People taking imipenem-cilastatin together with ganciclovir have experienced seizures. Avoid this combination.

• Mixing ganciclovir with other drugs that can be damaging to the kidneys may increase the rate and extent of kidney damage.

• Probenecid interferes with ganciclovir release through the kidneys and substantially increases blood levels of ganciclovir.

• Mixing ganciclovir with the anti-HIV drugs didanosine or zidovudine (AZT) may increase didanosine or AZT levels and reduce ganciclovir levels. Because AZT and ganciclovir both cause anemia and low white-blood-cell counts, many people cannot tolerate this combination.

Food Interactions

High-fat, high-calorie meals can increase the amount of ganciclovir absorbed into the blood. Take this drug with food.

Usual Dose

Adult and Child (age 13 and over): 3000 mg a day, divided into 3 or 6 equal doses. People with reduced kidney function will need to have their dosage reduced accordingly, possibly to as little as 500 mg 3 times a week.

Child (under age 13): not recommended.

Overdosage

Little is known about the effects of ganciclovir overdose. As much as 6000 mg a day has been taken with only temporary lowering of white-blood-cell count. Call your hospital emergency room for instructions in case of ganciclovir overdose.

Special Information

Ganciclovir does not cure CMV eye infection, and immunocompromised people taking this drug may find their disease worsening. Dosage reductions or discontinuation of the drug may be necessary if white-blood-cell or platelet counts get too low.

Ganciclovir may cause infertility in men and women. Pregnant women taking this drug should use effective contraception. Men should use a condom while taking the drug and for at least 90 days afterward to avoid passing the drug to their partners.

Good dental hygiene is important while taking ganciclovir to minimize the risk of infection. If you have dental work done while taking this drug, expect the healing process to take longer.

Regular blood tests are necessary to watch for white-blood-cell or platelet-level alterations.

It is very important to take ganciclovir exactly as directed. If you forget a dose, take it as soon as you remember and continue with your regular schedule. If you take ganciclovir 3 times a day and it is almost time for your next dose, take one dose immediately, another in 6 hours, and then continue with your regular schedule. If you take it 6 times a day and it is almost time for your next dose, skip the dose you forgot and continue with your regular schedule.

Special Populations

Pregnancy/Breast-feeding
Animal studies showed ganciclovir to be toxic to the fetus. There is no reliable information about its effect in pregnant women, but it should be taken only when the possible benefits outweigh the risks. Women who are likely to become pregnant while taking this drug should use reliable contraception.

It is not known if ganciclovir passes into breast milk, but the possible side effects of this drug on a nursing infant should be kept in mind. Nursing mothers who must take this drug should bottle-feed.

Seniors
Seniors often have reduced kidney function; dosage adjustments may be needed.

Generic Name

Gefitinib (gef-IT-in-ib)

Brand Name
Iressa

Type of Drug
Cancer chemotherapeutic.

Prescribed For
Non-small-cell lung cancer in people who have not responded to other treatments; also used for breast, colorectal, and prostate cancers.

General Information

Gefitinib is known as a signal transduction inhibitor. It works in a different way from traditional chemotherapy and hormonal therapy. On the surface of many types of cancer cells are structures known as epidermal growth factor receptors (EGFRs). These receptors allow epidermal growth factor—a body protein—to attach to them. When EGF attaches to the receptor, it causes a chemical called tyrosine kinase to trigger chemical processes inside the cell to make it grow and divide. Gefitinib attaches itself to the EGFRs inside the cell, blocking the activation of tyrosine kinase. This switches off the signals from the EGFR and therefore has the potential to stop the cancer cells from growing. This drug is taken alone, not with other chemotherapeutic medicines.

Cautions and Warnings

In studies, 1 of every 100 people taking gefitinib developed **severe and sometimes fatal lung disease**. Symptoms can develop from a minor cough to severe lung disease very quickly. Report any change in your health status to your doctor immediately. People with pre-existing lung disease are more likely to experience a decline in health while taking gefitinib than those without pre-existing lung conditions.

Do not take gefitinib if you are **sensitive** or **allergic** to it.

Gefitinib can cause **liver irritation** and increases in liver enzymes. This effect can be severe enough to discontinue drug use.

People with severe **kidney disease** should use caution when taking gefitinib since its effect on kidney disease is not known.

Possible Side Effects

The risk of drug side effects increases when taking high doses of gefitinib.

▼ Most common: diarrhea, rash, acne, dry skin, nausea, and vomiting.

▼ Common: itching, appetite loss, and weakness.

▼ Less common: weight loss, swelling in the arms or legs, poor vision in one eye, conjunctivitis, mild rash, mouth ulcers, and difficulty breathing, with or without cough and fever, that may become severe in a very short period of time.

Possible Side Effects *(continued)*

▼ Rare: eye pain, erosion of the cornea, eye ulcer, unusual eyelash growth, bleeding in the eye, severe skin reaction, and allergic reaction.

Drug Interactions

• Rifampicin and phenytoin reduce the amount of gefitinib in the blood by 85%. Your doctor may increase your dose to 500 mg a day to account for this effect.

• Itraconazole and ketoconazole increase the amount of gefitinib in the body by 88% by interfering with its breakdown in the liver. Your doctor should adjust your drug dosage if you must take both medicines together.

• Any drug that reduces the acid content of the stomach, such as ranitidine, cimetidine, or omeprazole, interferes with the absorption of gefitinib. Do not combine these medicines with gefitinib.

• Gefitinib can increase the effect of warfarin, causing bleeding episodes. Your doctor must check your blood regularly and may have to adjust your warfarin dose while you are taking gefitinib.

Food Interactions

You may take this drug without regard to food or meals.

Usual Dose

250 mg once a day.

Overdosage

Little is known about the effects of gefitinib overdose. Likely overdose symptoms include diarrhea and skin rash. Symptoms should be treated individually but it is particularly important to pay attention to severe diarrhea. In case of overdose, call your local poison control center or a hospital emergency room. If you seek treatment, ALWAYS bring the prescription bottle or container.

Special Information

If you forget to take a dose of gefitinib, take it as soon as you remember on the same day. If it is almost time for your next dose, skip the forgotten dose and continue with your regular schedule. Do not take a double dose.

Call your doctor at once if you develop cough, wheezing, or difficulty breathing and fever. You may have to stop taking gefitinib until the reason for your symptoms is discovered. These symptoms are fatal in one-third of people who develop them.

Other reasons to call your doctor right away are severe or persistent diarrhea, nausea, appetite loss, vomiting, eye irritation, or any other new symptom. If your diarrhea is severe, your doctor may have you discontinue the drug for 2 weeks to rest your gastrointestinal system.

Special Populations

Pregnancy/Breast-feeding

Gefitinib enters the fetal circulation. Women who are pregnant should not take it. Women who become pregnant while taking gefitinib must notify their doctor at once.

It is not known if this drug passes into breast milk. Nursing mothers who must take it should bottle-feed.

Seniors

Seniors may use this drug without special precaution.

Generic Name

Gemfibrozil (jem-FI-broe-zil) G

Brand Name

Lopid

Type of Drug

Anti-hyperlipidemic (blood-fat reducer).

Prescribed For

High blood triglycerides.

General Information

Gemfibrozil consistently reduces blood triglycerides and reduces the risk of heart disease in people with high levels of triglycerides, low levels of high-density lipoprotein (HDL) cholesterol, and high levels of low-density lipoprotein (LDL) cholesterol. It works by affecting the breakdown of body fats and by reducing the amount of triglyceride manufactured by the liver. It is usually prescribed only for people with very high blood-fat levels who have not responded to dietary changes or other therapies. Gemfibrozil usually has little effect on blood-cholesterol levels, although it may reduce blood cholesterol in some people.

Cautions and Warnings

Do not take gemfibrozil if you are **allergic** to it or have severe **liver or kidney disease**. Some people taking gemfibrozil have experienced worsening of kidney function. Gemfibrozil users may have an increased risk of developing **gallbladder disease** and **gallstones**. People taking gemfibrozil may develop **muscle aches and inflammation**. Tell your doctor if you experience muscle tenderness or weakness.

Estrogen drugs may cause massive increases in triglyceride levels. Stopping estrogen therapy in these cases may reduce triglyceride levels to normal.

Gemfibrozil may cause a moderate rise in **blood sugar** and mild decreases in **white-blood-cell counts**.

Possible Side Effects

▼ Most common: abdominal and stomach pain, fatigue, heartburn, gas, diarrhea, nausea, and vomiting.

▼ Less common: rash, itching, dizziness, blurred vision, anemia, reduced levels of white blood cells, increased blood sugar, and muscle pain—especially in the arms or legs.

▼ Rare: dry mouth, constipation, appetite loss, upset stomach, sleeplessness, tingling in the hands or feet, ringing or buzzing in the ears, back pain, painful muscles or joints, swollen joints, feeling unwell, reduction in blood potassium, and abnormal liver function.

Drug Interactions

• Gemfibrozil increases the effects of oral anticoagulant (blood-thinning) drugs. Your anticoagulant dosage must be reduced when starting gemfibrozil.

• Combining gemfibrozil with a statin cholesterol-lowering drug (atorvastatin, cerivastatin, fluvastatin, lovastatin, pravastatin, or simvastatin) has led to the destruction of skeletal muscles. This effect may begin as early as 3 weeks after you start taking the combination or may not appear for months.

• Combining gemfibrozil and sulfonylurea antidiabetes drugs or repaglinide may cause unexpectedly low blood sugar levels. The sulfonylurea drug dosage may need adjustment.

• Gemfibrozil can substantially increase the amount of glitazone antidiabetes drugs in the blood. Glitazone dosages may need to be adjusted.

• Combining gemfibrozil and cyclosporine may decrease the effectiveness of cyclosporine. This combination should only be used if it is absolutely necessary and the lowest possible dose of gemfibrozil is used.

Food Interactions

Gemfibrozil is best taken on an empty stomach 30 minutes before meals but may be taken with food if it upsets your stomach. It is important that you follow your doctor's dietary instructions.

Usual Dose

1200 mg a day, divided into 2 doses taken 30 minutes before breakfast and dinner.

Overdosage

Little is known about the effects of gemfibrozil overdose. Symptoms may include severe side effects. Induce vomiting with ipecac syrup—available at any pharmacy—but call your doctor or local poison control center before doing this. If you go to a hospital emergency room, ALWAYS bring the prescription bottle or container.

Special Information

Your doctor should perform periodic blood counts during the first year of gemfibrozil treatment to check for anemia or other changes in blood components. Liver-function tests are also necessary. Blood-sugar levels should be checked periodically while you are taking gemfibrozil, especially if you are diabetic or have a family history of diabetes.

Gemfibrozil may cause dizziness or blurred vision. Be careful when driving or doing any task that requires concentration.

Gemfibrozil is less effective if you are greatly overweight.

Call your doctor if side effects become severe or intolerable, especially diarrhea, nausea, vomiting, or stomach pain or gas. These may disappear if your doctor reduces the dosage.

If you forget a dose, take it as soon as you remember. If it is almost time for your next dose, skip the one you forgot and continue with your regular schedule. Do not take a double dose.

Special Populations

Pregnancy/Breast-feeding
The safety of using gemfibrozil during pregnancy is not known. When this drug is considered crucial by your doctor, its potential benefits must be carefully weighed against its risks.

This drug passes into breast milk and should not be taken by a nursing mother.

Seniors
Seniors are more likely to develop drug side effects due to normal declines in kidney function.

Generic Name

Glatiramer (glah-TYE-ram-er)

Brand Name

Copaxone

Type of Drug

Relapsing-remitting multiple sclerosis (MS) therapy.

Prescribed For

MS.

General Information

Glatiramer is a mixture of several amino acids. It is thought to work by modifying the immune processes responsible for MS. In studies, people who took the drug for over a year were twice as likely to be relapse-free as those who took a placebo (sugar pill).

Cautions and Warnings

Do not use this drug if you are **allergic** to it or mannitol.

About 10% of people who self-administer glatiramer experience a **post-injection reaction** with symptoms that include flushing, chest pain, heart palpitations, anxiety, breathing difficulties, closing of the throat, and an itchy rash. These symptoms usually go away without treatment. This reaction generally occurs after several months of drug therapy, though it may occur earlier.

About 25% of the people who took glatiramer in drug studies had **chest pain,** but the exact relationship of this pain to use of glatiramer could not be determined. Report any chest pain to your doctor at once.

Glatiramer may make you more sensitive to **sunlight.**

Because it interferes with immune response, glatiramer may increase your risk of developing **infections** and **tumors.**

Glatiramer may interfere with **kidney function.**

Possible Side Effects

▼ Most common: infections, weakness, pain, chest pain, flu-like symptoms, back pain, flushing, heart palpitations, anxiety, muscle stiffness or spasticity, an urgent need to urinate, swollen lymph glands, injection-site reactions (including pain, inflammation, itching, an unknown mass at the injection site, welts, skin marks, and bleeding), breathing difficulties, runny nose, and joint pain.

▼ Common: fever, neck pain, facial swelling, bacterial infection, migraine, fever, rapid heartbeat, tremors, fainting, appetite loss, vomiting, general stomach disorders, vaginal infection, painful menstruation, black-and-blue marks, swelling in the arms or legs, bronchial irritation, spasm of the larynx, and ear pain.

▼ Less common: chills, cysts, agitation, foot drop, nervousness, rolling eyeballs, confusion, speech problems, cold sores, redness, itchy rash, skin nodules, stomach pain and irritation, weight gain, and eye disorders.

▼ Rare: Rare side effects can occur in almost any part of the body. Contact your doctor if you experience any side effect not listed above.

Food and Drug Interactions

None known.

Usual Dose

Adult (age 18 and over): 20 mg a day by injection under the skin.

Child: not recommended.

Overdosage

Little is known about the effects of glatiramer overdose. Call you local poison control center or a hospital emergency room for information. If you seek treatment, ALWAYS bring the prescription bottle or container.

Special Information

Store unused glatiramer in the refrigerator before it is mixed with the diluent supplied by the manufacturer. Do not use any other diluent. The mixed injection must be used right away.

Suggested injection sites are the arms, abdomen, hips, and thighs. Be sure to rotate injection sites.

If you forget to administer a dose, do so as soon as you remember. If it is almost time for your next dose, skip the dose you forgot and continue with your regular schedule. Do not take a double dose. Call your doctor if you miss more than 2 doses in a row.

Special Populations

Pregnancy/Breast-feeding

The safety of using glatiramer during pregnancy is not known. When this drug is considered crucial by your doctor, its potential benefits must be carefully weighed against its risks.

It is not known if glatiramer passes into breast milk. Nursing mothers who must take it should consider bottle-feeding.

Seniors

Seniors may use glatiramer without special restriction.

Type of Drug

Glitazone Antidiabetes Drugs

(GLIT-uh-zone)

Brand Names

Generic Ingredient: Pioglitazone
Actos

Generic Ingredient: Rosiglitazone
Avandia

Combination Products

Generic Ingredients: Rosiglitazone + Metformin
Avandamet

Prescribed for

Type 2 diabetes.

General Information

The glitazones reduce the amount of sugar produced by the liver and increase insulin sensitivity of muscle, liver, and fat cells. They may also help to control blood-fat levels, which are often elevated in diabetes. Glitazones only work when insulin is present. They do not increase the amount of insulin made in the pancreas. Glitazones work by affecting genes responsible for the control of sugar and fat use in the body, making cells more sensitive to insulin. They are effective for people with type 2 diabetes, who generally have enough insulin but whose cells do not respond to it. Glitazones can be used alone or combined with other diabetes drugs.

Cautions and Warnings

Do not take this drug if you are **sensitive** or **allergic** to it or related drugs. Glitazones are broken down in the liver; people with **liver disease** should not take them. Liver enzyme monitoring is recommended for all people taking a glitazone. People taking pioglitazone and rosiglitazone have experienced **liver failure**, though no direct causal effect of the drug has been established.

Glitazones may raise blood levels of **cholesterol** and other blood fats.

Glitazones may cause fluid retention, worsening **heart failure**.

These drugs can trigger **ovulation**. Premenopausal women who are not ovulating may be at risk of becoming pregnant.

Glitazones can cause **weight gain,** which increases with dosage.

Women may achieve maximum benefit with smaller dosages.

Possible Side Effects

Pioglitazone

In studies, the side effects of pioglitazone were about the same as those for a placebo (sugar pill).

▼ Most common: upper respiratory infections, headaches, and sinus irritation.

▼ Common: muscle aches, tooth problems, and sore throat.

▼ Less common: anemia and swollen legs or arms.

▼ Rare: yellowing of the skin or whites of the eyes, hepatitis, liver failure, and death.

Rosiglitazone

▼ Common: upper respiratory infections, accidental injuries, and headache.

▼ Less common: swelling, back pain, high blood sugar, fatigue, sinus irritation, and diarrhea.

▼ Rare: anemia and low blood sugar.

For additional side effects of Avandamet, see Metformin, page 685.

Drug Interactions

• Ketoconazole may significantly increase the amount of pioglitazone in the body. Other drugs that may have a similar effect but have not yet been studied include itraconazole, erythromycin, calcium channel blockers, corticosteroids, cyclosporine, protease inhibitor anti-HIV drugs, statin cholesterol-lowering drugs, tacrolimus, triazolam, and trimetrexate.

• Glitazones may reduce the effectiveness of oral contraceptives ("the pill") containing norethindrone and ethinyl estradiol. Higher-dose contraceptives or another contraceptive method may be needed.

• Pioglitazone may stimulate the breakdown of other drugs also metabolized in the liver.

• Taking rosiglitazone and insulin may increase the risk of fluid retention and heart failure.

For additional drug interactions for Avandamet, see Metformin, page 685.

Food Interactions

Grapefruit juice may interfere with the breakdown of pioglitazone in the liver. Otherwise, these drugs may be taken with or without food.

Usual Dose

Pioglitazone
Adult: 15–45 mg once a day.
Child: not recommended.

Rosiglitazone
Adult (age 18 and older): 4 mg–8 mg once a day or in divided doses.
Child: not recommended.

Avandamet
Adult: 2 mg/500 mg–4 mg/500 mg twice a day.
Child: not recommended.

Overdosage

Little is known about the effects of glitazone overdose. Take the victim to a hospital emergency room. ALWAYS bring the prescription bottle or container.

Special Information

Diet, calorie control, exercise, and weight loss are essential to controlling type 2 diabetes. Do not depend solely on this drug to manage your condition.

Alcohol, smoking, age, and race do not affect the way that glitazones are processed in the body.

Call your doctor if you develop symptoms of liver disease, including nausea, vomiting, abdominal pain, fatigue, appetite loss, or dark-colored urine.

See your doctor for regular monitoring of blood sugar, glycosylated hemoglobin (a more sensitive indicator of long-term diabetes control), and liver function.

If you forget a dose, take it as soon as you remember. If it is almost time for your next dose, skip the dose you forgot and continue with your regular schedule.

Special Populations

Pregnancy/Breast-feeding

The safety of using glitazones during pregnancy is not known. Most experts recommend that diabetes be controlled with insulin during pregnancy.

It is not known if glitazones pass into breast milk. Nursing mothers who must take it should consider bottle-feeding.

Seniors

Seniors may take this drug without special precaution.

Glucophage XR see Metformin, page 685

Glucotrol XL see Sulfonylurea Antidiabetes Drugs, page 1003

Brand Name

Glucovance (GLEW-ko-vance)

Generic Ingredients

Glyburide + Metformin

Type of Drug

Antidiabetic.

Prescribed For

Type 2 diabetes.

General Information

Metformin lowers the amount of glucose produced by the liver, reduces the amount of glucose you absorb from food, and helps cells use glucose. Metformin can also moderately lower body fats. Glyburide stimulates the release of insulin from the pancreas. Glucovance is a combination of these two antidiabetic drugs.

Cautions and Warnings

Do not take Glucovance if you are **allergic** to it or have **heart failure**. People with **kidney disease** should not take this drug.

Mild stress, such as **infection, minor surgery,** or **emotional upset,** reduces the effectiveness of Glucovance. You must be under your doctor's continuous care while taking it.

People taking oral antidiabetes drugs are generally more likely to develop **heart disease,** compared with people taking insulin or those treated by diet alone.

Glucovance is not a form of **oral insulin** or a substitute for insulin. It does not lower blood sugar by itself.

This drug can cause **low blood sugar** (see "Overdosage") that may require medical attention.

Glucovance should be used with care if you have serious **liver, kidney, or endocrine disease;** monitor your blood sugar very closely.

Very rarely, Glucovance can cause a serious complication known as **lactic acidosis**. Lactic acidosis is fatal about half of the time. The risk of lactic acidosis increases with age, the presence of heart failure, and worsening kidney function. This disease is often subtle, and is accompanied only by non-specific symptoms such as not feeling well, muscle aches, breathing difficulties, tiredness, and nonspecific upset stomach. Low body temperature, low blood pressure, and slow heartbeat can develop with more severe acidosis. Call your doctor at once if you develop these symptoms.

Regular monitoring of kidney function minimizes the risk of developing lactic acidosis, as does using the minimum effective dosage of Glucovance. People with acidosis, including those with diabetic ketoacidosis, should not take Glucovance.

People with **liver disease** should not take Glucovance because of the increased risk of lactic acidosis.

Possible Side Effects

People who are stabilized on Glucovance should not consider gastrointestinal (GI) symptoms to be related to the drug unless other causes or lactic acidosis have been excluded.

▼ Most common: diarrhea, nausea, vomiting, stomach upset, abdominal bloating, gas, appetite loss and weakness or tingling in the hands and feet. These symptoms tend to occur when you first start taking Glucovance but are generally transient and resolve on their own. Occasionally, temporary dosage reduction is useful.

▼ Less common: abnormally low blood sugar levels.

▼ Rare: an unpleasant or metallic taste in the mouth, low blood levels of vitamin B12, yellowing of the skin or whites of the eyes, itching, and rash. Usually these reactions will disappear in time. If they persist, contact your doctor.

Drug Interactions

• The following drugs may increase your need for Glucovance: beta blockers, calcium channel blockers, cholestyramine, corticosteroids, diazoxide, estrogens, isoniazid, nicotinic acid, oral contraceptives, phenothiazines, phenytoin and other hydantoin drugs, rifampin, stimulants, thiazide diuretics, thyroid replacement drugs, charcoal tablets, and anything that makes your urine less acidic.

• The following drugs may reduce your need for Glucovance: androgens (male hormones), aspirin and other salicylates, bishydroxycoumarin, chloramphenicol, cimetidine, ciprofloxacin, clofibrate, dicumarol, famotidine, fenfluramine, fluconazole, gemfibrozil, itraconazole, ketoconazole, magnesium-containing products, methyldopa, miconazole, monoamine oxidase inhibitor (MAOI) drugs, nizatidine, oxyphenbutazone, phenylbutazone, probenecid, phenyramidol, ranitidine, sulfa drugs, sulfinpyrazone, tricyclic antidepressants, warfarin, large doses of vitamin C, and citrus fruits and other foods that make your urine more acidic.

• Cimetidine, nifedipine, and furosemide can cause a large increase in Glucovance blood levels and possible side effects. Furosemide levels are reduced by Glucovance.

• Glucovance may interfere with amiloride, digoxin, morphine, procainamide, quinine, quinidine, triamterene, trimethoprim, and vancomycin.

• Mixing insulin with Glucovance may lead to severely low blood sugar. This combination must be used only under a doctor's supervision.

• Glucovance may alter the effectiveness of oral anticoagulant (blood-thinning) drugs. Dosage may have to be adjusted by your doctor.

• Glucovance may increase the effects of digitalis drugs.

• Mixing this drug with alcohol can cause flushing and breathlessness. Other possible effects are throbbing pain in the head and neck, breathing difficulties, nausea, vomiting, increased sweating, excessive thirst, chest pains, palpitations, lowered blood pressure, weakness, dizziness, blurred vision, and confusion. If you experience any of these reactions, contact your doctor immediately. Alcohol also increases the risk of developing lactic acidosis while taking Glucovance.

• The stimulants in many over-the-counter cough, cold, and allergy remedies may affect your blood sugar; avoid them unless your doctor advises otherwise.

• If you are having surgery or an X-ray that requires the injection of an iodine-based contrast material, you should temporarily stop taking Glucovance because the combination could result in acute kidney problems.

Food Interactions

Take with food or meals to reduce upset stomach.

Usual Dose

Adult: 1.25/250 mg to 20/2000 mg once or twice a day.
Child: not recommended.

Overdosage

A mild overdose causes low blood sugar (symptoms include tingling of the lips and tongue, nausea, lethargy, yawning, confusion, agitation, nervousness, rapid heartbeat, increased sweating, tremors, and hunger). Eating sugar in such forms as candy, orange juice, or glucose tablets can treat these symptoms. Ultimately, low blood sugar may lead to convulsions, stupor, and coma. Lactic acidosis has occurred in some cases. Call your doctor, local poison control center, or hospital emergency room to find out if the overdose victim should be taken to a hospital emergency room. ALWAYS bring the prescription bottle or container.

Special Information

Diet and exercise are the mainstays of diabetes treatment. Be sure to follow your doctor's directions in these areas while taking your medication.

Alcohol increases the risk of developing lactic acidosis while taking Glucovance. Lactic acidosis is a medical emergency. Glucovance treatment must be stopped immediately if you develop it.

Call your doctor if you develop low blood sugar (see "Overdosage") or high blood sugar (symptoms include excessive thirst or urination and sugar or ketones in the urine), if you are not feeling well, or if you have symptoms such as itching, rash, yellowing of the whites of the eyes, abnormally light-colored stools, a low-grade fever, sore throat, diarrhea, or unusual bruising or bleeding.

Stomach and intestinal side effects may be reduced by gradually increasing your dosage and by taking your medication with meals.

Call your doctor if you have severe diarrhea or vomiting. You may need to temporarily stop your medication.

Do not stop taking this drug except under your doctor's supervision. If you forget a dose, take it as soon as you remember. If it is almost time for your next dose, skip the one you forgot and continue with your regular schedule. Do not take a double dose.

Special Populations

Pregnancy/Breast-feeding
The safety of Glucovance during pregnancy is not known. Pregnant women with diabetes should take insulin.

Glucovance passes into breast milk. Nursing mothers who must take it should consider bottle-feeding.

Seniors
Seniors should not receive the maximum dose of this drug because of the risk that low blood sugar may develop.

Generic Name

Guanabenz (GWAN-uh-benz) Ⓖ

Brand Name

Wytensin

Type of Drug

Antihypertensive.

Prescribed For

High blood pressure.

General Information

Guanabenz acetate works by depressing the central nervous system by stimulating certain receptors. Initially, guanabenz reduces blood pressure without a major effect on blood vessels; however, long-term use of guanabenz may result in the dilation (widening) of blood vessels and a slight slowing of pulse rate. Guanabenz may be taken alone or with a thiazide diuretic.

Cautions and Warnings

Do not take guanabenz if you are **sensitive** or **allergic** to it.

People with severe **kidney or liver disease** should take this drug with caution. Guanabenz should also be used with caution by people who have had a recent **heart attack** or **stroke**.

Possible Side Effects

Risk and severity of side effects increase with dosage.

▼ Most common: drowsiness, sedation, dry mouth, dizziness, weakness, and headache.

▼ Less common: chest pain; swelling in the hands, legs, or feet; heart palpitations or abnormal heart rhythms; stomach or abdominal pain or discomfort; nausea; diarrhea; vomiting; constipation; anxiety; poor muscle control; depression; difficulty sleeping; stuffy nose; blurred vision; muscle aches and pains; breathing

---

Possible Side Effects *(continued)*

difficulties; frequent urination; impotence; unusual taste in the mouth; and swollen and painful breasts in men.

Drug Interactions

• Other blood-pressure-lowering agents increase the effect of guanabenz.

• The sedating effects of guanabenz are increased by combining it with tranquilizers, sleeping pills, or other central nervous system (CNS) depressants, including alcohol.

• People taking this drug for high blood pressure should avoid over-the-counter drugs that might aggravate their condition, including decongestants, cold and allergy remedies, and diet pills—all of which may contain stimulants.

Food Interactions

This drug is best taken on an empty stomach, but it may be taken with food if it upsets your stomach.

Usual Dose

4 mg twice a day to start; increased gradually to a maximum dose of 32 mg twice a day—though doses this large are rarely needed.

Overdosage

Overdose causes sleepiness, lethargy, low blood pressure, irritability, pinpoint pupils, and reduced heart rate. Overdose victims should be made to vomit with ipecac syrup—available at any pharmacy—but call your doctor or poison control center first. If you must go to a hospital emergency room, ALWAYS bring the prescription bottle or container.

Special Information

Take guanabenz exactly as prescribed for maximum benefit. If any side effect becomes severe or intolerable, contact your doctor.

Guanabenz often causes tiredness or dizziness; avoid alcohol because it increases these effects. Take care when driving or doing anything that requires concentration.

Do not stop taking guanabenz without your doctor's approval. Suddenly stopping this drug may cause a rapid increase in blood pressure. Dosage must be gradually reduced by your doctor.

If you forget a dose, take it as soon as you remember. If it is almost time for your next dose, skip the one you forgot and continue with your regular schedule. Do not take a double dose. Call your doctor if you miss 2 or more consecutive doses.

Special Populations

Pregnancy/Breast-feeding

Guanabenz may affect the fetus. It should be avoided by women who are or might be pregnant. When guanabenz is considered crucial by your doctor, its potential benefits must be carefully weighed against its risks.

It is not known if guanabenz passes into breast milk. Nursing mothers who must take this drug should bottle-feed.

Seniors

Seniors are more sensitive to the sedating and blood-pressure-lowering effects of guanabenz.

Generic Name

Haloperidol (hal-oe-PER-ih-dol) Ⓖ

Brand Name

Haldol

Type of Drug

Butyrophenone antipsychotic.

Prescribed For

Psychotic disorders, including Tourette's syndrome; severe behavioral problems in children; short-term treatment of hyperactive children; chronic schizophrenia; vomiting; treatment of acute psychiatric situations; and phencyclidine (PCP) psychosis.

General Information

Haloperidol is one of many nonphenothiazine agents used to treat psychosis. These drugs are equally effective when given in therapeutically equivalent doses. The major differences are in the type and severity of side effects. Some people may respond well to one and not at all to another. Haloperidol acts on a portion of the brain called the hypothalamus. It affects parts of the hypothalamus that control metabolism, body temperature, alertness, muscle tone, hormone balance, and vomiting. Haloperidol is available in liquid form for those who have trouble swallowing tablets.

Cautions and Warnings

Haloperidol should not be used by people who are **allergic** to it.

People with very **low blood pressure, Parkinson's disease,** or **blood, liver, heart, or kidney disease** should avoid this drug.

If you have **glaucoma, epilepsy, ulcers,** or **difficulty urinating,** haloperidol should be used with caution and under strict supervision of your doctor.

Avoid **exposure to extreme heat** because this drug can upset your body's temperature-regulating mechanism.

Haloperidol may cause **dystonia, tardive dyskinesia,** or **neuroleptic malignant syndrome,** all serious conditions.

Possible Side Effects

▼ Most common: drowsiness, especially during the first or second week of therapy. If the drowsiness becomes troublesome, contact your doctor.

▼ Less common: jaundice (yellowing of the whites of the eyes or skin), which may occur in the first 2 to 4 weeks. The jaundice usually goes away when the drug is discontinued, but there have been cases in which it did not. If you notice this effect, develop fever, or generally feel unwell, contact your doctor immediately. Other less common side effects are changes in components of the blood, including anemias; raised or lowered blood pressure; abnormal heartbeat; heart attack; and feeling faint or dizzy.

▼ Rare: neurological effects such as spasms of the neck muscles, severe stiffness of the back muscles, rolling back of the eyes, convulsions, difficulty in swallowing, and symptoms associated with Parkinson's disease. These

---

Possible Side Effects *(continued)*

effects usually disappear after the drug has been withdrawn; however, symptoms of the face, tongue, or jaw
may persist for years, especially in seniors with a long history of brain disease. If you experience any of these effects,
contact your doctor immediately. Other rare side effects
can occur in almost any part of the body. Contact your doctor if you experience any side effect not listed above.

Drug Interactions

• Be cautious about taking haloperidol with barbiturates,
sleeping pills, narcotics or other tranquilizers, alcohol, or any
other medication that may produce a depressive effect.

• Anticholinergic drugs may reduce the effectiveness of
haloperidol and increase the risk of side effects.

• The blood-pressure-lowering effect of guanethidine may
be counteracted by haloperidol.

• Taking lithium together with haloperidol may lead to disorientation, loss of consciousness, or uncontrolled muscle
movements.

• Combining methyldopa with haloperidol may increase
the effects of haloperidol.

• Combining beta-blockers such as propranolol or diuretics
and haloperidol may lead to unusually low blood pressure
and other problems.

• Combining antidepressant drugs and haloperidol can
lead to antidepressant side effects.

• Haloperidol may increase the effects of antihypertensive
drugs.

• Haloperidol may affect phenytoin and carbamazepine
levels, as well as levels of other anitpsychotic drugs.

Food Interactions

Haloperidol is best taken on an empty stomach, but you may
take it with food if it upsets your stomach.

Usual Dose

Psychotic disorders
    Adult: starting dose—0.5–2 mg 2 or 3 times a day. Some
patients may need 3–5 mg 2 or 3 times a day. Rarely, some
patients may require up to 100 mg a day.

Child (age 3–12 or 33–88 lbs.): starting dose—0.5 mg a day. Dosage may be increased in 0.5-mg steps every 5–7.

Child (under age 3): not recommended.

Tourette's syndrome
  Adult: starting dose—0.5–2 mg 3 times a day; up to 10 mg a day may be needed.

  Child (age 3–12 or 33–88 lbs.): 0.02–0.03 mg per lb. a day. The same dosages apply to children with behavioral disorders or hyperactivity.

Overdosage

Symptoms of overdose are depression, extreme weakness, tiredness, desire to sleep, coma, lowered blood pressure, uncontrolled muscle spasms, agitation, restlessness, convulsions, fever, dry mouth, and abnormal heart rhythm. The patient should be taken to a hospital emergency room immediately. ALWAYS bring the prescription bottle or container.

Special Information

This medication may cause drowsiness. Use caution when driving or operating hazardous equipment; also, avoid alcoholic beverages while taking it.

  Haloperidol may cause unusual sensitivity to the sun. It may also turn your urine reddish-brown or pink.

  If dizziness occurs, avoid sudden changes in posture and avoid climbing stairs. Use caution in hot weather. This medication may make you more prone to heat stroke.

  If you forget to take a dose of haloperidol, take it as soon as you remember. Take the rest of the day's doses evenly spaced throughout the day. Do not take a double dose.

Special Populations

Pregnancy/Breast-feeding
Serious problems have been seen in pregnant animals given large amounts of haloperidol. Although haloperidol has not been studied in pregnant women, you should avoid this drug if you are or might be pregnant.

  Haloperidol passes into breast milk. Nursing mothers who must use this medication should bottle-feed.

Seniors
Seniors are more sensitive to the effects of this medication and usually require ½ to ¼ the usual adult dose. Seniors are also more likely to develop side effects.

Brand Name

Helidac

Generic Ingredients

Bismuth Subsalicylate + Metronidazole + Tetracycline

Type of Drug

Antibacterial combination.

Prescribed For

Duodenal ulcers.

General Information

Research has shown that the bacterium *Helicobacter pylori* is usually present in ulcer disease and some forms of gastritis. This discovery changed the treatment of these diseases. Drugs used to treat the *H. pylori* infection are now prescribed along with a drug that alleviates ulcer symptoms by blocking stomach acid. Doctors have developed a variety of approaches to treating ulcers by using combinations of various antibiotic and acid-blocking drugs. Helidac combines 3 drugs with antibacterial or antibiotic action. This combination generally works by disrupting the cell walls of the bacterium and interfering with its ability to make proteins or duplicate itself. It is often prescribed together with ranitidine, cimetidine, or another acid blocker. Other treatments use other drug combinations.

Cautions and Warnings

Do not take Helidac if you are **sensitive** or **allergic** to any of its ingredients.

Rarely, bismuth causes severe **nervous-system toxicity**. Symptoms go away after the drug is stopped. Bismuth subsalicylate can cause dark stools or darkening of the tongue. This darkening of stools is not dangerous; however, be aware that blood in the stool often manifests as blackening of the stool.

Children or teenagers who have or are recovering from chickenpox should not use Helidac because it contains a small amount of salicylate, which is related to aspirin.

Children or teenagers who take aspirin or a salicylate may develop Reye's syndrome, symptoms of which include nausea and vomiting.

Metronidazole can cause convulsive **seizures** and **nervous system effects** including numbness or tingling in the arms, legs, hands, or feet. The risk of developing these effects increases with dosage and duration of use. Call your doctor at once if you experience any of these effects.

Metronidazole should be taken with caution by people who have had **blood diseases.**

Candida infections may worsen while you are taking metronidazole. People with **liver disease** may require reduced dosage.

Tetracycline should be avoided by people with severe **kidney disease.** Other infections, called superinfections, can develop while you are taking tetracycline. If this happens, your doctor will discontinue Helidac and prescribe a different drug to treat your *H. pylori* infection, as well as another drug to treat the superinfection. People taking tetracycline can develop **pseudotumor cerebri** (pressure inside the brain), the symptoms of which are usually headache and blurred vision. Symptoms usually go away when the drug is stopped, but permanent damage can result. Tetracycline may increase your **sensitivity to the sun;** use sunscreen and wear protective clothing.

Possible Side Effects

For more information on possible side effects, see Metronidazole, page 703 and Tetracycline Antibiotics, page 1043.

▼ Most common: nausea and diarrhea.

▼ Less common: abdominal pain, blood in the stool, headache, anal discomfort, appetite loss, dizziness, tingling in the hands or feet, vomiting, muscle weakness, constipation, sleeplessness, pain, and respiratory infections.

Drug Interactions

• Tetracycline antibiotics, which are bacteriostatic, may interfere with the action of bactericidal (bacteria-killing) agents such as penicillin. You should not take both kinds of antibiotics for the same infection.

• Antacids, mineral supplements, and multivitamins containing bismuth, calcium, zinc, magnesium, and iron can reduce the effectiveness of tetracycline. Separate doses of your antacid, mineral supplement, vitamin with minerals, or sodium bicarbonate and Helidac by at least 2 hours.

• Tetracycline and metronidazole may each increase the effect of anticoagulant (blood-thinning) drugs such as warfarin. An adjustment in the anticoagulant dosage may be required.

• Cimetidine can increase metronidazole blood levels. Your metronidazole dosage may be reduced if you are also taking cimetidine.

• Tetracycline may increase blood levels of digoxin in a small number of people, leading to possible digoxin side effects. In some people this interaction with digoxin can occur for months after tetracycline has been stopped. If you are taking this combination, watch carefully for digoxin side effects and call your doctor if any develop.

• Tetracycline may reduce diabetic insulin requirements. If you are using this combination, be sure to carefully monitor your blood-sugar level.

• Tetracycline may increase or decrease lithium blood levels. Metronidazole raises lithium blood levels, effects, and toxicity.

• Combining alcohol and metronidazole may cause abdominal cramps, nausea, vomiting, headaches, and flushing. Modification of the taste of alcohol has also been reported. Metronidazole should not be used if you are taking disulfiram (a drug used to maintain alcohol abstinence) because the combination can cause confusion and psychotic reactions.

• Phenobarbital and other barbiturates can decrease metronidazole's effectiveness.

• Drugs that cause nervous system toxicity, such as mexiletine, ethambutol, isoniazid, lincomycin, lithium, pemoline, quinacrine, and long-term high-dose pyridoxine (vitamin B_6) should not be taken with metronidazole because of the increased risk of nervous system side effects.

• Metronidazole may increase phenytoin blood levels and the risk of phenytoin side effects; your doctor may need to adjust your phenytoin dosage.

Food Interactions

Do not take this drug with milk or dairy products. Helidac should be taken with meals and at bedtime.

Usual Dose

Adult: Each dose consists of 4 pills. Take all 4 pills, 4 times a day for 14 days. Take your acid blocker according to your doctor's directions.

Child: not recommended.

Overdosage

All 3 ingredients in Helidac can be dangerous if taken in overdose, but salicylate poisoning is the most threatening. Symptoms of salicylate toxicity are rapid or heavy breathing, nausea, vomiting, ringing or buzzing in the ears, high fever, lethargy, rapid heartbeat, and confusion. Other more serious symptoms may develop. Take the victim to a hospital emergency room at once. ALWAYS bring the prescription bottle or container.

Special Information

Each Helidac dose consists of 2 pink, round, chewable tablets (bismuth subsalicylate); 1 white tablet (metronidazole); and 1 pale orange and white capsule (tetracycline). Chew the 2 bismuth tablets and then swallow the other 2 pills with a full glass (8 oz.) of water. Take the acid blocker according to your doctor's directions.

Tetracycline can reduce the effectiveness of oral contraceptives ("the pill"); you should use backup contraception while taking Helidac. Breakthrough bleeding is also possible.

Bismuth can cause a temporary darkening of your tongue or stool. This is a harmless effect. Stool darkening should not be confused with blood in the stool, which turns it black.

Avoid alcohol while taking Helidac and for 1 day after you stop taking it.

Call your doctor if you develop ringing in the ears. This can be a sign of salicylate toxicity from the bismuth subsalicylate.

If you forget a dose, take it as soon as you remember. If it is almost time for your next dose, skip the dose you forgot and continue with your regular schedule. Never take a double dose. If you have any doses left after 14 days, continue to take them at your regular times until you have used up all the medication. Call your doctor if you forget more than 4 doses in 14 days.

Special Populations

Pregnancy/Breast-feeding

Helidac should not be taken by pregnant women. Tetracycline affects bone and tooth development in the fetus.

Tetracycline and metronidazole pass into breast milk. Tetracycline interferes with the development of the child's skull, bones, and teeth, and metronidazole also may cause side effects in the baby. Nursing mothers who must take Helidac should bottle-feed.

Seniors

Seniors may take this drug without special restriction.

Humalog   *see Insulin, page 572*

Humulin 70/30   *see Insulin, page 572*

Humulin N   *see Insulin, page 572*

Generic Name

Hydralazine (hye-DRAL-uh-zene) G

Brand Names

Apresoline

Type of Drug

Antihypertensive.

Prescribed for

High blood pressure, aortic insufficiency after heart valve replacement, and congestive heart failure (CHF).

General Information

Although its mechanism of action is not completely understood, hydralazine hydrochloride is believed to lower blood pressure by relaxing vascular smooth muscles throughout the body. This also helps to improve heart function and blood flow to the kidneys and brain.

Cautions and Warnings

Do not use hydralazine if you are **sensitive** or **allergic** to it.

Long-term administration of more than 200 mg a day of hydralazine may produce the symptoms of **lupus erythematosus** (a chronic condition affecting the body's connective tissue), including muscle and joint pain, skin reactions, fever, kidney inflammation, and anemia, although they usually disappear when the drug is discontinued. Report any fever, chest pain, feelings of ill health, or other unexplained symptoms to your doctor. The risk of developing lupus increases with higher dosages; approximately 5 out of 100 and 10% of people taking 200 mg a day of hydralazine develop lupus.

Hydralazine may actually improve kidney blood flow and kidney function in people who have below-normal function. It should be used with caution in people with advanced **kidney damage**.

Hydralazine may worsen heart problems and should be used with care in people with a history of **heart disease**. It can cause **angina pain** and may cause **heart attacks**. This medication should also be used with caution in people with **pulmonary hypertension**.

Tingling in the hands or feet caused by hydralazine may be relieved by taking pyridoxine (vitamin B6).

People taking hydralazine may develop **reduced hemoglobin and red-blood-cell counts. Reduced white-blood-cell and platelet counts** may also occur. Periodic blood counts are recommended while taking hydralazine.

Possible Side Effects

▼ Most common: headache, appetite loss, nausea, vomiting, diarrhea, rapid heartbeat, and chest pain.

▼ Less common: stuffy nose, flushing, tearing of the eyes, itching or redness of the eyes, numbness or tingling in the hands or feet, dizziness, tremors, muscle cramps,

---

Possible Side Effects *(continued)*

---

depression, disorientation, anxiety, itching, rash, fever, chills, occasional hepatitis (symptoms include yellowing of the skin or whites of the eyes), constipation, urinary difficulties, and adverse effects on normal blood composition.

Drug Interactions

• Taking hydralazine with the beta blockers, metoprolol, or propranolol may result in increased blood levels of both hydralazine and the beta blocker.

• Indomethacin may reduce the effects of hydralazine.

• Do not use over-the-counter cough, cold, or allergy medications, or appetite suppressants. These products often contain stimulant ingredients that can increase blood pressure.

Food Interactions

Take hydralazine with food.

Usual Dose

Adult: 10 mg 4 times day for the first 2–4 days; increased to 25 mg 4 times a day for the rest of the first week. Dosage is then increased until the maximum effect is seen.

Child: 0.34 mg per lb. of body weight a day divided in 4 doses; increased up to 200 mg a day.

Overdosage

Symptoms include extreme lowering of blood pressure, rapid heartbeat, headache, flushing, chest pain, and abnormal heart rhythms. If you experience any of these symptoms, contact your doctor immediately. If you go to a hospital emergency room, ALWAYS bring the prescription bottle or container.

Special Information

Take hydralazine exactly as prescribed.

Call your doctor if you experience prolonged and unexplained tiredness, fever, muscle or joint aching, or chest pain while taking this drug.

If you forget a dose, take it as soon as you remember. If it is almost time for your next dose, skip the one you forgot and continue with your regular schedule. Do not take a double dose.

Special Populations

Pregnancy/Breast-feeding

High doses of hydralazine caused birth defects in animal studies, and temporary blood-related problems have been seen in newborns whose mothers took hydralazine during pregnancy. Women who are or might be pregnant should not take hydralazine unless its possible benefits have been carefully weighed against its risks.

Hydralazine passes into breast milk. Nursing mothers who must take this drug should consider bottle-feeding.

Seniors

Seniors are more sensitive to the blood-pressure-lowering effects of hydralazine and its side effects, especially low body temperature.

Generic Name

Hydroxyzine (hye-DROK-suh-zene) G

Brand Names

Atarax   Vistaril

Type of Drug

Antihistamine and antianxiety agent.

Prescribed For

Nausea, vomiting, anxiety, tension, agitation, itching caused by allergy, and sedation.

General Information

Hydroxyzine is an antihistamine with antianxiety, muscle-relaxing, antiemetic (antivomiting), bronchial-dilation, pain-relieving, and antispasmodic properties. Hydroxyzine has been used to treat a variety of problems including stress related to dental or other minor surgical procedures, acute emotional problems, anxiety associated with stomach and digestive disorders, skin problems, and behavioral difficulties in children.

Cautions and Warnings

Hydroxyzine should not be used if you are **sensitive** or **allergic** to it or to cetirizene.

Changes in **heart rhythm** have occurred in people taking this drug to relieve anxiety.

Hydroxyzine may worsen **porphyria**, a rare condition. People with this condition should not take hydroxyzine.

Because hydroxyzine controls nausea and vomiting, it may hide the symptoms of **appendicitis** or **overdoses** of other drugs.

Possible Side Effects

Wheezing, chest tightness, and breathing difficulties are signs of a drug-sensitivity reaction.

▼ Most common: dry mouth and drowsiness. These usually disappear after a few days of continuous use or when the dose is reduced.

▼ Rare: occasional tremors or convulsions at higher doses.

Drug Interactions

• This drug should not be taken with a monomine oxidose inhibitor (MAOI) antidepressant.

• Hydroxyzine depresses the nervous system, producing drowsiness and sleepiness. Do not take this drug with alcohol, tranquilizers, sedatives, or other antihistamines or central nervous system (CNS) depressants. When hydroxyzine is taken with one of these drugs, the dose of the latter should be cut in half.

Food Interactions

Take hydroxyzine with food if it upsets your stomach.

Usual Dose

Adult: 25–100 mg 3–4 times a day.
Child (age 6 and over): 5–25 mg 3–4 times a day.
Child (under age 6): 5–10 mg 3–4 times a day.

Overdosage

The most common sign of overdose is sleepiness. Overdose victims should be taken to a hospital emergency room for treatment. ALWAYS bring the prescription bottle or container.

Special Information

Hydroxyzine may cause drowsiness: Be careful when driving, operating hazardous machinery, or doing anything that requires concentration.

The dry mouth associated with taking hydroxyzine may increase your risk of dental cavities and decay. Pay attention to dental hygiene while taking this drug.

Call your doctor if you develop a drug-sensitivity reaction to hydroxyzine (symptoms include wheezing, chest tightness, and breathing difficulties).

If you forget a dose of hydroxyzine, take it as soon as you remember. If it is almost time for your next dose, skip the one you forgot and continue with your regular schedule. Do not take a double dose.

Special Populations

Pregnancy/Breast-feeding

Animal studies have shown that regular treatment with hydroxyzine during the first few months of pregnancy may cause birth defects. Do not take this drug without your doctor's knowledge if you are or might be pregnant.

Hydroxyzine may reduce the amount of breast milk you produce and may pass into breast milk. Nursing mothers who must take hydroxyzine should bottle-feed.

Seniors

Seniors are more sensitive to side effects and may require lower dosages.

Hyzaar   *see Angiotensin II Blockers, page 84*

Generic Name

Ibuprofen (eye-bue-PROE-fen) G

Brand Names

Advil*	Children's Advil*
Bayer Select Pain Relief	Children's Motrin*
Formula	Genpril

Haltran   Midol
IBU   Midol-IB
Ibuprin   Motrin*
Ibuprohm   Motrin IB
Infants' Motrin*   Nuprin
Menadol   Pediacare Fever

The information in this profile also applies to the following drug:

Generic Ingredient: Diclofenac
Cataflam   Voltaren
Solareze Gel   Voltaren-XR

Combination Products

Generic Ingredients: Diclofenac + Misoprostol
Arthrotec

The information in this profile also applies to the following drugs:

Generic Ingredient: Sulindac G
Clinoril

Generic Ingredient: Tolmetin Sodium G
Tolectin   Tolectin DS

Generic Ingredient: Diflunisal
Dolobid

Generic Ingredient: Fenoprofen G
Nalfon

Generic Ingredient: Flurbiprofen G
Ansaid

Generic Ingredient: Ketoprofen G
Orudis KT   Oruvail

Generic Ingredient: Meclofenamate G
Meclomen

Generic Ingredient: Mefenamic Acid
Ponstel

Generic Ingredient: Oxaprozin G
Daypro   Daypro ALTA

Some products in this brand-name group are alcohol- or sugar-free. Consult your pharmacist.

Type of Drug

Nonsteroidal anti-inflammatory drug (NSAID).

Prescribed For

Rheumatoid arthritis, osteoarthritis, fever, mild to moderate pain, juvenile rheumatoid arthritis, sunburn, menstrual pain, and other inflammatory conditions.

General Information

NSAIDs are used to relieve pain and inflammation. We do not know exactly how NSAIDs work, but they may achieve their effects by blocking the body's production of a hormone called prostaglandin and the action of other body chemicals known as COX-1 and COX-2 enzymes. Pain relief comes within 1 hour after taking the first dose of these medicines, but their anti-inflammatory effects take several days to 2 weeks to become apparent and may take a month or more to reach their maximum effect.

Cataflam, a newer version of diclofenac, has no sodium and is preferred for menstrual pain and cramps. Voltaren, the older version of diclofenac, has sodium. Women taking Cataflam for menstrual problems should not switch to Voltaren. The combination of diclofenac and misoprostol is used to protect against stomach and intestinal irritation and ulcer. NSAID eyedrops are used during eye surgery to prevent movement of the eye muscles and for itching and redness due to seasonal allergies. After cataract surgery, they are used to prevent inflammation.

Cautions and Warnings

People **allergic** to any NSAID and those with a history of **asthma** attacks brought on by an NSAID, iodides, or aspirin should not take these medicines.

These drugs may cause **gastrointestinal (GI) tract bleeding, ulcers, and perforation**. This can occur at any time, with or without warning, in people who take ibuprofen regularly. People with a history of active GI bleeding should be cautious about taking any NSAID. Alcoholism may increase the risk of bleeding. People who develop these symptoms and continue NSAID treatment should be aware of the possibility of developing more serious side effects.

Ibuprofen can affect platelets and **blood clotting** at high doses and should be avoided by people with clotting problems and those taking warfarin.

People with **heart problems** who use ibuprofen may experience swelling in their arms, legs, or feet.

People taking ibuprofen, especially those with a **collagen disease such as systemic lupus erythematosus**, may experience an unusually severe drug-sensitivity reaction. Report any unusual symptoms to your doctor at once.

Ibuprofen may cause severe toxic effects to the **kidney**. Report any unusual side effects to your doctor, who might need to periodically test your kidney function.

Diflunisal is a chemical similar to aspirin and should not be given to children or teens. It may cause a serious complication called Reye's syndrome.

Ibuprofen may make you **unusually sensitive to the effects of the sun**.

Ibuprofen may affect your **liver**, sometimes with serious or fatal results.

Possible Side Effects

▼ Common: diarrhea, nausea, vomiting, constipation, dizziness, rash, and minor stomach upset, distress, or gas, especially during the first few days of treatment.

▼ Less common: stomach ulcers, GI bleeding, appetite loss, hepatitis, gallbladder attacks, painful urination, poor kidney function, kidney inflammation, blood and protein in the urine, fainting, nervousness, depression, hallucinations, confusion, disorientation, tingling in the hands or feet, light-headedness, itching, sweating, dry nose and mouth, heart palpitations, chest pain, breathing difficulties, and muscle cramps.

▼ Rare: severe allergic reactions including closing of the throat, fever and chills, changes in liver function, jaundice (yellowing of the skin and whites of the eyes), and kidney failure. These must be treated in a hospital

Possible Side Effects *(continued)*

emergency room or doctor's office. NSAIDs have caused severe skin reactions; see your doctor immediately if this happens to you.

Diclofenac Eyedrops
▼ Most common: temporary burning, stinging, or other minor eye irritation.
▼ Less common: nausea, vomiting, vital infections, and eye allergies including persistent redness, burning, itching, or tearing.
▼ Rare: The risk of developing bleeding problems or other systemic (whole body) side effects is low because only a small amount of the drug is absorbed into the bloodstream.

Drug Interactions

• These drugs may increase the effects of oral anticoagulant (blood-thinning) drugs such as warfarin. Your anticoagulant dose may need to be reduced.
• These drugs may reduce the blood-pressure-lowering effect of beta-blockers, ACE inhibitors, and diuretics.
• Combining these drugs with cyclosporine may increase the kidney-related side effects of both drugs.
• Ibuprofen may increase digoxin blood levels and toxicity.
• Ibuprofen may increase phenytoin side effects.
• Lithium blood levels and side effects may be increased by ibuprofen.
• Methotrexate side effects may be increased in people also taking ibuprofen.
• Blood levels of these drugs may be affected by cimetidine.
• Probenecid may increase the risk of NSAID side effects.
• Aspirin and other salicylates should never be combined with an NSAID in the treatment of arthritis.

Food Interactions

Take these drugs with food or a magnesium/aluminum antacid if it upsets your stomach.

Usual Dose

Diclofenac Tablets
  Adult: 100–200 mg a day.
  Senior: starting dose—⅓–½ the usual dosage.

Diclofenac Eyedrops
  1 drop 4 times a day for 2 weeks, beginning 24 hours after cataract surgery.

Diclofenac and Misoprostol
  Adult: one 50/200 tablet 3 or 4 times a day or one 75/200 tablet 3 times a day. For seniors, taking the combination product 4 times a day provides better ulcer protection, but arthritis relief does not improve.

Sulindac
  Adult (age 18 and over): 150–200 mg twice a day.

Tolmetin
  Adult (age 18 and over): 12.5–50 mg once a day.
  Child (under age 18): not recommended.

Diflunisal
  Starting dosage—500–1000 mg. Maintenance dosage—250–500 mg every 8–12 hours. Do not take more than 1500 mg a day. Do not crush or chew diflunisal tablets.

Fenoprofen
  Adult: mild to moderate pain—200 mg every 4–6 hours. Arthritis—300–600 mg 3–4 times a day to start, individualized to your needs. Total daily dose should not exceed 3200 mg.
  Child: not recommended.

Flurbiprofen
200–300 mg a day in divided doses.

Ibuprofen
  Adult: 200–800 mg 4 times a day depending on the condition being treated; follow your doctor's directions. 200 mg every 4–6 hours is appropriate for mild to moderate pain.
  Child: juvenile arthritis—9–18 mg per lb. of body weight a day, divided into several doses.

Ketoprofen
50–75 mg 3–4 times a day. Do not exceed 300 mg a day. Seniors and people with kidney problems should start with ⅓–½ of the usual dose.

Ketoprofen ER
200 mg once a day.

Meclofenamate
   Adult and Child (age 14 and over): 200–400 mg a day in divided doses.
   Child (under age 14): not recommended.

Mefenamic Acid
   Adult and Child (age 14 and over): 500 mg to start, then 250 mg every 6 hours in divided doses.
   Child (under age 14): not recommended.

Oxaprozin
600–1800 mg once a day. Do not exceed 12 mg per lb. of body weight daily.

Overdosage

People have died from NSAID overdoses. Common signs of overdose are drowsiness, nausea, vomiting, diarrhea, abdominal pain, rapid breathing, rapid heartbeat, sweating, ringing or buzzing in the ears, confusion, disorientation, stupor, and coma. Take the victim to a hospital emergency room at once for treatment. ALWAYS bring the prescription bottle or container.

Special Information

Take each dose with a full glass of water and do not lie down for 15 to 30 minutes afterward.
   NSAIDs may make you drowsy or tired: Be careful when driving or operating hazardous equipment. Do not take OTC products containing aspirin while taking ibuprofen. Avoid alcohol.
   Contact your doctor if you develop rash, itching, visual disturbances, weight gain, breathing difficulties, fluid retention, hallucinations, black stools, persistent headache, or any unusual or intolerable side effect.
   If you forget a dose of any of these drugs, take it as soon as you remember. If you take several doses a day and it is within 4 hours of your next dose, skip the dose you forgot and continue with your regular schedule. Do not take a double dose.

Special Populations

Pregnancy/Breast-feeding

NSAIDs may affect the developing fetal heart during the last half of pregnancy. Women who are or might become pregnant should not take ibuprofen without their doctor's approval. When the drug is considered crucial by your doctor, its potential benefits must be carefully weighed against its risks.

NSAIDs may pass into breast milk. There is a possibility that a nursing mother taking ibuprofen could affect her baby's heart or cardiovascular system. Nursing mothers who must take this drug should bottle-feed.

Seniors

Seniors, especially those with poor kidney or liver function, may be more susceptible to side effects.

Generic Name

Imatinib (ih-MAH-tin-ib)

Brand Name

Gleevec

Type of Drug

Anticancer.

Prescribed For

Chronic myeloid leukemia (CML), gastrointestinal tumors, and other cancers.

General Information

Imatinib is a product of new genetic and protein research. It works by inhibiting a specific enzyme that is produced only by a specific chromosome in diseased cells. Imatinib can be considered a revolutionary approach to cancer treatment because it targets only cancerous cells and has a minimal effect on healthy cells. In clinical studies, up to 88% of patients taking imatinib responded to treatment and 30% of patients in the chronic phase of CML responded completely to treatment with no evidence of disease remaining.

Cautions and Warnings

Do not take imatinib if you are **sensitive** or **allergic** to it.

Imatinib can cause **fluid retention and swelling** that can be serious and cause an unusual and rapid weight gain. This can be a special problem for people with heart failure, pulmonary edema, liver disease, and other conditions. The chances of retaining fluid increases with rising drug dose and increasing age.

Imatinib can affect **blood platelets** and some **white blood cells**. Your doctor will take blood counts once a week during the first month, twice a month in the second month, and every 2–3 months afterward.

Imatinib can cause **liver** toxicity. Your doctor will monitor liver function and may make dosage adjustments based on these results.

Some people have experienced **bleeding,** particularly in the GI tract, while taking imatinib.

There is no information on the long-term effects of imatinib, but animal studies suggest that the **kidney, liver, and immune system** may be affected.

Possible Side Effects

Most side effects are mild to moderate, but are very common in patients experiencing a myeloid blast crisis. As many as 5% of people taking the drug in clinical studies stopped because of side effects. Women taking imatinib are likely to develop more swelling around the eyes, headache, and fatigue.

▼ Most common: nausea, vomiting, swelling around the eyes, leg swelling and muscle cramps, diarrhea, and upset stomach.

▼ Common: muscle pain, fever, cough, rash, and difficulty breathing.

▼ Less common: headache, fatigue, severe joint pain, weight gain, abdominal pain, appetite loss, constipation, irritation of the nose or nasal cavity, night sweats, and weakness.

▼ Rare: severe fluid retention, bleeding, easy bruising, and pneumonia.

Drug Interactions

Imatinib exerts a potent effect on several liver enzymes that play an important role in the breakdown of other drugs. It is likely that new imatinib drug interactions will be discovered as a result of this action.

• Drugs that increase the amount of imatinib in the blood are ketoconazole, erythromycin, itraconazole, and clarithromycin. Mixing ketoconazole with imatinib can increase the amount of imatinib in the blood by as much as 40%.

• Drugs that can decrease the amount of imatinib in the blood are dexamethasone, phenytoin, carbamazepine, rifampin, St. John's wort, and phenobarbital.

• Imatinib stimulates enzymes in the liver that break down phenytoin. Patients taking this combination may need to increase their phenytoin dosage to maintain seizure control.

• Imatinib increases the amount of simvastatin in the bloodstream by up to 350%. Other statin drugs may also be affected. Cyclosporine, pimozide, the benzodiazepine tranquilizers and sedatives, and some calcium channel blockers are similarly affected.

• Imatinib will interfere with the metabolism of warfarin, a potent anticoagulant. People taking warfarin who must also take imatinib should be switched to a heparin (injectable) product by their doctor.

Food Interactions

Imatinib can cause stomach and intestinal irritation. Take each dose with food and a glass of water to minimize this side effect.

Usual Dose

400–800 mg a day. Treatment should be continued for as long as the patient continues to benefit. Drug dosage should be reduced or stopped if severe liver or other problems develop until they resolve.

Overdosage

There is little experience with imatinib doses larger than 800 mg a day, the maximum human dose. Overdose victims should be taken to a hospital emergency room for treatment. ALWAYS bring the medicine bottle or container.

Special Information

Report any unusual or rapid weight gain to your doctor at once. This can be a sign of fluid retention that should be treated.

Imatinib can cause liver toxicity. Symptoms of liver toxicity may include yellowing of the skin or whites of the eyes.

If you forget a dose, take it as soon as you remember. If it almost time for your next dose, space out the remaining doses for the day to allow you to take your total prescribed dosage for the day. Contact your doctor if you forget more than one dose in a row.

Special Populations

Pregnancy/Breast-feeding

Women taking imatinib should not become pregnant because the drug may cause birth defects. In animal studies, doses of imatinib approximately equal to the maximum human dose produced severe birth defects.

It is estimated that about 1.5% of each imatinib dose passes into breast milk. Nursing mothers who must take this drug should bottle-feed.

Seniors

Seniors may take this drug with no special restriction. Fluid retention is more likely in this population.

Generic Name

Imiquimod (ih-MIH-kwih-mod)

Brand Name

Aldara

Type of Drug

Immune modifier.

Prescribed For

Genital warts, perianal warts, and condyloma acuminata.

General Information

Imiquimod has no direct antiviral activity. Animal studies suggest that imiquimod stimulates the skin to produce cytokines, potent natural chemicals that fight the warts, but its actual effect on genital warts and condyloma is not known. In studies of the drug, 50% of people who used it had complete clearance of their warts. But imiquimod is not a cure for genital warts—

new ones may develop while others are being treated. Only minimal amounts of imiquimod enter the bloodstream.

Cautions and Warnings

Do not use this product if you are **sensitive** or **allergic** to it.

Imiquimod has not been studied in other viral diseases of the skin, such as papilloma virus, and should not be used to treat them, since its effect is unknown.

Do not apply imiquimod to any area until it has healed from any previous drug or surgery. Imiquimod can worsen skin that is already inflamed.

Possible Side Effects

▼ Most common: redness, itching, erosion of the skin, burning, flaking, abrasions, swelling, and fungal infections in women.

▼ Common: pain, marks on the skin, ulcers, skin scabbing, and headache.

▼ Less common: skin soreness, flu-like symptoms, skin discoloration, muscle aches, fungal infections in men, and diarrhea.

Drug Interactions

• Do not apply imiquimod with other drugs that may cause skin irritation.

Usual Dose

Adult: Apply a thin layer of the cream to external warts and rub it in until the cream disappears. Leave it on the skin for 6–10 hours, then remove the cream with mild soap and water. Do this 3 times a week—for example, Monday, Wednesday, and Friday. Continue treatment for up to 16 weeks or until the warts go away.

Child (under age 18): not recommended.

Overdosage

Overdose is not likely because such a small amount of imiquimod is absorbed through the skin. Accidental ingestion of imiquimod may cause low blood pressure. Anyone who has swallowed imiquimod should be taken to a hospital emergency room. ALWAYS bring the prescription bottle or container.

Special Information

Wash your hands before each application of imiquimod.

Most skin reactions are mild. If you develop a severe skin reaction to imiquimod, call your doctor and remove the cream with a mild soap and water. You can resume treatment with imiquimod after the reaction has completely subsided.

Imiquimod may weaken condoms and vaginal diaphragms. These birth control methods may prove undependable while you are using imiquimod cream. Avoid sexual contact while the cream is on your skin.

Uncircumcised men who use imiquimod to treat warts under the foreskin should retract the foreskin and cleanse the area every day.

Imiquimod is meant to be applied to the skin only. Do not let it get into your eyes, mouth, nose, or other mucous membranes. If you forget to apply a dose of imiquimod, do it as soon as you remember. If you don't remember until your next scheduled application, space the remaining doses equally throughout the rest of the week and continue with your regular schedule.

Special Populations

Pregnancy/Breast-feeding

The safety of using imiquimod during pregnancy is not known. When this drug is considered crucial by your doctor, its potential benefits must be carefully weighed against its risks.

It is not known if imiquimod passes into breast milk. Nursing mothers who must use this drug should consider bottle-feeding.

Seniors

Seniors may use this drug without special precaution.

Imitrex   see Triptan-Type Antimigraine Drugs, page 1120

Inderal LA   see Propanolol, page 898

Generic Name

Indinavir (in-DIN-uh-vere)

Brand Name

Crixivan

Type of Drug

Protease inhibitor.

Prescribed For

Human immunodeficiency virus (HIV) infection.

General Information

Part of the multidrug cocktail responsible for the most important gains in the fight against acquired immunodeficiency syndrome (AIDS), indinavir sulfate belongs to a group of anti-HIV drugs called protease inhibitors. Triple-drug cocktails were considered responsible for the first overall reduction in the AIDS death rate, recorded in 1996. Protease inhibitors work in a unique way but are not a cure for HIV infection or AIDS. When the HIV virus attacks a cell, it must be converted into viral DNA. Older drugs, known as reverse transcriptase inhibitors, interfere with this step, but they need help in fighting HIV. Protease inhibitors work at the end of the HIV reproduction process, when proteins are "cut" into strands of exactly the right size to duplicate HIV. The protein is cut by a protease enzyme. Protease inhibitors prevent the mature HIV virus from being formed by interfering with this cutting process. Proteins that are cut to the wrong length or that remain uncut are inactive.

Protease inhibitors are always taken with 1 or 2 other nucleoside antiviral drugs such as AZT, ddI, ddC, or 3TC. Protease inhibitors revolutionized HIV treatment because, when taken in combination, they reduce the amount of HIV virus in the bloodstream to levels that are undetectable by current methods—CD_4 cell (immune system cell) counts and viral load (amount of virus in the blood) measurements. Multiple drug therapy has changed the current view of HIV from a fatal disease to a manageable chronic illness.

Newer approaches are exploring multiple protease-inhibitor treatment.

People taking a protease inhibitor may still develop infections or other conditions associated with HIV disease. Because of this, it is very important for you to remain under the care of a doctor or other health care provider. The long-term effects of indinavir are not known. You may be able to pass the HIV virus to others even if you are on triple-drug therapy.

Cautions and Warnings

Do not take indinavir if you are **allergic** to it. People with mild or moderate **liver disease** or **cirrhosis** break down indinavir more slowly than those with normal liver function and may be more likely to develop side effects. People with cirrhosis should receive a reduced dose of indinavir.

About 4 of every 100 people taking indinavir can develop a **kidney stone,** indicated by pain in the middle to lower abdomen or back, or painful urination. Drinking at least 6 full glasses of liquid—48 oz.—a day will reduce your risk of developing a stone.

Indinavir may **raise blood sugar,** worsen diabetes, or bring out latent diabetes. Diabetics who take indinavir may have to have the dose of their antidiabetes medication adjusted against this effect.

Possible Side Effects

▼ Most common: nausea, abdominal pain, and headache.

▼ Common: kidney stones, itching, weakness or fatigue, pain in the side, diarrhea, vomiting, changes in sense of taste, acid regurgitation, and sleeplessness.

▼ Less common: dizziness, drowsiness, and back pain.

▼ Rare: Rare side effects can occur in almost any part of the body. Contact your doctor if you experience any side effect not listed above.

Drug Interactions

• Rifampin reduces the amount of indinavir in the blood. Do not combine these drugs.

• Indinavir should not be used with amiodarone, as amiodarone toxicity may result.

• Indinavir interferes with the liver's ability to break down terfenadine, triazolam, and midazolam. Do not combine indinavir with any of these drugs, as severe side effects may result.

• Combining indinavir with clarithromycin or with zidovudine increases the amount of each drug in the blood. Combining indinavir with isoniazid increases the amount of isoniazid in the blood.

• Combining indinavir with rifabutin can reduce the amount of indinavir absorbed into the blood by ⅓ and double the amount of rifabutin absorbed.

• Didanosine (ddI) interferes with the absorption of indinavir into the body. If you need both of these medications, take them at least 1 hour apart.

• Combining fluconazole with indinavir reduces the amount of indinavir in the blood by about 20%.

• Combining indinavir with ketoconazole increases the amount of indinavir in the blood by about 65%.

• Combining indinavir with quinidine raises indinavir levels by about 10%.

• Taking indinavir with zidovudine and lamivudine results in ⅓ more zidovudine in the blood and small decreases in lamivudine blood levels.

• Indinavir raises the amount of stavudine absorbed into the blood by 25% and the amount of trimethoprim by about 20%.

• Delaviridine increases the effects of indinavir.

• St. John's wort and efavirenz decrease the effects of indinavir.

• Indinavir increases the effects of ritonavir, sildenafil, tadalafil, vardenafil, and fentanyl.

• Combining indinavir with oral contraceptives can result in higher blood hormone levels. This may lead to an excess of hormone-related side effects. If this happens to you, your doctor may be able to lower the dose of your contraceptive pills.

Food Interactions

Indinavir is best taken with water—or liquids such as skim milk, juice, coffee—at least 1 hour before or 2 hours after a meal. You should not eat meals that are high in calories, fat, and protein from 1 hour before to 2 hours after taking indinavir. You may take indinavir with a light meal.

Usual Dose

Adult: 800 mg every 8 hours, around the clock. People with cirrhosis should take 600 mg every 8 hours.

Child: not recommended.

Overdosage

Little is known about the effects of indinavir overdose except that it may cause severe drug side effects. Take overdose victims to a hospital emergency room at once. ALWAYS bring the prescription bottle or container.

Special Information

Indinavir does not cure HIV. It will not prevent you from transmitting HIV to another person; you must still practice safe sex.

It is imperative to take your HIV medication exactly as prescribed. Missing doses of indinavir makes you more likely to become resistant to the drug and to lose the benefits of therapy.

Call your doctor if you develop pains in the middle to lower abdomen, back pain, or painful urination. Drink at least 48 oz. of liquid each day—for example, six 8-oz. glasses.

Stay in close touch with your doctor while taking indinavir and report anything unusual.

If you forget a dose of indinavir, take it as soon as you remember. If it is almost time for your next dose, skip the dose you forgot and continue with your regular schedule. Do not take a double dose.

Special Populations

Pregnancy/Breast-feeding

There is little information on how indinavir affects pregnant women and their fetuses. Pregnant women should take this drug with caution.

Indinavir passes into breast milk. Women with HIV and nursing mothers who must take indinavir should bottle-feed.

Seniors

Seniors may take indinavir without special restriction.

Generic Name

Indomethacin (IN-doe-METH-uh-sin) Ⓖ

Brand Names

Indochron E-R   Indocin SR
Indocin

Type of Drug

Nonsteroidal anti-inflammatory drug (NSAID).

Prescribed For

Rheumatoid arthritis; osteoarthritis; ankylosing spondylitis; menstrual pain; tendinitis; bursitis; painful shoulder; gout—except Indocin SR; sunburn; migraine and cluster headache—except Indocin SR. Indomethacin has been used to prevent premature labor, to treat a rare condition in premature infants called patent ductus arteriosus, and (in eyedrop form) to treat a severe and unusual inflammation in the retina.

General Information

Indomethacin and other NSAIDs are used to relieve pain and inflammation. We do not know exactly how NSAIDs work, but they may achieve their effects by blocking the body's production of a hormone called prostaglandin and the action of other body chemicals. Pain relief comes about 30 minutes after taking the first dose of indomethacin and lasts for 4 to 6 hours, but its anti-inflammatory effect takes a week to become apparent and may take 2 weeks to reach maximum effect. Indomethacin is broken down in the liver and eliminated through the kidneys.

Cautions and Warnings

People **allergic** to indomethacin or any other NSAID and those with a history of **asthma** attacks brought on by an NSAID, iodides, or aspirin should not take indomethacin.

Indomethacin may cause **gastrointestinal (GI) bleeding, ulcers,** and **stomach perforation,** which can occur at any time, with or without warning, in people who take indomethacin regularly. People with a history of active GI bleeding should be cautious about taking any NSAID. People who develop bleeding or ulcers and continue NSAID treatment may develop more serious side effects.

Indomethacin may affect platelets and **blood clotting** at high doses and should be avoided by people with clotting problems and those taking warfarin.

People with **heart problems** who use indomethacin may experience swelling in their arms, legs, or feet.

Indomethacin should not be used by people who have had **ulcers or other stomach lesions**.

Indomethacin may worsen **depression or other psychiatric disorders, epilepsy, and parkinsonism**.

Indomethacin should never be used as "first therapy" for any disorder, with the possible exception of ankylosing spondylitis, because of the severe side effects associated with this drug.

Indomethacin may cause severe toxic effects to the **kidney**. Report any unusual side effects to your doctor, who might need to periodically test your kidney function.

Indomethacin may make you **unusually sensitive to the effects of the sun**.

Possible Side Effects

▼ Most common: headache, dizziness, diarrhea, nausea, vomiting, constipation, stomach gas, stomach upset or irritation, and appetite loss, especially during the first few days of treatment.

▼ Less common: stomach ulcers, GI bleeding, hepatitis, gallbladder attacks, painful urination, poor kidney function, kidney inflammation, blood and protein in the urine, dizziness, fainting, nervousness, depression, hallucinations, confusion, disorientation, tingling in the hands or feet, light-headedness, itching, increased sweating, dry nose and mouth, heart palpitations, chest pain, breathing difficulties, and muscle cramps.

▼ Rare: severe allergic reactions including closing of the throat, fever and chills, changes in liver function, jaundice (yellowing of the skin or whites of the eyes), and kidney failure. People who experience such effects must be promptly treated in a hospital emergency

Possible Side Effects *(continued)*

room or doctor's office. NSAIDs have caused severe skin reactions; if this happens to you, see your doctor immediately.

Drug Interactions

• Indomethacin may increase the effects of oral anticoagulant (blood-thinning) drugs such as warfarin. Your anticoagulant dose may need to be reduced.

• Indomethacin may reduce the effects of thiazide diuretics.

• Combining diflunisal and indomethacin has resulted in fatal GI hemorrhage.

• Indomethacin may reduce the blood-pressure-lowering effect of beta blockers, angiotensin-converting enzyme (ACE) inhibitor drugs, and loop diuretics.

• Taking indomethacin with cyclosporine may increase the kidney-related side effects of both drugs. Methotrexate side effects may be increased in people also taking indomethacin.

• Indomethacin may increase digoxin levels in the blood.

• Indomethacin may increase the body's absorbtion of penicillamine.

• Combining indomethacin with phenylpropanolamine—found in many over-the-counter (OTC) drug products—may cause an increase in blood pressure.

• Combining indomethacin and dipyridamole may increase water retention.

• Indomethacin may increase phenytoin's side effects.

• Lithium blood levels may be increased by indomethacin.

• Indomethacin blood levels may be affected by cimetidine.

• Cholestyramine may decrease the effectiveness of indomethacin.

• Probenecid may increase the risk of indomethacin side effects.

• Aspirin and other salicylates should never be combined with indomethacin to treat arthritis.

Food Interactions

Take indomethacin with a glass of water, food, or a magnesium/aluminum antacid to avoid an upset stomach.

Usual Dose

Adult and Child (age 15 and over): 50–200 mg a day, individualized to your needs.

Child (under age 15): not recommended.

Overdosage

People have died from NSAID overdoses. Common signs of overdose are drowsiness, nausea, vomiting, diarrhea, abdominal pain, rapid breathing, rapid heartbeat, increased sweating, ringing or buzzing in the ears, confusion, disorientation, stupor, and coma. Take the victim to a hospital emergency room at once. ALWAYS bring the prescription bottle or container.

Special Information

Take each dose with a full glass of water and do not lie down for 15 to 30 minutes afterward.

Indomethacin can make you drowsy or tired: Be careful when driving or operating hazardous equipment. Do not take any OTC products containing acetaminophen or aspirin while taking indomethacin. Avoid alcohol.

Contact your doctor if you develop rash or itching, visual disturbances, weight gain, breathing difficulties, fluid retention, hallucinations, black or tarry stools, persistent headache, or any unusual or intolerable side effect.

If you forget a dose of indomethacin, take it as soon as you remember. If you take indomethacin once a day and it is within 8 hours of your next dose, or if you take several doses a day and it is within 4 hours of your next dose, skip the dose you forgot and continue with your regular schedule. Never take a double dose.

Special Populations

Pregnancy/Breast-feeding

Indomethacin may affect the developing fetal heart if used during the second half of pregnancy. Pregnant women should not take indomethacin without their doctor's approval. When the drug is considered crucial by your doctor, its potential benefits must be carefully weighed against its risks.

Indomethacin may pass into breast milk. There is a possibility that the heart of a nursing baby could be affected by indomethacin. Nursing mothers who must take indomethacin should bottle-feed.

Seniors

Seniors may be more susceptible to side effects, especially ulcer disease.

Generic Name

Infliximab (in-FLIX-ih-mab)

Brand Name

Remicade

Type of Drug

Monoclonal antibody.

Prescribed For

Crohn's disease and rheumatoid arthritis.

General Information

High levels of tumor necrosis factor (TNFα), which plays an important role in the inflammatory process, are linked to the worsening of Crohn's disease and rheumatoid arthritis. Infliximab neutralizes TNFα so that it cannot exert its effects. TNFα levels have been found to correlate with the severity of Crohn's disease.

Cautions and Warnings

Do not take infliximab if you are **allergic** to it.

The safety and effectiveness of more than 3 infliximab infusions are not known.

People taking infliximab may develop **serious infections** such as tuberculosis and fungal infections.

Infliximab may cause **allergic reactions** including itching, breathing difficulties, and low blood pressure (symptoms include dizziness and fainting). These reactions may require emergency treatment. **Lupus erythematosus** may develop but goes away once drug treatment is stopped.

People with **compromised immune systems** should be cautious about using this drug because it can suppress immune function and result in serious infections.

People with **congestive heart failure** should take infliximab with caution because it may worsen heart function.

People with **nervous system disorders** or **seizures** should take infliximab with caution.

Possible Side Effects

Most people (8 of 10) experience more than 1 side effect. Sixteen percent develop a reaction to the drug within 2 hours. Those reactions include fever, chills, itching, rash, chest pain, changes in blood pressure, and breathing difficulties.

▼ Most common: headache, nausea, upper respiratory infection, abdominal pain, fatigue, and fever.

▼ Common: sore throat, vomiting, pain, dizziness, bronchitis, rash, runny nose, chest pain, coughing, itching, sinus inflammation, muscle aches, back pain, and fungus infection.

▼ Less common: Less common side effects can occur in almost any part of the body. Contact your doctor if you experience any side effect not listed above.

Drug Interactions

• Infliximab should not be combined with any drug infused into the bloodstream.

Food Interactions

None known.

Usual Dose

Adult: 1.35–2.25 mg per lb. of body weight. Another dose may be given 2 and 6 weeks after the first injection, then every 8 weeks.

Child: not recommended.

Overdosage

Symptoms may include drug side effects. Take the victim to a hospital emergency room.

Special Populations

Pregnancy/Breast-feeding

The safety of taking infliximab during pregnancy is not known. When this drug is considered crucial by your doctor, its potential benefits must be carefully weighed against its risks.

It is not known if infliximab passes into breast milk. Nursing mothers who must take it should bottle-feed.

Seniors

Seniors may be more likely to develop infections while taking this drug.

Generic Name

Insulin (IN-suh-lin)

Most Common Brand Names

Generic Ingredient: Regular Insulin

Humulin R	Novolin R
Iletin II	Velosulin BR

Generic Ingredient: Insulin Aspart

Novolog   Novolog Mix 70/30

Generic Ingredient: Insulin Glargine

Lantus

Generic Ingredient: Insulin Lispro

Humalog	Humalog Mix 50/50
Humalog Mix 75/25	

Generic Ingredient: NPH Insulin

NPH Iletin II	Novolin N
Humulin N	

Generic Ingredients: NPH Insulin + Insulin

Humulin 70/30	Novolin 70/30
Humulin 50/50	

Generic Ingredient: Lente Insulin

Lente Iletin II	Novolin L
Humulin L	

Generic Ingredient: Ultralente Insulin
Humulin U

Type of Drug

Antidiabetic.

Prescribed For

Type 1 and type 2 diabetes mellitus; also prescribed for hyperkalemia (very high blood-potassium levels) and for severe complications of diabetes such as ketoacidosis or diabetic coma. Insulin may be prescribed in combination with oral antidiabetes drugs for people with type 2 diabetes who do not respond to pills alone.

General Information

Insulin, a hormone made in the pancreas, helps the body turn sugar into energy. Insulin works by helping sugar enter body cells. Also, insulin helps us store energy that we can use later. Between meals, insulin helps us use the fat, sugar, and protein we have stored. In type 1 diabetes, the body does not make enough insulin to meet its needs. Type 2 diabetics may actually overproduce insulin, but do not properly utilize it. Without insulin, glucose cannot get into body cells and the cells will not work properly. Insulin dosage must be balanced against the amount and type of food eaten and the amount of exercise you do. Blood glucose can drop too low or rise too high if diet and/or exercise change without modifying insulin dosage. The most widely used variety is human insulin. It is identical to natural human insulin but it is manufactured by semisynthetic or recombinant DNA methods. Older semisynthetic insulins start with an animal product and may contain some impurities. Of these types, only insulin obtained from pork pancreas glands is available in the U.S. All types of insulin must be injected because insulin is destroyed by stomach acid. An inhalable insulin is being developed.

People whose diabetes is well controlled by insulin derived from pork should not automatically be switched to a human insulin product, but people newly diagnosed with type 1 diabetes are usually treated with highly purified synthetic human insulin. Human insulin is also the product of choice for people allergic to other insulin products, pregnant women with diabetes, and people who require insulin only during surgery or for short periods of time.

Rapid-acting insulins: Regular insulin starts to work in 30 to 60 minutes and lasts only 8 to 12 hours. Prompt Insulin Zinc Suspension—also called Semilente Insulin—is also considered rapid-acting. It starts to work in 60 to 90 minutes and lasts 12 to 16 hours. Lispro insulin starts working in 15 minutes and lasts for 2 to 5 hours. Insulin aspart starts working in 15 minutes and lasts for 3 to 5 hours.

Intermediate-acting insulins: NPH insulin starts working in 60 to 90 minutes and lasts for 24 hours. Lente insulin starts working in 1 to 2 ½ hours and lasts for 24 hours.

Long-acting insulins: Insulin glargine starts working in about an hour and lasts for at least 24 hours. Protamine Zinc Insulin Suspension and Ultralente insulin start working in 4 to 8 hours and last for 20 to 36 hours. Other factors that influence insulin response include diet, exercise, and the use of other drugs.

Cautions and Warnings

Low blood sugar (see "Overdosage" for symptoms) can result from taking too much insulin, doing excess physical work or exercise without eating, not absorbing food normally because meals are postponed or skipped, or because of illness with vomiting, fever, or diarrhea. You may be able to correct the imbalance by eating sugar, food with sugar, or a commercial 40% glucose product. The symptoms of low blood sugar are less pronounced if you are taking human insulin.

Hypersensitivity reactions to insulin can develop at the site of injection, such as redness, swelling, and itching, and may indicate a need to change the type of insulin you use. Reactions such as difficulty catching your breath, feeling your throat closing, fast pulse, sweating, low blood pressure with or without fainting, and skin eruptions may be life-threatening.

Skin depressions can develop at the injection sites unless you rotate the locations. This can interfere with the absorption of the insulin.

Thyroid disease can affect the clearance of insulin from the body.

Possible Side Effects

▼ Most common: high or low blood sugar, allergic reactions, salt and water retention, itching, rash, and accumulation of fat under the skin from repeatedly using the same injection site.

Drug Interactions

• Drugs that reduce the effect of insulin include acetazolamide, AIDS antivirals, albuterol, asparaginase, calcitonin, oral contraceptives, corticosteroids, cyclophosphamide, danazol, dextrothyroxine, diazoxide, diltiazem, dobutamine, epinephrine, estrogens, ethacrynic acid, isoniazid, lithium carbonate, morphine, niacin, nicotine, phenothiazines, phenytoin, somatropin, terbutaline, thiazide diuretics, and thyroid hormones. Dosage increases may be required.

• Drugs that increase the effects of insulin include oral antidiabetes drugs, ACE inhibitors, alcohol, anabolic steroids, beta blockers, calcium, chloroquine, clofibrate, clonidine, disopyramide, fluoxetine, guanethidine, lithium carbonate, monoamine oxidase (MAO) inhibitors, mebendazole, pentamidine, phenylbutazone, propoxyphene, pyridoxine, salicylates, sulfinpyrazone, sulfa drugs, and tetracycline. Dosage reductions may be required.

• Beta-blocking drugs can mask the symptoms of low blood sugar and thus increase the risk of taking insulin.

• Quitting smoking—regardless of whether you are using a nicotine patch or gum, or another smoking deterrent—can also lower blood sugar. Lowering insulin dosage may be necessary if you stop smoking.

• Insulin may affect blood-potassium levels and digitalis drugs.

Food Interactions

Follow your doctor's directions for diet restrictions.

Usual Dose

Dosage must be individualized. Insulin is generally injected 30 minutes before meals; lispro is injected 15 minutes before meals; and the longer-acting forms are taken a half hour before breakfast. Glargine is taken once a day at bedtime.

Insulin is typically self-administered under the skin. Hospitalized patients may receive insulin injection directly into a vein.

Overdosage

Accidental ingestion has little or no effect. Injecting too much insulin causes an insulin reaction or low blood sugar. Symptoms occur suddenly and include weakness, fatigue, nervousness, confusion, headache, double vision, convulsions, dizziness, psychoses, unconsciousness, rapid and shallow breathing, numbness or tingling around the mouth, hunger, nausea, loss of skin color, dry skin, and pulse changes. Overdose victims should eat chocolate, candy, or another sugar source at once to raise blood-sugar levels.

Special Information

Use the same brand and strength of insulin and insulin syringes or administration devices to avoid dosage errors. Rotate injection sites to prevent fat loss at the site.

Low blood sugar develops suddenly. Symptoms are fatigue, weakness, nervousness, confusion, headache, double vision, convulsions, psychosis, dizziness, fainting, rapid and shallow breathing, hunger, nausea, tingling or numbness around your mouth, pale skin, thin skin that may be either moist or dry, and change in pulse rate. Go to an emergency room or contact your doctor immediately if these symptoms develop.

Ketoacidosis develops over hours or days. Symptoms are drowsiness, dim vision, a feeling of not getting enough air, thirst, nausea, vomiting, breath that smells like acetone (nail polish remover), abdominal pain, loss of appetite, dry and red skin, and rapid pulse. Go to an emergency room or contact your doctor immediately if these symptoms develop.

Mix insulins according to your doctor's directions; do not change the method or order of mixing.

Take the exact dose of insulin prescribed. Too much insulin will excessively lower blood sugar, and too little will not control diabetes. Follow the diet prescribed by your doctor and avoid alcohol.

You may develop low blood sugar (see "Overdosage" for symptoms) if you take too much insulin, work or exercise more strenuously than usual, skip a meal, take insulin too long before a meal, or vomit before a meal. To help raise low blood sugar, eat a candy bar or lump of sugar, which you should carry with you at all times. If the signs of low blood sugar do not clear up within 30 minutes, call your doctor. You may need further treatment.

Your insulin requirements may change if you get sick, especially if you vomit or have a fever.

If your insulin is in suspension form, you must gently rotate the vial and turn it over several times to evenly distribute the particles throughout the liquid before withdrawing the dose. Do not shake the vial.

People with diabetes must maintain good dental hygiene because of their increased risk of developing oral infections. Be sure your dentist knows you have diabetes. Visit your doctor every 6 months and have your eyes checked regularly.

Read and follow all patient information provided with insulin products. Monitor your blood and urine regularly for sugar and ketones.

Insulin products are generally stable at room temperature for about 2 years. They must be kept away from direct sunlight and extreme temperatures. Most manufacturers recommend that insulin be stored in a refrigerator or another cool place though it should not be put in a freezer. Partly used vials of insulin should be thrown away after several weeks if not used. Do not use any insulin that looks any different from the way it did when you purchased it.

Insulin products can be mixed only if you have been so directed by your doctor. Your pharmacist may also mix your insulins to ensure accuracy.

If you forget a dose, take it as soon as you remember. If it is almost time for your next dose, or if you completely forget 1 or more doses, call your doctor for exact instructions.

Special Populations

Pregnancy/Breast-feeding
Human insulin is the preferred method for controlling diabetes in pregnant women. These women must follow their doctor's directions for insulin use exactly, because insulin requirements normally decrease during the first half of pregnancy and then increase during the second half.

Insulin does not pass into breast milk. Breast-feeding can reduce your insulin needs, so your doctor should closely monitor your insulin dosage during this period.

Seniors

Seniors may use insulin without special restriction.

Generic Name

Interferon Alfa (in-ter-FEER-on AL-fuh)

Brand Name

Alferon N
Infergen
Intron A

PegIntron
Roferon-A

Type of Drug

Antiviral.

Prescribed For

Hepatitis C, hairy cell leukemia, malignant melanoma, and AIDS-related Kaposi's sarcoma; also used to treat laryngeal papillomatosis (growths in the respiratory tract) in children and genital warts, bladder cancer, carcinoid tumors, chronic myelocytic leukemia, kidney cancer, non-Hodgkin's lymphoma, multiple myeloma, mycosis fungoides, ovarian cancer, polycythemia vera (a cancer of the blood), skin cancer, and thrombocytosis.

General Information

Interferon alfa attaches to the surface of an infected cell and stimulates a complicated set of reactions. These reactions lead to the production of enzymes inside the cell that prevent the hepatitis C virus, for example, from reproducing. Other causes of hepatitis do not respond to interferon treatment.

Cautions and Warnings

People taking this drug must be closely monitored by their doctors and receive periodic blood tests and liver and thyroid function tests.

Serious and life-threatening **allergic or drug-sensitivity reactions** can develop including an itchy rash, swelling, and breathing difficulties.

People with **kidney or heart disease** should use this drug with caution. If heart disease worsens during treatment, the drug should be discontinued.

Interferon alfa may worsen **liver disease**.

Interferon alfa can affect the nervous system in many ways, including **seizures, coma, dizziness, memory loss, agitation, psychosis,** and **complete loss of sensation**. These effects generally go away when the drug is stopped.

Interferon alfa may cause **menstrual problems** or interfere with **ovulation**.

People who develop **severe side effects** or become **depressed** while taking this drug should have their dosage temporarily lowered. The drug should be stopped if depression is severe.

It is not known if this drug is safe for **children**.

Possible Side Effects

▼ Most common: anxiety, sleep disturbances, depression, hair loss, nausea, diarrhea, abdominal pain, muscle or joint pain, weakness, headache, fever, chills, injection-site reactions, back pain, and generalized pain.

▼ Common: dizziness, confusion, abnormal thought patterns, memory loss, tingling in the hands or feet, rash, dry skin, sweating, vomiting, appetite loss, weight loss, cough, bronchitis, breathing difficulties, pneumonia, pleurisy, lung problems, runny nose, and sore throat.

▼ Less common: poor vision, abnormal heart rhythms, high blood pressure, chest pain, high blood sugar, thyroid problems, urinary infection, low sex drive, accidental injury, liver problems, migraine, increased sensitivity to the sun, psoriasis, attempted suicide, seizures, and a ruptured spleen.

▼ Rare: blood in the urine, eye problems, rheumatoid arthritis, lupus and other autoimmune conditions, painful spasms of blood vessels in the legs, and worsening of diabetes and thyroid problems.

Drug Interactions

• Interferon alfa may interfere with the breakdown of vinblastine, zidovudine (also known as AZT), and theophylline.

Food Interactions

None known.

Usual Dose

Alferon N

0.05 ml (250,000 IU) per wart twice weekly for up to 8 weeks. The maximum recommended dose per treatment session is 0.5 ml (2.5 million IU).

Infergen

9 mcg in a single subcutaneous injection 3 times a week for 24 weeks. Allow at least 2 days between doses.

Intron A

2–5 million units by subcutaneous or intramuscular injection 3 times a week for 6 to 18 months. Larger doses (10–20 million units) are given by intravenous infusion.

PegIntron

1–1.5 mcg for every 2.2 pounds of body weight by subcutaneous injection once a week for one year.

Roferon A

3 million units by subcutaneous or intramuscular injection 3 times a week. Length of treatment depends on the specific condition.

Overdosage

Symptoms may include increased side effects and changes in lab test results. Seizures have occurred at high dosages. Repeated overdose may cause lethargy or coma. Call your local poison control center or a hospital emergency room for more information. If you seek treatment, ALWAYS bring the prescription bottle or container.

Special Information

This drug does not prevent you from giving hepatitis C to others through unprotected sex or contact with blood or other body fluids.

People who have a seizure disorder or other nervous system problem, low white-blood-cell or blood-platelet count, or asthma or other breathing problems, or who take drugs that depress bone marrow function may be especially sensitive to the effects of interferon alfa.

This medication is given by injection under the skin. For information on how to properly administer this drug, see page 1188.

Ibuprofen, aspirin, and other anti-inflammatory drugs may alleviate some of the discomfort associated with starting interferon alfa.

Your doctor may instruct you to drink extra fluids while taking interferon alfa. This will help prevent low blood pressure due to excess loss of water.

This drug must be stored in the refrigerator and protected from light. Do not shake or freeze it.

Special Populations

Pregnancy/Breast-feeding

Animal studies suggest that interferon alfa may harm the fetus and cause spontaneous abortion. When this drug is considered crucial by your doctor, its potential benefits must be carefully weighed against its risks.

It is not known if this drug passes into breast milk. Nursing mothers who must take it should bottle-feed.

Seniors

Seniors with liver, kidney, or heart conditions should use this drug with caution.

Generic Name

Interferon Beta (in-ter-FEER-on BAY-tuh)

Brand Names

Avonex (interferon beta-1a)   Rebif (interferon beta-1a)
Betaseron (interferon beta-1b)

Type of Drug

Multiple sclerosis (MS) therapy; biological response modifier.

Prescribed For

MS; also used for AIDS, AIDS-related Kaposi's sarcoma, metastic renal-cell carcinoma, herpes of the lips or genitals, malignant melanoma, cutaneous T-cell lymphoma, and acute non-A/non-B hepatitis.

General Information

The interferons are a family of natural proteins produced in response to viral infection and other biological inducers. Three major classes of interferons have been identified: Alfa, beta, and gamma; they each have overlapping, yet distinct, biologic activities. Interferon beta has antiviral effects, slows cell growth, and helps regulate the immune system. The way it works in MS is not clearly understood. However, it is known that interferon beta interacts with specific receptors on the surface of human cells. Binding causes the production of a number of gene products believed to mediate the biological actions of interferon beta.

Cautions and Warnings

Do not take interferon beta if you are **sensitive** or **allergic** to it or human albumin.

The safety and benefit of interferon beta in **chronic progressive MS** is unproven.

People taking interferon beta in studies had potentially severe **depression** and **suicidal tendencies**. Depressed patients should use any interferon product with caution and report any changes in their outlook to a doctor.

People with **seizure** disorders may be more likely to develop a seizure while taking interferon beta.

Up to 75% of people who take interferon beta are likely to develop **flu-like symptoms** including fever, chills, muscle aches, sweating, and feeling unwell. These symptoms may prove stressful to people with **heart disease**.

Interferon beta may cause **increased sensitivity to the sun**. Wear protective clothing and use sunscreen.

In rare cases, severe **liver disease** has occured while taking interferon beta. People with liver disease should not use this drug.

Possible Side Effects

In general, interferon beta-1a has fewer side effects than interferon beta-1b.

Interferon Beta-1a
▼ Most common: respiratory infection, sinusitis, headache, fever, weakness, chills, dizziness, muscle aches, abdominal pain, flu-like symptoms, painful menstruation, diarrhea, nausea, upset stomach, and sleeping difficulties.
▼ Less common: swelling, pelvic pain, cyst, thyroid goiter, heart palpitations, bleeding, laryngitis, breathing

---

Possible Side Effects *(continued)*

difficulties, joint pain, stiffness, tiredness, speech problems, convulsions, uncontrolled movements, hair loss, urinary urgency, and cystitis. Pain, burning, or stinging at the injection site may also occur.

▼ Rare: Rare side effects can occur in almost any part of the body. Contact your doctor if you experience any side effect not listed above.

Interferon Beta-1b

▼ Most common: pain, burning, or stinging at the injection site, sinusitis, headache, migraine, fever, weakness, chills, muscle ache, abdominal pain, flu-like symptoms, menstrual disorders, painful menstruation, constipation, diarrhea, vomiting, liver inflammation, sweating, and reduced white-blood-cell count.

▼ Less common: itching, swelling, pelvic pain, cyst, thyroid goiter, heart palpitations, high blood pressure, rapid heartbeat, bleeding, laryngitis, breathing difficulties, muscle weakness, stiffness, tiredness, speech problems, convulsions, uncontrolled movements, visual disturbances or conjunctivitis (pinkeye), urinary urgency, cystitis, breast pain, cystic breast disease, breast cancer, and weight changes.

▼ Rare: Rare side effects can occur in almost any part of the body. Contact your doctor if you experience any side effect not listed above.

Food and Drug Interactions

None known.

Usual Dose

Avonex
30 mcg into a large muscle once a week.

Betaseron
The usual dose is 0.25 mg injected under the skin every other day. Patients are started at $1/4$ of the usual dose and increased gradually over 7 weeks to the regular dose. Betaseron comes with a special solution with which to mix the product before injection.

Rebif

The usual dose is 44 mcg injected 3 times a week, 2 days apart, usually late in the day. Patients are started on injections of 8.8 mcg 3 times weekly. Dosage is increased over 4 weeks to the usual dose.

Overdosage

Little is known about the effects of interferon beta overdose. Symptoms may include exaggerated side effects. Call your local poison control center or a hospital emergency room for more information. If you seek treatment, ALWAYS bring the prescription bottle or container.

Special Information

Interferon beta-1a and interferon beta-1b may be associated with severe depression. Mood swings or changes, lack of interest in daily activities, excessive sleep, and other possible signs of depression should be reported to your doctor at once.

If you forget to administer a dose, do so as soon as you remember. If it is almost time for your next dose, skip the one you forgot and continue with your regular schedule. Do not take a double dose.

Special Populations

Pregnancy/Breast-feeding

Animal studies show that interferon beta may cause abortion. Women who are or might be pregnant should not use this drug.

It is not known if interferon beta passes into breast milk. Nursing mothers who must take it should consider bottle-feeding.

Seniors

Seniors may use this drug without special restriction.

Generic Name

Ipratropium (ipe-ruh-TROE-pee-um) Ⓖ

Brand Name

Atrovent

Combination Products

Generic Ingredients: Ipratropium Bromide + Albuterol Sulfate
Combivent   DuoNeb

The information in this profile also applies to the following drugs:

Generic Ingredient: Tiotropium Bromide
Spiriva

Type of Drug

Anticholinergic.

Prescribed For

Bronchospasm associated with bronchitis, emphysema, and other chronic lung diseases; also prescribed for runny nose.

General Information

Ipratropium bromide is related to atropine sulfate, another anticholinergic drug. Ipratropium works against natural acetylcholine in the bronchial muscles, causing them to dilate. It has little effect on other parts of the body. Much of each inhaled dose is swallowed and passes out of the body in the stool. Like all anticholinergic drugs, ipratropium has a drying effect; the nasal spray provides relief from runny nose.

Cautions and Warnings

Do not use ipratropium if you are **allergic** to atropine, soya lecithin, or to any related product. It should be used with caution if you have **glaucoma, prostate disease,** or **bladder obstruction.**

Ipratropium is not meant for the treatment of acute bronchospasm. This drug should be used only to prevent bronchospasm associated with chronic lung diseases.

Patients may experience a temporary blurring of vision or worsening of narrow-angle glaucoma if the solution comes into direct contact with the eyes.

Possible Side Effects

Generally, ipratropium side effects are infrequent and mild.

Inhalation

▼ Most common: bronchitis, upper respiratory infection, nervousness, dizziness, headache, nausea, upset stomach, blurred vision, sensitivity to bright light, dry mouth, throat irritation, cough, worsening of symptoms, heart palpitations, rash, and mouth irritation.

▼ Less common: rapid heartbeat, urinary difficulties, tingling in the hands or feet, poor coordination, itching, hives, flushing, loss of hair, constipation, tremors, fatigue or sleeplessness, and hoarseness.

▼ Rare: worsening of glaucoma, eye pain, low blood pressure, and severe skin reactions.

Nasal Spray

▼ Most common: headache, upper respiratory infection, nosebleeds, and nasal dryness.

▼ Less common: dry mouth or throat and stuffed nose.

▼ Rare: changes in sense of taste, nasal burning, red and itchy eyes, coughing, dizziness, hoarseness, heart palpitations, rapid heartbeat, thirst, ringing or buzzing in the ears, blurred vision, and difficulty urinating.

Drug Interactions

None known.

Food Interactions

Do not inhale a dose of ipratropium if you have any food in your mouth.

Usual Dose

Inhalation

Adult and Child (age 12 and over): 2 inhalations—36 mcg—4 times a day; no more than 12 inhalations every 24 hours. For DuoNeb, 1 vial 4 times a day.

Child (under age 12): not recommended.

Nasal Spray

Adult and Child (age 5 and over): 2 sprays of 0.03% solution per nostril up to 2–3 times a day; the 0.06% solution frequency is 3–4 times a day.

Overdosage

The risk of overdose is small because very little ipratropium is absorbed into the bloodstream. Ipratropium accidentally sprayed into the eye will cause blurred vision. ALWAYS bring the prescription bottle or container with you if you go to an emergency room for treatment.

Special Information

Use this product according to your doctor's instructions. Do not stop taking ipratropium without your doctor's approval even if you feel well.

Call your doctor if you develop rash or hives, sores on the mouth or lips, blurred vision, or other side effects that are bothersome or persistent.

Call your doctor if you stop responding to your usual dose of ipratropium: This may be a sign that your condition has worsened.

Prolonged use of ipratropium may decrease or stop the flow of saliva produced in your mouth. This can expose you to an increased chance of cavities, gum disease, oral infections, and other problems. Dry mouth can be relieved with hard candies or regular fluids. Increased attention to dental hygiene is important.

If, in addition to ipratropium, you use a corticosteroid inhaler or cromolyn sodium for lung disease, use the ipratropium about 5 minutes before the other inhaler.

If you take ipratropium and albuterol, metaproterenol, or another beta-stimulating aerosol product for bronchial disease, use the beta stimulator about 5 minutes before ipratropium unless otherwise instructed by your doctor. Ipratropium solution for inhalation can be mixed with albuterol or metaproterenol for inhalation so long as the mixture is used within 1 hour. The combination product Combivent (a mixture of ipratropium and albuterol) is also available.

The first use of each ipratropium nasal pump requires 7 pumps to prime the spray. Regular use of the spray should prevent the need to prime the pump again. If you do not use the spray for a day, you will have to pump twice to prime the spray. If you do not use the spray for a week, you will have to prime the spray again with 7 pumps.

If you forget to administer a dose of ipratropium, do so as soon as you remember. If it is almost time for your next dose, skip the one you forgot and continue with your regular schedule. Do not take a double dose.

Store this product at room temperature—59° to 86°F—and avoid freezing. Unused vials of the solution for inhalation should be stored in their foil wrapper.

Special Populations

Pregnancy/Breast-feeding
Massive oral doses of ipratropium have caused birth defects in animals. Ipratropium should be used during pregnancy only if clearly needed.

It is not known if ipratropium passes into breast milk. Nursing mothers who must take this drug should consider bottle-feeding.

Seniors
Seniors, especially those with prostate disease, may be more sensitive to the side effects of this drug and may require a dosage adjustment.

Type of Drug

Iron Supplements

Brand Names

Generic Ingredient: Carbonyl Iron, 100% Iron

Feosol   Ircon
Icar

Generic Ingredient: Ferrous Fumarate G , *33% Iron*

Femiron   Hemocyte
Feostat   Nephro-Fer S
Ferretts   Vitron-C S

Generic Ingredient: Ferrous Gluconate G , *12% Iron*

Fergon

Generic Ingredient: Ferrous Sulfate G , *20% to 30% Iron*

ED-IN-SOL   Fer-Gen-Sol
Feosol   Fer-In-Sol
Feratab   Slow-FE

Generic Ingredient: Polysaccharide Iron Complex

Ferrex 150	Niferex-150
Hytinic	Nu-Iron
Niferex $	Nu-Iron 150

Prescribed For

Iron-deficiency anemia.

General Information

Iron supplements are used to treat anemias that result from iron deficiency. Iron is incorporated into red blood cells, which carry oxygen throughout the body. Iron is absorbed only in a small section of the gastrointestinal (GI) tract called the duodenum, the upper part of the small intestine. Sustained-release iron products should be used only to help minimize the stomach discomfort that iron supplements can cause, as some of the drug in these forms may bypass the duodenum and not be absorbed. Other products combining iron with vitamins or special extracts may also be used to treat iron-deficiency anemia. Iron supplements are available in many different forms and they all have different amounts of iron. When choosing an iron supplement, you must be sure to take one that gives you the amount of elemental iron you need.

Cautions and Warnings

Do not take an iron supplement if you are allergic or sensitive to any ingredient or if you have **hemochromatosis, hemosiderosis,** or a **hemolytic anemia**.

Do not take iron supplements if you have a history of **stomach problems, peptic ulcer,** or **ulcerative colitis**. People with normal iron levels should not take any iron product on a regular basis.

Possible Side Effects

▼ Common: stomach upset or irritation, nausea, diarrhea, constipation, appetite loss, and darkened stools.

Drug Interactions

• Iron and tetracycline interfere with each other. Separate doses of these by at least 2 hours.

• Iron interferes with the absorption of levodopa, methyldopa, penicillamine, and quinolone antibacterials.

• Antacids and cimetidine interfere with iron absorption.

• Ascorbic acid (vitamin C) and chloramphenicol increase the amount of iron absorbed.

• Iron reduces the effectiveness of levothyroxine, a thyroid replacement hormone. Combining these 2 drugs may lead to symptoms of hypothyroidism (underactive thyroid gland).

Food Interactions

Iron supplements are best taken on an empty stomach, but they may be taken with food if they upset your stomach. Eggs and milk interfere with iron absorption. Coffee or tea consumed with a meal or within an hour of eating reduces the amount of iron absorbed into the blood. Do not take iron products together with calcium supplements and food. If you need both iron and calcium, take calcium carbonate (Tums) and use it between meals.

Usual Dose

Iron dosage is the same regardless of type. Read the product label to determine iron content.

Adult and Child (age 13 and over): 0.9–1.4 mg per lb. of body weight a day, divided in 3 doses.

Pregnant Women: 30 mg a day. Do not take with food or meals.

Child (age 3–12): 0.45–0.7 mg per lb. of body weight a day, divided in 3–4 doses.

Child (age 6 months–2 years): up to 2.7 mg per lb. of body weight a day, divided in 3–4 doses.

Child (under age 2): 10–25 mg a day, divided in 3–4 doses.

Overdosage

Iron overdosage can be fatal. Overdose symptoms usually appear after 30 minutes to several hours; they include tiredness, vomiting, diarrhea, upset stomach, weak and rapid pulse, and lowered blood pressure—or, after massive doses, shock, black and tarry stools due to massive bleeding in the stomach or intestine, and pneumonia. In case of overdose, call your local poison control center of a hospital emergency room. You may be told to induce vomiting with ipecac syrup—available at any pharmacy—and to give the victim eggs and milk before seeking treatment. Time is a critical factor in emergency care: Stomach pumping should not be performed after the first hour of iron ingestion due to the risk of stomach perforation. If you seek treatment ALWAYS bring the prescription bottle or container.

Special Information

Iron often causes black discoloration of stools and is slightly constipating. However, stools that are black or tarry may also indicate bleeding in the stomach or intestine. If you experience this symptom, discuss it with your doctor at once.

Do not chew or crush sustained-release iron products. Liquid iron products may stain your teeth. Mix water or juice with them and sip the iron through a straw to prevent tooth contact.

If you forget a dose, take it as soon as you remember. If it is almost time for your next dose, skip the one you forgot and continue with your regular schedule. Do not take a double dose.

Special Populations

Pregnancy/Breast-feeding
This drug is safe for use during pregnancy and breast-feeding and is frequently prescribed for pregnant and nursing women. If you are pregnant, however, you should check with your doctor before taking any medication.

Seniors
Seniors may require larger dosages.

Generic Name

Isosorbide Dinitrate

(eye-soe-SORE-bide dih-NYE-trate) G

Brand Names

Dilatrate-SR	Isordil Titradose
Isochron	Sorbitrate
Isordil Tembids	

The information in this profile also applies to the following drug:

Generic Ingredient: Isosorbide Mononitrate [G]

Imdur	Isotrate ER
ISMO	Monoket

Type of Drug

Antianginal agent.

Prescribed For

Heart or chest pain associated with angina pectoris; also prescribed in congestive heart failure (CHF) and similar conditions to prevent the recurrence of chest or heart pain and to reduce stress on the heart.

General Information

Isosorbide dinitrate and other nitrates are used to treat pain associated with heart problems. While the exact nature of their action is not fully understood, they are believed to relax vascular smooth muscles. Isosorbide dinitrate sublingual tablets begin working in 2 to 5 minutes and last for 1 to 3 hours. The regular tablets begin working in 20 to 40 minutes and continue for 4 to 6 hours. The sustained-release form may take up to 4 hours to begin working and lasts for 6 to 8 hours. Isosorbide mononitrate begins working in 30 to 60 minutes and lasts for an undetermined period of time.

Cautions and Warnings

If you are **allergic** or **sensitive** to this drug or to other drugs used for heart pain such as nitroglycerin, do not use it.

If you have or recently have had a **head injury,** use this drug with caution.

This drug may be inappropriate for you if you have had a recent **heart attack** or have severe **anemia, glaucoma,** severe **kidney** or **liver disease, overactive thyroid, cardiomyopathy** (loss of blood-pumping ability due to damaged heart muscle), **glaucoma,** or **low blood pressure,** especially postural low blood pressure (symptoms include dizziness or fainting when rising from a sitting or lying position).

Possible Side Effects

▼ Common: headache and flushing, which should disappear after your body adjusts to the drug. You may

---

Possible Side Effects *(continued)*

experience dizziness and weakness during this process. There is a risk of blurred vision and dry mouth; if either occurs, stop taking the drug and call your doctor.

▼ Less common: rapid heartbeat, low blood pressure, fainting, nausea, vomiting, weakness, trouble urinating, bronchitis, sweating, and rash with itching, redness, and peeling. If these symptoms appear, discontinue the medication and consult your doctor.

Drug Interactions

• If you take isosorbide dinitrate, do not self-medicate with over-the-counter appetite suppressants and cough, cold, and allergy remedies, since many contain ingredients that may aggravate heart disease.

• Taking this drug with large amounts of alcohol may rapidly lower blood pressure, resulting in weakness, dizziness, and fainting.

• Nitrates raise dihydroergotamine blood levels, which may elevate blood pressure or block isosorbide's effects.

• Aspirin and calcium channel blockers can increase isosorbide blood levels and the risk of side effects.

• Do not take sildenafil, vardenafil, or taldenafil if you are taking isosorbide or another nitrate drug. The combination can result in a rapid and potentially fatal drop in blood pressure.

Food Interactions

Take isosorbide on an empty stomach with a glass of water unless you get a persistent headache. If this occurs, the drug can be taken with meals.

Usual Dose

Isosorbide Dinitrate: Initially, 5–20 mg every 6 hours; maintain at 10–40 mg every 6 hours. Sustained release initial dose is 40 mg; maintenance at 40–80 mg every 8–12 hours.

Isosorbide Mononitrate: 20 mg twice a day, with the 2 doses taken 7 hours apart. Usually, the first dose is taken upon waking and the second dose is taken 7 hours later. Extended-release tablets should begin with 30–60 mg once a day; after several days this may be increased to 120 mg once a day, though rarely 240 mg may be required.

Overdosage

Overdose can result in low blood pressure; very rapid heartbeat; flushing; perspiration followed by cold, bluish, and clammy skin; headache; heart palpitations; blurred vision and other visual disturbances; dizziness; nausea; vomiting; difficult, slow breathing; slow pulse; confusion; moderate fever; and paralysis. Take the victim to a hospital emergency room at once. ALWAYS bring the prescription bottle or container.

Special Information

If you take this drug sublingually (under the tongue), be sure the tablet is fully dissolved before you swallow the drug. Do not crush or chew sustained-release capsules or tablets. Avoid alcohol.

Do not switch brands of isosorbide without consulting your doctor or pharmacist—they may not be equivalent.

Call your doctor if you develop a persistent headache, dizziness, facial flushing, blurred vision, or dry mouth.

If you take isosorbide on a regular schedule and forget a dose, take it as soon as you remember. If you take isosorbide more than once a day and it is within 2 hours of your next dose, skip the dose you forgot and continue with your regular schedule. If you take the sustained-release form once a day and it is within 6 hours of your next dose, skip the dose you forgot and continue with your regular schedule. Never take a double dose.

Special Populations

Pregnancy/Breast-feeding

Isosorbide crosses into the fetal circulation. When this drug is considered crucial by your doctor, its potential benefits must be carefully weighed against its risks.

This drug passes into breast milk. Nursing mothers who must take it should consider bottle-feeding.

Seniors

Seniors may take isosorbide without special restriction.

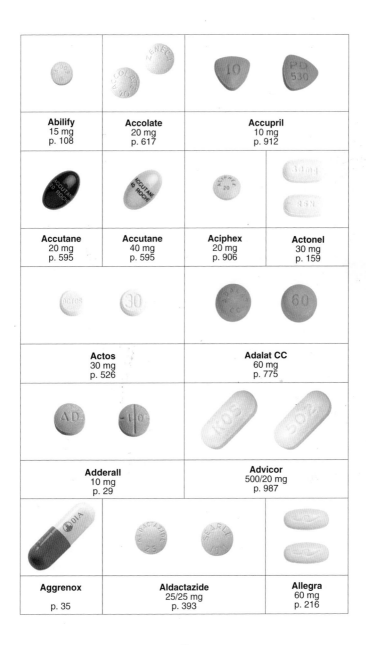

Abilify 15 mg p. 108	**Accolate** 20 mg p. 617	**Accupril** 10 mg p. 912
Accutane 20 mg p. 595	**Accutane** 40 mg p. 595	**Aciphex** 20 mg p. 906	**Actonel** 30 mg p. 159

Actos
30 mg
p. 526

Adalat CC
60 mg
p. 775

Adderall
10 mg
p. 29

Advicor
500/20 mg
p. 987

Aggrenox
p. 35

Aldactazide
25/25 mg
p. 393

Allegra
60 mg
p. 216

A

Allegra-D p. 96	Altace 2.5 mg p. 913	Altace 5 mg p. 913
Amaryl 2 mg p. 1003	Ambien 5 mg p. 1178	
Ambien 10 mg p. 1178	Amoxil 250 mg p. 825	Amoxil 500 mg p. 825
Ancobon 500 mg p. 492	Ansaid 50 mg p. 550	Antivert 12.5 mg p. 366
Aricept 5 mg p. 239	Aricept 10 mg p. 239	

B

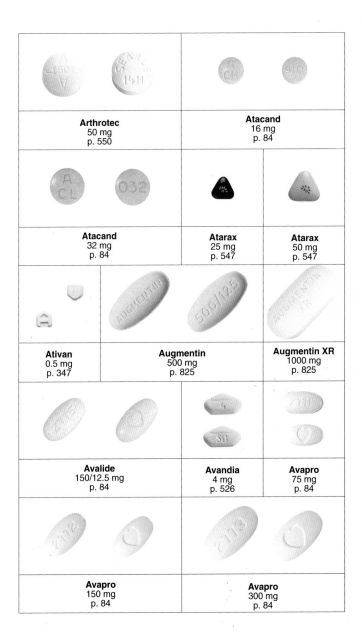

Arthrotec
50 mg
p. 550

Atacand
16 mg
p. 84

Atacand
32 mg
p. 84

Atarax
25 mg
p. 547

Atarax
50 mg
p. 547

Ativan
0.5 mg
p. 347

Augmentin
500 mg
p. 825

Augmentin XR
1000 mg
p. 825

Avalide
150/12.5 mg
p. 84

Avandia
4 mg
p. 526

Avapro
75 mg
p. 84

Avapro
150 mg
p. 84

Avapro
300 mg
p. 84

C

Avelox 400 mg p. 495	**Axert** 6.25 mg p. 1120	**Axid** 150 mg p. 793
Bactrim DS p. 974	**Bentyl** 10 mg p. 351	**Bentyl** 20 mg p. 351
Bextra 10 mg p. 206	**Bextra** 20 mg p. 206	
Biaxin 250 mg p. 250	**Biaxin** 500 mg p. 250	**Biaxin XL** 500 mg p. 250
Blocadren 10 mg p. 1069	**Blocadren** 20 mg p. 1069	

D

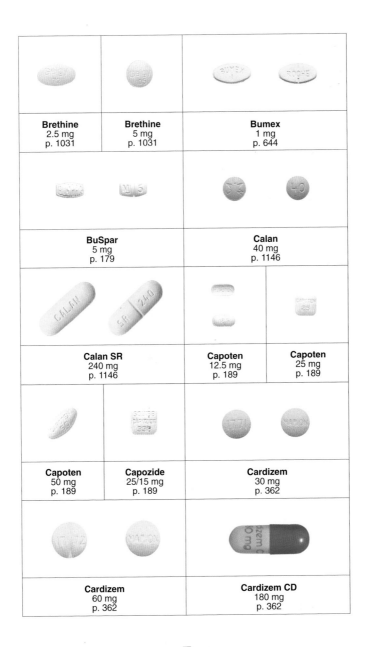

Brethine 2.5 mg p. 1031	**Brethine** 5 mg p. 1031	**Bumex** 1 mg p. 644
BuSpar 5 mg p. 179		**Calan** 40 mg p. 1146
Calan SR 240 mg p. 1146	**Capoten** 12.5 mg p. 189	**Capoten** 25 mg p. 189
Capoten 50 mg p. 189	**Capozide** 25/15 mg p. 189	**Cardizem** 30 mg p. 362
Cardizem 60 mg p. 362		**Cardizem CD** 180 mg p. 362

E

Cardizem SR 60 mg p. 362	**Cardizem SR** 90 mg p. 362	**Cardura** 2 mg p. 384	
Cartia XT 180 mg p. 363	**Cartia XT** 240 mg p. 363	**Cartrol** 2.5 mg p. 199	**Cartrol** 5 mg p. 199
Catapres 0.1 mg p. 265	**Catapres** 0.2 mg p. 265	**Ceclor** 500 mg p. 210	**Ceftin** 125 mg p. 211
Cefzil 500 mg p. 211		**Celebrex** 100 mg p. 206	**Celexa** 20 mg p. 965
CellCept 250 mg p. 741	**Cialis** 20 mg p. 430	**Cipro** 250 mg p. 495	**Cipro** 500 mg p. 495

F

Cipro 750 mg p. 495	**Cipro XR** 500 mg p. 495	**Clarinex** 5 mg p. 651

Clinoril 150 mg p. 550	**Clozaril** 100 mg p. 278

Colazal 750 mg p. 169	**Compazine** 10 mg p. 886	**Compazine Spansule** 15 mg p. 886

Comtan 200 mg p. 418	**Concerta** 18 mg p. 691	**Cordarone** 200 mg p. 63

Corgard 40 mg p. 1069	**Corgard** 80 mg p. 1069

G

Coumadin
5 mg
p. 1150

Covera HS
180 mg
p. 1146

Cozaar
25 mg
p. 84

Cozaar
50 mg
p. 84

Dalmane
30 mg
p. 504

Darvocet-N
100 mg
p. 895

Daypro
600 mg
p. 551

Deconamine SR

p. 95

Deltasone
10 mg
p. 311

Demerol
50 mg
p. 674

Depakote
125 mg
p. 1139

Depakote
250 mg
p. 1139

Depakote ER
500 mg
p. 1139

Depakote Sprinkle
125 mg
p. 1139

Desyrel
50 mg
p. 1096

Desyrel
100 mg
p. 1096

H

Desyrel Dividose 150 mg p. 1096	**Detrol** 2 mg p. 1082	**Detrol LA** 2 mg p. 1082
DiaBeta 5 mg p. 1003	**Diabinese** 100 mg p. 1003	**Diabinese** 250 mg p. 1003
Diflucan 100 mg p. 1107	**Diflucan** 150 mg p. 1107	

Dilacor XR 120 mg p. 363	**Dilacor XR** 180 mg p. 363	**Dilacor XR** 240 mg p. 363	**Dilantin** 100 mg p. 854
Diovan 80 mg p. 85		**Diovan** 160 mg p. 85	

Diovan HCT p. 85	**Ditropan** 5 mg p. 812

Ditropan XL p. 812	**Diuril** 500 mg p. 1053	**Doral** 15 mg p. 1103

Duricef 500 mg p. 210	**Dyazide** p. 393	**Dynabac** 250 mg p. 372	**DynaCirc** 2.5 mg p. 775

E.E.S. 400 mg p. 437	**Effexor** 25 mg p. 1143	**Effexor** 37.5 mg p. 1143	**Effexor** 50 mg p. 1143

Effexor 75 mg p. 1143	**Effexor** 100 mg p. 1143

J

Effexor XR 75 mg p. 1143	**Elmiron** 100 mg p. 830	**Ery-Tab** 250 mg p. 437

Ery-Tab 333 mg p. 437	**Erythrocin Stearate** 250 mg p. 437

Erythrocin Stearate 500 mg p. 437	**Eskalith** 300 mg p. 639	**Eskalith CR** 450 mg p. 639

Estrace 1 mg p. 445	**Estratest** p. 445	**Eulexin** 125 mg p. 507	**Evista** 60 mg p. 919

Exelon 6 mg p. 239	**Famvir** 500 mg p. 463	**Feldene** 20 mg p. 865

K

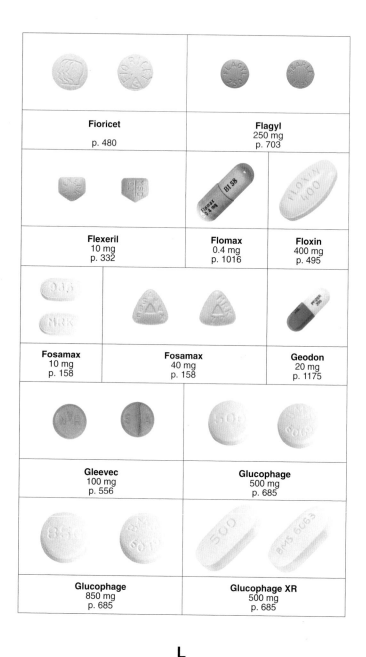

Fioricet

p. 480

Flagyl
250 mg
p. 703

Flexeril
10 mg
p. 332

Flomax
0.4 mg
p. 1016

Floxin
400 mg
p. 495

Fosamax
10 mg
p. 158

Fosamax
40 mg
p. 158

Geodon
20 mg
p. 1175

Gleevec
100 mg
p. 556

Glucophage
500 mg
p. 685

Glucophage
850 mg
p. 685

Glucophage XR
500 mg
p. 685

L

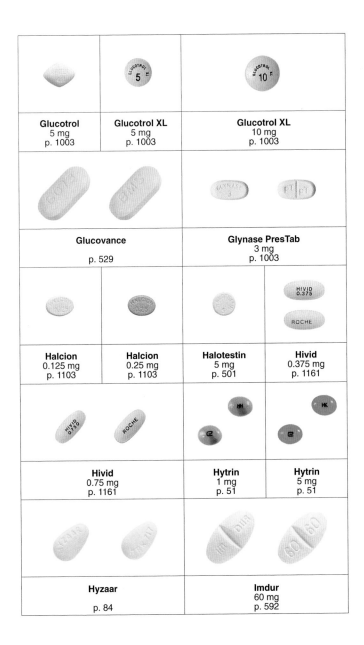

Glucotrol 5 mg p. 1003	**Glucotrol XL** 5 mg p. 1003	**Glucotrol XL** 10 mg p. 1003

Glucovance p. 529	**Glynase PresTab** 3 mg p. 1003

Halcion 0.125 mg p. 1103	**Halcion** 0.25 mg p. 1103	**Halotestin** 5 mg p. 501	**Hivid** 0.375 mg p. 1161

Hivid 0.75 mg p. 1161	**Hytrin** 1 mg p. 51	**Hytrin** 5 mg p. 51

Hyzaar p. 84	**Imdur** 60 mg p. 592

M

Imdur 120 mg p. 592	**Imitrex** 25 mg p. 1120
Inderal 40 mg p. 898	**Inderal** 80 mg p. 898
Inderal LA 60 mg p. 898 — **Inderal LA** 120 mg p. 898	**Inderide** 40/25 mg p. 898
Inderide 80/25 mg p. 898	**Indocin** 50 mg p. 566 — **Indocin SR** 75 mg p. 566
Isordil Titradose 10 mg p. 591 — **Isordil Titradose** 40 mg p. 591	**Kaletra** p. 947

N

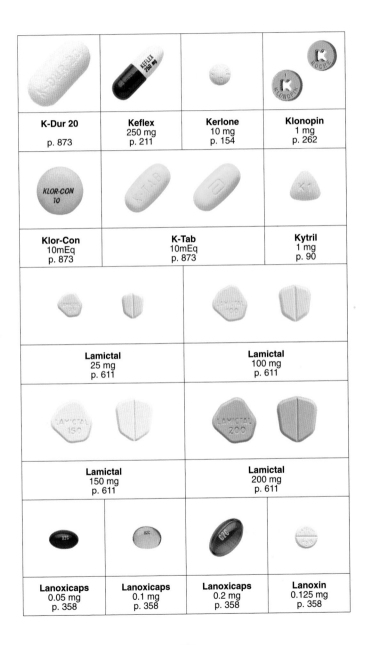

K-Dur 20 p. 873	**Keflex** 250 mg p. 211	**Kerlone** 10 mg p. 154	**Klonopin** 1 mg p. 262
Klor-Con 10mEq p. 873	**K-Tab** 10mEq p. 873		**Kytril** 1 mg p. 90
Lamictal 25 mg p. 611		**Lamictal** 100 mg p. 611	
Lamictal 150 mg p. 611		**Lamictal** 200 mg p. 611	
Lanoxicaps 0.05 mg p. 358	**Lanoxicaps** 0.1 mg p. 358	**Lanoxicaps** 0.2 mg p. 358	**Lanoxin** 0.125 mg p. 358

O

Lanoxin 0.25 mg p. 358	**Lanoxin** 0.5 mg p. 358

Lasix
40 mg
p. 644

Lasix
80 mg
p. 644

Lescol
20 mg
p. 986

Lescol
40 mg
p. 986

Levaquin
500 mg
p. 495

Levatol
20 mg
p. 698

Levitra
10 mg
p. 430

Levoxyl
25 mcg
p. 1058

Levoxyl
50 mcg
p. 1058

Levoxyl
100 mcg
p. 1058

Levoxyl
125 mcg
p. 1058

Lexapro
10 mg
p. 965

P

Lexapro 20 mg p. 965	**Lexxel** p. 629	**Librium** 10 mg p. 222
Lipitor 40 mg p. 986	**Lipitor** 80 mg p. 986	
Lodine 300 mg p. 455	**Lodine XL** 500 mg p. 455	**Lopid** 600 mg p. 520
Lopressor 100 mg p. 698	**Lorabid** 400 mg p. 211	**Lorcet Plus** p. 833
Lotensin 5 mg p. 139		**Lotensin HCT** p. 139

Q

Lotrel p. 653	**Lozol** 2.5 mg p. 1053	**Luvox** 50 mg p. 965
Luvox 100 mg p. 965	**Macrobid** p. 785	**Macrodantin** 50 mg p. 785
Maxaquin 400 mg p. 495	**Mellaril** 25 mg p. 229	**Meridia** 5 mg p. 980
Metaglip 2.5/500 mg p. 1003	**Metaglip** 5/500 mg p. 1003	
Mevacor 20 mg p. 986	**Mevacor** 40 mg p. 986	**Micro-K Extencaps** 10 mEq p. 873 **Micronase** 1.25 mg p. 1003

R

Mifeprex 1.25 mg p. 711	**Minipress** 1 mg p. 879	**Minipress** 2 mg p. 879	**Minizide 1** p. 879
Minizide 2 p. 879	**Minocin** 50 mg p. 1043	**Minocin** 100 mg p. 1043	**Mirapex** 0.125 mg p. 876

Mirapex
0.25 mg
p. 876

Mirapex
1 mg
p. 876

Mirapex
1.5 mg
p. 876

Mobic
15 mg
p. 668

Moduretic

p. 393

Monopril
10 mg
p. 511

S

Nalfon 200 mg p. 550	**Nalfon** 300 mg p. 500	**Naprosyn** 375 mg p. 748
Neurontin 300 mg p. 1063	**Nexium** 40 mg p. 906	**Nizoral** 200 mg p. 1107
Nolvadex 10 mg p. 1013		**Noroxin** 400 mg p. 495

Norpace 100 mg p. 374	**Norpace CR** 100 mg p. 374	**Norpramin** 50 mg p. 1113	**Norvasc** 5 mg p. 69
Omnicef 300 mg p. 210	**Orudis** 50 mg p. 550	**Orudis** 75 mg p. 550	**Oruvail** 200 mg p. 550

T

Pamelor
25 mg
p. 1113

Pamelor
75 mg
p. 1113

Parafon Forte DSC
500 mg
p. 233

Paxil
12.5 mg
p. 965

Paxil
20 mg
p. 965

Paxil CR
25 mg
p. 965

Paxil CR
37.5 mg
p. 965

PCE
333 mg
p. 437

PCE
500 mg
p. 437

Pepcid
20 mg
p. 465

Phenergan
25 mg
p. 890

Plavix
75 mg
p. 269

Plendil

p. 471

U

Pletal 50 mg p. 244	**Pletal** 100 mg p. 244	**Ponstel** 250 mg p. 550	**Prandin** 1 mg p. 931
Pravachol 10 mg p. 987		**Premarin** 0.625 mg p. 445	**Premarin** 1.25 mg p. 445
Prevacid 15 mg p. 906	**Prevacid** 30 mg p. 906	**Prilosec** 20 mg p. 906	**Prinivil** 20 mg p. 636
ProAmatine 2.5 mg p. 709		**ProAmatine** 5 mg p. 709	
Procardia 10 mg p. 775	**Procardia XL** 30 mg p. 775	**Procardia XL** 60 mg p. 775	**Procardia XL** 90 mg p. 775

V

Prograf 1 mg p. 1008	**Prograf** 5 mg p. 1008	**Prolixin** 5 mg p. 229	**Prolixin** 10 mg p. 229

Prometrium 100 mg p. 664	**Proscar** 5 mg p. 477	**Protonix** 40 mg p. 906

Provera 2.5 mg p. 664	**Provera** 5 mg p. 664	**Prozac** 10 mg p. 965	**Prozac** 20 mg p. 965

Prozac Weekly 90 mg p. 965	**Quinidex Extentabs** 300 mg p. 916	**Reglan** 10 mg p. 695

Relafen 500 mg p. 745	**Remeron** 30 mg p. 720

W

Reminyl 8 mg p. 239	**Restoril** 30 mg p. 1104	**Retrovir** 100 mg p. 1170
Risperdal 2 mg p. 943	**Risperdal** 3 mg p. 943	
Risperdal 4 mg p. 943	**Ritalin-SR** 20 mg p. 692	**Sandimmune** 25 mg p. 335
Sandimmune 100 mg p. 335	**Sectral** 200 mg p. 9	**Sectral** 400 mg p. 9

Septra DS p. 974	**Serax** 10 mg p. 347	**Serax** 30 mg p. 347	**Seroquel** 25 mg p. 909

X

Seroquel 100 mg p. 909	**Seroquel** 200 mg p. 909	**Serzone** 100 mg p. 752
Serzone 150 mg p. 752		**Serzone** 200 mg p. 752
Serzone 250 mg p. 752		**Sinemet** 10/100 mg p. 983
Sinemet 25/250 mg p. 983		**Sinemet CR** 50/200 mg p. 983
Singulair 10 mg p. 617		**Skelaxin** 400 mg p. 682

Y

Slow-K 600 mg p. 873	**Sonata** 5 mg p. 1165	**Sorbitrate** 5 mg p. 591	

Sorbitrate 10 mg p. 591	**Sorbitrate** 40 mg p. 591

Starlix 60 mg p. 931	**Strattera** 10 mg p. 123	**Strattera** 25 mg p. 123

Strattera 40 mg p. 123	**Sumycin** 250 mg p. 1044	**Surmontil** 25 mg p. 1114	**Surmontil** 50 mg p. 1114

Surmontil 100 mg p. 1114	**Synthroid** 25 mcg p. 1058	**Synthroid** 75 mcg p. 1058	**Synthroid** 125 mcg p. 1058

Z

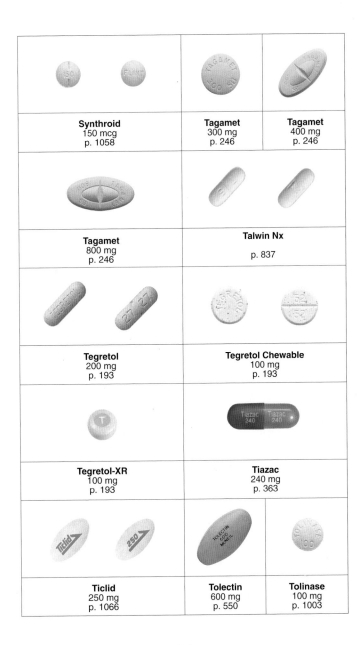

Synthroid 150 mcg p. 1058	**Tagamet** 300 mg p. 246	**Tagamet** 400 mg p. 246
Tagamet 800 mg p. 246	**Talwin Nx** p. 837	
Tegretol 200 mg p. 193	**Tegretol Chewable** 100 mg p. 193	
Tegretol-XR 100 mg p. 193	**Tiazac** 240 mg p. 363	
Ticlid 250 mg p. 1066	**Tolectin** 600 mg p. 550	**Tolinase** 100 mg p. 1003

AA

Tolinase 500 mg p. 1003	**Topamax** 25 mg p. 1084	**Toprol-XL** 50 mg p. 698
Toprol-XL 100 mg p. 698	**Tranxene T-Tab** 15 mg p. 272	**Tricor** 54 mg p. 474
Trileptal 300 mg p. 807	**Trimox** 250 mg p. 825	**Trimox** 500 mg p. 825
Trizivir p. 1128	**Tylenol with Codeine #2** p. 833	
Tylenol with Codeine #3 p. 833	**Tylox** p. 832	

BB

Univasc 7.5 mg p. 730	**Univasc** 15 mg p. 730
Valium 5 mg p. 347	**Valium** 10 mg p. 347
Valtrex 500 mg p. 1137	**Vaseretic** 10/25 mg p. 412
Vasotec 5 mg p. 412	**Vasotec** 10 mg p. 412

Vasotec 20 mg p. 412	**Veetids** 250 mg p. 826	**Veetids** 500 mg p. 826

Verelan 240 mg p. 1146	**Viagra** 50 mg p. 430	**Vibramycin** 50 mg p. 1043
Vibramycin 100 mg p. 1043	**Vibra-Tabs** 100 mg p. 1043	**Vicodin** p. 833
Vicodin-ES p. 833	**Vioxx** 25 mg p. 951	**Welchol** 625 mg p. 235

Wellbutrin 75 mg p. 175	**Wellbutrin** 100 mg p. 175	**Wellbutrin SR** 150 mg p. 175	**Wellbutrin XL** 150 mg p. 175
Wellbutrin XL 300 mg p. 175	**Xanax** 0.25 mg p. 55	**Xanax** 0.5 mg p. 55	**Xanax** 1 mg p. 55

DD

Xenical 120 mg p. 802	**Zanaflex** 4 mg p. 1074
Zantac 150 mg p. 922	**Zantac** 300 mg p. 922

Zaroxolyn
10 mg
p. 1053

Zebeta
5 mg
p. 154

Zerit
15 mg
p. 993

Zerit
20 mg
p. 993

Zerit
30 mg
p. 993

Zerit
40 mg
p. 993

Zestoretic 10-12.5

p. 636

Zestoretic 25

p. 636

Zestril
5 mg
p. 636

EE

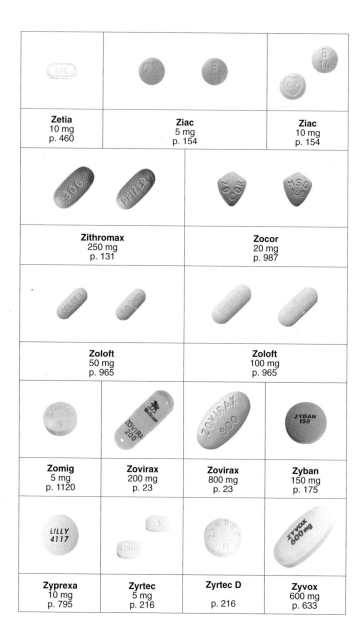

Zetia 10 mg p. 460	**Ziac** 5 mg p. 154	**Ziac** 10 mg p. 154

Zithromax 250 mg p. 131	**Zocor** 20 mg p. 987

Zoloft 50 mg p. 965	**Zoloft** 100 mg p. 965

Zomig 5 mg p. 1120	**Zovirax** 200 mg p. 23	**Zovirax** 800 mg p. 23	**Zyban** 150 mg p. 175

Zyprexa 10 mg p. 795	**Zyrtec** 5 mg p. 216	**Zyrtec D** p. 216	**Zyvox** 600 mg p. 633

FF

Generic Name

Isotretinoin (eye-soe-TRET-ih-noin)

Brand Name

Accutane   Sotret
Claravis

Type of Drug

Antiacne.

Prescribed For

Severe cystic acne that has not responded to other treatment.

General Information

It is not known exactly how isotretinoin, which is related to vitamin A, works in cases of severe cystic acne. It reduces the amount of sebum (the skin's natural oily lubricant), shrinks the skin glands that produce sebum, and inhibits keratinization (hardening of the skin cells)—key to the problem of severe acne because it leads to the buildup of sebum within skin follicles and causes the formation of closed comedones (whiteheads). Sebum production may be permanently reduced after isotretinoin treatment.

Isotretinoin is also being studied as a treatment for keratinization and mycosis fungoides.

Cautions and Warnings

People **allergic** or **sensitive to vitamin A** (or any vitamin A product) or to paraben preservatives—used in isotretinoin—should not use isotretinoin.

Isotretinoin greatly increases the risk of **severe birth defects, abortion,** and **premature birth**. Women who are pregnant or nursing must not take isotretinoin.

Isotretinoin has been associated with **depression, psychosis,** and **suicidal thoughts or attempts**. Use with caution if you have a history of psychiatric disorders.

Isotretinoin has been associated with **pseudotumor cerebri** (increased pressure in the brain). The symptoms of this condition include severe headaches, nausea, vomiting, and visual disturbances.

Isotretinoin may cause an increased risk for **pancreatitis,** sometimes fatal, and **low white-blood-cell counts.**

Diabetics taking this drug may have their diabetes drugs re-evaluated by their doctors. Some new cases of diabetes were found in people taking isotretinoin, but no direct relationship to drug therapy has been found.

Isotretinoin may cause temporary opaque spots on the cornea of your eye, causing **visual disturbances.** These are usually gone by 2 months after the drug is stopped.

Difficulty seeing at night or in the dark can develop suddenly while taking isotretinoin.

Several cases of **severe bowel inflammation** (symptoms include abdominal discomfort and pain, severe diarrhea, or bleeding from the rectum) have developed in people taking isotretinoin.

About 25% of people who take isotretinoin develop **high blood-triglyceride levels.** Fifteen percent have lower high-density lipoprotein (HDL)—"good" cholesterol—and 7% have higher total cholesterol.

Several cases of **hepatitis** have been linked to this drug. Fifteen percent of people who take it develop signs of **liver inflammation**.

Isotretinoin may worsen **osteoporosis,** cause **low bone density,** and **slow bone healing**. Long-term treatment or multiple courses of therapy may worsen these problems.

Possible Side Effects

Side effects increase with dosage.

▼ Most common: dry, chapped, or inflamed lips; dry mouth; dry nose; nosebleeds; eye irritation; conjunctivitis (pinkeye); dry or flaky skin; rash; itching; peeling skin on the face, palms, or soles; unusual sensitivity to the sun; temporary skin discoloration; brittle nails; inflammation of the nailbed or bone under toes or fingernails; temporary hair thinning; nausea; vomiting; abdominal pain; tiredness; lethargy; sleeplessness; headache; tingling in the hands or feet; dizziness; protein, blood, or white blood cells in the urine; urinary difficulties; blurred vision; bone and joint aches or pains; and muscle pain or stiffness. Isotretinoin causes extreme elevations of blood-triglyceride levels and milder elevations of other blood-fat levels

Possible Side Effects (continued)

including cholesterol. It also can raise blood-sugar or uric-acid levels and can increase liver-function-test values.

▼ Less common: wound crusting caused by an exaggerated healing response stimulated by the drug, hair problems other than thinning, appetite loss, upset stomach or intestinal discomfort, severe bowel inflammation, stomach or intestinal bleeding, weight loss, visual disturbances, contact lens intolerance, pseudotumor cerebri, mild bleeding or easy bruising, fluid retention, and lung or respiratory system infection. Several people taking isotretinoin have developed widespread herpes simplex infections.

Drug Interactions

• Vitamin A supplements increase isotretinoin's side effects and must be avoided while taking this drug. Avoid alcohol because this combination can severely raise blood-triglyceride levels.

• Combining tetracycline antibiotics and isotretinoin may increase the risk of pseudotumor cerebri.

• Isotretinoin may reduce the amount of carbamazepine (an anticonvulsant) in the blood.

• Isotretinoin may decrease the effectiveness of oral contraceptives. Use an additional form of contraception.

Food Interactions

Isotretinoin should be taken with food or meals. Avoid eating beef or chicken liver while taking isotretinoin, because liver contains very large amounts of vitamin A. Limit your intake of foods containing moderate to large amounts of vitamin A.

Usual Dose

Adult and Child (age 13 and over): 0.22–0.9 mg per lb. of body weight a day in 2 divided doses for 15–20 weeks. Lower doses may be effective, but relapses are more common. Isotretinoin, like vitamin A, dissolves in body fat. People weighing more than 155 lbs. may need doses at the high end of the usual range.

If the total acne lesion count drops by 70% in 15–20 weeks, the drug may be discontinued. Stop taking isotretinoin for 2 months after 15–20 weeks of treatment. A second course of treatment may be needed if the acne does not clear.

Overdosage

Isotretinoin overdose is likely to cause nausea, vomiting, facial flushing, abdominal pain, lethargy, and other common drug side effects. Overdose victims must be made to vomit with ipecac syrup—available at any pharmacy—to remove any remaining drug from the stomach. Call your doctor or poison control center before doing this. If you must go to a hospital emergency room, ALWAYS bring the prescription bottle or container.

Special Information

Women of childbearing age should not take isotretinoin unless their severe, disfiguring acne has not responded to any other treatment, they are using effective contraception, they understand that it causes serious birth defects, and they have had two negative pregnancy tests during the 2 cycles before taking isotretinoin and after the last incidence of unprotected sex. You should start taking isotretinoin on day 2 or 3 of your next period. Be sure your doctor knows if you are breast-feeding, diabetic, taking a vitamin A supplement—as a multivitamin or vitamin A alone—or if you or any family member has a history of high blood-triglyceride levels. Continue using contraceptives for at least one month after stopping isotretinoin.

Your skin may become unusually sensitive to the sun while you are taking this drug. Use sunscreen and wear protective clothing until your doctor can determine if you are likely to develop this effect.

Call your doctor if you develop any severe or unusual side effects, such as abdominal pain; bleeding from the rectum; severe diarrhea; headache; nausea or vomiting; visual difficulties; severe muscle, bone, or joint aches or pains; or unusual sensitivity to sunlight or to ultraviolet light.

Your acne may worsen when isotretinoin treatment begins, but then it should improve. Do not be alarmed if this happens, but tell your doctor.

Do not donate blood during isotretinoin treatment—or for at least 30 days after you have stopped—because of the risk to the fetus of a pregnant woman who may receive the blood.

If you forget a dose of isotretinoin, take it as soon as you remember. If it is almost time for your next dose, skip the one you forgot and continue with your regular schedule. Do not take a double dose.

Special Populations

Pregnancy/Breast-feeding
Pregnant women should NEVER take isotretinoin because it will injure the fetus. Your doctor will confirm that you are not pregnant before starting isotretinoin (see "Special Information"). Accidental pregnancy during isotretinoin therapy may be grounds for an abortion due to the severe birth defects this drug will cause. Call your doctor immediately.

It is not known if isotretinoin passes into breast milk. Nursing mothers should not take isotretinoin because of the possibility that it will affect the nursing infant.

Seniors
Seniors may take this medication without special restriction.

Generic Name

Ketorolac (kee-TOE-roe-lak) G

Brand Names

Acular Eyedrops   Toradol

Type of Drug

Nonsteroidal anti-inflammatory drug (NSAID).

Prescribed For

Moderately severe pain. The eyedrops are prescribed for eye redness and inflammation caused by seasonal allergies and for inflammation following cataract surgery.

General Information

Ketorolac tromethamine and other NSAIDs are used to relieve pain and inflammation. We do not know exactly how NSAIDs work, but they may achieve their effects by blocking the body's production of a hormone called prostaglandin and the action of other body chemicals. Pain relief comes within 1 hour after taking the first dose of ketorolac. Unlike other NSAIDs, ketorolac is a potent drug with serious risks. Taking more ketorolac than is prescribed only increases risk; it does not offer better results. People who have first been treated with ketorolac injection should only take ketorolac tablets. Total treatment with injectable and oral ketorolac should not exceed 5 days.

NSAID eyedrops may be used during eye surgery to prevent movement of the eye muscles.

Cautions and Warnings

People **allergic** to ketorolac or any other NSAID and those with a history of **asthma** attacks brought on by an NSAID, iodides, or aspirin should not take ketorolac.

Ketorolac may cause **gastrointestinal (GI) bleeding**, **ulcers**, and **stomach perforation**. This can occur at any time, with or without warning, in people who take ketorolac regularly. People with a history of active GI bleeding should be cautious about taking any NSAID. People who develop bleeding or ulcers and continue NSAID treatment should be aware of the possibility of developing more serious side effects.

Ketorolac may affect platelets and **blood clotting** at high doses and should be avoided by people with clotting problems and those who take warfarin.

People with **heart problems** who use ketorolac may experience swelling in their arms, legs, or feet.

Ketorolac may actually cause **headaches**. If this happens, you might have to stop taking this drug or switch to another NSAID.

Ketorolac may cause severe toxic effects to the **kidney**. Report any unusual side effects to your doctor, who might need to periodically test your kidney function.

People taking ketorolac on a regular basis should have their **liver function** checked periodically.

Ketorolac may make you **unusually sensitive to the effects of the sun**.

Possible Side Effects

Injection and Tablets

▼ Most common: diarrhea, nausea, vomiting, constipation, minor stomach upset or distress, gas, and appetite loss, especially during the first few days of treatment.

▼ Less common: stomach ulcers, GI bleeding, hepatitis, gallbladder attacks, painful urination, poor kidney function, kidney inflammation, blood and protein in the urine, dizziness, fainting, nervousness, depression, hallucinations, confusion, disorientation, tingling in the

Possible Side Effects *(continued)*

hands or feet, light-headedness, itching, increased sweating, dry nose and mouth, heart palpitations, chest pain, breathing difficulties, and muscle cramps.

▼ Rare: severe allergic reactions including closing of the throat, fever and chills, changes in liver function, jaundice (yellowing of the skin or whites of the eyes), and kidney failure. People who experience such effects must be promptly treated in a hospital emergency room or doctor's office. NSAIDs have caused severe skin reactions; if this happens to you, see your doctor immediately.

Eyedrops

▼ Most common: temporary burning, stinging, or other minor eye irritation.

▼ Less common: nausea, vomiting, viral infections, and eye reactions including persistent redness, burning, itching, or tearing. The risk of developing bleeding problems or other systemic (whole-body) side effects with ketorolac eyedrops is low because only a small amount of the drug is absorbed into the blood.

Drug Interactions

Injection and Tablets

• Ketorolac may increase the effects of oral anticoagulant (blood-thinning) drugs such as warfarin. Your anticoagulant dose may need to be reduced.

• Taking ketorolac with cyclosporine may increase the kidney-related side effects of both drugs. Methotrexate side effects may be increased in people also taking ketorolac.

• Ketorolac may reduce the blood-pressure-lowering effect of beta blockers and loop diuretics.

• Ketorolac may increase phenytoin side effects. Lithium blood levels may be raised by ketorolac.

• Ketorolac blood levels may be affected by cimetidine.

• Probenecid may increase the risk of ketorolac side effects.

• Aspirin and other salicylates should never be combined with ketorolac.

Eyedrops
None known.

Food Interactions

Take ketorolac with food or a magnesium/aluminum antacid if it upsets your stomach.

Usual Dose

Tablets: Up to 40 mg a day for no more than 5 consecutive days.

Eyedrops: 1 drop 4 times a day for itching and irritation due to seasonal allergies.

Overdosage

People have died from NSAID overdoses. Common signs of overdose are drowsiness, nausea, vomiting, diarrhea, abdominal pain, rapid breathing, rapid heartbeat, increased sweating, ringing or buzzing in the ears, confusion, disorientation, stupor, and coma. Take the victim to a hospital emergency room at once. ALWAYS bring the prescription bottle or container.

Special Information

Injection and Tablets: Take each dose with a full glass of water and do not lie down for 15 to 30 minutes afterward.

Ketorolac can make you drowsy or tired: Be careful when driving or operating hazardous equipment. Do not take any over-the-counter products containing acetaminophen or aspirin while taking ketorolac. Avoid alcoholic beverages.

Contact your doctor if you develop rash or itching, visual disturbances, weight gain, breathing difficulties, fluid retention, hallucinations, black or tarry stools, persistent headache, or any unusual or intolerable side effect.

If you forget a dose of ketorolac tablets, take it as soon as you remember. If you take ketorolac once a day and it is within 8 hours of your next dose, or if you take several doses a day and it is within 4 hours of your next dose, skip the dose you forgot and continue with your regular schedule. Never take a double dose.

Eyedrops: To prevent possible infection, do not allow the dropper to touch your fingers, eyelids, or any surface. Wait at least 5 minutes before using any other eyedrops.

If you forget to administer a dose of ketorolac eyedrops, do so as soon as you remember. If it is almost time for your next dose, skip the dose you forgot and continue with your regular schedule. Do not take a double dose.

Special Populations

Pregnancy/Breast-feeding
Ketorolac should not be taken by pregnant women because it may affect fetal blood circulation and prevent normal labor.

Ketorolac may pass into breast milk. There is a possibility that a nursing mother taking ketorolac could affect her baby's heart or cardiovascular system. Nursing mothers who must take this drug should bottle-feed.

Seniors
Seniors may be more susceptible to side effects, especially ulcer disease.

Generic Name

Ketotifen (kee-toe-TIH-fen)

Brand Name

Zaditor Eyedrops

The information in this profile also applies to the following drug:

Generic Ingredient: Lodoxamide
Alomide Eyedrops

Type of Drug

Antihistamine.

Prescribed For

Conjunctivitis (pinkeye) caused by allergies.

General Information

Ketotifen relieves and prevents eye itchiness and irritation associated with seasonal allergies. Lodoxamide only prevents itchiness and allergies. They achieve their effects by stabilizing mast cells in the eye, which prevents the release of chemicals such as histamine that cause redness and irritation during an allergic reaction. Ketotifen starts working within minutes after administering the drops. This drug has not been studied in children under age 3. Lodoxamide may be used in children age 2 and over.

Cautions and Warnings

Do not use this drug if you are **sensitive** or **allergic** to it.

Possible Side Effects

▼ Most common: eye redness, headache, and runny nose.

▼ Less common: a burning or stinging sensation in the eye, eye discharge, tearing, increased sensitivity to bright light, dilation of the pupil, allergic reactions, rash, flu-like symptoms, and sore throat.

Drug Interactions

• If you use more than 1 eyedrop medication, separate doses of these drugs by at least 1 hour.

Usual Dose

Ketotifen: Adults and children age 3 and over—1 drop in affected eye every 8–12 hours.

Lodoxamide: Adults and children age 2 and over—1 drop in affected eye 4 times a day.

Overdosage

Accidental ingestion of an entire bottle of ketotifen is unlikely to cause side effects since it contains less than 2 mg of medicine. Call your local poison control center or a hospital emergency room for more information. If you seek treatment, ALWAYS bring the prescription bottle or container.

Special Information

Do not wear contact lenses if your eyes are red because they may worsen the irritation.

Ketotifen does not alleviate eye irritation caused by contact lenses.

Remove your soft contact lenses before using ketotifen eyedrops; you may replace them 10 minutes after a dose.

To prevent contamination, do not allow the eyedropper to touch your fingers, eyelids, or any surface.

If you forget to administer a dose, do so as soon as you remember. If it is almost time for your next dose, skip the dose you forgot and continue with your regular schedule. Do not take a double dose.

Special Populations

Pregnancy/Breast-feeding
In animal studies, very large dosages of ketotifen caused bone malformations in the fetus. When this drug is considered crucial by your doctor, its potential benefits must be carefully weighed against its risks.

Though unlikely, ketotifen may pass into breast milk. Nursing mothers who must use this drug should consider bottle-feeding.

Seniors
Seniors may use this drug without special precaution.

Generic Name

Labetalol (luh-BET-uh-lol) [G]

Brand Names

Normodyne   Trandate

Type of Drug

Adrenergic blocker and antihypertensive.

Prescribed For

Hypertension (high blood pressure).

General Information

Labetalol hydrochloride is unique because it selectively blocks both alpha- and beta-adrenergic impulses. This combination of actions contributes to its ability to reduce blood pressure. Other drugs can increase or decrease heart rate; labetalol has an advantage over other beta blockers because it rarely affects heart rate.

Cautions and Warnings

People with **asthma, chronic bronchitis, emphysema,** severe **heart failure, reduced heart rate,** and **heart block** (disruption of the electrical impulses that control heart rate) should not take labetalol. People with **angina** who take labetalol for hypertension risk aggravating their angina if they suddenly stop taking the drug. These people should have their dosage reduced gradually over 1 to 2 weeks. Labetalol should be used with caution if you have **liver disease**.

Possible Side Effects

Side effects develop early and increase with dosage.

▼ Most common: dizziness, tingling of the scalp, nausea, vomiting, upset stomach, distortion in the sense of taste, fatigue, sweating, impotence, urinary difficulties, diarrhea, bile-duct blockage, bronchial spasm, breathing difficulties, muscle weakness, cramps, dry eyes, blurred vision, rash, facial swelling, and hair loss.

▼ Less common: aggravation of lupus erythematosus (chronic condition affecting the body's connective tissue), stuffy nose, depression, confusion, disorientation, loss of short-term memory, emotional instability, colitis, drug allergy (symptoms include fever, sore throat, and breathing difficulties), and a reduction in levels of white blood cells and blood platelets.

Drug Interactions

• Labetalol may suppress normal signs of low blood sugar and interfere with the action of oral antidiabetes drugs.

• Combining labetalol and a tricyclic antidepressant may cause tremor.

• Labetalol may interfere with the effect of some anti-asthma drugs, especially ephedrine, isoproterenol, and other beta stimulants.

• Cimetidine increases the amount of labetalol absorbed into the bloodstream from oral tablets.

• Glutethimide decreases the amount of labetalol in the blood.

• Labetalol may increase the blood-pressure-lowering effect of nitroglycerin.

• Use caution when combining labetol with calcium channel blockers.

Food Interactions

This drug may be taken with food if it upsets your stomach. Food increases the amount of labetalol absorbed into the blood.

Usual Dose

Starting dosage—100 mg twice a day; may be increased gradually to as much as 1200 mg twice a day. Maintenance dosage—200–400 mg twice a day.

Overdosage

Overdose slows heart rate and causes an excessive drop in blood pressure. The possible consequences of these effects can be treated only in a hospital emergency room. ALWAYS bring the prescription bottle or container.

Special Information

You may experience scalp tingling, especially when you first start taking labetalol.

Labetalol is meant to be taken on a continuing basis. Do not stop this drug unless instructed to do so by your doctor.

Weakness; swelling of your ankles, feet, or legs; breathing difficulties; or other side effects should be reported to your doctor as soon as possible. Most side effects are not serious, but about 7% of people have to switch to another drug because of them.

If you forget a dose, take it as soon as possible. If it is within 8 hours of your next dose, skip the dose you forgot and go back to your regular schedule. Do not take a double dose.

Special Populations

Pregnancy/Breast-feeding

Labetalol enters the fetal circulation. Women who are or might be pregnant should not take this drug without their doctor's approval. When the drug is considered crucial by your doctor, its possible benefits must be carefully weighed against its risks.

This drug passes into breast milk. Nursing mothers who must take labetalol should consider bottle-feeding.

Seniors

Seniors may be more sensitive to the effects of labetalol. Your dosage must be individually adjusted by your doctor, especially if you have liver disease. Seniors may be more likely to suffer from cold hands and feet, reduced body temperature, chest pain, feeling unwell, sudden breathing difficulties, sweating, or changes in heartbeat.

Generic Name

Lamivudine (lam-IV-ue-dene)

Brand Name

Epivir   Epivir-HBV

Combination Products

Generic Ingredients: Lamivudine + Zidovudine
Combivir

Type of Drug

Antiviral.

Prescribed For

Human immunodeficiency virus (HIV) infection, in combination with other anti-HIV drugs; and hepatitis B.

General Information

Lamivudine, also known as 3-TC, is a nucleoside-type antiviral that works on the HIV virus in the same way as zalcitibine, zidovudine (AZT), stavudine, and other drugs of this type. It is generally given in combination with other antiviral drugs. Lamivudine is eliminated primarily through the kidneys.

Cautions and Warnings

Do not take lamivudine if you are **sensitive** or **allergic** to it.

People with **kidney disease** need less lamivudine than people with normal kidney function.

In some cases, **lactic acidosis** (a potentially fatal metabolic imbalance) and severe **liver enlargement** has been reported with the use of lamivudine. Patients with liver disease should use this drug with caution.

The zidovudine in Combivir has been associated with **low white-blood-cell counts** and severe **anemia.**

Possible Side Effects

Because this drug is always taken with AZT, the listed side effects are those of the drugs in combination. The long-term effects of lamivudine are not known.

▼ Most common: headache, not feeling well, fever, chills, rash, nausea, vomiting, diarrhea, appetite loss, abdominal pain or cramps, nervous system problems including tingling and poor coordination, sleeplessness, dizziness, depression, stuffy or runny nose, cough, and muscle pain.

▼ Common: upset stomach, joint pain, and tingling in the hands or feet in children. Lamivudine may affect the results of a variety of blood tests.

▼ Rare: pancreas irritation, more often seen in children than adults.

Drug Interactions

• Lamivudine increases maximum blood levels of AZT by 39%, which is helpful in fighting the HIV virus.

• Trimethoprim-sulfamethoxazole, taken for opportunistic AIDS-related infections, increases the amount of lamivudine in the blood.

• Lamivudine should not be taken with zalcitabine, as they decrease each other's effectiveness.

Food Interactions

Lamivudine is absorbed more slowly when taken with food, but not enough to affect the total amount of drug that reaches the blood.

Usual Dose

Lamivudine
Adult and Child (age 16 and over): 150 mg twice a day in combination with other antiretroviral agents. Adults who weigh less than 110 lbs. should receive about 1 mg per lb. of body weight twice a day. Dosage is reduced as kidney function decreases. For hepatitis B, take 100 mg once a day.

Child (age 3 months–16 years): about 1.4–2 mg per lb. of body weight twice a day, no more than 150 mg per dose.

Lamivudine-Zidovudine

Adult and Child: 1 tablet—lamivudine 150 mg plus zidovudine 300 mg—twice a day. Poor kidney or liver function requires reducing the dosage of both drugs. In this situation, it is preferable to take the individual drugs separately so that you retain maximum dosage flexibility.

Overdosage

Little is known about the effects of lamivudine overdose. Call your local poison control center for more information.

Special Information

Lamivudine does not cure AIDS. It will not prevent you from transmitting the HIV virus to another person; you must still practice safe sex. People taking this drug will still develop opportunistic infections and other complications of AIDS.

It is very important to take lamivudine exactly as prescribed. If you forget a dose, take it as soon as you remember. If it is almost time for your next dose, skip the dose you forgot and continue with your regular schedule. Call your doctor if you forget 2 or more doses in a row.

Call your doctor at once if your child develops signs of pancreas inflammation while taking lamivudine. Symptoms include very severe abdominal pain, tense abdominal muscles, sweating, feeling very ill, shallow and rapid breathing, fever, and possible fainting.

Special Populations

Pregnancy/Breast-feeding

Lamivudine passes into the blood circulation of the fetus. Some animal studies of lamivudine indicate that it may be dangerous to the fetus, but others showed no effect. There is no information about the effect of lamivudine in pregnant women. Like all drugs, lamivudine should be taken during pregnancy only if absolutely necessary.

It is not known if lamivudine passes into breast milk. Nursing mothers who must take lamivudine should bottle-feed. In any case, nursing mothers who are HIV positive should bottle-feed to avoid transmitting the virus through their milk.

Seniors

Seniors may require a smaller dose of lamivudine, depending on their kidney function. Otherwise, seniors may take this drug without special restriction.

Generic Name

Lamotrigine (lam-OE-trih-jene)

Brand Names

Lamictal   Lamictal CD

Type of Drug

Anticonvulsant.

Prescribed For

Adult epilepsy and partial seizure; also prescribed for tonic-clonic, absence, and myoclonic seizures, bipolar disorder, and for infants and children with Lennox-Gastaut syndrome.

General Information

Much like phenytoin and carbamazepine, lamotrigine stabilizes voltage-dependent channels in the brain. This prevents the release of chemicals that would stimulate the nervous system and lead to seizure. It reaches maximum blood concentration in 1½ to 5 hours. Lamotrigine is eliminated from the body by the liver.

Cautions and Warnings

Lamotrigine may cause severe and possibly **life-threatening rashes,** nearly always within 2 to 8 weeks of use. Minor rashes also occur, but it is not possible to tell which ones may become life threatening. If you develop a rash while taking this drug, call your doctor at once.

Twenty sudden and **unexplained deaths** occurred among 4700 people taking lamotrigine before it was approved for general use. These deaths are thought to be unrelated to lamotrigine.

Five people taking lamotrigine died from acute **liver failure** or **multi-organ failure** before the drug was approved for general use. It is not known if the drug played a role in these deaths.

Lamotrigine is not recommended for general use in **children under age 16**.

Lamotrigine binds to melanin, a body hormone found in the skin and eyes. The long-term effects of lamotrigine on the eyes are not known.

When you stop taking lamotrigine, the dose should be reduced gradually over a period of 2 weeks or more to prevent **withdrawal seizures**.

Status epilepticus, a severe seizure disorder, and **worsening of existing seizure disorders** may develop in a small number of people taking lamotrigine.

People with **heart disease** or severe **kidney or liver disease** should use this drug with caution.

Lamotrigine may cause unusual **sensitivity to the sun**. Wear protective clothing and use sunscreen.

Possible Side Effects

▼ Most common: headache, dizziness, nausea, weakness, tiredness, runny nose, double vision, and blurred vision.

▼ Common: accidental injury, flu-like symptoms, abdominal pain, vomiting, infection, neck pain, feeling unwell, worsening of seizure, diarrhea, upset stomach, constipation, dental problems, loss of coordination, sleeplessness, tremors, depression, anxiety, convulsions, irritability, itching, visual difficulties, painful menstruation, and vaginal irritation.

▼ Less common: chills, hot flashes, heart palpitations, appetite loss, dry mouth, joint ache, muscle weakness, speech disorders, sore throat, coughing, speech problems involving the tongue, memory loss, confusion, loss of concentration, sleep disorders, emotional upset, fainting, racing thoughts, rolling of the eyes, muscle spasm, breathing difficulties, hair loss, acne, ear pain, ringing or buzzing in the ears, and missed periods.

▼ Rare: Rare side effects can occur in almost any part of the body. Contact your doctor if you experience any side effect not listed above.

Drug Interactions

• Combining lamotrigine and sodium valproate doubles lamotrigine concentrations in the blood and reduces those of valproate by ¼. Dosage adjustments are necessary. Combining these drugs also increases the risk of rash.

• Combining carbamazepine and lamotrigine increases carbamazepine blood levels, possibly leading to side effects, and reduces the amount of lamotrigine in the blood by 40%.

• Combining acetaminophen and lamotrigine can slightly increase the rate at which lamotrigine is broken down, but occasional use of the two drugs together is not likely to be a problem. Regular acetaminophen users may require more lamotrigine.

• Anti-folate drugs—often used in cancer treatment—can increase the effects of lamotrigine.

• Phenobarbital and primidone may reduce the effects of lamotrigine.

• Phenytoin reduces the amount of lamotrigine in the blood by about ½.

• Rifamycins, succinimides, oral contraceptives, progestins, and oxcarbazepine may reduce the effectiveness of lamotrigine.

Food Interactions

None known.

Usual Dose

Adult and Child (age 12 and over): starting dosage—25 or 50 mg a day. Increase gradually to a maximum daily dosage of 500 mg. Lamotrigine is usually taken twice a day; be sure to take your doses 12 hours apart.

Child (under age 12): consult your physician.

Overdosage

Symptoms include dizziness, headache, sleepiness, and coma. Take the victim to a hospital emergency room at once. ALWAYS bring the prescription bottle or container.

Special Information

Dosage increases may be required if your liver starts breaking down the drug faster over time. Periodic monitoring of lamotrigine blood levels is necessary to determine this.

People with impaired kidney or liver function may require smaller dosages.

Call your doctor at once if you develop a rash, but do not change your lamotrigine dosage or stop taking it.

Lamotrigine may cause drowsiness, dizziness, or blurred vision, effects that are increased by alcohol. Be careful while driving or engaging in any activity requiring concentration, alertness, and coordination.

If you take acetaminophen while you are taking lamotrigine, especially for a lamotrigine headache, do not take more acetaminophen than is recommended on the package.

If you take lamotrigine once a day and forget a dose, take it as soon as you remember. If it is within 8 hours of your next dose, skip the one you forgot and continue with your regular schedule. Do not take a double dose.

After the first 2 weeks of treatment, most people take lamotrigine twice a day. If you take it twice a day, be sure to take your medication every 12 hours. If you forget a dose, take it as soon as you remember. If it is within 4 hours of your next dose, take 1 dose as soon as you remember and another in 5 or 6 hours, then go back to your regular schedule.

Special Populations

Pregnancy/Breast-feeding

Animal studies suggest that lamotrigine causes fetal injury. It reduces the amount of folate in the fetus, an effect that is associated with birth defects. Seizure disorder itself also increases the risk of birth defects. Pregnant women should take lamotrigine only after discussing with their doctors its potential benefits and risks.

Lamotrigine passes into breast milk. Nursing mothers who must take it should bottle-feed.

Seniors

Seniors may take lamotrigine without special restriction.

Lanoxin   *see Digoxin, page 358*

Lantus   *see Insulin page 572*

Generic Name

Leflunomide (leh-FLUE-noe-mide)

Brand Name

Arava

Type of Drug

Anti-inflammatory and antiproliferative (cell growth slower).

Prescribed For

Rheumatoid arthritis.

General Information

Leflunomide can help relieve symptoms of rheumatoid arthritis and slow the structural damage and erosion of tissues in affected joints. In studies, it was found to be as effective as methotrexate and sulfasalazine. It takes about a month for leflunomide to begin working and it reaches maximum effect in 3 to 6 months. The maximum effect is retained for as long as you take this medicine. Leflunomide is broken down in the liver.

Cautions and Warnings

Leflunomide should not be taken during **pregnancy.**

People who are **sensitive** or **allergic** to leflunomide should not take it.

Leflunomide causes **liver irritation** and an increase in certain liver enzymes. Your dosage may have to be reduced or the drug discontinued if the effect is severe. People with **hepatitis B or C** should not take this drug. People with **kidney problems** should use it with caution.

Leflunomide is not recommended for people with severely **depressed immune systems, abnormal bone marrow,** or severe and uncontrolled **infection.**

Use of **live-virus vaccines** is not recommended while taking leflunomide.

Possible Side Effects

▼ Most common: diarrhea, high blood pressure, nausea, hair loss, rash, and respiratory infection.

▼ Common: headache, upset stomach, stomach or abdominal pain, abnormal liver function, bronchitis,

Possible Side Effects *(continued)*

generalized pain, back pain, urinary infection, and accidents or injuries.

▼ Less common: chest pain, dizziness, tingling in the hands or feet, eczema, mouth ulcer, tooth disorder, itching, dry skin, appetite loss, vomiting, low blood potassium, weight loss, muscle pain, leg cramps, inflamed tendons, arthritis, cough, sore throat, pneumonia, runny nose, sinus irritation, allergic reaction, weakness, flu-like symptoms, and infections.

▼ Rare: Rare side effects can occur in almost any part of the body. Contact your doctor if you experience any side effect not listed above.

Drug Interactions

• Cholestyramine and charcoal rapidly reduce leflunomide blood levels.

• Rifampin increases the amount of leflunomide in the blood by 40%.

• Leflunomide can increase the liver toxicity of other drugs that are toxic to the liver, such as methotrexate.

• Leflunomide increases blood levels of nonsteroidal anti-inflammatory drugs (NSAIDs). The importance of this effect is unclear.

• Leflunomide increases the amount of tolbutamide (an antidiabetes drug) in the blood by up to 50%. The importance of this effect is unclear.

Food Interactions

Leflunomide may be taken without regard to food or meals.

Usual Dose

Adult: 100 mg a day for 3 days, then 20 mg once a day.
Child: not recommended.

When you stop taking leflunomide, it is recommended that you follow a drug elimination procedure: Take 8 g of cholestyramine (ordinarily used to help lower blood cholesterol) 3 times a day for 11 days. Without this procedure, it may take up to 2 years to eliminate the drug and its breakdown products from your body.

Overdosage

Symptoms are likely to include drug side effects. Take the victim to a hospital emergency room at once. ALWAYS bring the prescription bottle or container.

Special Information

Your liver function must be monitored regularly while you take this drug.

If you forget a dose, take it as soon as you remember. If it is almost time for your next dose, skip the one you forgot and continue with your regular schedule.

Special Populations

Pregnancy/Breast-feeding

Leflunomide causes birth defects and should not be used during pregnancy. Women of childbearing age must be tested for pregnancy before taking leflunomide and use effective contraception during treatment. Women who plan to become pregnant after discontinuing the drug must follow the drug elimination procedure (see "Usual Dose").

Leflunomide may pass into breast milk. Nursing mothers who must take it should bottle-feed.

Seniors

Seniors may take this drug without special precaution.

Type of Drug

Leukotriene Antagonists/Inhibitors

(LUE-koe-treen)

Brand Names

Generic Ingredient: Montelukast
Singulair

Generic Ingredient: Zafirlukast
Accolate

Generic Ingredient: Zileuton
Zyflo

Prescribed For

Asthma.

General Information

Leukotrienes play an important role in the body's allergic response. They are associated with the swelling of tissues and tightening of muscles in the throat that cause the throat to close during an asthma attack. Leukotriene receptor antagonists (montelukast and zafirlukast) help to prevent attacks by blocking leukotriene from binding to special tissue receptors. Zileuton interferes with the formation of leukotriene and has no effect on the receptor. When taken on a regular basis, these drugs can reduce the number of asthma attacks you experience but do not treat them once they occur; other drugs must be used to treat attacks.

Cautions and Warnings

Do not take any of these drugs if you are **allergic** or **sensitive** to them. It may be possible to be sensitive to one drug and tolerate another.

Avoid aspirin and other nonsteroidal anti-inflammatory drugs (NSAIDs) if they have triggered an asthma attack in the past. These drugs may not offer protection against **NSAID-related asthma attacks**.

Keep your regular inhalants and other asthma drugs handy at all times in case you have an asthma attack. These drugs do not prevent all attacks.

People age 56 and older taking zafirlukast reported more mild to moderate **respiratory infections** than those taking a placebo (sugar pill). Infections were more common in people taking larger dosages of zafirlukast and among those who took zafirlukast with an inhaled corticosteroid.

People with **cirrhosis of the liver** may require lower dosages of zafirlukast and montelukast.

People taking zileutron should have their liver enzymes measured periodically by their doctor.

Possible Side Effects

▼ Most common: headache.

▼ Less common: flu, dizziness, upset stomach, gastroenteritis (inflammation of the mucous lining of the

Possible Side Effects *(continued)*

stomach and intestine), cough, stuffy nose, abdominal pain, hypersensitivity reactions, dream abnormalities, drowsiness, irritability, and restlessness.

▼ Rare: dental pain, rash, fever, injuries, weakness, and tiredness.

Zafirlukast
▼ Most common: headache.
▼ Less common: nausea, diarrhea, and infections.
▼ Rare: dizziness, abdominal pain, vomiting, generalized pain, weakness, accidental injury, muscle aches, fever, back pain, liver inflammation, and upset stomach.

Zileuton
▼ Most common: headache.
▼ Common: general pains, upset stomach, nausea, and liver inflammation.
▼ Less common: abdominal pain, weakness, accidental injury, and muscle aches.
▼ Rare: joint pain, chest pain, eye redness, constipation, dizziness, fever, gas, muscle stiffness, sleeplessness, swollen lymph glands, feeling unwell, neck pain or rigidity, nervousness, itching, tiredness, urinary infections, vaginal inflammation, vomiting, and jaundice.

Drug Interactions

Montelukast
• Phenobarbital and rifampin can reduce blood levels of montelukast, but dosage adjustment is not needed.

Zafirlukast
• Aspirin increases the amount of zafirlukast in the blood by 45%.
• Zafirlukast may increase the effects of other drugs broken down in the liver.
• Erythromycin, terfenadine, and theophylline may reduce zafirlukast's effectiveness.
• Zafirlukast increases the effects of astemizole, carbamazepine, cyclosporine, felodipine, isradipine, nicardipine, nifedipine, nimodipine, phenytoin, tolbutamide, and warfarin.

Zileuton
• Alcohol use and liver disease may increase the risk of serious side effects.
• Zileuton increases the effects of astemizole, beta-blockers, cisapride, cyclosporine, felodipine, isradipine, nicardipine, nifedipine, nimodipine, theophylline, and warfarin. Dosage adjustments are necessary.

Food Interactions

Zileuton and montelukast may be taken with or without food. For optimal effectiveness, take each dose of zafirlukast at least 1 hour before or 2 hours after meals.

Usual Dose

Montelukast
  Adult and Child (age 15 and over): 10 mg every evening.
  Child (age 6–14): 5-mg chewable tablet every evening.

Zafirlukast
  Adult and Child (age 12 and over): 20 mg 2 times a day. Take this medication on an empty stomach, at least 1 hour before or 2 hours after meals.
  Child (age 5–11): 10 mg 2 times a day.
  Child (age 2–5): 4-mg chewable tablet every evening.

Zileuton
  Adult and Child (age 12 and over): 600 mg 4 times a day.
  Child (under age 12): not recommended.

Overdosage

Little is known about the effects of overdose. Call your local poison control center or a hospital emergency room for more information. If you seek treatment, ALWAYS bring the prescription bottle or container.

Special Information

These drugs must be taken on a regular basis to prevent asthma attacks. You should continue taking them even if you are having an asthma attack, unless instructed by your doctor to stop.

Your dosage of inhaled corticosteroids, commonly used for asthma prevention, may be gradually reduced if you take these drugs. This reduction should be gradual and occur only under your doctor's supervision. Do not stop using your corticosteroid inhaler without your doctor's knowledge.

Call your doctor if, after starting on leukotriene antago-nist/inhibitor, your need for your regular asthma drug increases.

If you forget a dose, take it as soon as you remember. If it is almost time for your next dose, skip the one you forgot and continue with your regular schedule. Do not take a double dose.

Special Populations

Pregnancy/Breast-feeding

Montelukast passes into fetal circulation. Zafirlukast and zileuton have harmed the fetus in animal studies. When any of these drugs is considered crucial by your doctor, its potential benefits must be carefully weighed against its risks.

These drugs may pass into breast milk. Nursing mothers who must take any of these drugs should bottle-feed.

Seniors

In studies, people age 55 and older who took zafirlukast reported more infections (see "Cautions and Warnings"). Seniors taking this drug may require reduced dosage.

Generic Name

Levamisole (lee-VAM-ih-sole)

Brand Name

Ergamisol

Type of Drug

Immune-system modulator.

Prescribed For

Duke's stage-C colon cancer, together with fluorouracil; also prescribed for malignant melanoma after surgery in people in whom the disease has not metastasized (spread).

General Information

Levamisole hydrochloride can restore depressed immune function. It stimulates the formation of antibodies to various agents, enhances T-cell response by stimulating and activating these important immune-system cells, and stimulates the infection-fighting and other functions of white blood cells. The exact way that it works in concert with fluorouracil is not known. In a clinical study of levamisole and Duke's stage-C colon cancer, survival rates were improved by 27% for levamisole plus fluorouracil and 28% for levamisole alone. The reduced recurrence rate for the disease was 36% for the drug combination and 28% for levamisole alone. Another study showed 33% improved survival and 41% reduction in disease recurrence for the 2 drugs. Levamisole is broken down in the liver.

Cautions and Warnings

Do not take levamisole if you are **allergic** to it.

People taking levamisole may develop **agranulocytosis** (a drastic reduction in the number of white blood cells) suddenly and without warning. Common symptoms of agranulocytosis are fever, chills, and flu-like symptoms. Regular blood monitoring is necessary while you are on levamisole: Your doctor may suddenly stop treatment if blood tests indicate the development of this problem, which may go away when you stop the drug.

Possible Side Effects

Virtually everyone taking fluorouracil and levamisole experiences side effects, which are due to either or both drugs. Some people decide to stop drug treatment because of side effects such as rash, joint and muscle aches, fever, white-blood-cell reduction, urinary infection, and cough.

▼ Most common: nausea, vomiting, diarrhea, mouth sores, appetite loss, abdominal pain, constipation, a metallic taste, joint and muscle aches, dizziness, headache, tingling in the hands or feet, white-blood-cell reduction, rash, hair loss, fatigue, sleepiness, fever, chills, and infection.

▼ Less common: reduced platelet levels, itching, upset stomach, gas, changes in sense of smell, depression, nervousness, sleeplessness, anxiety, blurred vision, and eye redness.

▼ Rare: peeling rash, swelling around the eyes, vaginal bleeding, severe allergic reaction (symptoms include

---

Possible Side Effects *(continued)*

breathing difficulties, rash, intense itching, and elevated pulse), confusion, convulsions, hallucinations, loss of concentration, and kidney failure.

Drug Interactions

• Combining levamisole and alcohol may cause severe side effects.

• Combining phenytoin with fluorouracil and levamisole may increase phenytoin blood levels and the risk of side effects.

Food Interactions

None known.

Usual Dose

Colon Cancer: 50 mg every 8 hours for 3 days starting 7–30 days after surgery; then 50 mg every 8 hours for 3 days every 2 weeks.

Malignant Melanoma: 2.5 mg once daily for 2 consecutive days each week.

Overdosage

Levamisole overdose is potentially fatal. The most likely symptoms are severe side effects including those that affect the blood system, stomach, and intestines. Take the victim to a hospital emergency room at once. ALWAYS bring the prescription bottle or container.

Special Information

Call your doctor if you develop any side effects, especially fever, chills, or flu-like symptoms.

Taking more than the recommended dosage of levamisole increases side-effect risk without improving the drug's effectiveness. Carefully follow your doctor's directions.

If you forget a dose, call your doctor. Do not take the dose you forgot and do not take a double dose.

Special Populations

Pregnancy/Breast-feeding

Animal studies indicate that levamisole may injure the fetus. When this drug is considered crucial by your doctor, its potential benefits must be carefully weighed against its risks. Use effective contraceptive measures to be sure that you do not become pregnant while taking levamisole and fluorouracil.

Levamisole may pass into breast milk. Nursing mothers who must take levamisole should bottle-feed.

Seniors

Seniors may take this drug without special restriction.

Levaquin *see Fluoroquinolone Anti-Infectives,*

page 495

Generic Name

Levetiracetam (leh-veh-tir-ASS-eh-tam)

Brand Name

Keppra

Type of Drug

Antiepileptic.

Prescribed For

Partial onset seizures.

General Information

Levetiracetam works differently than other antiepileptic drugs. While it does not affect any pathway known to either block or stimulate nerve transmissions, research shows that it can help prevent seizures in adults with epilepsy. Levetiracetam is always prescribed in combination with other antiepileptics.

Cautions and Warnings

Do not take this drug if you are **sensitive** or **allergic** to it. People with **kidney problems** require reduced dosage.

Levetiracetam is a **nervous system depressant** and can cause **fatigue, sleepiness, poor coordination,** and **behavioral changes** (including psychosis), most commonly during the first 4 weeks of treatment.

Levetiracetam can cause **reductions in white- and red-blood-cell counts**. Your doctor will evaluate your blood components periodically.

People with **impaired kidney function** should use levetiracetam with caution.

Possible Side Effects

▼ Most common: tiredness, weakness, dizziness, and infection.

▼ Common: pain and sore throat.

▼ Less common: appetite loss, memory loss, anxiety, poor muscle coordination, depression, emotional upset, hostility, nervousness, tingling in the hands or feet, fainting, cough, runny nose, sinus irritation, and double vision.

▼ Rare: muscle aches, diarrhea, constipation, stomach problems, chest pain, black and blue marks, fever, flu-like symptoms, convulsions, sleeplessness, rash, middle ear infection, tremors, swollen gums, and weight gain.

Food and Drug Interactions

None known.

Usual Dose

Adult: 500–1500 mg twice a day.

Overdosage

Symptoms may include drowsiness. Call your local poison control center or a hospital emergency room for more information. If you seek treatment, ALWAYS bring the prescription bottle or container.

Special Information

Levetiracetam must be discontinued gradually. Stopping the drug too suddenly can lead to "withdrawal seizures."

Levetiracetam causes dizziness and tiredness. Be careful when driving or performing any task that requires concentration.

Call your doctor if you become pregnant or are planning on becoming pregnant while taking this medication.

If you forget a dose, take it as soon as you remember. If it is almost time for your next dose, skip the one you forgot and continue with your regular schedule. Do not take a double dose.

Special Populations

Pregnancy/Breast-feeding

Animal studies show that levetiracetam can cause birth defects. When this drug is considered crucial by your doctor, its potential benefits must be carefully weighed against its risks.

This drug may pass into breast milk. Nursing mothers who must take it should bottle-feed.

Seniors

Seniors should receive lower dosages.

Generic Name

Levodopa (lee-voe-DOE-puh) G

Brand Names

Dopar   Larodopa

Type of Drug

Antiparkinsonian.

Prescribed For

Parkinson's disease, restless leg syndrome, and herpes zoster (shingles).

General Information

When levodopa—also known as L-dopa—enters the brain, it is converted to dopamine, a chemical found in the central nervous system and deficient in people with Parkinson's disease. Some people who take levodopa develop the "on-off" phenomenon, in which they suddenly lose all drug effect and then regain it minutes or hours later. About 15% to 40% of people with Parkinson's disease develop this phenomenon after 2 to 3 years of levodopa treatment. The on-off effect becomes more frequent after 5 years and may result in a gradual decline in drug effect.

Cautions and Warnings

People with a history of **heart attacks,** severe **heart or lung disease, glaucoma, asthma,** or **kidney, liver, or hormone disease** should be cautious about using this drug. Do not take it if you have a history of stomach **ulcer.** People with a history of **psychosis** must be treated with extreme care; this drug can cause depression with suicidal tendencies. Levodopa may activate an existing **malignant melanoma:** People with a family history of melanoma or suspicious skin lesions should not take this drug.

Possible Side Effects

▼ Most common: muscle spasms or inability to control arm, leg, or facial muscles; appetite loss; nausea; vomiting, with or without stomach pain; dry mouth; drooling; difficulty eating due to poor muscle control; tiredness; hand tremors; headache; dizziness; numbness; weakness or a faint feeling; confusion; sleeplessness; grinding of the teeth; nightmares; euphoria (feeling "high"); hallucinations; delusions; agitation; anxiousness; and feeling unwell.

▼ Less common: heart irregularities or palpitations; dizziness when standing or rising, particularly in the morning; changes in mental state, including depression with or without suicidal tendencies, paranoia, and loss of intellectual function; difficulty urinating; muscle twitching; burning sensation on the tongue; bitter taste in the mouth; diarrhea; constipation; unusual breathing patterns; blurred or double vision; hot flashes; weight gain or loss; darkening of the urine; and increased perspiration.

▼ Rare: stomach bleeding, ulcer, high blood pressure, convulsions, adverse effects on the blood, difficulty

Possible Side Effects *(continued)*

controlling eye muscles, stimulation, hiccups, hair loss, hoarseness, decreasing size of male genitalia, and fluid retention.

Drug Interactions

• Anticholinergic drugs such as trihexyphenidyl decrease levodopa's effects. Other drugs that may interfere with levodopa are benzodiazepine-type tranquilizers and sedatives, phenothiazine antipsychotic medication, phenytoin, methionine, papaverine, pyridoxine, and tricyclic antidepressants.

• Antacids may increase levodopa's effects.

• Metoclopramide may increase levodopa blood levels, levodopa may reduce metoclopramide's effects on the stomach. Levodopa may interact with drugs for high blood pressure to further reduce pressure. Dosage adjustments in the high-blood-pressure medication may be required. Methyldopa (an antihypertensive) may increase levodopa's effects.

• People taking monoamine oxidase inhibitor (MAOI) antidepressants should stop taking them at least 2 weeks before starting on levodopa.

Food Interactions

Take each dose with food to avoid upset stomach. A low-protein diet may help to minimize variations in drug response that occur in some people. Do not take vitamin preparations that contain vitamin B_6 (pyridoxine), which decreases the effectiveness of levodopa.

Usual Dose

0.5–8 g a day.

Overdosage

Take the victim to a hospital emergency room immediately. ALWAYS bring the prescription bottle or container.

Special Information

Be careful when driving or performing any task that requires concentration.

Call your doctor immediately if you experience: fainting, dizziness, or light-headedness; abnormal results in diabetic urine tests; uncontrollable movements of the face, eyelids, mouth, tongue, neck, arms, hands, or legs; mood changes; palpitations or irregular heartbeats; difficulty urinating; or severe nausea or vomiting.

If you forget a dose, take it as soon as possible. If it is within 2 hours of your next dose, skip the dose you forgot and go back to your regular schedule. Do not take a double dose.

Special Populations

Pregnancy/Breast-feeding
Animal studies indicate that levodopa may interfere with fetal development. Pregnant women should take levodopa only when it is absolutely necessary.

Levodopa may pass into breast milk. Nursing mothers who must take it should bottle-feed.

Seniors
Seniors may require smaller dosages and are more likely to experience abnormal heart rhythms and other cardiac effects, especially if they have heart disease.

Lexapro *see Selective Serotonin Reuptake Inhibitors (SSRIs) , page 965*

Brand Name

Lexxel

Generic Ingredients
Enalapril + Felodipine

Type of Drug
Antihypertensive combination.

Prescribed For
Hypertension (high blood pressure).

General Information

Lexxel contains 5 mg of felodipine, a calcium channel blocker, and 5 mg of enalapril, an angiotensin-converting enzyme (ACE) inhibitor. The two drugs in this combination belong to widely prescribed groups of hypertension medication. Lexxel is not meant for the initial treatment of hypertension. Most people taking this product have taken one of the ingredients as an individual pill and need more medication to control their blood pressure.

Felodipine works by blocking the passage of calcium into heart and smooth-muscle tissue, especially the smooth muscle found in arteries. Since calcium is an essential factor in muscle contraction, any drug that affects calcium in this way will interfere with the contraction of these muscles. This causes the veins to dilate (widen), reducing blood pressure. Also, the amount of oxygen used by these muscles is reduced.

ACE inhibitors such as enalapril work by preventing the conversion of a hormone called angiotensin I to another hormone called angiotensin II, a potent blood-vessel constrictor. Preventing this conversion relaxes blood vessels and helps to reduce blood pressure and relieve the symptoms of heart failure. Enalapril's effect on other hormones may also help to promote blood-vessel dilation. It begins working about 1 hour after you take it and continues to work for 24 hours.

Cautions and Warnings

Do not take Lexxel if you are **sensitive** or **allergic** to either ingredient. Rarely, it causes **very low blood pressure**. It may also affect your **kidneys,** especially if you have **congestive heart failure (CHF).** Your doctor should check your urine for protein content during the first few months of treatment.

Enalapril may affect **white-blood-cell counts,** possibly increasing your susceptibility to **infection.** Your doctor should monitor your blood counts periodically.

People taking a beta-blocking drug who begin taking felodipine may develop **heart failure** or increased **angina pain**. Angina pain may also increase if your felodipine dosage is increased. People with severe **liver disease** break down felodipine much more slowly than those with less severe disease or normal livers.

A sudden, painless **swelling** in the hands, face, feet, lips, tongue, or throat may develop while you are taking any ACE inhibitor. If this happens, you must call your doctor and stop taking the medication at once. This condition usually goes away on its own, though antihistamines may also prove helpful.

Possible Side Effects

Calcium-channel-blocker side effects are generally mild. Side effects are more common with higher dosages and increasing age.

▼ Most common: swelling in the ankles, feet, and legs; dizziness; light-headedness; muscle weakness or cramps; facial flushing; headache; fatigue; nausea; and chronic (long-term) cough. The cough usually goes away a few days after you stop taking the medication.

▼ Less common: respiratory infection, cough, tingling in the hands or feet, upset stomach, abdominal pain, chest pain, nausea, constipation, diarrhea, heart palpitations, sore throat, runny nose, back pain, rash, angina (condition characterized by brief attacks of chest pain), dizziness when rising from a sitting or lying position, fainting, vomiting, bronchitis, urinary tract infection, breathing difficulties, and weakness.

▼ Rare: Rare side effects can affect your heart, muscles and joints, stomach and intestines, sexual function, kidney or liver, and other body parts. Contact your doctor if you experience any side effect not listed above.

Drug Interactions

• The blood-pressure-lowering effect of Lexxel adds to that of diuretic (agent that increases urination) drugs or beta blockers. Any other drug that causes a rapid blood-pressure drop should be used with caution if you are taking Lexxel.

• Lexxel may raise blood-potassium levels, especially when taken with Dyazide or other potassium-sparing diuretics.

• Lexxel may increase the effects of lithium; this combination should be used with caution.

• Capsaicin may cause or aggravate the cough associated with Lexxel therapy.

- Indomethacin may reduce the blood-pressure-lowering effect of Lexxel.
- Phenothiazine tranquilizers and antiemetics may increase the effects of Lexxel.
- Rifampin may reduce the effects of Lexxel.
- Combining allopurinol with Lexxel increases the risk of an adverse drug reaction.
- Cimetidine and ranitidine increase the amount of felodipine in the blood, causing a slight increase in the drug's effect.
- Phenytoin and other hydantoin anti-seizure drugs, carbamazepine, and barbiturate sleeping pills and sedatives may decrease the amount of felodipine in the blood, reducing its effect.
- Erythromycin may increase the side effects of felodipine.
- Felodipine may increase the effects of theophylline (a drug used to treat asthma and other respiratory problems) and oral anticoagulant (blood-thinning) drugs.
- Felodipine may interact with quinidine (an antiarrhythmic) to produce low blood pressure, very slow heart rate, abnormal heart rhythms, and swelling in the arms or legs.

Food Interactions

Lexxel may be taken without regard to food or meals; you may take it with food if it upsets your stomach. Avoid grapefruit juice while you are on Lexxel.

Usual Dose

1 tablet a day.

Overdosage

Overdose may cause low blood pressure. In case of overdose, call your doctor or go to a hospital emergency room. ALWAYS bring the prescription bottle or container.

Special Information

Call your doctor if you develop a sore throat, mouth sores, abnormal heartbeat, chest pain, a persistent rash, loss of taste perception, constipation, nausea, very low blood pressure, breathing difficulties, increased heart pain, dizziness, lightheadedness, or any bothersome or persistent side effect.

Continue taking your medication and follow any instructions for diet restriction or other treatments to help maintain lower blood pressure, even if you feel well. Hypertension may be present without symptoms.

Do not break or crush Lexxel tablets.

Maintain good dental hygiene while taking Lexxel and use extra care when brushing or flossing because of the increased risk of oral infection associated with Lexxel.

Avoid over-the-counter diet pills, decongestants, and stimulants while taking Lexxel; they may raise blood pressure.

If you forget a dose, take it as soon as you remember. If it is almost time for your next dose, skip the dose you forgot and continue with your regular schedule. Do not take a double dose.

Special Populations

Pregnancy/Breast-feeding

Women who are or might be pregnant should not take Lexxel. ACE inhibitors have caused low blood pressure, kidney failure, slow skull formation, and death in the fetus when taken during the last 6 months of pregnancy. Women of childbearing age who must take Lexxel must use an effective contraceptive method. If you become pregnant, stop taking the medication and call your doctor immediately.

Small amounts of enalapril and felodipine pass into breast milk. Nursing mothers who must take Lexxel should consider bottle-feeding.

Seniors

Seniors, especially those with liver disease, may be more sensitive to the drug's effects.

Generic Name

Linezolid (lie-NEZ-oh-lid)

Brand Name

Zyvox

Type of Drug

Antibiotic.

Prescribed For

Staphylococcus, streptococcus, and enterococcus infections.

General Information

Linezolid is the first of a new group of antibiotics for infections that cannot be treated by other antibiotics. It does not kill bacteria, but rather interferes with their reproduction. The oral form of this antibiotic can be directly substituted for the intravenous form. This is helpful for people who may have been started on linezolid in a hospital or emergency room with an intravenous dose and who can then continue taking linezolid at home.

Cautions and Warnings

Colitis has been associated with nearly all antibiotic drugs, including linezolid. Mild colitis usually abates when the drug is stopped, but it is possible for drug-associated colitis to be fatal.

Low levels of different types of blood cells have developed in people taking linezolid, which leads to a higher risk of **bleeding**.

Possible Side Effects

▼ Common: diarrhea, headache, and nausea.

▼ Less common: bleeding due to low blood platelet counts, and vaginal fungus infection.

▼ Rare: dizziness, vomiting, abdominal or stomach pain, taste changes, tongue discoloration, and oral fungus infection.

Drug Interactions

• Linezolid inhibits the enzyme monamine oxidase (MAO). MAO is a key component of the nervous system and linezolid may interact with any stimulant or agent that activates the nervous system, such as dopamine or noradrenaline.

• People taking any antidepressant drugs should be extremely cautious about taking this medicine because of the risk of serious and even fatal reactions. This applies to both the SSRI antidepressants and the tricyclic antidepressants. Two weeks should elapse between stopping the antidepressant and starting linezolid.

• Mixing linezolid with anesthetics, barbiturates, antidiabetes drugs, beta blockers, bupropion, buspirone, carbamazepine, cyclobenzaprine, methyldopa, meperidine, rauwolfia drugs, sulfa drugs, sumatriptan, and diuretics can lead to severely exaggerated drug side effects.

• Mixing linezolid with dextromethorphan may lead to severe reactions including high fever, abnormal muscle movement, psychosis, coma, and low blood pressure.

• The stimulant and blood pressure effects of levodopa, pseudoephedrine, phenylephrine, and similar agents may be enhanced by linezolid.

Food Interactions

Avoid foods that have been fermented, pickled, aged, or smoked. These include pickles, tap beer, fava beans, cheddar cheese, red wine, soy sauce, sauerkraut, and smoked meats or fish. These foods contain tyramine and can cause very high blood pressure if mixed with linezolid.

Usual Dose

Adult: 800–1200 mg a day for 10–28 days.
Child: consult your physician.

Overdosage

Overdose symptoms may include vomiting, tremors, poor muscle coordination, and reduced activity. Overdose victims should be taken to a hospital emergency room. ALWAYS bring the prescription bottle or container.

Special Information

Be sure to tell your doctor if you have or have had high blood pressure.

Avoid foods that have been pickled, smoked, aged, or fermented.

Linezolid oral suspension contains phenylalanine. The intravenous and oral forms do not.

If you forget a dose of linezolid, take it as soon as you remember. If it is almost time for your next dose, skip the dose you forgot and continue with your regular schedule. Do not take a double dose.

Special Populations

Pregnancy/Breast-feeding

There is no information on the effect of linezolid during pregnancy. When it is considered crucial by your doctor, its potential benefits must be weighed against its risks.

Linezolid passes into the breast milk of laboratory animals

but it is not known if the drug passes into human breast milk. Nursing mothers should consider bottle-feeding.

Seniors

Seniors may take this medication without special restriction.

Lipitor *see Statin Cholesterol-Lowering Agents,*
page 986

Generic Name

Lisinopril (lih-SIN-oe-pril)

Brand Names

Prinivil   Zestril

Combination Products

Generic Ingredients: Lisinopril + Hydrochlorothiazide
Prinzide   Zestoretic

Type of Drug

Angiotensin-converting enzyme (ACE) inhibitor.

Prescribed For

Hypertension (high blood pressure), congestive heart failure, kidney protection in people with diabetes, and improving survival after a heart attack.

General Information

Lisinopril and other ACE inhibitors work by preventing the conversion of a hormone called angiotensin I to another hormone called angiotensin II, a potent blood-vessel constrictor. Preventing this conversion relaxes blood vessels, thus reducing blood pressure and relieving the symptoms of heart failure. Lisinopril also affects the production of other hormones and enzymes that participate in the regulation of blood vessel dilation. Lisinopril begins working about 1 hour after you take it and lasts for 24 hours.

Some people who start taking an ACE inhibitor after they are already on a diuretic (an agent that increases urination) experience a rapid drop in blood pressure after their first doses or when the dosage is increased. To prevent this from happening, you may be told to stop taking the diuretic 2 or 3 days before starting the ACE inhibitor or to increase your salt intake during that time. The diuretic may then be restarted gradually.

Cautions and Warnings

Do not take lisinopril if you have had an **allergic reaction** to it. Occasionally, severe allergic reactions have occurred in people undergoing desensitization treatments or certain kinds of kidney dialysis.

Lisinopril occasionally causes **very low blood pressure**.

Lisinopril can affect your **kidneys,** especially if you have congestive **heart failure**. Your doctor should check your urine for changes during the first few months of treatment. Dosage adjustment is required if you have reduced kidney function.

ACE inhibitors can affect white-blood-cell count, possibly increasing your susceptibility to **infection**. Blood counts should be monitored periodically.

Lisinopril can cause serious injury or death to the fetus if taken during **pregnancy**. Pregnant women should not take lisinopril.

Possible Side Effects

▼ Most common: headache, dizziness, fatigue, low blood pressure, nausea, diarrhea, and chronic cough. The cough is more common in women and usually goes away a few days after the medication is stopped.

▼ Less common: chest pain, vomiting, upset stomach, breathing difficulties, rash, and muscle weakness.

▼ Rare: Rare side effects can affect your muscles and joints, sex drive, liver, mental status, and respiratory tract. Contact your doctor if you experience any side effect not listed above.

Drug Interactions

• The blood-pressure-lowering effect of lisinopril is additive with diuretic drugs and beta blockers. Any other drug that can reduce blood pressure should be used with caution if you are taking an ACE inhibitor.

• Combining 325 mg a day or more of aspirin with lisinopril carries a higher risk of death than taking lower doses (less than 160 mg a day). People taking aspirin to prevent a heart attack should take lower doses of aspirin.

• Lisinopril may increase your blood potassium levels, especially when taken with Dyazide or other potassium-sparing diuretics.

• Lisinopril may increase the effects of lithium; this combination should be used with caution.

• Antacids and lisinopril should be taken at least 2 hours apart.

• Capsaicin may trigger or aggravate lisinopril cough.

• Indomethacin and other NSAIDs may reduce the blood-pressure-lowering effect of lisinopril.

• Phenothiazine tranquilizers and antiemetics may increase the effects of lisinopril.

• The combination of allopurinol and lisinopril increases the chance of side effects.

• Lisinopril may increase or decrease blood levels of digoxin, possibly increasing the chance of digoxin-related side effects.

• Combining lisinopril with antidiabetes drugs or insulin may increase the risk of hypoglycemia.

Food Interactions

None known.

Usual Dose

5–40 mg a day. People with severe kidney disease should begin with 2.5 mg a day; dosage may then be increased up to 5–20 mg a day.

Overdosage

The principal effect of lisinopril overdose is a rapid drop in blood pressure, as evidenced by dizziness or fainting. Take the overdose victim to a hospital emergency room immediately. ALWAYS remember to bring the prescription bottle or container.

Special Information

Unexplained swelling of the face, lips, hands, and feet can also affect the larynx (throat) and tongue and interfere with breathing. If this happens, the victim should be taken to a hospital emergency room at once for treatment. Also, call your doctor if you develop a sore throat, mouth sores, abnormal heartbeat, chest pain, persistent rash, or loss of taste perception.

You may get dizzy if you rise quickly from a sitting or lying position.

Avoid strenuous exercise and very hot weather because heavy sweating or dehydration can cause a rapid drop in blood pressure.

Avoid over-the-counter diet pills, decongestants, and other stimulants that can raise blood pressure.

If you forget to take a dose of lisinopril, take it as soon as you remember. If it is within 8 hours of your next dose, skip the one you forgot and continue with your regular schedule. Do not take a double dose.

Special Populations

Pregnancy/Breast-feeding
ACE inhibitors can cause fetal injury or death. Women who are or might be pregnant should not take lisinopril. Stop taking the medication and contact your doctor if you become pregnant.

It is not known if lisinopril passes into breast milk. Nursing mothers who must take this drug should consider bottle-feeding.

Seniors
Seniors may be more sensitive to the effects of lisinopril due to age-related kidney impairment.

Generic Name

Lithium Carbonate

(LITH-ee-um CAR-buh-nate) Ⓖ

Brand Names

Eskalith	Lithobid
Eskalith CR	Lithonate
Lithane	Lithotabs

The information in this profile also applies to the following drug:

Generic Ingredient: Lithium Citrate [G]
Only available in generic form.

Type of Drug

Antipsychotic and antimanic.

Prescribed For

Bipolar (manic-depressive) disorder, especially suppression of manic attacks or reduction in their number and intensity; also prescribed for cancer and acquired immunodeficiency syndrome (AIDS), premenstrual tension, bulimia, postpartum depression, overactive thyroid, and alcoholism, especially in people who are also depressed. Lithium lotion has been used for genital herpes and dandruff.

General Information

Lithium carbonate and lithium citrate are the only effective antimanic drugs. They reduce the levels of manic episodes and may produce normal activity within the first 3 weeks of treatment. Typical manic symptoms include rapid speech, elation, hyperactive movements, little need for sleep, grandiose ideas, poor judgment, aggressiveness, and hostility.

Cautions and Warnings

Lithium should not be taken by people with **heart or kidney disease, dehydration, low blood sodium,** or those taking **diuretic drugs**. If such people require lithium carbonate, they must be very carefully monitored by their doctors, and hospitalization may be needed until the lithium carbonate dose is stabilized.

A few people treated with both lithium carbonate and haloperidol or another antipsychotic have developed **encephalopathic syndrome** (symptoms include weakness, tiredness, fever, confusion, tremulousness, and uncontrollable muscle spasms). In addition, your doctor may find laboratory indicators of liver or kidney disease. Rarely, this combination of symptoms is followed by irreversible brain damage.

Up to 20% of people on long-term lithium carbonate treatment develop **structural changes in their kidneys** and **reduced kidney function**.

Long-term use of this drug may lead to **reduced thyroid activity, enlargement of the thyroid gland,** and **increased**

blood levels of thyroid-stimulating hormone. All of these conditions may be treated with thyroid hormone replacement therapy. **Overactive thyroid** has occasionally occurred.

Frequent urination and thirst associated with lithium carbonate may be a sign of a condition known as diabetes insipidus, in which the kidney stops responding to a hormone called vasopressin. This causes the kidney to reabsorb water and make concentrated urine. Lithium carbonate may reverse the kidneys' ability to perform this function, but things usually go back to normal when lithium carbonate treatment is stopped, dosage is reduced, or small doses of a thiazide diuretic are taken.

Your lithium carbonate dosage may have to be temporarily reduced if you develop an infection or fever.

Some lithium carbonate products contain tartrazine dyes for coloring purposes. Tartrazine can stimulate allergic responses in some people, including asthma.

Possible Side Effects

Side effects of lithium carbonate are directly related to the amount of drug in the bloodstream.

▼ Most common: fine hand tremor, thirst, and excessive urination, especially when treatment is first started; mild nausea and discomfort during the first few days of treatment.

▼ Less common: diarrhea, vomiting, drowsiness, muscle weakness, poor coordination, giddiness, ringing or buzzing in the ears, and blurred vision.

▼ Rare: Rare side effects can affect muscles and nerves (blackouts, seizures, and dizziness), stomach and intestines, kidneys and urinary tract, skin, and thyroid function. Contact your doctor if you experience any side effect not listed above. Lithium carbonate can also affect tests used to monitor heart and brain function.

Drug Interactions

• When lithium carbonate is combined with haloperidol, weakness, tiredness, fever, or confusion may result. In some people, these symptoms have been followed by permanent brain damage. Also, haloperidol may increase the effect of lithium carbonate.

• Combining lithium carbonate and chlorpromazine may reduce the effect of chlorpromazine and increase the lithium carbonate effect.

• Lithium may interfere with the effectiveness of phenothiazine drugs. Combining these drugs can have serious side effects.

• Lithium carbonate is counteracted by sodium bicarbonate, acetazolamide, urea, mannitol, urinary alkalinizers, and theophylline drugs. Verapamil can lower blood levels of lithium carbonate and reduce the risk of toxicity.

• Lithium's effect may be increased by methyldopa, fluoxetine and other SSRIs, carbamazepine, thiazide and loop diuretics, and nonsteroidal anti-inflammatory drugs (NSAIDs).

• Lithium carbonate may increase the effects of tricyclic antidepressant medications.

• Lithium may interfere with the effectiveness of stimulant drugs.

• Lithium may increase the effects of neuromuscular blocking agents, which can lead to severe respiratory side effects.

Food Interactions

Lithium carbonate should be taken immediately after meals or with food or milk.

Usual Dose

Dosage must be individualized. Most people respond to 1800 mg a day at first in 2 or 3 divided doses. Once the person has responded, daily lithium dosage is reduced to the lowest effective level, usually 300 mg 3–4 times a day.

Overdosage

Toxic blood levels of lithium carbonate are only slightly above the levels required for treatment. Signs of drug toxicity may be diarrhea, vomiting, nausea, tremors, drowsiness, poor coordination, giddiness, weakness, blurred vision, ringing or buzzing in the ears, dizziness, fainting, confusion, muscle twitching, uncontrollable muscle movements, loss of bladder control, worsening of manic symptoms, overactive reflexes, and painful muscles or joints. If any of these symptoms occur, stop taking the medication and call your doctor immediately. ALWAYS bring the prescription bottle or container with you when you go to an emergency room.

Special Information

Lithium carbonate may cause drowsiness. Be cautious while driving or operating hazardous machinery.

Lithium carbonate causes your body to lose sodium (salt). You must maintain a well-balanced diet and drink 8 to 12 glasses of water a day while taking this drug. Excessive sweating or diarrhea may make you more sensitive to side effects.

Call your doctor if you develop diarrhea, vomiting, unsteady walking, tremors, drowsiness, or muscle weakness.

To avoid side effects, your doctor may need to reduce your dosage once manic symptoms decline.

If you forget to take a dose of lithium carbonate, take it as soon as possible. However, if it is within 2 hours of your next dose, or 6 hours if you take the long-acting form, skip the missed dose and go back to your regular schedule. Do not take a double dose. Call your doctor if you miss more than 1 dose.

Special Populations

Pregnancy/Breast-feeding
Lithium can cause heart and thyroid birth defects, especially if taken during the first 3 months of pregnancy. Talk with your doctor about the risks of taking lithium during pregnancy.

Lithium carbonate passes into breast milk. It may cause weak muscle tone, low body temperature, bluish discoloration of the skin, and abnormal heart rhythm in an infant. You should bottle-feed your baby while taking this medication.

Seniors
Seniors are more sensitive to the effects of lithium carbonate. It is potentially toxic to the central nervous system in older adults, even when lithium carbonate blood levels are in the desired range. Seniors are also more likely to develop an underactive thyroid.

Type of Drug

Loop Diuretics

Brand Names

Generic Ingredient: Bumetanide Ⓖ
Bumex

Generic Ingredient: Ethacrynic Acid
Edecrin

Generic Ingredient: Furosemide Ⓖ
Lasix

Generic Ingredient: Torsemide
Demadex

Prescribed For

Congestive heart failure (CHF), cirrhosis of the liver, fluid accumulation in the lungs, kidney dysfunction, high blood pressure, and other conditions where it may be desirable to rid the body of excess fluid. Bumetanide can be used to treat people who urinate frequently at night.

General Information

Stronger than thiazide diuretics, loop diuretics work in a similar fashion. Not only do they affect the same part of the kidney as thiazide diuretics, they also act in another portion called the "loop of Henle." This dual action is what makes loop diuretics so potent. All 4 loop diuretics can be used for the same purposes, but their dosages vary.

Cautions and Warnings

Do not take these drugs if you are **sensitive** or **allergic** to them. People allergic to sulfa drugs may also be allergic to furosemide, torsemide, or bumetanide.

Loop diuretics can cause **depletion of water and electrolytes**. They should not be taken without constant medical supervision. Frequent lab evaluations of electrolytes should be performed during therapy and periodically thereafter. You should not take these drugs if your urine production has been decreased abnormally by kidney disease.

Excessive use of loop diuretics results in **dehydration** or **reduction in blood volume**, and may cause **circulatory collapse** or other related problems, particularly in older adults.

Ringing or buzzing in the ears, hearing loss, deafness, fainting, and a **sensation of fullness in the ears** can occur with these drugs. Hearing usually returns within 24 hours, but some loss may be permanent.

These drugs may worsen systemic **lupus erythematosus. Diarrhea** may occur with ethacrynic acid or furosemide solution. Rarely people taking bumetanide develop **thrombocytopenia** (low blood-platelet count).

People taking a loop diuretic may develop increased levels of total **cholesterol**, low-density lipoprotein (LDL) cholesterol, and triglycerides.

Possible Side Effects

▼ Common: Changes may occur in blood levels of potassium or other electrolytes. Hypokalemia (low blood potassium), may cause dry mouth, excessive thirst, weakness, lethargy, drowsiness, restlessness, muscle pain or cramps, muscular tiredness, low blood pressure, decreased frequency of urination and urine volume, abnormal heart rate, and upset stomach, including nausea and vomiting. Loop diuretics may alter sugar metabolism. If you have diabetes mellitus, you may develop high blood sugar or sugar in the urine. To treat this problem, the dosage of your antidiabetes drugs must be increased.

▼ Less common: abdominal discomfort, nausea, vomiting, diarrhea, rash, dizziness, light-headedness, headache, blurred vision, fatigue, weakness, jaundice (symptoms include yellowing of the skin or whites of the eyes), acute gout attacks, dermatitis and other skin reactions, tingling in the extremities, dizziness upon rising quickly from a sitting or lying position, and anemia.

▼ Rare: a sweet taste in the mouth, a burning sensation in the stomach or mouth, excessive thirst, increased perspiration, and frequent urination.

Drug Interactions

• Loop diuretics increase the effects of other blood-pressure-lowering drugs. This is beneficial and is frequently used to help lower blood pressure in people with hypertension.

• Combining a loop diuretic and digitalis drugs or adrenal corticosteroids increases the risk of developing electrolyte imbalances. Potassium loss caused by loop diuretics significantly increases the toxicity of digitalis.

• Loop diuretics may increase the effect of oral anticoagulants (blood thinners); a dosage adjustment may be needed.

• The dosage of an oral antidiabetes drug—except metformin—may need to be altered if you start taking a loop diuretic.

• The effect of theophylline may be altered by any loop diuretic. Your doctor should check your theophylline levels after you have started on a loop diuretic.

• If you are taking lithium carbonate, you should probably not take a diuretic, which greatly increases the risk of lithium side effects.

• People taking chloral hydrate as a nighttime sedative may, in rare cases, experience hot flashes, high blood pressure, sweating, abnormal heart rhythms, weakness, and nausea when they also take a loop diuretic.

• Periodic hearing loss or ringing or buzzing in the ears may occur if a loop diuretic is taken with cisplatin (an anticancer drug) or an aminoglycoside antibiotic. Make sure your doctor knows you are taking a loop diuretic before giving you an injection of either of these.

• Clofibrate and thiazide diuretics increase the effect of loop diuretics.

• Charcoal tablets, phenytoin, probenecid, and aspirin and other salicylate drugs, or nonsteroidal anti-inflammatory drugs (NSAIDs) may decrease the effectiveness of loop diuretics.

• If you are taking a loop diuretic for high blood pressure or CHF, avoid over-the-counter (OTC) cough, cold, and allergy products, which often contain stimulant drugs that can raise your blood pressure. Check with your pharmacist before taking any OTC drug if you are taking a loop diuretic.

Food Interactions

Furosemide should be taken on an empty stomach at least 1 hour before or 2 hours after meals. The other loop diuretics may be taken with food if they upset your stomach.

Usual Dose

Bumetanide
Generally, 0.5–2 mg a day, up to 10 mg a day. It may also be taken every other day for 3–4 consecutive days followed by 1–2 days off the drug.

Ethacrynic Acid
   Adult: 50–200 mg taken every day or every other day.
   Child: starting dose—25 mg; increase slowly.

Furosemide
   Adult: 20–80 mg a day. Dosages of 600 mg or more a day have been prescribed.
   Child: 0.9 mg per lb. of body weight in a single daily dose. If therapy is not successful, the dosage may be increased in small steps up to 2.7 mg per lb. a day.

Torsemide
   Adult: 5–20 mg once a day. Dosages up to 200 mg may be prescribed.
   Child: not recommended.

Maintenance dosages for all of the loop diuretics are adjusted to individual needs.

Overdosage

Symptoms include dehydration, reduced blood volume, high urine volume, weakness, dizziness, confusion, appetite loss, tiredness, vomiting, circulatory collapse, and cramps. Take the victim to a hospital emergency room. ALWAYS bring the prescription bottle or container.

Special Information

If the amount of urine you produce each day is dropping, or if you suffer from cramps, significant appetite loss, muscle weakness, tiredness, or nausea, contact your doctor immediately.

Loop diuretics are usually taken once a day after breakfast. If a second dose is needed, it should be taken no later than 2 p.m. to avoid nighttime urination.

To avoid the dizziness associated with these drugs, rise slowly and carefully from a sitting or lying position.

Loop diuretics can increase blood sugar. People with diabetes may need their medication adjusted.

Loop diuretics rob your body of potassium. To counteract this effect, be sure to eat high-potassium foods such as bananas, citrus fruits, melons, and tomatoes.

Loop diuretics can increase your sensitivity to the sun. Use sunscreen and wear protective clothing.

If you forget a dose, take it as soon as you remember. If it is almost time for your next dose, skip the one you forgot and

continue with your regular schedule. Do not take a double dose.

Special Populations

Pregnancy/Breast-feeding

Loop diuretics have been used to treat specific conditions in pregnancy, but they should be used only when absolutely necessary.

Furosemide passes into breast milk, and the other loop diuretics may pass into breast milk. Nursing mothers who must take any of these drugs should bottle-feed.

Seniors

Seniors are more sensitive to the effects of these drugs.

Generic Name

Loperamide (loe-PER-uh-mide) Ⓖ

Brand Name

Imodium   Imodium A-D

Type of Drug

Antidiarrheal.

Prescribed For

Acute and chronic diarrhea; also prescribed to reduce the amount of discharge in an ileostomy (surgical procedure in which a hole is made in the small intestine, usually through the abdominal wall).

General Information

Loperamide hydrochloride, which relieves diarrhea but does not address the underlying cause, should be used only for short periods. It works by slowing intestinal movement and affecting the movement of water and salts in the intestines. In some cases antidiarrheals should not be used at all; these drugs may harm people with bowel, stomach, or other diseases. Loperamide is available over-the-counter (OTC) under a variety of brand names. OTC loperamide products are used to treat acute diarrhea and traveler's diarrhea.

Cautions and Warnings

Do not use loperamide if you are **allergic** or **sensitive** to it, if you suffer from diarrhea associated with **colitis,** or if you have an **intestinal infection** of *Escherichia coli, Salmonella,* or *Shigella.*

If you have **ulcerative colitis** and start taking loperamide, stop the drug at once and call your doctor if you develop abdominal problems of any kind.

Possible Side Effects

Incidence of side effects is low. They are most likely to occur when loperamide is taken over longer periods to treat chronic diarrhea.

▼ Most common: stomach and abdominal pain, bloating or other discomfort, constipation, dry mouth, dizziness, tiredness, nausea and vomiting, and drug-sensitivity reactions, including rash.

Drug Interactions

• Loperamide increases the sedative effects of sleeping pills, tranquilizers, and alcohol. Avoid these combinations.

• Loperamide should not be taken with clindamycin or lincomycin, agents that can cause severe and possibly fatal colitis.

Food Interactions

Loperamide should be taken on an empty stomach.

Usual Dose

Acute Diarrhea

Adult and Child (age 12 and over): 4 mg to start, followed by 2 mg after each loose stool, up to 16 mg a day maximum. Improvement should be seen in 2 days.

Child (age 9–12): 2 mg 3 times a day to start, followed by 1 mg per 22 lbs. of body weight after each loose stool, up to 6 mg a day maximum.

Child (age 6–8): 2 mg twice a day to start, followed by 1 mg per 22 lbs. of body weight after each loose stool, up to 4 mg a day maximum.

Child (age 2–5): 1 mg 3 times a day to start, followed by 1 mg per 22 lbs. of body weight after each loose stool, up to 3 mg a day maximum.

Chronic Diarrhea

Adult and Child (age 12 and over): 4 mg to start, followed by 2 mg after each loose stool, until symptoms are controlled. Then dosage should be tailored to individual needs—usually 4–8 mg a day. Loperamide is usually effective within 10 days or not at all.

Overdosage

Symptoms include constipation, irritation of the stomach, and tiredness. Large doses usually cause vomiting. Take the victim to a hospital emergency room immediately. ALWAYS bring the prescription bottle or container.

Special Information

Loperamide depresses the central nervous system (CNS), which may cause drowsiness: Be careful when driving or performing any task that requires concentration.

Loperamide may cause dry mouth. Drink plenty of water or other clear fluids to prevent dehydration due to diarrhea. It is important to maintain a proper diet and drink plenty of fluids to restore normal bowel function.

Call your doctor if diarrhea persists after a few days of loperamide treatment or if you develop abdominal discomfort or pain, fever, or any bothersome or persistent side effect.

If you forget a dose, skip it and go back to your regular schedule. Do not take a double dose.

Special Populations

Pregnancy/Breast-feeding

Loperamide has not been found to cause birth defects; however, women who are or might be pregnant should not take this drug without their doctor's approval. When loperamide is considered crucial by your doctor, its potential benefits must be carefully weighed against its risks.

It is not known if loperamide passes into breast milk. Nursing mothers who must take this drug should consider bottle-feeding.

Seniors

Seniors may be more sensitive to the constipating effects of loperamide.

Generic Name

Loratadine (lor-AH-tuh-dene) G

Brand Names

Alavert   Claritin Reditabs
Claritin   Tavist ND

The information in this profile also applies to the following drug:

Generic Ingredient: Desloratadine
Clarinex   Clarinex RediTabs

Type of Drug

Antihistamine.

Prescribed For

Stuffy and runny nose, itchy eyes, and scratchy throat caused by seasonal allergy and for other symptoms of allergy such as rash, itching, and hives; also prescribed for asthma.

General Information

Antihistamines generally work by blocking the release of histamine (chemical released by body tissue during an allergic reaction) from cells at the H_1 histamine receptor site, drying up secretions of the nose, throat, and eyes. Loratadine causes less sedation than most antihistamines and appears to be just as effective.

Cautions and Warnings

Do not take loratadine if you are **allergic** to it.
   People with **liver disease** and **kidney disease** require reduced dosage.

Possible Side Effects

▼ Less common: headache, dry mouth, drowsiness, and fatigue.
▼ Rare: Rare side effects can occur in almost any part of the body. Contact your doctor if you experience any side effect not listed above.

Drug Interactions

• Loratadine may interact with ketoconazole, ery-thromycin, and theophylline, but the evidence for this inter-action is inconclusive.

• Cimetidine can substantially increase the amount of loratadine in the bloodstream.

• Combine loratadine with MAOIs with caution, as it can increase side effects.

• Combining loratadine with alcohol or nervous system depressants can cause increased nervous system depres-sion.

Food Interactions

Loratadine is best taken on an empty stomach 1 hour before or 2 hours after eating; it may be taken with food or milk if it upsets your stomach. Desloratadine may be taken with or without food.

Usual Dose

Loratadine

Adult and Child (over age 6): 10 mg once a day. People with liver disease should take 10 mg every other day.

Child (age 2–5): 1 tsp. (5 ml) a day of loratadine syrup. Chil-dren with liver disease should take 1 tsp. every other day.

Desloratadine

Adult and Child (age 12 and over): 5 mg once a day. People with liver disease should take one 5 mg tablet every other day.

Child (under age 12): not recommended.

Overdosage

Overdose is likely to cause drowsiness, headache, rapid heartbeat, or severe side effects. Overdose victims should be given ipecac syrup—available at any pharmacy—to make them vomit and should be taken to a hospital emergency room for treatment. Call your local poison control center or hospital emergency room for instructions. ALWAYS bring the prescription bottle or container.

Special Information

Dizziness or fainting may be the first sign of a serious side effect. Call your doctor at once if this happens to you. Also report sore throat; unusual bleeding, bruising, tiredness, or weakness; or any other unusual side effect.

If you forget to take a dose of loratadine, take it as soon as you remember. If it is almost time for your next dose, skip the one you forgot and continue with your regular schedule. Do not take a double dose.

Rapidly disintegrating loratadine tablets must be used as soon as they are removed from their foil package. Place on you tongue and allow to dissolve. You may drink water or another liquid with it but it is not necessary.

Special Populations

Pregnancy/Breast-feeding

Do not take any antihistamine without your doctor's knowledge if you are or might be pregnant—especially during the last 3 months of pregnancy—because newborns may have severe reactions to antihistamines.

Loratadine passes into breast milk. Nursing mothers who must take loratadine should bottle-feed.

Seniors

Seniors are unlikely to experience nervous-system effects with loratadine as opposed to the older, more sedating antihistamines. However, seniors, especially those with liver disease, are more likely to experience side effects than are younger adults. Seniors should take the smallest effective dose.

Lotensin *see Benazepril, page 139*

Brand Name

Lotrel

Generic Ingredients

Amlodipine + Benazepril Hydrochloride

Type of Drug

Antihypertensive.

Prescribed For

High blood pressure.

General Information

Lotrel combines the calcium channel blocker amlodipine with the angiotensin-converting enzyme (ACE) inhibitor benazepril. Both drugs are often prescribed individually for hypertension. Lotrel is not intended as a first treatment for hypertension. You should take Lotrel only after you have tried an ACE inhibitor or calcium channel blocker alone and your doctor feels you need an additional drug to control your blood pressure. (See the "Amlodipine" and "Benazepril" profiles for more information.)

Cautions and Warnings

Do not take Lotrel if you are **sensitive** or **allergic** to any of its ingredients or to any other ACE inhibitor. People taking any ACE inhibitor may experience severe **drug reactions,** including swelling of the face, throat, lips, tongue, hands, and feet—this reaction occurs in about 5 in 1000 people.

Lotrel should not be taken by **pregnant women.**

In rare instances, people taking a calcium channel blocker who have severe **heart disease** develop increased **angina pain** or a **heart attack.**

In people with **heart failure,** ACE inhibitors may cause **very low blood pressure, kidney failure,** and **death.** People with heart failure who start Lotrel must be under a doctor's care.

This medication may cause **high blood potassium,** especially in people with diabetes or kidney disease, which can lead to abnormal heart rhythms.

Another ACE inhibitor has caused **depression of bone marrow** and **reduced white-blood-cell counts,** especially in people with **kidney failure.** Fever and chills can be a sign of this problem.

Lotrel should be used with caution by people with **kidney** or **liver disease.**

In rare instances, people taking ACE inhibitors have developed **liver failure.**

All ACE inhibitors may cause a persistent **cough.**

Possible Side Effects

Side effects are generally mild and temporary.

▼ Most common: cough, headache, dizziness, and swelling.

▼ Less common: allergic reactions, weakness, fatigue, dry mouth, nausea, abdominal pain, constipation, diarrhea, upset stomach, throat irritation, low blood-potassium levels, back pain, muscle cramps and pain, sleeplessness, nervousness, anxiety, tremors, reduced sex drive, sore throat, flushing, hot flashes, rash, impotence, and frequent urination.

▼ Rare: inflammation of the pancreas, hemolytic anemia, chest pain, abnormal heart rhythms, gout, neuritis, and ringing or buzzing in the ears, and hair loss.

Drug Interactions

• Combining a diuretic and Lotrel lowers blood pressure, possibly excessively.

• Combining potassium supplements or a potassium-sparing diuretic such as spironolactone, amiloride, or triamterene and benazepril increases the risk of high blood potassium. High blood-potassium levels may lead to abnormal heart rhythms.

• Combining lithium with benazepril may increase blood-lithium levels and lithium side effects.

Food Interactions

Food does not affect individual tablets of amlodipine and benazepril, but the effects of food on Lotrel have not been studied. Until more information is available, take Lotrel on an empty stomach at least 1 hour before or 2 hours after meals.

Usual Dose

Adult: Daily doses range from 2.5 mg of amlodipine and 10 mg of benazepril to 5 mg of amlodipine and 20 mg of benazepril. Dosage depends on your need for each of the 2 ingredients. Small or frail people or those with liver failure should follow dosage recommendations for seniors.

Senior: Start with 2.5 mg of amlodipine and 10 mg of benazepril a day and increase gradually. You may need to take amlodipine and benazepril in separate pills until your daily needs are established.

Overdosage

Little is known about the effects of Lotrel overdose. Call your local poison control center for more information. Overdose victims should be taken to a hospital emergency room for treatment. ALWAYS bring the prescription bottle or container.

Special Information

Continue taking your medication and follow all instructions including diet restriction and other treatments, even if you feel well. Hypertension may be present without symptoms.

Call your doctor if you develop swelling in the hands, feet, face, or throat; sudden breathing difficulties; a sore throat; mouth sores; abnormal heartbeat; increased chest pain; persistent rash; constipation; nausea; weakness; dizziness; loss of the sense of taste; or any bothersome or persistent side effect.

You may get dizzy if you rise to your feet quickly from a sitting or lying position.

Avoid strenuous exercise and very hot weather because heavy sweating or dehydration may lead to a rapid drop in blood pressure.

Avoid over-the-counter stimulants that can raise blood pressure, including diet pills and decongestants.

Maintain good dental hygiene while taking Lotrel and use extra care when brushing or flossing because of the increased risk of oral infection associated with Lotrel.

If you forget a dose, take it as soon as you remember. If it is within 8 hours of your next dose, skip the one you forgot and continue with your regular schedule. Do not take a double dose.

Special Populations

Pregnancy/Breast-feeding

ACE inhibitors may cause fetal damage or death. Lotrel should not be taken by pregnant women. If you are taking Lotrel and become pregnant, see your doctor at once about changing drugs.

Small amounts of both active ingredients pass into breast milk. Nursing mothers who must take Lotrel should bottle-feed.

Seniors

Seniors should begin with the lowest strength of Lotrel available—2.5 mg of amlodipine and 10 mg of benazepril.

Brand Name

Lotrisone

Generic Ingredients

Betamethasone Dipropionate + Clotrimazole Ⓖ

Type of Drug

Corticosteroid and antifungal combination.

Prescribed For

Severe fungal infection.

General Information

The corticosteroid in Lotrisone is betamethasone dipropionate; the antifungal is clotrimazole. Lotrisone is used to relieve the symptoms of itching, rash, or skin inflammation associated with a severe fungal infection. It may also treat the underlying cause of the skin problem by killing the fungus. Improvement usually occurs within the first week of treatment. Creams that contain only clotrimazole or only betamethasone—as betamethasone diproprionate or in a slightly different form called betamethasone valerate—may be more effective than a combination product for certain skin conditions.

Cautions and Warnings

Do not use Lotrisone if you are **sensitive** or **allergic** to either of its ingredients.

Do not apply Lotrisone near or in your **eyes**. Avoid using this product on the **ear** if the eardrum is perforated, unless specifically directed to do so by your doctor.

Do not use an old tube of Lotrisone for a new skin problem without your doctor's knowledge.

Lotrisone may cause viral skin infections such as **chicken pox** and **herpes** to spread. It may also worsen **tuberculosis (TB) of the skin, bacterial skin infections, skin diseases** that affect circulation, and **diaper rash**. Do not use this medication on children under the age of 2 without your doctor's approval.

Lotrisone may **increase glucose levels** in the blood or urine, especially in people with severe **diabetes**.

Possible Side Effects

▼ Most common: itching, stinging, burning, peeling skin, and swelling.

Drug Interactions

None known.

Usual Dose

Adult and Child (age 12 and over): Gently rub a thin film onto the affected area and surrounding skin 2 times a day for 2–4 weeks.

Child (age 2–12): as instructed by your doctor.

Child (under age 2): not recommended.

Overdosage

Accidental ingestion of Lotrisone may cause nausea and vomiting. Call your local poison control center or a hospital emergency room for more information. If you seek treatment, ALWAYS bring the prescription bottle or container.

Special Information

Washing or soaking the skin before applying the medication may increase the amount that penetrates into your skin.

Applying this drug to the face, underarms, groin, genitals or genital areas, abdomen, or between the toes for more than a few days may result in stretch marks.

Do not wear tight clothing after applying Lotrisone, especially when applied to the genitals or genital areas.

Stop using the medication and call your doctor if Lotrisone causes itching, burning, or skin irritation.

Although prolonged treatment with Lotrisone is not recommended, it is important to take this drug for the entire period prescribed by your doctor, even if you are no longer experiencing symptoms.

Call your doctor if you develop acne or oily skin, bruising, white spots, increased hair growth, or inflammation of hair follicles.

If you do not see results after 1–2 weeks, your doctor may need to prescribe a different medication.

If you forget a dose, apply it as soon as you remember. If it is almost time for your next application, skip the dose you forgot and continue with your regular schedule.

Special Populations

Pregnancy/Breast-feeding

Lotrisone can adversely affect fetal development. Pregnant women should not apply Lotrisone over large areas of skin or use it for a prolonged period. When this drug is considered crucial by your doctor, its potential benefits must be weighed against its risks.

The ingredients in Lotrisone may pass into breast milk when applied to the breast. Nursing mothers who must apply it there should bottle-feed.

Seniors

Seniors may use Lotrisone without special restriction.

Type of Drug

Luteinizing Hormone Inhibitors

Brand Names

Generic Ingredient: Cetrorelix
Cetrotide

Generic Ingredient: Ganirelix
Antagon

Prescribed For

Infertility.

General Information

Luteinizing hormone inhibitors are prescribed as part of a treatment program offered by fertility specialists to help stimulate the development of follicles into mature eggs in women who have had difficulty becoming pregnant. These drugs block the release of gonadotropin-releasing hormones (GnRH), which stimulate the production and release of two other hormones: luteinizing hormone (LH) and follicle stimulating hormone (FSH). LH and FSH levels return to normal within 48 hours after treatment is stopped.

A luteinizing hormone inhibitor may be taken once a day by subcutaneous (under the skin) injection during the several days after FSH is given, specifically on day 2 or 3 of the cycle.

Treatment with an LH inhibitor continues until chorionic gonadotropin (hCG)—the final drug in the sequence—is given. Your doctor will determine when enough follicles have reached an adequate size by ultrasound. In some cases hCG is given to help the follicles develop into mature eggs.

Cautions and Warnings

Do not use luteinizing hormone inhibitors if you are **sensitive** or **allergic** to them.

People with a **latex allergy** may react adversely to ganirelix.

People who are allergic to **mannitol** should not use cetrorelix.

People who are allergic to **gonadotropin releasing hormone** must be monitored carefully after the first injection. A severe reaction associated with cough, rash, and hypotension occurred in 1 patient after 7 months of treatment with cetrorelix, when taken at a dosage of 10 mg a day, in a study for a use unrelated to infertility.

Possible Side Effects

▼ Less common: abdominal pain, headache, miscarriage, hyperstimulation of the ovary, vaginal bleeding, injection site allergy (symptoms include redness, rash, bruising, itching, and swelling), and nausea.

Food and Drug Interactions

None known.

Usual Dose

Cetrorelix

Single dose—one 3 mg subcutaneous dose, usually on stimulation day 7 (range: day 5–9). If hCG is not given within 4 days after injection of 3 mg cetrorelix, then cetrorelix 0.25 mg once daily is prescribed until the day of hCG administration.

Multiple-dose program—0.25 mg of cetrorelix, on either stimulation day 5 (morning or evening) or day 6 (morning). Continue every day until the day of hCG administration.

Ganirelix
250 mcg once daily after starting FSH therapy on day 2 or 3 of the cycle. Treatment is continued until the day of hCG administration.

Overdosage

Very high doses of these medicines have been employed in clinical trials without serious side effects. Call your local poison center or a hospital emergency room for more information. If you seek treatment, ALWAYS bring the prescription bottle or container.

Special Information

This drug is given by injection under the skin. For more information on how to properly administer this drug, see page 1188.

Cetrorelix injection requires more manipulation than cetrotide, which comes in pre-filled syringes. You must dissolve the powder with sterile water provided by the manufacturer before it is injected. Follow the directions for dilution in the package.

Special Populations

Pregnancy/Breast-feeding
Women who are pregnant should not take these drugs because they may harm a developing fetus.

It is not known if these drugs pass into breast milk. Nursing mothers who must use luteinizing hormone inhibitors should bottle-feed.

Seniors
These medicines are not intended for use by seniors.

Macrobid *see Nitrofurantoin, page 785*

Generic Name

Malathion (MAL-uh-thye-on)

Brand Name

Ovide

Type of Drug

Scabicide.

Prescribed For

Head lice.

General Information

Originally used as an agricultural insecticide, malathion is effective against common lice and the eggs they leave behind in the scalp. Malathion works by interfering with the breakdown of acetylcholine, a neurohormone that carries nervous-system impulses. The excess acetylcholine produced by malathion kills lice and their eggs. Once applied to the hair, malathion binds with the hair shaft within 6 to 12 hours, providing some protection against future infestations.

Cautions and Warnings

Malathion is extremely **toxic** if swallowed (see "Overdosage").

People with malathion **sensitivity** should not use it. Normally, about 89% of the malathion applied to the skin is absorbed into the bloodstream; more may be absorbed if it is applied to **broken skin or open sores**—this may cause a toxic reaction.

Malathion **lotion is flammable**. Do not expose the lotion or hair that is still wet with the lotion to an open flame or an electric dryer because of the risk of fire. Allow hair to dry naturally after application.

Malathion can **damage the eyes** and cause conjunctivitis. If it gets into your eyes, flush them with water immediately.

People who have had a recent **heart attack** or who have any of the following conditions should be cautious when using malathion because it can precipitate an attack or worsen your condition: **asthma,** very **slow heartbeat, low blood pressure, stomach spasms or ulcer,** or **Parkinson's disease**.

Do not use malathion in **children under age 2,** as they may absorb too much of it through the scalp.

Malathion can worsen the following conditions: **severe anemia, dehydration, insecticide exposure effects, liver disease** or **cirrhosis, malnutrition, myasthenia or other neuromuscular diseases,** and **seizure** disorders.

People with recent **brain surgery** should be cautious about using this product because it can initiate toxic nervous-system effects, including seizures.

Possible Side Effects

▼ Common: scalp irritation.

▼ Rare: Convulsions and other side effects can occur if too much of the drug is absorbed into the blood through the scalp (see "Overdosage").

Drug Interactions

• Large dosages of malathion may interact with aminogly-cosides (injectable antibiotics) to cause breathing problems, with local anesthetics to cause systemic side effects, and with glaucoma eyedrops—physostigmine, echothiophate, deme-carium, and isoflurophate—to cause side effects.

• Combining malathion and anticholinesterase muscle stimulants used to treat myasthenia gravis may lead to increased side effects.

Usual Dose

Adult and Child (age 2 and over): Sprinkle the lotion onto dry hair and rub it in until the hair and scalp are wet. Pay special attention to the back of your head and neck. Avoid contact with the eyes. Immediately after applying the lotion, wash your hands. Allow the treated hair to dry naturally; do not cover it or use an electric dryer or other heat source. After 8 to 12 hours, wash your hair with a plain shampoo. Remove dead lice and eggs from the scalp with a fine-toothed comb. Repeat after 7–9 days if necessary.

Overdosage

Accidental ingestion or absorbing too much drug through the skin is serious and potentially fatal. Symptoms of malathion toxicity include abdominal cramps; anxiety; restlessness; clumsiness or unsteadiness; confusion; depression; diarrhea; dizziness; drowsiness; increased sweating; watery eyes or mouth; loss of bowel or bladder control; muscle twitching in the eyelids, face, or neck; pinpointed pupils; difficulty breathing; seizures; slow heartbeat; trembling; and weakness. People who swallow this drug may not experience toxic effects for up to 12 hours. In case of accidental ingestion induce vomiting with ipecac syrup—available at any pharmacy. Take the victim to a hospital emergency room. ALWAYS bring the prescription bottle or container.

Special Information

Follow your prescription exactly.

Pregnant women should not handle this medication or apply it to others.

Avoid exposure to other insecticides while being treated with malathion.

Special Populations

Pregnancy/Breast-feeding

Malathion may enter the fetal bloodstream and affect the fetus. Pregnant women should not use it or apply it to others.

Malathion may pass into breast milk. Nursing mothers who must use it should bottle-feed.

Seniors

Seniors may use this drug without special restriction.

Generic Name

Medroxyprogesterone Acetate

(med-rok-see-proe-JES-ter-one) G

Brand Names

Amen
Curretab
Cycrin

Depo-Provera
Provera

The information in this profile also applies to the following drugs:

Generic Ingredient: Norethindrone Acetate G
Aygestin

Generic Ingredient: Progesterone
Crinone

Prometrium

Type of Drug

Progestin.

Prescribed For

Absence of menstruation, abnormal uterine bleeding caused by fibroids or uterine cancer, and menopausal changes in the lining of the uterus—in conjunction with estrogen replacement therapy (ERT); also prescribed to stimulate breathing in people who suffer from sleep apnea and for other conditions in which breathing rate is abnormally slow or stops completely for short periods of time. Norethindrone acetate may be used for endometriosis. Progesterone has been used to treat premenstrual syndrome (PMS), prevent spontaneous abortion or premature labor, and support embryo implantation and help maintain pregnancy in some assisted reproductive technology (ART) procedures.

General Information

Progesterone is the principal hormone involved in the process of pregnancy. It helps to prepare the womb to accept the fertilized egg and maintain the growth and development of the fetus. The decision to take medroxyprogesterone acetate on a regular basis should be made carefully by you and your doctor because of this drug's risks.

Another progestin called megestrol (Megace) is used in breast and endometrial cancer, and for weight loss and decreased appetite in people living with AIDS.

Cautions and Warnings

Do not take this drug if you are **sensitive** or **allergic** to it or any progestin or have a history of **stroke, blood clots or similar disorders, varicose veins, liver disease,** known or suspected **breast or genital cancer,** undiagnosed **vaginal bleeding,** or **miscarriage.** Medroxyprogesterone and other progestins should not be used regularly to avoid weight loss.

Although progestins have been used to prevent spontaneous abortion, such treatment can harm a fetus if given during the first 4 months of pregnancy.

Medroxyprogesterone acetate use should be carefully considered if you have had **asthma, cardiac insufficiency, epilepsy, HIV infection, migraine, kidney problems, ectopic pregnancy, high blood cholesterol,** or **depression.** People with **diabetes** may experience a decrease in glucose tolerance, worsening their condition.

Possible Side Effects

There is a strong relationship between the use of progestin drugs and the development of blood clots in the veins, lungs, or brain.

Medroxyprogesterone Acetate and Norethindrone Acetate

▼ Most common: breakthrough bleeding, spotting, changes in or loss of menstrual flow, water retention, weight loss or gain, breast tenderness, jaundice, acne, rash with or without itching, and depression.

▼ Common: changes in sex drive, changes in appetite and mood, headache, nervousness, dizziness, tiredness, backache, loss of scalp hair, hair growth in unusual quantities or places, itching, symptoms similar to those of a urinary infection, and unusual rashes.

▼ Rare: allergy, fatigue, fever, flu-like symptoms, bloating, asthma, back or leg pain, sinus inflammation, respiratory infection, upset stomach, stomach gas or noise, emotional instability, sleeplessness, acne, itching, painful urination, and urinary infections.

Progesterone Gel

Side effects are less common if you use this drug once a day.

▼ Most common: pelvic or abdominal pain or cramps, sleepiness, tiredness, headache, nervousness, depression, reduced sex drive, constipation, nausea, breast enlargement, and nighttime urination.

▼ Common: bloating, dizziness, diarrhea, vomiting, painful intercourse, joint pain, itching, and vaginal infection or discharge.

Drug Interactions

• Rifampin and aminoglutethimide reduce medroxyprogesterone acetate's effectiveness.

Food Interactions

You may take this drug with food if it upsets your stomach.

Usual Dose

Medroxyprogesterone Acetate: 5–10 mg a day for 5–10 days.

Norethindrone Acetate: For endometriosis—5 mg a day for 14 days, then increased gradually up to 15 mg a day; treatment may continue for 6–9 months. For abnormal periodic bleeding or no period—2.5–10 mg a day for 5–10 days during the second half of the menstrual cycle.

Progesterone Capsules: 5-10 mg a day for 6–8 days.

Progesterone Gel: Apply a single-use disposable unit once or twice a day.

Overdosage

Symptoms may include severe side effects, though small overdoses generally do not cause unusual symptoms. Call your local poison control center or a hospital emergency room for more information. If you seek treatment, ALWAYS bring the prescription bottle or container.

Special Information

Your need for this drug should be evaluated at least every 6 months.

This drug may make you drowsy. Be careful when driving or performing any tasks that require concentration.

Stop taking this drug immediately and call your doctor if you experience sudden, partial, or complete loss of vision; double vision; sudden falling; calf pain, swelling, and redness; numbness in an arm or leg; leg cramp; water retention; unusual vaginal bleeding; migraine or a sudden and severe headache; depression; or if you think you have become pregnant.

Medroxyprogesterone acetate may increase your sensitivity to the sun. Use sunscreen and wear protective clothing.

Medroxyprogesterone acetate may mask symptoms of menopause.

If you forget a dose, take it as soon as you remember. If it is almost time for your next dose, skip the one you forgot and continue with your regular schedule. Do not take a double dose.

Special Populations

Pregnancy/Breast-feeding

Medroxyprogesterone acetate and norethindrone may cause birth defects or interfere with fetal development; it can double the rate of certain birth defects if used during the first 4 months of pregnancy. It is not considered safe for use during pregnancy, except under very specific circumstances. Progesterone gel is used to support embryo implantation and help maintain pregnancies in some ART procedures.

Medroxyprogesterone acetate passes into breast milk. It may also increase the amount of milk produced and the duration of milk production when taken after childbirth. Nursing mothers who must use this drug should consider bottle-feeding.

Seniors

Seniors with severe liver disease are more sensitive to the effects of this drug.

Generic Name

Meloxicam (mel-OX-ih-kam)

Brand Name

Mobic

Type of Drug

Nonsteroidal anti-inflammatory drug (NSAID).

Prescribed For

Osteoarthritis. Other NSAIDs like meloxicam are also prescribed for rheumatoid arthritis, mild to moderate pain, juvenile rheumatoid arthritis, sunburn, menstrual pain, tendinitis, bursitis, migraine headache, resistant acne, PMS, and fever.

General Information

NSAIDs work by blocking the body's production of a hormone called prostaglandin. They also block both known types of cyclooxygenase, COX-1 and COX-2, though the degree to which individual NSAIDs block COX-1 and COX-2 vary tremendously. Meloxicam inhibits both COX-1 and COX-2. Inhibition of COX-1 can cause irritation of the gastrointestinal (GI) tract. Half of each meloxicam dose is broken down in the liver and the other half is eliminated through the kidneys.

Cautions and Warnings

People **allergic** to any NSAID and those with a history of **asthma** attacks brought on by an NSAID, iodides, or aspirin should not take meloxicam.

Meloxicam may cause **gastrointestinal (GI) tract bleeding, ulcers, and perforation**. This can occur at any time, with or without warning, in people who take meloxicam regularly. People with a history of active GI bleeding should be cautious about taking any NSAID. People who develop these symptoms and continue meloxicam treatment should be aware of the possibility of developing more serious side effects.

Meloxicam can affect platelets and **blood clotting** at high doses, and should be avoided by people with clotting problems and those taking warfarin.

People with **heart problems** who take meloxicam may experience swelling in their arms, legs, or feet.

People taking meloxicam, especially those with a collagen disease such as **systemic lupus erythematosus,** may experience an unusually severe drug-sensitivity reaction. Report any unusual symptoms to your doctor at once.

Meloxicam can be toxic to the **kidney**. Report any unusual side effects to your doctor, who might need to periodically test your kidney function.

Meloxicam can make you **unusually sensitive to the effects of the sun**.

Possible Side Effects

▼ Common: diarrhea, nausea, vomiting, constipation, and minor stomach upset, distress, or gas, especially during the first few days of treatment.

▼ Less common: stomach ulcers, GI bleeding, appetite loss, hepatitis, gallbladder attacks, headache, sleeplessness, painful urination, poor kidney function, kidney inflammation, blood and protein in the urine, dizziness, fainting, nervousness, depression, hallucinations, confusion, disorientation, tingling in the hands or feet, lightheadedness, itching, sweating, dry nose and mouth, heart palpitations, chest pain, breathing difficulties, and muscle cramps.

Possible Side Effects *(continued)*

▼ Rare: severe allergic reactions including closing of the throat, fever and chills, changes in liver function, jaundice (yellowing of the skin and whites of the eyes), and kidney failure. These people must be treated in a hospital emergency room or doctor's office. NSAIDs have caused severe skin reactions; see your doctor immediately if this happens to you.

Drug Interactions

• Meloxicam may increase the effects and side effects of digoxin, lithium, phenytoin, and oral anticoagulant (blood-thinning) drugs such as warfarin.

• Meloxicam may reduce the blood-pressure-lowering effect of beta-blocker drugs and diuretics.

• Colestipol, cholestyramine, rifampin, and phenobarbital reduce the amount of meloxicam in the bloodstream.

• Fluconazole, probenecid, and ritonavir may increase blood levels of meloxicam.

• Combining meloxicam with cyclosporine may increase the kidney-related side effects of both drugs.

• Aspirin, acetaminophen, ketorolac, and other salicylates should never be combined with meloxicam in the treatment of arthritis. Some people may take low-dose aspirin for heart attack prevention, but even low doses can increase NSAID irritation.

• Meloxicam may reduce the blood-pressure-lowering effects of ACE inhibitors.

• Mixing meloxicam with dipyridamole may worsen water retention.

Food Interactions

Take meloxicam with food or a magnesium and aluminum antacid if it upsets your stomach.

Usual Dose

Adult (age 18 and over): 7.5–15 mg once a day.
Child (under age 18): not recommended.

Overdosage

People have died from NSAID overdose. Common signs of overdose are drowsiness, nausea, vomiting, diarrhea, abdominal pain, rapid breathing, rapid heartbeat, sweating, ringing or buzzing in the ears, confusion, disorientation, stupor, and coma. Take the overdose victim to a hospital emergency room at once. ALWAYS bring the prescription bottle or container.

Special Information

Take each dose with a full glass of water and do not lie down for 15 to 30 minutes afterward.

Meloxicam may make you drowsy or tired; be careful when driving or operating hazardous equipment. Do not take OTC products containing acetaminophen or aspirin while taking NSAIDs. Avoid alcohol.

Contact your doctor if you develop a rash, itching, visual disturbances, weight gain, breathing difficulties, fluid retention, hallucinations, black stools, persistent headache, or any unusual or intolerable side effect.

If you forget a dose of meloxicam, take it as soon as you remember. If you take several doses a day and it is within 4 hours of your next dose, skip the dose you forgot and continue with your regular schedule. Do not take a double dose.

Special Populations

Pregnancy/Breast-feeding

Meloxicam may affect the developing fetal heart during the last half of pregnancy. Women who are or might become pregnant should not take meloxicam without their doctor's approval. When your doctor considers the drug crucial, its potential benefits must be carefully weighed against its risks.

Meloxicam may pass into breast milk. There is a possibility that a nursing mother taking meloxicam could affect her baby's heart or cardiovascular system. Nursing mothers who must take this drug should bottle-feed.

Seniors

Seniors, especially those with poor kidney or liver function, may be more susceptible to side effects.

Generic Name

Memantine (meh-MAN-teen)

Brand Name

Namenda

Type of Drug

NMDA receptor inhibitor.

Prescribed For

Moderate to severe Alzheimer's disease (AD).

General Information

Over stimulation of NMDA receptors in the brain is thought to be one cause of Alzheimer's disease (AD) symptoms. Memantine blocks NMDA receptors but it does not stop the nerve degeneration that is a normal part of AD. Thus, the drug can be expected to improve the symptoms of AD for several weeks and prolong a patient's mental decline. Memantine is the first medicine to be approved in the United States for moderate to severe AD. It has been available in other countries since 1982. Memantine is not a cure for AD. Other available AD treatments work differently and are only approved for mild to moderate AD though they have been studied in people with severe AD.

Cautions and Warnings

Do not take this drug if you are **sensitive** or **allergic** to it.

People with **kidney disease** may retain more memantine in their bodies. People with severe kidney disease should not use this drug.

Memantine has not been studied in people with **seizure disorders**. A very small number of people taking memantine in drug studies had seizures, but the number was similar to that which occurred in people taking an inactive placebo.

Possible Side Effects

In most cases, memantine side effects reported in clinical studies were similar to those reported by people who took an inactive placebo.

▼ Common: dizziness, headache, and constipation.

▼ Less common: confusion, fatigue, hallucinations, vomiting, difficulty breathing, high blood pressure, back pain, and fatigue.

▼ Rare: Rare side effects can occur in almost any part of the body. Contact your doctor if you experience any side effect not listed above.

Drug Interactions

• Carbonic anhydrase inhibitors (such as acetazolamide) and bicarbonate of soda (or "baking soda") can cause the body to retain memantine. The importance of these interactions is not known.

• Memantine does not interfere with the ability of donepezil and other cholinesterase inhibitors to function. In fact, studies adding memantine to donepezil have shown an improved response with the combination than with donepezil alone.

• Dextromethorphan, a common ingredient in over-the-counter cough medicines, should be avoided if you are taking memantine. The effect of combining memantine and other NMDA antagonists—including amantadine and ketamine—is unknown.

• Memantine is released through the kidneys by the same system as other drugs including hydrochlorthiazide, triamterene, cimetidine, ranitidine, quinidine, and nicotine. Combining these drugs could change the pattern of their elimination, but more research on this possibility is needed.

Food Interactions

This drug can be taken without regard to food or meals.

Usual Dose

Starting dose—5 mg a day. Dose is increased weekly in 5 mg increments up to 20 mg a day.

Overdosage

Symptoms include restlessness, psychosis, hallucinations, sleepiness, stupor, and loss of consciousness. Take the victim to a hospital emergency room. ALWAYS bring the prescription bottle or container.

Special Information

Patient caregivers that are responsible for ensuring that medicines are taken correctly must understand how memantine is taken and its dosage regimen.

Special Populations

Pregnancy/Breast-feeding

Animal studies with memantine revealed no danger to a developing fetus, even at the highest dosage. When this drug is considered crucial by your doctor, its potential benefits must be carefully weighed against its risks.

It is not known if memantine passes into breast milk. Nursing mothers who must take it should bottle-feed.

Seniors

Seniors may use this drug without special precaution. Those with kidney disease may require lower doses.

Generic Name

Meperidine (muh-PER-ih-dine) G

Brand Name

Demerol

Type of Drug

Narcotic analgesic (pain reliever).

Prescribed For

Moderate to severe pain.

General Information

Meperidine hydrochloride is a potent narcotic analgesic and cough suppressant. It is also used before surgery to reduce anxiety and help bring the patient into early stages of anesthesia. Meperidine is probably the most widely used narcotic in American hospitals. It compares favorably with morphine sulfate, the standard for narcotic analgesics.

It is useful for mild to moderate pain; 25 to 50 mg of meperidine are approximately equal in pain-relieving effect to two 325-mg aspirin tablets. Meperidine may be less effective than aspirin for pain associated with inflammation because aspirin reduces inflammation but meperidine does not. Meperidine suppresses the cough reflex but does not cure the underlying cause of the cough.

Cautions and Warnings

Do not take meperidine if you are **allergic** or **sensitive** to it. Use this drug with extreme caution if you suffer from **asthma or other breathing problems**. Meperidine should be used with caution if you have **kidney or liver disease, head injuries, brain disease,** a history of **seizures, hypothyroidism** (underactive thyroid gland), **inflammatory bowel disease, gallstones or gallbladder disease, enlarged prostate,** or **urinary difficulties**.

Meperidine may cause postural **low blood pressure** (symptoms include dizziness or fainting when rising from a sitting or lying position).

Chronic (long-term) use of meperidine may cause drug dependence or **addiction**.

Meperidine is a respiratory depressant and affects the central nervous system (CNS), producing **sleepiness, tiredness,** and an **inability to concentrate. Alcohol** may increase the CNS depression caused by this drug.

Possible Side Effects

▼ Most common: light-headedness, dizziness, sleepiness, nausea, vomiting, appetite loss, and increased sweating. These side effects usually disappear if you lie down. More serious side effects of meperidine are shallow breathing or breathing difficulties.

▼ Less common: euphoria (feeling "high"), weakness, headache, agitation, uncoordinated muscle movement, minor hallucinations, disorientation, visual disturbances, dry mouth, constipation, flushing of the face, rapid heartbeat, palpitations, faintness, urinary difficulties or hesitancy, reduced sex drive or potency, itching, rash, anemia, lowered blood sugar, and yellowing of the skin or whites of the eyes. Narcotic analgesics may aggravate convulsions in those who have had them.

Drug Interactions

• Because of its depressant effect and potential effect on breathing, meperidine should be taken with extreme caution in combination with alcohol, sleeping medications, antihistamines, tranquilizers, or other depressant drugs.

• People taking cimetidine and a narcotic analgesic may experience confusion, disorientation, depression, seizure, or breathing difficulties.

• Combining meperidine and a monoamine oxidase inhibitor (MAOI) antidepressant may lead to breathing difficulties; blood pressure changes; bluish discoloration of the lips, fingernails, or skin; coma; or death. Do not take meperidine within 2 weeks of your last dose of an MAOI.

• Combining meperidine and the antipsychotic drug chlorpromazine (Thorazine) or thioridazine may lead to serious side effects.

• Meperidine may decrease the effectiveness of hydantoin anticonvulsant drugs.

• Combining meperidine and a protease inhibitor may increase the risk of CNS depressant and breathing difficulties.

Food Interactions

Meperidine may be taken with food to reduce upset stomach.

Usual Dose

Adult: 50–150 mg every 3–4 hours as needed.

Child: 0.5–0.8 mg per lb. of body weight every 3–4 hours as needed, up to the adult dosage.

Overdosage

Symptoms include slow breathing, extreme tiredness progressing to stupor and then coma, pinpointed pupils, no response to pain stimulation, cold or clammy skin, slow heartbeat, low blood pressure, convulsions, and cardiac arrest. The victim should be taken to a hospital emergency room immediately. ALWAYS bring the prescription bottle or container.

Special Information

Be extremely careful when driving or doing any task that requires concentration. Avoid alcohol.

Call your doctor if you develop nausea, vomiting, constipation, breathing difficulties, or any bothersome or persistent side effect.

Ask your doctor to consider lowering your meperidine dosage if you experience light-headedness, dizziness, sleepiness, nausea, vomiting, appetite loss, or increased sweating.

If you have been taking meperidine for more than a few weeks, do not stop taking it without your doctor's instruction. Suddenly stopping this drug may lead to withdrawal symptoms.

If you forget a dose, take it as soon as you remember. If it is almost time for your next dose, skip the one you forgot and continue with your regular schedule. Do not take a double dose.

Special Populations

Pregnancy/Breast-feeding

Large amounts of meperidine taken during pregnancy may cause addiction in newborns. Narcotics may also cause breathing difficulties in newborns if taken just before delivery. When this drug is considered crucial by your doctor, its potential benefits must be carefully weighed against its risks.

Meperidine passes into breast milk. Nursing mothers who must take this drug should bottle-feed.

Seniors

Seniors are more likely to experience side effects and should take the smallest effective dosage.

Generic Name

Meprobamate (meh-proe-BUH-mate) G

Brand Names

Equanil   Probate
Meprospan   Trancot
Miltown   Tranmep
Neuramate

Type of Drug

Antianxiety agent.

Prescribed For

Short-term anxiety and tension.

General Information

Meprobamate works by directly affecting several areas of the brain. It can relax you, relieve anxiety, and act as a muscle relaxant, anticonvulsant, or sleeping pill. This drug should be used for less than 4 months.

Cautions and Warnings

Do not take meprobamate if you are **allergic** to it or a related drug such as carbromal, carisoprodol, felbamate, or mebutamate, or if you have **intermittent porphyria**. People with epilepsy should use this drug with caution because it may cause **seizures**. Meprobamate should be used with caution by people with **kidney disease,** who may need to take lower dosages.

Some people taking meprobamate have developed severe physical and psychological **drug dependence.** This drug can produce **chronic intoxication** after prolonged use or if used in greater than recommended doses: Symptoms include slurred speech, dizziness, general sleepiness, and depression. Suddenly stopping meprobamate after prolonged and excessive use may result in drug withdrawal symptoms, including severe anxiety, vomiting, appetite loss, sleeplessness, tremors, muscle twitching, confusion, hallucinations, and convulsions. Withdrawal symptoms usually begin 12 to 48 hours after meprobamate has been stopped and may last 1 to 4 days. When stopping treatment with meprobamate, the drug should be reduced gradually over 1 or 2 weeks.

Possible Side Effects

▼ Most common: drowsiness, sleepiness, dizziness, slurred speech, poor muscle coordination, headache, weakness, tingling in the arms and legs, and euphoria (feeling "high").

▼ Less common: nausea, vomiting, diarrhea, abnormal heart rhythm, excitement or overstimulation, low blood pressure, itching, rash, and changes in blood components.

▼ Rare: allergic reactions, including high fever, chills, bronchospasm (closing of the throat), and reduced urinary function.

Drug Interactions

• Combining meprobamate with central nervous system (CNS) depressants, including alcohol, other tranquilizers, narcotics, barbiturates, sleeping pills, or antihistamines, can cause excess tranquilization, depression, sleepiness, or fatigue.

Food Interactions

Take this drug with food if it upsets your stomach.

Usual Dose

Adult and Child (age 13 and over): 1200–1600 mg a day in 3–4 doses; maximum daily dose, 2400 mg.

Child (age 6–12): 100–200 mg 2–3 times a day.
Child (under age 6): not recommended.

Overdosage

Overdose symptoms include extreme drowsiness, lethargy, stupor, and coma, with possible shock and respiratory collapse. If alcohol or another depressant has also been taken, small overdoses can be fatal. After a large overdose, the victim will go to sleep very quickly, and blood pressure, pulse, and breathing levels will drop rapidly. The overdose victim must immediately be taken to a hospital emergency room. ALWAYS bring the prescription bottle or container.

Special Information

Take this drug according to your doctor's direction. Do not change your dose without your doctor's approval. Do not crush or chew meprobamate tablets.

This drug causes drowsiness and poor concentration. Be careful when driving or performing complex activities. Avoid alcohol and other CNS depressants because they increase these effects.

Call your doctor if you develop fever, sore throat, rash, mouth sores, nosebleeds, unexplained black-and-blue marks, or easy bruising or bleeding, or if you become pregnant.

If you forget a dose and remember within about 1 hour of your regular time, take it right away. If you do not remember until later, skip the dose you forgot and go back to your regular schedule. Do not take a double dose.

Special Populations

Pregnancy/Breast-feeding

Meprobamate increases the risk of birth defects, particularly during the first 3 months of pregnancy. Inform your doctor immediately if you are taking this drug and are pregnant. When this drug is considered crucial by your doctor, its potential benefits must be carefully weighed against its risks, although there are few good reasons for pregnant women to take meprobamate.

Large amounts of meprobamate pass into breast milk. Nursing mothers who must take this drug should bottle-feed.

Seniors

Seniors are more sensitive to the sedative and other effects of this drug and should take the lowest effective dosage.

Generic Name

Metaproterenol (meh-tuh-proe-TER-uh-nol) [G]

Brand Name

Alupent   Tornalate

Type of Drug

Bronchodilator.

Prescribed For

Asthma, bronchospasm, and emphysema.

General Information

Metaproterenol sulfate can be taken both by mouth as a tablet or syrup and by inhalation. This drug may be used with other drugs to produce relief from asthma symptoms. Oral metaproterenol begins working 15 to 30 minutes after a dose; its effects may last for up to 4 hours. Metaproterenol inhalation begins working in 5 to 30 minutes and lasts for 2 to 6 hours.

Cautions and Warnings

This drug should be used with caution by people with a history of **angina pectoris, heart disease, high blood pressure, stroke, seizures, diabetes, thyroid disease, prostate disease,** or **glaucoma.** Excessive use of metaproterenol could lead to worsening of your condition. Using excessive amounts of metaproterenol can lead to increased breathing difficulties rather than relief. In the most extreme cases, people have had heart attacks after using excessive amounts of inhalant.

Possible Side Effects

▼ Common: heart palpitations, rapid heartbeat, tremors, convulsions, shakiness, nervous tension, dizziness, fainting, headache, heartburn, upset stomach, nausea and vomiting, cough, dry or sore and irritated throat, muscle cramps, and urinary difficulties.

Possible Side Effects *(continued)*

▼ Less common: high blood pressure, abnormal heart rhythms, and angina. Metaproterenol inhalation is less likely to cause these effects than some of the older asthma drugs. It can also cause diarrhea, unusual tastes or smells, dry mouth, drowsiness, hoarseness, stuffy nose, worsening of asthma, backache, fatigue, and rash.

Drug Interactions

• The effect of this drug may be increased by antidepressant drugs, some antihistamines, levothyroxine, and monoamine oxidase inhibitors (MAOIs).

• The risk of cardiac toxicity may be increased in people combining metaproterenol and theophylline.

• Beta-blocking drugs such as propanolol antagonize metaproterenol. Metaproterenol may antagonize the effects of blood-pressure-lowering drugs, especially reserpine, methyldopa, and guanethidine.

Food Interactions

If the tablets upset your stomach, they may be taken with food.

Usual Dose

Tablets or Syrup
Adult and Child (age 10 and over or 60 lbs.): 60–80 mg a day.
  Child (age 6–9 or under 60 lbs.): 30–40 mg a day.
  Child (under age 6): 0.6–1.2 mg per lb. of body weight a day. Children this age should be treated only with metaproterenol syrup.

Inhalation
Adult and Child (age 12 and over): 2–3 puffs every 3–4 hours. Each canister contains about 300 inhalations. Do not use more than 12 puffs a day.
  Child (under age 12): not recommended.

Overdosage

Symptoms include palpitations, abnormal heart rhythm, rapid or slow heartbeat, chest pain, high blood pressure, fever, chills, cold sweat, blanching of the skin, nausea, vomiting, sleeplessness, delirium, tremor, pinpoint pupils, convulsions, coma, and collapse. The victim should see a doctor or be taken to a hospital emergency room. ALWAYS bring the prescription bottle or container.

Special Information

Be sure to follow your doctor's instructions for using metaproterenol. Using more than the amount prescribed can lead to drug tolerance and actually worsen your symptoms. If your condition worsens rather than improves after taking metaproterenol, stop taking it and call your doctor.

Metaproterenol inhalation should be breathed in during the second half of your inward breath, since this allows it to reach more deeply into your lungs.

Call your doctor immediately if you develop chest pain, palpitations, rapid heartbeat, muscle tremors, dizziness, headache, facial flushing, or urinary difficulty, or if you still have trouble breathing after using this medication.

If you miss a dose of metaproterenol, take it as soon as possible. Take the rest of that day's dose at regularly spaced time intervals. Go back to your regular schedule the next day.

Special Populations

Pregnancy/Breast-feeding

Metaproterenol has caused birth defects when given in large amounts to pregnant animals. When this drug is considered crucial by your doctor, its potential benefits must be carefully weighed against its risks.

It is not known if metaproterenol passes into breast milk. Nursing mothers who must use it should consider bottle-feeding.

Seniors

Seniors are more sensitive to the effects of this drug.

Generic Name

Metaxalone (meh-TAX-uh-lone)

Brand Name

Skelaxin

Type of Drug

Skeletal muscle relaxant.

Prescribed For

Muscle spasms.

General Information

Metaxalone is prescribed as part of a coordinated program of rest, physical therapy, and other measures for the relief of acute, painful spasm conditions. Exactly how metaxalone works is unknown.

Cautions and Warnings

Metaxalone should be taken with caution if you have had a **reaction** to it, have a tendency toward **anemia,** or have **poor kidney or liver function**.

Possible Side Effects

▼ Most common: nausea, vomiting, upset stomach, stomach cramps, drowsiness, dizziness, headache, nervousness, and irritability.

▼ Less common: rapid or pounding heartbeat, fainting, convulsions, hallucinations, depression, clumsiness or unsteadiness, constipation, diarrhea, heartburn, hiccups, black or tarry bowel movements, vomiting of material that resembles coffee grounds, agranulocytosis (symptoms include fever with or without chills, sore throat, and sores or white spots on the lips or mouth), uncontrolled eye movement, stuffy nose, stinging or burning eyes, bloodshot eyes, weakness, unusual tiredness, chest tightness, swollen glands, unusual bleeding or bruising, and breathing difficulties.

▼ Rare: liver inflammation, yellowing of the skin or whites of the eyes, and drug-sensitivity reactions (symptoms include rash, hives, itching, changes in facial color, and breathing difficulties).

Drug Interactions

• Tranquilizers, alcohol, and other nervous system depressants may increase the depressant effects of metaxalone.

Food Interactions

Metaxalone may be taken with food or meals if it upsets your stomach.

Usual Dose

Adult and Child (age 13 and over): 800 mg 3 or 4 times a day.
Child (under age 13): not recommended.

Overdosage

Symptoms are likely to be severe side effects but may include some less common reactions as well. Overdose victims should be taken to a hospital emergency room. ALWAYS bring the prescription bottle or container.

Special Information

Long-term metaxalone treatment may cause liver toxicity or damage. If you are using this medicine for an extended period, your doctor should check your liver function about every 1 to 2 months.

Metaxalone may cause tiredness, dizziness, and lightheadedness. Be careful when driving or performing tasks that require concentration and coordination.

Call your doctor if you develop breathing difficulties, unusual tiredness or weakness, fever, chills, cough or hoarseness, lower back or side pain, painful urination, yellowing of the skin or whites of the eyes, rash, hives, itching, redness, or any other bothersome or persistent symptom.

If you miss a dose of metaxalone, take it as soon as you remember. If it is almost time for your next dose, take 1 dose as soon as you remember, another in 3 or 4 hours, and then go back to your regular schedule. Do not take a double dose.

Special Populations

Pregnancy/Breast-feeding

As with all drugs, pregnant women should not use metaxalone unless its benefits have been carefully weighed against its risks.

It is not known if metaxalone passes into breast milk. Nursing mothers who must take it should consider bottle-feeding.

Seniors

Seniors with reduced kidney or liver function may require less medicine.

Generic Name

Metformin (met-FOR-min) Ⓖ

Brand Name

Glucophage   Glucophage XR

Type of Drug

Biguanide antihyperglycemic.

Prescribed For

Type 2 diabetes. It may also be prescribed for insulin-resistant and prediabetic conditions including impaired glucose tolerance, obesity, polycystic ovary syndrome, and metabolic abnormalities associated with HIV disease.

General Information

Metformin lowers the amount of glucose produced by the liver, reduces the amount of glucose you absorb from food, and helps cells use glucose. Generally, metformin is not prescribed until a sulfonylurea has been tried without a satisfactory response. If neither drug works alone, combining metformin with another antidiabetic drug may control your diabetes. Metformin can also moderately lower blood fats.

Cautions and Warnings

Do not take metformin if you are **allergic** to it or have **heart failure.** Metformin should not be taken by people with **kidney disease**. If you are having surgery or an x-ray that requires the injection of an iodine-based contrast material, you should temporarily stop taking metformin because the combination could result in acute kidney problems.

Metformin is related to an older antidiabetes drug that was removed from the market because of the risk of a very rare but serious complication known as **lactic acidosis**. Lactic acidosis is fatal about half of the time. It may also occur in association with a number of conditions, including diabetes mellitus. The risk of lactic acidosis increases with age, the presence of heart failure, and worsening kidney function. Regular monitoring of kidney function minimizes the risk of developing lactic acidosis, as does using the minimum effective dosage of metformin. Metformin should not be taken by people with acidosis, including those with diabetic ketoacidosis. Diabetic ketoacidosis should be treated with insulin.

People with **liver disease** should not take metformin because of the increased risk of lactic acidosis.

People taking oral antidiabetes drugs are generally more likely to develop **heart disease** compared with people taking insulin or those treated by diet alone.

Possible Side Effects

People who have been stabilized on metformin should not consider gastrointestinal (GI) symptoms to be related to the drug unless other causes or lactic acidosis have been excluded.

▼ Most common: diarrhea, nausea, vomiting, abdominal bloating, gas, and appetite loss. These symptoms tend to occur when you first start taking metformin but are generally transient and resolve on their own. Occasionally, temporary dosage reduction is useful.

▼ Rare: An unpleasant or metallic taste in the mouth (this usually resolves on its own) and low blood levels of vitamin B_{12}. Blood levels of vitamin B_{12} should be periodically checked, or you may take a B_{12} supplement.

Drug Interactions

• Metformin may reduce the effect of glyburide (a sulfonylurea) but this interaction is highly variable from one person to another.

• Alcohol increases the risk of developing lactic acidosis while taking metformin.

• Metformin may interfere with amiloride, digoxin, morphine, procainamide, quinine, quinidine, ranitidine, triamterene, trimethoprim, and vancomycin. Careful monitoring is necessary.

• Cimetidine, nifedipine, and furosemide can cause a large increase in metformin blood levels and possible side effects. Furosemide levels are reduced by metformin.

Food Interactions

Metformin may be taken with food to reduce upset stomach.

Usual Dose

Adult: 500 mg twice daily or 850 mg once daily, increased gradually to a maximum daily dosage of 2550 mg. Older adults should start with the regular dosage but generally are not given the maximum.

Child (age 10 and older)*:* Same adult dosage. Extended-release tablets should not be taken by those under age 17.

Overdosage

Lactic acidosis has occurred in some cases. Take the victim to a hospital emergency room at once. ALWAYS bring the prescription bottle or container.

Special Information

Diet and exercise are the mainstays of diabetes treatment. Be sure to follow your doctor's directions in these areas while taking your medication.

Alcohol increases the risk of developing lactic acidosis while taking metformin.

Lactic acidosis is a medical emergency. Metformin treatment must be stopped immediately if you develop it. This disease is often subtle and is accompanied only by nonspecific symptoms such as feeling unwell, muscle aches, breathing difficulties, tiredness, and nonspecific upset stomach. Low body temperature, low blood pressure, and slow heartbeat can develop with more severe acidosis. Call your doctor at once if you develop these symptoms.

Stomach and intestinal side effects may be reduced by gradually increasing your dosage and by taking metformin with meals.

Metformin should be temporarily stopped if you have severe diarrhea or vomiting. However, do not stop taking your medication without first consulting your doctor.

If you forget a dose, take it as soon as you remember. If it is almost time for your next dose, skip the dose you forgot and continue with your regular schedule. Do not take a double dose.

Special Populations

Pregnancy/Breast-feeding
The safety of using metformin during pregnancy is not known. Pregnant women with diabetes should take insulin.

Metformin passes into breast milk. Nursing mothers who must take it should consider bottle-feeding.

Seniors

Seniors may require reduced dosage.

Generic Name

Methyldopa (meth-ul-DOPE-uh) Ⓖ

Brand Name

Aldomet   Amodopa

Type of Drug

Antihypertensive.

Prescribed For

High blood pressure.

General Information

How methyldopa works is not well understood. It may lower blood pressure by stimulating receptors in the central nervous system (CNS), and by inhibiting or reducing levels of important pressure-regulating hormones such as norepinephrine and serotonin. It takes about 2 days for methyldopa to reach its maximal antihypertensive (blood-pressure-lowering) effect. It is usually prescribed with one or more other antihypertensive drugs or a diuretic.

Cautions and Warnings

Do not take methyldopa if you are **allergic** to it or any other ingredient in the formulation, including sulfites.

Do not take this drug if you have had a previous liver-related **reaction** to it, or if you have liver disease such as **hepatitis** or **cirrhosis**. People taking this drug may develop a **fever** with changes in liver function within the first 3 weeks of treatment. Some people develop **jaundice** (symptoms include yellowing of the skin or whites of the eyes) during the first 2 or 3 months of treatment. Your doctor should periodically evaluate your liver function during the first 3 months of methyldopa treatment, or if you develop an unexplained fever.

Methyldopa should be used with caution in people with severe **kidney disease,** who may need reduced dosage. Methyldopa may increase the risk of **hemolytic anemia.**

Possible Side Effects

Most people have little trouble with methyldopa, but it can cause temporary sedation in the first few weeks of treatment or when the dose is increased. Passing headache and weakness are other possible early side effects.

▼ Less common: dizziness; light-headedness; tingling in the extremities; muscle spasms or weakness; decreased mental acuity; psychological disturbances including nightmares, mild psychosis, and depression; rash; changes in heart rate; increased angina pain; water retention, resulting in weight gain; dizziness when rising suddenly from a sitting or lying position; nausea; vomiting; constipation; diarrhea; mild dry mouth; sore or black tongue; stuffy nose; male breast enlargement or pain; lactation in females; impotence or decreased sex drive in males; mild arthritis symptoms; and skin reactions.

▼ Rare: Methyldopa may affect white blood cells or blood platelets. It may also cause involuntary jerky movements, twitching, restlessness, and slow, continuous, wormlike movements of the fingers, toes, hands, or other body parts.

Drug Interactions

• Do not combine methyldopa and a monoamine oxidase inhibitor (MAOI) antidepressant. This combination can cause excessive stimulation.

• Methyldopa increases the effect of other blood-pressure-lowering drugs. This is a desirable interaction for people with hypertension. However, the combination of methyldopa and propranolol or nadolol—two beta blockers often prescribed for hypertension—has, rarely, caused an increase in blood pressure.

• Avoid over-the-counter cough medicines, cold and allergy remedies, and appetite suppressants. These products contain stimulant ingredients that can increase blood pressure.

• Methyldopa may increase the blood-sugar-lowering effect of tolbutamide or other sulfonylurea-type oral antidiabetic drugs.

• If methyldopa is combined with phenoxybenzamine, urinary incontinence (inability to control the bladder) may result.

• The effect of methyldopa may be reduced by barbiturates, tricyclic antidepressants, and iron.

• The combination of methyldopa and lithium may cause symptoms of lithium overdose—upset stomach, frequent urination, muscle weakness, tiredness, and tremors—even though blood levels of lithium have not changed.

• Methyldopa in combination with haloperidol may produce irritability, aggressiveness, assaultive behavior, or other psychiatric symptoms.

• Combining methyldopa and levodopa may increase the effects of both drugs.

• Combining methyldopa with stimulants or a phenothiazine-type drug may lead to a serious increase in blood pressure.

Food Interactions

Methyldopa is best taken on an empty stomach, but you may take it with food if it upsets your stomach.

Usual Dose

Adult: starting dosage—250 mg tablet 2–3 times a day for the first 2 days. Dosage may then be increased until lower blood pressure is achieved. Maintenance dose—500–2000 mg a day in 2–4 divided doses, depending on individual need.

Child: 4.5 mg per lb. of body weight a day in 2–4 divided doses, depending on individual need. Do not exceed 30 mg per lb. of body weight a day.

Overdosage

Symptoms include sedation, very low blood pressure, weakness, dizziness, light–headedness, fainting, slow heartbeat, constipation, abdominal gas or bulging, nausea, vomiting, and coma. Overdose victims should be made to vomit if they are still conscious by using ipecac syrup—available at any pharmacy—and then taken to a hospital emergency room. If some time has passed since the overdose was taken, take the victim directly to an emergency room. ALWAYS bring the prescription bottle or container.

Special Information

Take methyldopa exactly as prescribed to maintain maximum control of your hypertension. Do not stop taking this drug unless you are told to do so by your doctor.

A mild sedative effect is to be expected from methyldopa and will resolve within several days. Be careful when driving, operating hazardous machinery, or performing any task that requires concentration.

Your urine may darken if left exposed to air. This is normal and not a cause for alarm.

Call your doctor if you develop fever, prolonged general tiredness, or dizziness. If you develop involuntary muscle movements, fever, or jaundice, stop taking the drug and contact your doctor immediately. If these reactions are due to methyldopa, your temperature or liver abnormalities will begin to normalize as soon as you stop taking it.

If you forget a dose, take it as soon as you remember. If it is almost time for your next dose, skip the one you forgot and continue with your regular schedule. Do not take a double dose.

Special Populations

Pregnancy/Breast-feeding

Methyldopa crosses into the fetal circulation. When this drug is considered crucial by your doctor, its potential benefits must be carefully weighed against its risks.

Small amounts of methyldopa pass into breast milk. Nursing mothers who must take this drug should consider bottle-feeding.

Seniors

Seniors are more sensitive to the sedating and blood-pressure-lowering effects of methyldopa and may experience dizziness or fainting. Older adults should receive reduced dosage.

Generic Name

Methylphenidate (meth-ul-FEN-ih-date) G

Brand Names

Concerta   Methylin ER

Metadate	Ritalin
Metadate CD	Ritalin LA
Metadate ER	Ritalin-SR
Methylin	

The information in this profile also applies to the following drug:

Generic Ingredient: Dexmethylphenidate
Focalin

Type of Drug

Mild central-nervous-system stimulant.

Prescribed for

Attention-deficit hyperactivity disorder (ADHD); also prescribed for psychological, educational, or social disorders; narcolepsy; and mild depression in the elderly. Methylphenidate is also used in cancer treatment and stroke recovery and for treating hiccups after anesthesia.

General Information

Methylphenidate hydrochloride is prescribed for the treatment of ADHD in children. It should be used only after conducting a complete evaluation of the child. Frequency and severity of symptoms and their appropriateness for the age of the child—not solely the presence of certain behavioral characteristics—determine whether drug therapy is required. Many experts believe that methylphenidate offers only a temporary solution because it does not permanently change behavioral patterns. Psychological measures must also be taken to ensure successful treatment in the long term.

Cautions and Warnings

Chronic or abusive use of methylphenidate can lead to drug dependence or **addiction**. This drug can also cause severe psychotic episodes. Do not use methylphenidate for the prevention or treatment of normal fatigue.

Take methylphenidate with caution if you have **glaucoma or other visual problems, high blood pressure,** a **seizure** disorder, severe **depression, tics** or **Tourette's syndrome,** if you are extremely **tense or agitated,** or if you are **allergic** to this drug.

Stimulants like methylphenidate are not effective in children whose symptoms are related to environmental factors or to primary psychiatric conditions, including psychosis. Methylphenidate should not be used to treat a primary stress reaction.

Possible Side Effects

Adults

▼ Most common: nervousness and inability to sleep, which doctors generally control by reducing or eliminating the afternoon or evening dose.

▼ Rare: rash, itching, fever, symptoms resembling those of arthritis, appetite loss, nausea, dizziness, abnormal heart rhythm, headache, drowsiness, changes in blood pressure or pulse, chest pain, stomach pain, psychotic reactions, changes in blood components, and loss of some scalp hair.

Children

▼ Most common: appetite loss; stomach pain; weight loss, especially during prolonged therapy; sleeping difficulties; and abnormal heart rhythm.

Drug Interactions

• Methylphenidate reduces the effectiveness of guanethidine (an antihypertensive drug).

• Monoamine oxidase inhibitors (MAOIs) may significantly increase the effect of methylphenidate, which may lead to extreme high blood pressure. Use with caution.

• Methylphenidate may increase tricyclic antidepressant and SSRI blood levels and the risk of side effects.

• Methylphenidate may increase anticonvulsant blood levels.

• If you take methylphenidate regularly, avoid alcohol: This combination increases drowsiness.

Food Interactions

This medication is best taken 30 to 45 minutes before meals.

Usual Dose

Adult: Doses range from 10–30 mg a day but can be as high as 60 mg. The immediate-release drug is taken 2–3 times a day.

Child (age 6 and over): starting dosage—5 mg before breakfast and lunch. Increase by 5–10 mg each week as required, not to exceed 60 mg a day.

Child (under age 6): not recommended.

SR tablets and ER tablets are designed to last for 8 hours, and Concerta, Ritalin LA, and Metadate CD last 8–12 hours. These medications may be used in place of more frequent doses during the same period of time.

Overdosage

Symptoms include vomiting, agitation, uncontrollable twitching of the muscles, convulsions followed by coma, euphoria (feeling "high"), confusion, hallucinations, delirium, sweating, flushing, headache, high fever, abnormal heart rate, high blood pressure, and dryness of the mouth and nose. Take the victim to a hospital emergency room immediately. ALWAYS bring the prescription bottle or container.

Special Information

Methylphenidate can mask the signs of temporary drowsiness or fatigue: Be careful when driving or doing any task that requires concentration. Take your last daily dose no later than 6 p.m. to avoid sleeping difficulties.

Call your doctor if you develop any persistent or bothersome side effect. Do not increase your dosage without your doctor's knowledge.

Suppression of growth in children has been reported with long-term use of this drug. Contact your doctor if your child does not grow or gain weight as expected.

SR-tablets must be swallowed whole, never crushed or chewed.

If you miss a dose, take it as soon as possible. Space the remaining daily dosage evenly throughout the day. Go back to your regular schedule the next day.

Special Populations

Pregnancy/Breast-feeding

Methylphenidate crosses into the fetal circulation. When this drug is considered crucial by your doctor, its potential benefits must be carefully weighed against its risks.

Small amounts of methylphenidate may pass into breast milk. Nursing mothers who must take this drug should consider bottle-feeding.

Seniors
Seniors may take this drug without special restriction.

Generic Name

Metoclopramide (met-oe-KLOE-pruh-mide) Ⓖ

Brand Names

Clopra	Reclomide
Maxolon	Reglan*
Octamide	

*Some products in this brand-name group are alcohol- or sugar- free. Consult your pharmacist.

Type of Drug

Antiemetic and gastrointestinal (GI) stimulant.

Prescribed For

Nausea and vomiting; also prescribed for diabetic gastro-pareisis (stomach paralysis associated with diabetes), gas-troesophageal reflux disease (GERD), stomach ulcer, anorexia nervosa, and bleeding from blood vessels in the esophagus—often associated with severe liver disease. It also facilitates diagnostic x-ray procedures and improves the absorption of anti-migraine medication and narcotic pain relievers. Nursing mothers are occasionally given metoclo-pramide to increase milk production.

General Information

Metoclopramide stimulates movement of the upper GI tract without producing excess stomach acids or other secretions. Doctors believe that it prevents nausea and vomiting primar-ily by affecting dopamine receptors in the brain. Metoclo-pramide also affects the secretion of a variety of hormones and may improve the absorption of other drugs into the bloodstream.

Cautions and Warnings

People with **high blood pressure, Parkinson's disease, asthma, liver or kidney failure,** or **seizure disorders** should use metoclopramide with caution. Do not take this drug if you are **allergic** to it. Metoclopramide should not be used if you have a **bleeding ulcer** or any condition that makes stimulation of the GI tract dangerous.

Mild to severe **depression** has occurred with metoclopramide.

Uncontrollable motions similar to those associated with Parkinson's disease have developed as a side effect of this drug. These generally occur within 6 months after starting metoclopramide and subside within 2 to 3 months.

This drug may cause **extrapyramidal side effects** similar to those associated with phenothiazine drugs. These effects, which occur in 0.2–1% of the people taking the drug, include restlessness and involuntary movements of the arms and legs, face, tongue, lips, and other parts of the body. Do not combine metoclopramide with a phenothiazine drug because this may increase the risk of extrapyramidal effects.

Women taking this drug develop chronic elevations of the hormone prolactin. About 33% of breast tumors are prolactin-dependent, a factor that you should consider before taking metoclopramide.

Possible Side Effects

Mild side effects occur in 20% to 30% of people. Side effects increase with dosage or prolonged use.

▼ Most common: restlessness, drowsiness, fatigue, sleeplessness, dizziness, anxiety, loss of muscle control, headache, muscle spasm, confusion, severe depression, convulsions, and hallucinations.

▼ Less common: rash, diarrhea, blood-pressure changes, abnormal heart rhythms, slow heartbeat, oozing from the nipples, tender nipples, loss of regular menstrual periods, breast swelling and tenderness, impotence, reduced white-blood-cell counts, frequent urination, loss of urinary control, visual disturbances, and worsening of bronchial spasm.

▼ Rare: People taking this drug may develop a group of possibly fatal symptoms collectively called neuroleptic malignant syndrome. These symptoms include very high fever, semi-consciousness, rigid muscles, flushing of the face and upper body, and liver toxicity after high doses.

Drug Interactions

• Narcotics and anticholinergic drugs interfere with metoclopramide's effect on stomach acid.

• Metoclopramide may increase the effects of alcohol and cyclosporine.

• Metoclopramide may increase the sedative effects of nervous-system depressants including tranquilizers and sleeping pills.

• Metoclopramide and levodopa interfere with each other.

• Metoclopramide may reduce the effects of digitalis drugs and cimetidine.

• Combining metoclopramide and a monoamine oxidase inhibitor (MAOI) antidepressant may cause very high blood pressure.

Food Interactions

Take this drug 30 minutes before meals and at bedtime.

Usual Dose

Adult and Child (age 15 and over): 5–15 mg before meals and at bedtime. Single doses of 10–20 mg are used before x-ray diagnostic procedures.

Senior: starting dosage—5 mg.

Child (age 6–14): ¼–½ the adult dosage.

Child (under age 6): 0.05 mg per lb. of body weight per dose.

Overdosage

Symptoms of overdose include drowsiness, disorientation, restlessness, or uncontrollable muscle movement. These usually disappear within 24 hours after the drug has been stopped. Anticholinergic drugs help control overdose symptoms. Call your local poison control center or a hospital emergency room for more information.

Special Information

Call your doctor if you develop chills; fever; sore throat; dizziness; severe or persistent headache; feeling unwell; rapid or irregular heartbeat; difficulty speaking or swallowing; loss of balance; stiffness of the arms or legs; a shuffling walk; a mask-like face; lip-smacking or puckering; puffing of the cheeks; rapid, worm-like tongue movement; uncontrollable chewing movement; uncontrolled arm and leg movement; or any persistent or intolerable side effect.

Metoclopramide may cause dizziness, confusion, and drowsiness. Be careful when driving or doing any task that requires concentration. Avoid alcohol and be cautious about taking tranquilizers or sleeping pills.

If you forget a dose, take it as soon as you remember. If it is almost time for your next dose, skip the dose you forgot and continue with your regular schedule. Do not take a double dose.

Special Populations

Pregnancy/Breast-feeding

Metoclopramide enters the fetal circulation. When this drug is considered crucial by your doctor, its potential benefits must be carefully weighed against its risks.

This drug passes into breast milk. Nursing mothers occasionally receive metoclopramide to increase milk production. There appears to be no risk for the infant whose nursing mother takes 45 mg or less a day. Always consider possible effects on the nursing infant if breast-feeding while taking this drug.

Seniors

Seniors, especially women, are more sensitive to side effects (see "Cautions and Warnings"). Shuffling walk and shaking hands may be likely to occur in seniors after a prolonged use of metoclopramide.

Generic Name

Metoprolol (meh-TOPE-roe-lol)

Brand Names

Lopressor   Toprol-XL

The information in this profile also applies to the following drug:

Generic Ingredient: Penbutolol
Levatol

Type of Drug

Beta-adrenergic blocking agent.

Prescribed For

High blood pressure, angina pectoris, abnormal heart rhythms, prevention of second heart attack, migraine, tremors, aggressive behavior, side effects of antipsychotic drugs, improving cognitive performance, congestive heart failure, and bleeding from the esophagus.

General Information

Metoprolol is one of 15 beta-adrenergic-blocking drugs, or beta blockers, that interfere with the action of a specific part of the nervous system. Beta receptors are found all over the body and affect many body functions. Each beta blocker has particular characteristics that make it more suitable for certain conditions or people. Metoprolol is available in a sustained-release formulation, taken only once a day, that maintains a steady blood level of the drug for a full 24 hours.

Cautions and Warnings

Do not take metoprolol if you are **allergic** to beta blockers.

You should be cautious about taking metoprolol if you have **asthma,** a **very slow heart rate,** or **heart block** (disruption of the electrical impulses that control heart rate) because the drug may aggravate these conditions.

People with **angina** who take metoprolol for high blood pressure risk aggravating their angina if they suddenly stop taking the drug. These people should have their drug dosage reduced gradually over 1 to 2 weeks.

Metoprolol should be used with caution if you have **liver or kidney disease** because your ability to eliminate the drug from your body may be impaired.

Metoprolol reduces the amount of blood pumped by the heart with each beat. This reduction in blood flow may aggravate the condition of people with **poor circulation or circulatory disease**.

If you are undergoing **major surgery,** your doctor may want you to stop taking metoprolol at least 2 days before.

Possible Side Effects

Metroprolol side effects are relatively uncommon and usually mild.

▼ Less common: impotence, unusual tiredness or weakness, slow heartbeat, heart failure, dizziness,

Possible Side Effects *(continued)*

breathing difficulties, bronchospasm, depression, confusion, anxiety, nervousness, sleeplessness, disorientation, short-term memory loss, emotional instability, cold hands and feet, constipation, diarrhea, nausea, vomiting, upset stomach, increased sweating, urinary difficulties, cramps, blurred vision, rash, hair loss, stuffy nose, facial swelling, aggravation of lupus erythematosus, itching, chest pain, back or joint pain, colitis, drug allergy (symptoms include fever and sore throat), and liver toxicity.

Drug Interactions

• Metoprolol may interact with surgical anesthetics to increase the risk of heart problems during surgery. Some anesthesiologists recommend gradually stopping the drug by 2 days before surgery.

• Metoprolol may interfere with the normal signs of low blood sugar and with the action of oral antidiabetes medications.

• Metoprolol increases the blood-pressure-lowering effect of other blood-pressure-reducing agents, including clonidine, guanabenz, and reserpine, as well as calcium-channel blockers such as nifedipine.

• Aspirin-containing drugs, indomethacin, sulfinpyrazone, and estrogen drugs may interfere with the blood-pressure-lowering effect of metoprolol.

• Cocaine may reduce the effectiveness of all beta blockers.

• Metoprolol may worsen the problem of cold hands and feet associated with taking ergot alkaloids, which are used to treat migraine. Gangrene is a possibility in people taking both an ergot and metoprolol.

• The effect of benzodiazepine antianxiety drugs may be increased by metoprolol.

• Metoprolol will counteract thyroid hormone replacements.

• Combining metoprolol and prazosin may increase the risk of postural hypotension.

• SSRIs may increase the side effects of metoprolol.

• Calcium channel blockers, flecainide, hydralazine, oral contraceptives, propafenone, haloperidol, phenothiazine tranquilizers (molindone and others) quinolone antibacterials, and quinidine may increase the amount of metoprolol in the bloodstream and lead to increased metoprolol effects.

• Metoprolol should not be taken within 2 weeks of taking a monoamine oxidase inhibitor (MAOI) antidepressant.

• Aluminum salts, barbituates, calcium salts, cholestyramine, colestipol, ampicillin, and rifampin may reduce the effectiveness of metoprolol.

• Cimetidine increases the amount of metoprolol absorbed into the bloodstream from oral tablets.

• Metoprolol may interfere with the effectiveness of some asthma medications, including theophylline and aminophylline, and especially ephedrine and isoproterenol.

• Combining metoprolol with phenytoin or digitalis drugs may result in excessive slowing of the heart, possibly causing heart block.

• If you stop smoking while taking metoprolol, your dose may have to be reduced because your liver will break down the drug more slowly afterward.

Food Interactions

Sustained-release metoprolol—Toprol-XL—may be taken with food if it upsets your stomach. Because food increases the amount of short-acting metoprolol—Lopressor—absorbed into the blood, take the short-acting form without food.

Usual Dose

Metoprolol: 100–450 mg a day; dosage must be tailored to your specific needs.

Penbutolol: 20 mg once a day. Seniors may require more or less medication and must be carefully monitored by their doctors. People with liver problems may require lower dosage.

Overdosage

Symptoms include changes in heartbeat—unusually slow, unusually fast, or irregular—severe dizziness or fainting, breathing difficulties, bluish-colored fingernails or palms, and seizures. The victim should be taken to a hospital emergency room. ALWAYS bring the prescription bottle or container.

Special Information

Metoprolol should be taken continuously. When ending metoprolol treatments, dosage should be lowered gradually over a period of about 2 weeks. Do not stop taking this drug unless directed to do so by your doctor: Abrupt withdrawal may cause chest pain, breathing difficulties, increased sweating, and unusually fast or irregular heartbeat.

Call your doctor at once if you develop back or joint pain, breathing difficulties, cold hands or feet, depression, rash, or changes in heartbeat. This drug may produce an undesirable lowering of blood pressure, leading to dizziness or fainting; call your doctor if this happens to you. Call your doctor if you experience persistent or bothersome nausea or vomiting, upset stomach, diarrhea, constipation, impotence, headache, itching, anxiety, nightmares or vivid dreams, trouble sleeping, stuffy nose, frequent urination, unusual tiredness, or weakness.

Metoprolol can cause drowsiness, light-headedness, dizziness, or blurred vision. Be careful when driving or performing complex tasks.

It is best to take metoprolol at the same time each day. If you forget a dose, take it as soon as you remember. If you take metoprolol once a day and it is within 8 hours of your next dose, skip the dose you forgot and continue with your regular schedule. If you take it twice a day and it is within 4 hours of your next dose, skip the dose you forgot and continue with your regular schedule. Never take a double dose.

Special Populations

Pregnancy/Breast-feeding
Infants born to women who took a beta blocker while pregnant had lower birth weights, low blood pressure, and reduced heart rates. Metoprolol should be avoided by women who are or might be pregnant.

Small amounts of metoprolol pass into breast milk. Nursing mothers taking metoprolol should bottle-feed.

Seniors
Seniors require less of the drug to achieve results. Seniors taking metoprolol may be more likely to suffer from cold hands and feet, reduced body temperature, chest pain, general feelings of ill health, sudden breathing difficulties, increased sweating, or changes in heartbeat.

Generic Name

Metronidazole (meh-troe-NYE-duh-zole) Ⓖ

Brand Names

Flagyl
Flagyl ER
Metric 21
MetroCream

MetroGel
MetroLotion
Noritate
Protostat

Type of Drug

Amoebicide and antibiotic.

Prescribed For

Acute amoebic dysentery and infections of the vagina, bone, joint, brain, nervous system, urinary tract, abdomen, and skin; also prescribed for pneumonia, ulcers caused by *Helicobacter pylori,* inflammatory bowel disease, rosacea, colitis caused by other antibiotics, periodontal (gum) infection, and complications of severe liver disease. The gel may be used to treat acne, severe skin ulcers, and inflammation of the skin around the mouth. Metronidazole may be given by intravenous injection to prevent infectious complications of bowel surgery.

General Information

Metronidazole is effective against infections caused by a variety of fungi and some bacteria. Metronidazole kills these microorganisms by disrupting their DNA after they enter body cells. Metronidazole may be prescribed for symptomless diseases when the doctor feels that an underlying infection may be involved. For example, asymptomatic women may be treated with this drug when vaginal examination shows evidence of *Trichomonas*. Because vaginal trichomonal infection is a sexually transmitted disease, asymptomatic sexual partners should also be treated if the organism has been found in the woman's genital tract.

Cautions and Warnings

You should not use this drug if you have a history of **blood disease** or are **sensitive** or **allergic** to metronidazole.

People taking this medication have experienced **seizures** and **numbness or tingling in the hands or feet**. This effect is rare with low dosages but may be more common in people taking larger dosages for long periods, such as in Crohn's disease. If this occurs, stop taking the drug and call your doctor at once. Metronidazole should be taken with caution if you have active **nervous system disease,** including **epilepsy,** or severe **liver problems**.

Possible Side Effects

▼ Most common: gastrointestinal (GI) symptoms, including nausea that is sometimes accompanied by headache, dizziness, appetite loss, vomiting, diarrhea, vaginitis, upset stomach, abdominal cramping, and constipation. A sharp, unpleasant metallic taste is also associated with the use of this drug.

▼ Less common: numbness or tingling in the extremities, joint pain, confusion, irritability, depression, difficulty sleeping, and weakness. Itching and a sensation of pelvic pressure also have been reported.

▼ Rare: clumsiness or poor coordination, fever, increased urination, seizure, incontinence, and reduced sex drive.

Skin creams containing metronidazole may cause redness, itching, irritation, or worsening of rosacea.

Drug Interactions

• Avoid alcohol: Interaction with metronidazole may cause abdominal cramps, nausea, vomiting, headaches, and flushing. Modification of the taste of alcohol has also been reported. Metronidazole should not be used if you are taking disulfiram (a drug used to maintain alcohol abstinence) because the combination may cause confusion and psychotic reactions.

• Dosages of oral anticoagulants (blood-thinners) such as warfarin must be reduced because metronidazole increases their effect.

• Metronidazole increases lithium blood levels, effects, and side effects.

• Cimetidine may increase metronidazole blood levels. Metronidazole dosage may have to be reduced.

• Phenobarbital and other barbiturates may reduce metronidazole's effectiveness.

• Drugs that cause nervous system toxicity—such as mexiletine, ethambutol, isoniazid, lindane, lincomycin, lithium, pemoline, quinacrine, and long-term high-dose pyridoxine (vitamin B_6) should not be taken with metronidazole because nervous-system side effects may be increased.

• Metronidazole may increase blood levels of phenytoin and the risk of phenytoin side effects. Your doctor may need to adjust your phenytoin dosage.

Food Interactions

Take this drug with food to avoid upset stomach.

Usual Dose

Adult: amoebic dysentery—750 mg 3 times a day for 5–10 days. Trichomonal infection—250 mg 3 times a day for 7 days; or 2 g in 1 dose. *H.pylori*—250 mg 4 times a day. Reduced dosage may be necessary for seniors.

Child: amoebic dysentery—16–23 mg per lb. of body weight daily, divided in 3 equal doses for 10 days. Trichomonal infection—2.25 mg per lb. of body weight 3 times a day for 7 days.

Skin creams should be applied 1-2 times a day. Vaginal creams should be used 1-2 times a day for 5 days.

Overdosage

Symptoms include nausea, vomiting, clumsiness, unsteadiness, seizures, and pain or tingling in the hands or feet. Call your local poison control center or a hospital emergency room for more information. If you seek treatment, ALWAYS bring the prescription bottle or container.

Special Information

Call your doctor if you become dizzy or light-headed while taking this drug, or if you develop numbness, tingling, pain, or weakness in your hands or feet; seizures; clumsiness or unsteadiness; mood changes; unusual vaginal irritation, discharge, or dryness; frequent or painful urination; mood or mental changes; rash, hives, or itching; severe pain of the back or abdomen accompanied by vomiting, appetite loss, or nausea; or any bothersome or persistent side effect.

Metronidazole may cause darkening of your urine; this is probably not important, but inform your doctor if it happens.

Follow your doctor's dosage instructions exactly. Complete the full course of drug therapy.

Metronidazole may cause dry mouth, which usually can be relieved with ice, hard candy, or gum. Call your doctor or dentist if dry mouth persists for more than 2 weeks.

Avoid drinking alcohol while taking metronidazole.

If you forget a dose, take it as soon as you remember. If it is almost time for your next dose, skip the dose you forgot and continue with your regular schedule. Do not take a double dose.

Special Populations

Pregnancy/Breast-feeding

Metronidazole passes into the fetal circulation. This drug should not be taken during the first 3 months of pregnancy and should be used with caution during the last 6 months.

Metronidazole passes into breast milk. Nursing mothers who must take it should bottle-feed. After you have finished metronidazole treatment, express any milk produced while you were taking the drug and discard it along with any pumped breast milk you might have saved. Nursing can be resumed 1 or 2 days after stopping metronidazole.

Seniors

Seniors, particularly those with advanced liver disease, are more sensitive to the effects of this drug and may require lower dosages.

Generic Name

Miconazole (mye-KON-uh-zole) G

Brand Name

Monistat

The information in this profile also applies to the following drugs:

Generic Ingredient: Tioconazole G
Vagistat-1

Generic Ingredient: Butoconazole
Femstat

Type of Drug

Antifungal.

Prescribed For

Fungal infections of the vagina, skin, and blood.

General Information

Miconazole nitrate is used to treat a variety of fungal infections. Monistat-Derm cream and related products are applied directly to the skin to treat common fungal infections of the skin, including ringworm, athlete's foot, and jock itch. Monistat 3 and similar products are used to treat vaginal infections. Hospitalized patients may receive this drug by intravenous injection to ward off serious fungal infections. When used for vaginal or topical infections, it is also effective against several nonfungal organisms.

Cautions and Warnings

Do not use miconazole if you are **allergic** to it. Proper diagnosis is essential for effective treatment. Do not use this product without first consulting your doctor. If a reaction occurs while taking miconazole, (such as sensitivity or chemical irritation) discontinue use and consult your doctor.

Possible Side Effects

Intravenous Injection
▼ Common: vein irritation, itching, rash, nausea, vomiting, fever, drowsiness, diarrhea, loss of appetite, and flushing.

Vaginal Administration
▼ Common: itching, burning, and irritation.
▼ Less common: pelvic cramps, hives, rash, and headache.

Topical Application
▼ Less common: skin irritation, burning, and redness.

Drug Interactions

• Miconazole can increase the effect of warfarin (an antico-agulant drug) which may cause bleeding problems including nosebleeds, bleeding gums, and bruising.

Food Interactions

None known.

Usual Dose

Vaginal Suppositories and Cream: 1 applicatorful or supposi-tory into the vagina at bedtime for 1–7 days.

Topical Cream, Lotions, and Powder: Apply to affected areas 2 times a day, morning and evening, for up to 7 days, or as needed.

Overdosage

Accidental ingestion may cause upset stomach. Call your local poison control center or hospital emergency room for more information.

Special Information

When using the vaginal cream, insert the whole applicator of cream high into the vagina and be sure to complete the full course of treatment. Call your doctor if you develop burning or itching.

If you forget to administer a dose of miconazole, do so as soon as you remember. If it is almost time for your next dose, skip the dose you forgot and continue with your regular schedule. Do not take a double dose.

Special Populations

Pregnancy/Breast-feeding

Pregnant women should avoid using vaginal creams during pregnancy. It may be used if needed, but usage should begin during the first 3 months, and continue during the next 6 months only if absolutely necessary. Your doctor may want you to avoid using a vaginal applicator during pregnancy. Vaginal suppositories may be inserted by hand instead.

Miconazole has not been shown to cause problems in breast-fed infants.

Seniors

Seniors may take this medication without special restriction.

Generic Name

Midodrine (MYE-doe-dreen)

Brand Name

ProAmatine

Type of Drug

Alpha stimulant.

Prescribed For

Dizziness or fainting when rising from a sitting position. Midodrine is also used for poor urinary control and retrograde ejaculation.

General Information

Midodrine is recommended only if other treatments for dizziness or fainting have failed and symptoms are interfering with your daily routine. It stimulates nerve endings in small veins and arteries, "tightening" them slightly to raise blood pressure. This helps control dizziness and fainting caused by poor blood flow to the brain. Systolic blood pressure increases by 15 to 30 points 1 hour after taking 10 mg of midodrine. The effect lasts about 2 to 3 hours.

Cautions and Warnings

Do not take this drug if you **retain urine** or have severe **heart disease, kidney disease, diabetes, pheochromocytoma** (adrenal gland tumor), a severely **overactive thyroid gland, visual problems,** or excessive and persistent **high blood pressure** when lying down.

High blood pressure—especially when lying down—can be the most serious side effect of midodrine. This problem may be prevented by not completely reclining, or raising the head of your bed, when you sleep.

People with **kidney disease** require reduced dosage. People with **liver disease** should be cautious about using midodrine because it may be partially broken down in the liver. Your doctor should evaluate your kidney and liver function periodically.

Heart rate may decrease while taking midodrine.

Possible Side Effects

▼ Most common: tingling in the hands or feet, pain, itching, goosebumps, painful urination, high blood pressure when lying down, and chills.

▼ Less common: headache, sensation of pressure in the head, facial flushing, confusion, abnormal thinking, dry mouth, nervousness, anxiety, and rash.

▼ Rare: visual problems, dizziness, sensitive skin, sleeplessness, tiredness, canker sores, dry skin, urinary difficulties, weakness, backache, nausea, upset stomach, gas, heartburn, and leg cramps.

Drug Interactions

• Midodrine increases the effects of digoxin or digitoxin and similar drugs, psychoactive medications, beta blockers, and other stimulants. Be very cautious when combining any of these drugs and midodrine.

• People taking fludrocortisone must have their dosage reduced or salt intake lowered before starting midodrine.

• Alpha blockers such as prazosin, terazosin, and doxazosin can block midodrine's effects.

Food Interactions

None known.

Usual Dose

Dizziness or Fainting
    Adult: 10 mg 3 times a day. People with kidney failure should start with 2.5 mg.
    Child: not recommended.

Urinary Incontinence
    Adult: 2.5–5 mg 2–3 times a day.
    Child: not recommended.

Overdosage

Symptoms include high blood pressure, goosebumps, feeling cold, and difficulty urinating. Take the victim to a hospital emergency room. ALWAYS bring the prescription bottle or container.

Special Information

Your doctor may suggest that you take the medication about every 4 hours: when you get up, around noon, and in the late afternoon—no later than 6 p.m. The drug may also be taken every 3 hours to control symptoms. Do not take midodrine after dinner or less than 4 hours before you go to bed.

Continue taking midodrine only if it works for you. If you forget a dose, take it as soon as you remember. If it is almost time for your next dose, skip the dose you forgot and continue with your regular schedule. Call your doctor if you miss 2 or more doses in a row.

Special Populations

Pregnancy/Breast-feeding

Midodrine may pass into fetal circulation. When this drug is considered crucial by your doctor, its potential benefits must be carefully weighed against its risks.

It is not known if midodrine passes into breast milk. Nursing mothers who must take it should consider bottle-feeding.

Seniors

Seniors may take midodrine without special precaution.

Generic Name

Mifepristone (mif-ih-PRIS-tone)

Brand Name

Mifeprex

Type of Drug

Abortifacient.

Prescribed For

Termination of pregnancies of less than 7 weeks. Also used as a "morning after" contraceptive, for fetal deaths or fetuses that are not viable in the early stages of pregnancy, meningioma that cannot be treated surgically, endometriosis, and Cushing's syndrome.

General Information

Formerly known as RU-486, mifepristone is a prostaglandin that works by interrupting the supply of hormones that maintain the interior of the uterus where the fetus attaches to obtain nourishment and grow. Without these hormones, the uterus cannot support the pregnancy and the contents of the uterus are expelled. It is related to misoprostol, a drug used to prevent gastrointestinal tract ulcers from aspirin and other NSAID-type drugs.

Cautions and Warnings

Surgery may be needed if mifepristone treatment does not produce a complete termination. The same pre-surgical precautions should be taken with mifepristone as are taken with a surgical termination.

Vaginal bleeding or spotting should be expected for 9 to 16 days. Up to 8 percent of women who use mifepristone can bleed for 30 days or more, which may lead to anemia.

There is no information on the effect of this drug in liver or kidney disease. **Adrenal failure** may interfere with mifepristone's effectiveness.

Possible Side Effects

This drug is designed to produce the vaginal bleeding and cramping necessary to produce pregnancy termination. Nearly all women who use mifepristone can be expected to have at least 1 side effect.

▼ Most common: headache, abdominal cramps, uterine cramps, vaginal bleeding, nausea, vomiting, diarrhea, fatigue, and back pain.

▼ Common: Uterine hemorrhage.

▼ Less common: upset stomach, vaginitis, pelvic pain, fever, viral infection, shaking chills, weakness, leg pain, increased white blood cell count, sinus irritation, and fainting.

▼ Rare: Liver irritation.

Drug Interactions

• Mifepristone may be less effective if given within 2 days after taking mifepristol.

- Ketoconazole, itraconazole, erythromycin, and grapefruit juice may increase blood levels of mifepristone.
- Carbamazepine, dexamethasone, phenytoin, phenobarbital, rifampin, and St. John's wort may reduce the amount of mifepristone in the blood.
- Mifepristone stays in the body for a week or more and stimulates a particular liver enzyme involved in drug metabolism. This may lead to increases in blood levels of atorvastatin, benzodiazepine tranquilizers and sedatives, buspirone, caffeine, cocaine, codeine, lidocaine, calcium channel blockers, cerivastatin, clarithromycin, chlorpheniramine, cyclosporine, dapsone, dextromethorphan, erythromycin, estradiol, finasteride, haloperidol, hydrocortisone, indinavir, lovastatin, methadone, nelfinavir, ondansetron, pimozide, progesterone, propranolol, quinine, quinidine, ritonavir, salmeterol, saquinavir, sildenafil, simvastatin, tacrolimus, tamoxifen, testosterone, trazodone, vincristine, zaleplon, and zolpidem.
- Corticosteriods may interfere with mifepristone's effectiveness.

Food Interactions

Grapefruit juice may slow the breakdown of mifepristone in the liver, increasing drug levels in the blood.

Usual Dose

600 mcg on the first office visit. 400 mcg two days later if the termination has not occurred.

Overdosage

No serious symptoms were reported in men and non-pregnant women who took up to 3 times the recommended dose of mifepristone. Massive overdose may lead to adrenal gland failure.

Special Information

Be sure to read all written information given to you by your doctor and that all your questions are answered before proceeding.

Tell your doctor if you have any clotting or bleeding problems, or if you are anemic.

Surgery may be needed if mifepristone results in an incomplete termination. When using this drug, be sure you know exactly what to do and where to go if something goes wrong.

You may become pregnant again after your pregnancy has been terminated and before your next period. Contraception may be started as soon as your doctor has confirmed the pregnancy termination.

Special Populations

Pregnancy/Breast-feeding

Pregnant women who are not interested in pregnancy termination may not take this drug for any reason. Failed mifepristone treatment may lead to birth defects.

Mifepristone may pass into breast milk. Nursing mothers who must take this drug should bottle-feed for several days after taking mifepristone.

Generic Name

Miglitol (mig-LIH-tol)

Brand Name

Glyset

Type of Drug

Antidiabetic.

Prescribed For

Type 2 diabetes.

General Information

Miglitol works differently from other oral antidiabetes drugs, which control blood sugar levels by increasing the production of insulin or helping the body to use the hormone more efficiently. Miglitol delays the digestion of carbohydrates (sugars) by acting in the cells that line the small intestine, where sugar is absorbed. This results in less sugar being absorbed into the blood and, therefore, a lower blood-sugar level. Miglitol also has some effect against the enzyme lactase, but usually does not cause lactose intolerance. Hypoglycemia (very low blood sugar) is unlikely with miglitol because of the way the drug works in diabetes.

People taking miglitol should have their blood sugar checked periodically to see how well the drug is working. (Home glucose monitors are available.) Migitol may be prescribed with another antidiabetic drug if single-drug therapy is not enough to adequately control blood sugar levels.

Cautions and Warnings

Do not take miglitol if you are **sensitive** or **allergic** to it. Miglitol should be used with caution if you have **diabetic ketoacidosis, inflammatory bowel disease, ulcers in the colon, partial intestinal obstruction,** or **absorption or digestion disease**.

People with kidney disease retain higher levels of miglitol in the blood, but this does not affect the drug's action because it acts locally in cells lining the small intestine. Those with severe **kidney disease** should not take this drug because of drug retention in the blood.

Possible Side Effects

Most side effects of miglitol go away with continued use of the drug.
▼ Most common: gas, diarrhea, and abdominal pain.
▼ Common: rash and low blood iron.

Drug Interactions

• Miglitol may interfere with the absorption of several drugs into the blood, including propranolol, ranitidine, digoxin, glyburide, and metformin. Your doctor may need to adjust your dose of these drugs.

• Digestive enzymes, charcoal, and kaolin (an ingredient in Kaopectate) reduce the effects of miglitol.

• Miglitol may increase the risk of hypoglycemia if taken with a sulfonylurea-type antidiabetes drug.

Food Interactions

Miglitol must be taken with the first bite of each main meal.

Usual Dose

Adult: 25–100 mg with breakfast, lunch, and dinner.
Child: not recommended.

Overdosage

Unlike other antidiabetic medicines, a miglitol overdose does not cause hypoglycemia. Overdose symptoms are likely to include gas, diarrhea, and pain. Call your local poison control center or hospital emergency room for more information. If you seek treatment, ALWAYS bring the prescription bottle or container.

Special Information

Follow your doctor's instructions for diet, exercise, and blood-sugar testing.

Miglitol prevents the breakdown of table sugar. If you take this drug in combination with insulin or a sulfonylurea drug, be sure to have a quick source of glucose (dextrose) with you to treat hypoglycemia (symptoms include tiredness, increased hunger, increased heart rate, sweating, and numbness in the arms and legs).

Take your dose with the first bite of each meal. The drug has to be present in your intestine to prevent the absorption of sugar into your blood.

If you forget to take a dose of miglitol with your meal, skip the dose you forgot, since it cannot work unless there is food in your stomach. Continue with your regular dose at the beginning of your next meal.

Special Populations

Pregnancy/Breast-feeding

The safety of using miglitol during pregnancy is not known. When this drug is considered crucial by your doctor, its potential benefits must be carefully weighed against its risks. Diabetes that develops during pregnancy is usually treated with insulin.

Small amounts of miglitol pass into breast milk. Nursing mothers who must take this drug should bottle-feed.

Seniors

Seniors may take this drug without special precaution.

Generic Name

Minoxidil (mih-NOX-ih-dil) Ⓖ

Brand Names

Loniten

Rogaine

Type of Drug

Antihypertensive and hair-growth stimulant.

Prescribed For

Hypertension (high blood pressure), male-pattern baldness, and alopecia areata.

General Information

Oral minoxidil is prescribed for severe hypertension that has not responded to other drugs. It reduces blood pressure by dilating (widening) peripheral blood vessels, allowing more blood to flow through the arms and legs. This increased blood flow reduces resistance levels in central blood vessels—for example, in the heart, lungs, and kidneys—and therefore reduces blood pressure. Minoxidil's effect on blood pressure is seen 30 minutes after a dose is taken and lasts up to 3 days. Minoxidil, which is usually taken once or twice a day, reaches maximum effect in as little as 3 days if the dose is large enough—40 mg a day.

Topical minoxidil stimulates hair growth in men and women with hereditary hair loss. It is also used to treat alopecia areata, a condition in which patches of hair fall out all over the body. No one knows exactly how minoxidil produces this effect and it does not work for everyone. The ideal candidate is a man who has just started to lose hair. The drug is not effective unless hair in the balding area is at least ½ in. long, and it takes 4 to 6 months of applications before any effect can be expected. The application regimen must be followed carefully; stopping the drug will nullify its effects and new growth will be lost. In some men who used minoxidil for a year, hair loss was only slowed.

Cautions and Warnings

Oral minoxidil may cause severe **adverse effects on the heart,** including angina pain and fluid around the heart, which affects cardiac function. It is usually prescribed with a beta-blocking drug to prevent rapid heartbeat and a diuretic to prevent fluid accumulation. Hospitalization may be recommended for some people when they start minoxidil to avoid a rapid drop in blood pressure.

People with **pheochromocytoma** (adrenal gland tumor) should not use this drug.

This drug has not been carefully studied in people who have suffered a **heart attack** within a month of beginning minoxidil; cardiac side effects may be particularly serious in people with a history of **heart disease**. People who use minoxidil for hair growth must have a healthy scalp and no heart disease.

Possible Side Effects

Tablets
Water and sodium retention may develop (which can worsen heart failure) as well as fluid in the sacs surrounding the heart.

▼ Most common: 80% of people experience thickening, elongation, and darkening of body hair within 3 to 6 weeks, first noticed on the temples, between the eyebrows, on the forehead, or on the upper cheek. Later it may extend to the back, arms, legs, and scalp. This effect stops when the drug is stopped, and symptoms usually disappear in 1 to 6 months. Heart rhythm changes occur in 60% of people, but cause no symptoms. Some laboratory tests, such as blood, liver, and kidney tests, may be affected by minoxidil.

▼ Less common: bronchitis or other respiratory infections, sinus inflammation, rash, eczema, fungal infection, itching, redness, dry skin or scalp, flaking, worsening of hair loss, hair loss where none was present, diarrhea, nausea, vomiting, headache, dizziness, light-headedness, fainting, back pain, broken bones, tendinitis, aches and pains, swelling of the arms or legs, chest pain, blood-pressure changes, heart palpitations, pulse-rate changes, allergic reactions (symptoms include breathing difficulties, rash, and itching), hives, runny nose, facial swelling, conjunctivitis (pinkeye), ear infection, visual disturbances, weight gain, urinary infection, inflammation of the prostate or urethra, vaginal discharge, pain during sex, anxiety, depression, fatigue, menstrual

---

Possible Side Effects *(continued)*

changes, nonspecific breast symptoms, and pain, inflammation, or redness of the testes, vagina, or vulva.

Lotion
People using 2% minoxidil lotion may experience irritation or itching. Not enough minoxidil is absorbed into the blood to affect blood pressure or cause serious side effects.

Drug Interactions

• Minoxidil may interact with guanethidine to produce severe dizziness when rising from a sitting or lying position. These drugs should not be taken together.

• Do not take over-the-counter (OTC) products that contain stimulants.

• Do not use the lotion in conjunction with other topical drugs.

Food Interactions

None known.

Usual Dose

Tablets
   Adult and Child (age 12 and over): 5 mg a day to start; may be increased to 40 mg a day. Do not exceed 100 mg a day.
   Child (under age 12): 0.1 mg per lb. of body weight a day to start; may be increased to 0.5 mg per lb. of body weight a day. Do not exceed 50 mg a day.

Minoxidil is usually taken with a diuretic—such as 100 mg of hydrochlorothiazide, 50–100 mg of chlorthalidone, or 80 mg of furosemide daily; and a beta blocker—such as 80–160 mg a day of propranolol. People who cannot take beta blockers may take 500–1500 mg of methyldopa or 0.2–0.4 mg of clonidine daily.

Lotion
Apply to scalp twice a day.

Overdosage

Symptoms include dizziness, fainting, and rapid heartbeat. Call your local poison control center or a hospital emergency room for instructions. ALWAYS bring the prescription bottle or container if you seek treatment.

Special Information

Oral minoxidil is usually prescribed with 2 other drugs—a beta blocker and a diuretic; do not discontinue any of these drugs unless told to do so by your doctor. Take all medication exactly as prescribed.

The effect of this drug on body hair (see "Possible Side Effects") is more of a nuisance than a risk and is not a reason to stop taking it.

Call your doctor if you experience an increase in your pulse of 20 or more beats per minute; weight gain of more than 5 lbs.; swelling of your arms, legs, face, or stomach; chest pain; breathing difficulties; dizziness; or fainting spells.

If you forget a dose of oral minoxidil, take it as soon as you remember. If it is almost time for your next dose, skip the dose you forgot and continue with your regular schedule. Do not take a double dose.

Special Populations

Pregnancy/Breast-feeding

Oral minoxidil crosses into the fetal circulation. Women should avoid either form of minoxidil during pregnancy. When this drug is considered crucial by your doctor, its potential benefits must be carefully weighed against its risks.

Oral minoxidil passes into breast milk, as may the lotion. Nursing mothers who must take either form of minoxidil should bottle-feed.

Seniors

Seniors may be more sensitive to the blood-pressure-lowering effect of the drug due to loss of kidney function.

Generic Name

Mirtazapine (mur-TAZ-uh-pene)

Brand Name

Remeron   Remeron SolTab

The information in this profile also applies to the following drug:

Generic Ingredient: Maprotiline Ⓖ
Ludiomil

Type of Drug

Antidepressant.

Prescribed For

Depression, tremors, and panic disorder.

General Information

Mirtazapine blocks the passage of stimulant chemicals (serotonin and noradrenaline) in and out of nerve endings and has a sedative effect. It also moderately counteracts the effects of the neurohormone acetylcholine. Recent theory maintains that antidepressants work by causing long-term changes in the way nerve endings function. Mirtazapine can elevate mood, increase physical activity and mental alertness, and improve appetite and sleep patterns 2 to 4 weeks after you start taking it. Mirtazapine is useful in treating mild forms of depression associated with anxiety. It can also significantly reduce tremors associated with Parkinson's disease and other causes, though the effect is lost soon after drug treatment is stopped. Mirtazapine is broken down in the liver. Women clear the drug more slowly than men.

Cautions and Warnings

Do not take mirtazapine if you are **allergic** or **sensitive** to it.

Mirtazapine should be taken with care if you are recovering from a **heart attack**.

Take this drug with caution if you have a history of **epilepsy or other convulsive disorders, urinary difficulties, glaucoma, heart disease, liver disease,** or **hyperthyroidism.** Antidepressants may aggravate the condition of people who are **schizophrenic** or **paranoid** and may cause people with **bipolar (manic-depressive) disorder** to switch phase. These reactions are also possible when changing or stopping antidepressants.

Suicide is always a risk in severely depressed people, who should only be allowed to have minimal quantities of medication in their possession.

Seizures are rare and can be minimized by starting with a low mirtazapine dose and staying with the lowest effective dose. Dosage should be increased gradually and only after at least 2 weeks on the starting dose.

People taking mirtazapine may develop very **low white-blood-cell counts** leading to infections, fever, and related problems. Call your doctor at once if you develop a sore throat, fever, infection, or mouth sores while taking this drug.

Mirtazapine should be taken with care if you have severe **kidney or liver disease**.

Possible Side Effects

▼ Most common: tiredness, dizziness, dry mouth, constipation, abnormal dreams, increased appetite, weight gain, large increases in blood cholesterol or triglyceride levels, weakness, and flu symptoms.

▼ Less common: back pain, nausea, vomiting, muscle ache, abnormal dreaming or thinking, anxiety, agitation, confusion, tremors, itching, rash, breathing difficulties, and frequent urination.

▼ Rare: blood-pressure changes, weakness, hair loss, uncontrollable muscle spasms or movements, hallucinations, manic reactions, and liver function changes. Other rare side effects can occur in almost any part of the body. Contact your doctor if you experience any side effect not listed above.

Drug Interactions

Mirtazapine and Maprotiline

• Combining mirtazapine or maprotiline with a mono-amine oxidase inhibitor (MAOI) antidepressant may cause high fevers, convulsions, or death. Do not take an MAOI until at least 2 weeks after mirtazapine or maprotiline has been stopped. People who take either of these drugs and an MAOI require close medical observation.

• Mirtazapine and maprotiline increase the effects of alcohol, tranquilizers, and other sedative drugs.

Maprotiline

• Maprotiline interacts with guanethidine and clonidine (drugs used to treat high blood pressure). Tell your doctor if you are taking any drug for high blood pressure.

• Barbiturates may decrease the effectiveness of maprotiline. Combining maprotiline and thyroid medication enhances the effects of both drugs and may cause abnormal heart rhythms.

• Combining maprotiline and reserpine may cause over-stimulation.

• Oral contraceptives ("the pill") may reduce the effect of maprotiline, as may smoking. Charcoal tablets may block the absorption of maprotiline. Estrogen may increase or decrease the effect of maprotiline.

• Bicarbonate of soda, acetazolamide, quinidine, and procainamide increase the effect of maprotiline. Combining this drug and cimetidine, methylphenidate, or phenothiazine drugs such as Thorazine and Compazine may cause severe side effects.

Food Interactions

You may take mirtazapine with food if it upsets your stomach.

Usual Dose

Maprotiline
    Adult: 75–150 mg a day. Severely depressed patients may need up to 225 mg a day.
    Senior: usually 50–75 mg a day.

Mirtazapine
    Adult: 15 mg at bedtime to start. After the first 1–2 weeks of taking the drug, dosage may be increased up to 45 mg a day. Dosage must be tailored to your needs.

Overdosage

Symptoms of mirtazapine overdose include disorientation, drowsiness, memory loss, and rapid heartbeat. Symptoms of maprotiline overdose include confusion, inability to concentrate, hallucinations, drowsiness, lowered body temperature, abnormal heart rate, heart failure, enlarged pupils, seizures, convulsions, very low blood pressure, stupor, and coma; agitation, stiffening of muscles, vomiting, and high fever may also develop. The victim should be taken to a hospital emergency room immediately. ALWAYS bring the prescription bottle or container.

Special Information

Do not stop taking this drug without your doctor's knowledge. Abruptly stopping mirtazapine may cause nausea, headache, and feelings of ill health.

Mirtazapine may cause drowsiness and dizziness. Be careful when driving or doing any task that requires concentration. Avoid alcohol and other depressant drugs. Avoid prolonged exposure to the sun.

Be careful when taking over-the-counter (OTC) medications because mirtazapine may interact with sedative ingredients in OTC products.

Call your doctor at once if you develop chills, difficult or rapid breathing, fever, sweating, blood-pressure changes, muscle stiffness, loss of bladder control, or unusual tiredness or weakness.

If your symptoms are unchanged after 6 to 8 weeks of treatment with an antidepressant, contact your doctor.

If you forget a dose, skip it and go back to your regular schedule. Do not take a double dose.

Special Populations

Pregnancy/Breast-feeding

Mirtazapine crosses into the fetal circulation and may cause birth defects. When this drug is considered crucial by your doctor, its potential benefits must be carefully weighed against its risks.

It is not known if mirtazapine passes into breast milk. Nursing mothers who must take this drug should consider bottle-feeding.

Seniors

Seniors are more sensitive to side effects and may require reduced dosage. Older men may need less of the drug than women of the same age.

Generic Name

Misoprostol (mye-soe-PROS-tol)

Brand Name

Cytotec

Type of Drug

Anti-ulcer.

Prescribed For

Stomach ulcer and prevention of kidney rejection after transplant.

General Information

Like most anti-ulcer drugs, misoprostol suppresses stomach acid. It has a demonstrated ability to protect the stomach lining from damage, though the exact way misoprostol works is not known. It may increase production of stomach lining and the thickness of the protective gel layer lining the stomach. Misoprostol may also increase blood flow in and subsequent healing of the stomach lining in addition to increasing production of bicarbonate, a natural antacid found in the stomach.

Misoprostol is intended to prevent severe stomach irritation and ulcers in people taking a nonsteroidal anti-inflammatory drug (NSAID). It is helpful for seniors and others with a history of ulcer or stomach disease who require NSAID treatment for arthritis. It is often an effective ulcer treatment for people who do not respond to or cannot tolerate cimetidine, ranitidine, famotidine, or nizatidine. Misoprostol has also been studied as a vaginal abortion drug.

Cautions and Warnings

Misoprostol may reduce **fertility**. Do not take this drug if you are **allergic** to it or any prostaglandin agent, or if you are **pregnant.**

People with **kidney disease** may require reduced dosages.

People with **epilepsy** or **blood-vessel disease** in the heart or brain should be cautious about taking misoprostol, as should those with **heart disease.**

Possible Side Effects

▼ Most common: diarrhea and abdominal pain. Most cases of diarrhea are mild and last no more than 2 to 3 days.

▼ Less common: headache, nausea, vomiting, and stomach upset or gas.

▼ Rare: spotting, cramps, excessive menstrual bleeding, painful menstruation or other menstrual disorders, and vaginal bleeding.

Drug Interactions

• Misoprostol may interfere with the absorption of diazepam and theophylline.

• Rarely, antacids interfere with misoprostol's effectiveness. Magnesium-containing antacids may worsen misoprostol-induced diarrhea.

Food Interactions

Though food interferes with the absorption of this drug, it should be taken with or after meals (and at bedtime) to minimize gastrointestinal (GI) side effects.

Usual Dose

Adult: 100–200 mcg 4 times a day.

Overdosage

Symptoms include sedation; tremors; convulsions; breathing difficulties; stomach pain; diarrhea; fever; changes in heart rate—either very fast or very slow; and low blood pressure. Take the victim to a hospital emergency room. ALWAYS bring the prescription bottle or container.

Special Information

Do not stop taking misoprostol, or take it for more than 4 weeks, without your doctor's knowledge.

Call your doctor if side effects, especially diarrhea or abdominal or stomach pain, become severe or intolerable. Women who experience menstrual problems and postmenopausal women who experience vaginal bleeding should discuss these side effects with their doctors.

If you forget a dose, take it as soon as you remember. If it is almost time for your next dose, skip the dose you forgot and continue with your regular schedule. Do not take a double dose.

Special Populations

Pregnancy/Breast-feeding

PREGNANT WOMEN SHOULD NOT TAKE THIS DRUG. Women of childbearing age should take misoprostol only if they absolutely must take an NSAID and already have, or are at high risk of developing, stomach ulcers. Misoprostol causes spontaneous miscarriage. Within 2 weeks of starting treatment, you must receive a negative blood test result

for pregnancy—an over-the-counter urine test is not sufficient. Start taking misoprostol on day 2 or 3 of your period
and use effective contraception throughout drug therapy.

It is not known if misoprostol passes into breast milk,
though it is unlikely. Nursing mothers who must take this
drug should bottle-feed.

Seniors
Seniors should receive lower dosages if intolerable side
effects develop.

Generic Name

Modafinil (moe-DAF-ih-nil)

Brand Name
Provigil

Type of Drug
Stimulant.

Prescribed For
Narcolepsy (uncontrollable desire to sleep); also used to help
shift workers stay awake.

General Information
Modafinil promotes wakefulness. While some of its actions
are similar to those of amphetamine and methylphenidate, it
is not known exactly how modafinil achieves its effects. People being treated with this drug may experience euphoria
(feeling "high"), anxiety, and changes in mood, mental state,
and behavior.

Cautions and Warnings
Do not take modafinil if you are **allergic** or **sensitive** to it.

People with a history of **heart failure,** an **enlarged heart
ventricle, angina, chest pain, abnormal heart rhythms,** or
mitral valve prolapse should not take modafinil.

Modafinil has not been studied in people with **high blood
pressure**. People with high blood pressure who take this drug
must be closely monitored.

People with **cirrhosis of the liver** or **liver failure** may require reduced dosages.

People who regularly take large dosages (more than 400 mg a day) of modafinil may develop some **resistance** to its effects.

Possible Side Effects

▼ Most common: headache, nausea, and runny nose.

▼ Common: nervousness, dizziness, diarrhea, dry mouth, appetite loss, and sore throat.

▼ Less common: depression, anxiety, cataplexy (extreme muscle weakness, often precipitated by laughter, a surprised feeling, or emotions of fear or anger), sleeplessness, tingling in the hands or feet, unusual facial or mouth movements, muscle stiffness, blood pressure changes, liver function problems, vomiting, lung problems, breathing difficulties, vision problems, chest pain, neck pain, chills, and high white-blood-cell counts.

▼ Rare: confusion; memory loss; emotional instability; euphoria, changes in mood, manic behavior; flushing; fainting; dry skin; herpes infections; mouth sores; gum sores; thirst; difficulty urinating; abnormal urination; abnormal ejaculation; high blood sugar; nosebleeds; asthma; rigid neck; fever with chills; and joint problems.

Drug Interactions

• Combining modafinil and a monoamine oxidase inhibitor (MAOI) drug may increase the effects of both drugs. Use this combination with caution and only under your doctor's supervision.

• Methylphenidate can delay modafinil's effects.

• Carbamazepine, phenobarbital, rifampin, ketoconazole, and itraconazole may reduce modafinil's effects.

• Modafinil may reduce the effects of oral contraceptives ("the pill"), theophylline, and cyclosporine.

• Modafinil may elevate blood levels of clomipramine, clozapine, phenytoin, diazepam, propranolol, tricyclic antidepressants, and warfarin, increasing the risk of side effects—some of these can be very serious.

• Stimulants in over-the-counter (OTC) decongestants, diet pills, and asthma drugs may cause excessive stimulation when combined with modafinil.

Food Interactions

Food can slow the rate at which modafinil is absorbed into the blood but is unlikely to change its effect on your body.

Usual Dose

Adult: 200 mg every morning; 100 mg daily for people with cirrhosis or liver failure.

Senior: start with 100 mg daily and increase if needed.

Overdosage

Symptoms include excitation, sleeplessness, sleep disturbances, anxiety, irritability, aggressiveness, confusion, nervousness, tremors, heart palpitations, nausea, diarrhea, and bleeding. Take the victim to a hospital emergency room. ALWAYS bring the prescription bottle or container.

Special Information

Call your doctor if you develop a rash, hives, or other signs of a drug allergy.

Modafinil's beneficial effects on mood, thought, and perception may produce psychological dependence, though drug withdrawal symptoms have not been reported.

The stimulants in OTC decongestants, diet pills, and asthma drugs may cause excessive stimulation when combined with modafinil.

Be careful when driving or doing any task that requires concentration. Avoid alcohol.

Special Populations

Pregnancy/Breast-feeding

Modafinil causes fetal malformation in animal studies. When this drug is considered crucial by your doctor, its potential benefits must be carefully weighed against its risks.

This drug may pass into breast milk. Nursing mothers who must take it should consider bottle-feeding.

Seniors

Seniors with kidney or liver problems may require reduced dosage.

Generic Name

Moexipril (moe-EX-uh-pril)

Brand Name

Univasc

Combination Products

Generic Ingredients: Moexipril + Hydrochlorothiazide
Uniretic

Type of Drug

Angiotensin-converting enzyme (ACE) inhibitor.

Prescribed For

Hypertension (high blood pressure).

General Information

Moexipril hydrochloride and other ACE inhibitors work by preventing the conversion of a hormone called angiotensin I to another hormone called angiotensin II, a potent blood-vessel constrictor. Preventing this conversion relaxes blood vessels, thus reducing blood pressure and relieving the symptoms of heart failure. Moexipril also affects production of other hormones and enzymes that participate in the regulation of blood vessel dilation. Moexipril begins working about 1 hour after you take it and continues to work for 24 hours.

Some people who start taking an ACE inhibitor after they are already on a diuretic (an agent that increases urination) experience a rapid drop in blood pressure after their first doses or when the dosage is increased. To prevent this from happening, you may be told to stop taking the diuretic 2 or 3 days before starting the ACE inhibitor, or to increase your salt intake during that time. The diuretic may then be restarted gradually.

Cautions and Warnings

Do not take moexipril if you have had an **allergic reaction** to it.

Moexipril occasionally causes **very low blood pressure**.

Moexipril may cause a decline in **kidney function,** especially if you have congestive **heart failure.** Your doctor should check your urine for changes during the first few months of treatment. Dosage adjustment may be necessary.

Moexipril can occasionally affect white-blood-cell count, possibly increasing your susceptibility to **infection**. Blood counts should be monitored periodically.

Moexipril can cause injury and death to the fetus during pregnancy. **Pregnant women** should not take moexipril.

Possible Side Effects

▼ Most common: dizziness, tiredness, diarrhea, headache, nausea, low blood pressure, chest pain, and chronic cough. The cough usually goes away a few days after you stop taking the medicine.

▼ Less common: chest pain, angina, dizziness when rising from a sitting or lying position, fainting, abdominal pain, nausea, vomiting, bronchitis, urinary tract infection, breathing difficulties, weakness, and rash.

▼ Rare: Rare side effects can occur in almost any part of the body. Contact your doctor if you experience any side effect not listed above.

Drug Interactions

• The blood-pressure-lowering effect of moexipril is increased by taking diuretic drugs and beta blockers. Any other drug that causes a rapid drop in blood pressure should be used with caution if you are taking an ACE inhibitor.

• Combining 325 mg a day or more of aspirin with moexipril carries a higher risk of death than taking lower doses (less than 160 mg a day). People taking aspirin to prevent a heart attack should use the lower dose of aspirin.

• Moexipril may increase potassium levels in your blood, especially when taken with Dyazide or other potassium-sparing diuretics.

• Moexipril may increase the effects of lithium; this combination should be used with caution.

• Antacids and moexipril should be taken at least 2 hours apart.

• Capsaicin may trigger or aggravate the cough associated with moexipril therapy.

• Indomethacin may reduce the blood-pressure-lowering effect of moexipril.

• Phenothiazine tranquilizers and antiemetics may increase the effects of moexipril.

• The combination of allopurinol and moexipril increases the chance of side effects.

• Moexipril increases the levels of digoxin in the blood, possibly increasing the chance of digoxin-related side effects.

• Moexipril may decrease blood levels of tetracycline antibiotics.

Food Interactions

Moexipril should be taken 1 hour before meals.

Usual Dose

7.5–30 mg once a day. Some people may divide their daily dosage into 2 doses. People with poor kidney function should take half the usual dose.

Overdosage

The principal effect of moexipril overdose is a rapid drop in blood pressure, as evidenced by dizziness or fainting. Take the victim to a hospital emergency room immediately. ALWAYS bring the prescription bottle or container.

Special Information

Call your doctor if you develop swelling of the face or throat, if you have sudden difficulty in breathing, a sore throat, mouth sores, abnormal heartbeat, chest pain, a persistent rash, or loss of taste perception. Unexplained swelling of the face, lips, hands, and feet can also affect the larynx (throat) and tongue and interfere with breathing. If this happens, the victim should be taken to a hospital emergency room at once for treatment.

You may get dizzy if you rise to your feet quickly from a sitting or lying position.

Avoid strenuous exercise and very hot weather because heavy sweating or dehydration can cause a rapid blood pressure drop.

Avoid over-the-counter diet pills, decongestants, and other stimulants that can raise blood pressure.

If you take moexipril on a regular schedule and forget a dose, take it as soon as you remember. If you take it once a day and it is within 8 hours of your next dose, skip the one you forgot and continue with your regular schedule. If you take moexipril twice a day and it is within 4 hours of your next dose, take 1 dose as soon as you remember and another in 5 or 6 hours, then go back to your regular schedule. Never take a double dose.

Special Populations

Pregnancy/Breast-feeding

ACE inhibitors can cause fetal injury or death. Women who are or might be pregnant should not take moexipril. Stop taking the medication and contact your doctor if you become pregnant.

Small amounts of moexipril pass into breast milk. Nursing mothers who must take this drug should consider bottle-feeding.

Seniors

Seniors may be more sensitive to the effects of moexipril due to kidney impairment.

Monopril   see Fosinopril, page 511

Brand Name

Motofen

Generic Ingredients

Difenoxin + Atropine Sulfate

Type of Drug

Antidiarrheal.

Prescribed For

Acute and chronic diarrhea.

General Information

Difenoxin is an antidiarrheal agent related to meperidine, a narcotic analgesic (pain reliever) used in Demerol. Difenoxin, which can be addictive, works by slowing the contractions of intestinal-wall muscles. The atropine sulfate ingredient in Motofen guards against drug overdose or abuse by producing undesirable effects at small dosages, thus deterring users from taking larger amounts of Motofen. This drug, which relieves diarrhea but does not address the underlying cause, should only be used for short periods and in cases that do not respond to other treatment. Some people should not use this drug even if diarrhea is present. Antidiarrheal drugs may harm people with stomach, bowel, or other conditions.

Cautions and Warnings

Do not take Motofen if you are **allergic** to any of its ingredients or to Lomotil.

Avoid Motofen if you have advanced **liver disease** or have **jaundice** (symptoms include yellowing of the skin or whites of the eyes), or if your diarrhea was caused by taking clindamycin or another antibiotic.

People with **ulcerative colitis** should use Motofen with caution.

Possible Side Effects

▼ Most common: nausea, vomiting, dry mouth, dizziness, light-headedness, drowsiness, and headache.

▼ Less common: constipation, upset stomach, confusion, and tiredness or sleeplessness.

▼ Rare: a burning sensation in the eyes, blurred vision, dry skin, rapid heartbeat, elevated temperature, and urinary difficulties.

Drug Interactions

• Motofen may increase the effects of alcohol, barbiturates, tranquilizers, pain relievers, and other nervous-system depressants. Avoid these combinations.

• Monoamine oxidase inhibitor (MAOI) antidepressants may, in theory, produce a high-blood-pressure crisis in combination with Motofen. Do not use Motofen if you are taking an MAOI unless you are under a doctor's care.

Food Interactions

None known.

Usual Dose

Adult and Child (age 12 and over): 2 tablets to start, then 1 after each loose stool or every 3–4 hours, as needed; up to 8 tablets a day. Treatment for more than 2 consecutive days is usually not needed.

Child (under age 12): not recommended.

Overdosage

Symptoms include dry skin, mouth, and nose; flushing; fever; and rapid heartbeat. These symptoms may be followed by loss of reflexes, pinpointed pupils, droopy eyelids, breathing difficulty, and lethargy or coma. Take the victim to a hospital emergency room immediately. ALWAYS bring the prescription bottle or container.

Special Information

Motofen can make you tired, dizzy, or light-headed. Be careful when driving or doing any task that requires concentration. Alcohol, tranquilizers, and other nervous-system depressants increase the depressant effects of this drug.

Your doctor may prescribe fluid and salt mixtures to replace the body fluids you lose while taking Motofen.

Call your doctor if you develop heart palpitations or your symptoms do not clear up in 2 days. You may need a different dosage or drug.

If you forget a dose, take it as soon as you remember. If it is almost time for your next dose, skip the one you forgot and continue with your regular schedule. Do not take a double dose.

Special Populations

Pregnancy/Breast-feeding

Animal studies with very large dosages of Motofen showed an increase in stillbirths. When this drug is considered crucial by your doctor, its potential benefits must be carefully weighed against its risks.

The ingredients in Motofen may pass into breast milk. Nursing mothers taking Motofen should bottle-feed.

Seniors

Seniors with severe kidney or liver disease require reduced dosage.

Generic Name

Mupirocin (mue-PYE-roe-sin)

Brand Name

Bactroban   Centany

Type of Drug

Topical antibiotic.

Prescribed For

Impetigo (streptococcal skin infections), eczema, inflammation of the hair follicles, and minor bacterial skin infections. Mupirocin nasal is used to prevent resistant *Staphylococcus aureus* infections from spreading during outbreaks of the infection.

General Information

Mupirocin is a unique, non-penicillin drug that works against the common microorganisms that cause impetigo in children. It is used to supplement other treatments for impetigo, although many doctors prefer oral medication. Mupirocin works by interfering with bacteria's ability to make the proteins it needs for survival. Large amounts of mupirocin kill bacteria and smaller amounts stop the bacteria from growing. It may be effective against antibiotic-resistant bacteria.

Cautions and Warnings

Do not use a mupirocin product if you are **allergic** to any of its components. Mupirocin ointment is **not for use in the eye**.

Mupirocin nasal should be used only to treat *Staphylococcus aureus* infections, not to prevent them.

Large quantities of mupirocin ointment should **not be applied to an open wound** because polyethylene glycol—used as a base in mupirocin ointment—may be absorbed through the wound and damage the kidneys.

Long-term or chronic use of mupirocin may lead to **secondary infection** caused by drug-resistant bacteria or fungi.

Possible Side Effects

Ointment
- ▼ Less common: burning, pain, and itching.
- ▼ Rare: rash, stinging or pain where the ointment is applied, nausea, skin redness, dry skin, tenderness, swelling, and increased oozing from impetigo lesions.

Cream
- ▼ Less common: headache, rash, and nausea.
- ▼ Rare: abdominal pain, burning, irritation, inflammation, dizziness, itching, secondary infection, and mouth ulcer.

Possible Side Effects *(continued)*

Nasal Ointment
  ▼ Most common: headache and runny nose.
  ▼ Less common: respiratory congestion, sore throat, changes in sense of taste, burning or stinging, cough, and itching.
  ▼ Rare: eyelid inflammation, diarrhea, dry mouth, ear pain, nosebleeds, nausea, and rash.

Drug Interactions

• Do not use mupirocin nasal at the same time as any other prescription or over-the-counter nasal drug product.
• Taking other antibiotics while using mupirocin can lead to the development of resistant bacteria.

Usual Dose

Ointment and Cream: Apply a small amount to the affected area 3 times a day. Cover with gauze if desired.

Nasal Ointment: Put half the ointment from a single-use tube in each nostril morning and evening for 5 days. After the ointment is applied, gently squeeze your nostrils closed and allow them to open again. Repeat this continuously for about 1 minute.

Overdosage

Little is known about the effects of accidental ingestion. Call your local poison control center or a hospital emergency room for more information. If you seek treatment, ALWAYS bring the prescription bottle or container.

Special Information

Call your doctor if this medication does not work within 3 to 5 days or if any of the following symptoms develop: dry skin or redness, rash, itching, stinging, pain, or other possible drug reactions.

If you forget a dose, apply it as you remember. If it is almost time for your next dose, skip the one you forgot and continue with your regular schedule. Do not apply a double dose.

Special Populations

Pregnancy/Breast-feeding

The safety of using mupirocin during pregnancy is not known. When this drug is considered crucial by your doctor, its potential benefits must be carefully weighed against its risks.

It is not known if mupirocin passes into breast milk. Nursing mothers who must take this drug should bottle-feed.

Seniors

Seniors may use mupirocin without special restriction.

Generic Name

Muromonab-CD3 (muh-ROE-moe-nab)

Brand Name

Orthoclone OKT3

Type of Drug

Immunosuppressant.

Prescribed For

Kidney, heart, and liver transplantation.

General Information

Muromonab-CD3 is an important alternative to cyclosporine in preventing organ transplant rejection. By blocking the activity of T-cells, which protect the body against invading microorganisms or foreign substances, this drug suppresses the immune system and prevents organ rejection. The drug starts working in minutes and continues working for as long as it is used. T-cells rapidly return to normal within 1 week after the medication is stopped.

Cautions and Warnings

This drug should not be used by people with untreated **heart failure, fluid overload,** or a history of **seizures.**

Muromonab-CD3 is made in cells from mouse tissue and causes the development of **anti-mouse antibodies** in humans.

People who have received other drugs made in this way may already have high levels of this kind of antibody in their blood and, if they do, should not be treated with muromonab-CD3. Your doctor will test for antibody levels.

People who receive this drug usually develop **cytokine release syndrome (CRS)** from 30 minutes to 2 days after the first dose is given. CRS symptoms range from mild, flu-like symptoms such as fever, chills, joint aches, weakness, and headaches, to a less common, life-threatening shock-like reaction that involves the heart and nervous system. Some of the more severe symptoms of CRS are shortness of breath; high fever—up to 107°F; wheezing; rapid heartbeat; chest pain; respiratory collapse or failure; heart attack; severe drug reactions; seizures; confusion; hallucinations; stiff neck; brain swelling; and headache. People who are at risk for more severe forms of CRS include those with a recent heart attack or uncontrolled angina pectoris, heart failure, fluid in the lungs, serious lung disease, and a history of seizure or shock. CRS may be prevented or minimized by giving methylprednisolone 1 to 4 hours before the first dose of muromonab-CD3.

People receiving this drug are more likely to develop **infection**. Preventive antibiotic therapy is sometimes used to reduce the risk of infection.

Possible Side Effects

More than 90% of people receiving muromonab-CD3 experience some form of CRS, though it is usually mild (see "Cautions and Warnings").

▼ Rare: Rare side effects can occur in almost any part of the body. Contact your doctor if you experience any bothersome or persistent side effect.

Drug Interactions

• Other immunosuppressants (corticosteroids, cyclosporine, and azathioprine) and indomethacin increase the effect of muromonab-CD3, in turn increasing the risk of CRS.

Food Interactions

Muromonab-CD3 may be taken without regard to food.

Usual Dose

Adult and Child (age 12 and over): 5 mg intravenously a day for 10–14 days.

Child (under age 12): 0.1 mg intravenously for every 2.2 lbs. of body weight a day for 10–14 days.

Overdosage

Little is known about the effects of muromonab-CD 3 overdose. Call your local poison control center or a hospital emergency room for information.

Special Information

Call your doctor at the first sign of rash, itching, rapid heartbeat, difficulty swallowing, breathing difficulties, unusual swelling, allergic reaction, or if you experience any bothersome or persistent side effect. It is essential to maintain close contact with your doctor while taking muromonab-CD3.

Mild reactions due to CRS may be treated by taking acetaminophen or antihistamines. Your body temperature should be no higher than 100°F when each dose is given.

Avoid exposure to bacterial infection and immunizations while you are taking this drug. If an infection develops, your doctor will have to stop muromonab-CD3 therapy and treat the infection.

Maintain good dental hygiene while taking muromonab-CD3 and use extra care when brushing and flossing because this drug increases your risk of oral infection. See your dentist regularly.

This drug may cause confusion or interfere with your alertness, dexterity, or coordination. Be careful when driving or doing any task that requires concentration.

It is essential to complete the full course of treatment. This medication should not be stopped unless an infection or other severe side effect develops. If you miss a dose, take it as soon as you remember and call your doctor.

Special Populations

Pregnancy/Breast-feeding

Muromonab-CD3 may cross into the fetal circulation. When this drug is considered crucial by your doctor, its potential benefits must be carefully weighed against its risks.

It is not known if muromonab-CD3 passes into breast milk. Nursing mothers who must take this drug should bottle-feed.

Seniors

Seniors may use this drug without special restriction.

Generic Name

Mycophenolate (mye-coe-FEN-oe-late)

Brand Name

CellCept

Type of Drug

Immunosuppressant.

Prescribed For

Kidney, liver, and heart transplantation.

General Information

Mycophenolate mofetil is used with corticosteroids and cyclosporine to prevent the rejection of transplanted kidneys and other organs. In the body, the drug is metabolized into MPA, the active form of mycophenolate. MPA blocks the activity of T and B lymphocytes, which protect the body against invading microorganisms or foreign substances. MPA also suppresses antibody formation and may act directly on inflammation and organ rejection sites to prevent tissue rejection.

Cautions and Warnings

Do not take mycophenolate if your are **allergic** to it, or **sensitive** to mycophenolic acid or to polisorbate 80. As with other immunosuppressants, people taking mycophenolate are at increased risk of **infections** or developing a **lymphoma or other malignancy**. The risk increases with the degree of immune suppression and the length of time that the drug is taken.

About 2 in 100 people receiving mycophenolate develop a severe **reduction in white-blood-cell count**. Call your doctor if you develop symptoms of viral infection or other unusual symptoms.

About 3 in 100 people who take this drug develop **stomach or intestinal bleeding,** though many of these people are also taking other drugs that may affect the gastrointestinal (GI) tract. People with stomach or intestinal disease should take this drug with caution.

People with **kidney disease** should receive lower dosages. People who experience post-transplant reduction in liver function may develop kidney damage.

Mild to moderate **hypertension** (high blood pressure) is a common side effect of mycophenolate and may be a sign of kidney damage. People taking this drug should measure their blood pressure regularly.

Possible Side Effects

▼ Most common: general pain, abdominal pain, fever, headache, infection, blood infection, weakness, chest pain, back pain, hypertension, anemia, reduced white-blood-cell and platelet counts, urinary infection, blood in the urine, swelling of the arms or legs, diarrhea, anxiety, numbness or tingling, constipation, nausea, vomiting, upset stomach, oral fungus infection, respiratory infection, cough, breathing difficulties, and tremors.

▼ Common: kidney damage, urinary tract problems, high blood cholesterol, low blood-phosphate levels, fluid retention, changes in blood-potassium levels, high blood sugar, sore throat, pneumonia, bronchitis, acne, rash, sleeplessness, and dizziness.

▼ Less common: painful urination, impotence, frequent urination, pyelonephritis, urinary disorder, angina pain, heart palpitations, low blood pressure, dizziness when rising from a sitting or lying position, cardiovascular disorders, appetite loss, gas, stomach irritation or bleeding, gum irritation or enlargement, liver irritation, mouth ulcer, asthma, lung disorder, stuffy or runny nose, sinus irritation, hair loss, itching, sweating, skin ulcer, anxiety, depression, stiff muscles, tingling in the hands or feet, joint or muscle pain, leg cramps, double vision, cataracts, conjunctivitis (pinkeye), chills and fever, abdominal enlargement, facial swelling, cysts, flu-like

Possible Side Effects (continued)

symptoms, bleeding, hernia, feeling sick, pelvic pain, and black-and-blue marks.

▼ Rare: lymphoma, skin cancer—not melanomas—and other malignancies, herpes, chickenpox or shingles, fungus infection, and pneumocystis and other opportunistic infections that usually only develop in people with suppressed immune systems.

Drug Interactions

• Combining mycophenolate and acyclovir or ganciclovir (antiviral drugs) increases blood levels of both drugs.

• Cholestyramine and aluminum/magnesium antacids decrease mycophenolate blood levels and should be separated from mycophenolate by at least 1 hour.

• Azathioprine (an immune-system suppressant) should not be combined with mycophenolate because of the risk of excess immune-system suppression.

• Probenecid may double or triple mycophenolate blood levels. Aspirin also increases mycophenolate blood levels.

• Mycophenolate may moderately increase phenytoin and theophylline blood levels.

• Mycophenolate may reduce the effectiveness of some oral contraceptives.

• Mycophenolate should not be combined with iron supplements, as iron decreases blood levels of mycophenolate.

Food Interactions

Mycophenolate should be taken at least 1 hour before or 2 hours after meals.

Usual Dose

Adult: 2–3 g a day divided into 2 doses.
Child: not recommended.

Overdosage

Overdose is likely to cause side effects—especially those relating to the stomach and intestines—and blood abnormalities. Take the victim to a hospital emergency room. ALWAYS bring the prescription bottle or container.

Special Information

It is extremely important to take this drug exactly as prescribed. If you forget a dose, take it as soon as you remember. If it is almost time for your next dose, skip the dose you forgot and continue with your regular schedule. Do not take a double dose. Call your doctor if you forget 2 or more doses in a row.

Because this drug causes birth defects in animals, take extra caution when handling the capsules. Do not open or crush them. Avoid inhaling the powder or allowing it to touch your skin or the inside of your mouth or nose. If such contact does occur, wash thoroughly with soap and water. If the powder gets into your eyes, rinse them thoroughly with plain water.

People taking mycophenolate require regular testing to monitor their progress.

Call your doctor at the first sign of fever; sore throat; tiredness; weakness; nervousness; unusual bleeding or bruising; tender or swollen gums; convulsions; irregular heartbeat; confusion; numbness or tingling of your hands, feet, or lips; breathing difficulties; severe stomach pain with nausea; or blood in the urine. Other side effects are less serious but should be brought to your doctor's attention, particularly if they are bothersome or persistent.

Maintain good dental hygiene while taking mycophenolate and use extra care when brushing or flossing because this drug increases your risk of oral infection. See your dentist regularly.

This drug should be continued for as long as prescribed by your doctor. Do not stop taking it because of side effects or other problems without your doctor's knowledge.

Special Populations

Pregnancy/Breast-feeding

Animal studies show that mycophenolate may be highly toxic to the fetus. Women of childbearing age should have a negative pregnancy test at least 1 week before treatment is started. They should either use 2 effective contraceptive methods before treatment is started and continue until 6 weeks after mycophenolate is discontinued, or they should practice abstinence during this period. Should you accidentally become pregnant during mycophenolate treatment, discuss with your doctor the advisability of continuing the pregnancy. When this drug is considered crucial by your doctor, its potential benefits must be carefully weighed against its risks.

Mycophenolate passes into breast milk. Nursing mothers who must take this drug should bottle-feed.

Seniors

Seniors may require reduced dosage due to loss of kidney function.

Generic Name

Nabumetone (nah-BUE-meh-tone) G

Brand Name

Relafen

Type of Drug

Nonsteroidal anti-inflammatory drug (NSAID).

Prescribed For

Rheumatoid arthritis and osteoarthritis.

General Information

Nabumetone and other NSAIDs are used to relieve pain and inflammation. They may achieve their effects by blocking the body's production of a hormone called prostaglandin and the action of other body chemicals. Pain relief generally comes within 1 hour after taking the first dose of nabumetone, but its anti-inflammatory effect takes several days to 2 weeks to become apparent and may take a month or more to reach maximum effect. Nabumetone is broken down in the liver.

Cautions and Warnings

People who are **allergic** to nabumetone or any other NSAID and those with a history of **asthma** attacks brought on by an NSAID, iodides, or aspirin should not take nabumetone.

Nabumetone can cause **gastrointestinal (GI) bleeding, ulcers,** and **stomach perforation**. This can occur at any time, with or without warning, in people who take nabumetone regularly. People with a history of active GI bleeding should be cautious about taking any NSAID. People who develop bleeding or ulcers and continue NSAID treatment should be aware of the possibility of developing more serious side effects.

Nabumetone can affect platelets and **blood clotting** at high doses and should be avoided by people with clotting problems and those taking warfarin.

People with **heart problems** who use nabumetone may experience swelling in their arms, legs, or feet.

Nabumetone can cause severe toxic effects to the **kidney**. Report any unusual side effects to your doctor, who may need to periodically test your kidney function.

Nabumetone can make you **unusually sensitive to the effects of the sun.**

Possible Side Effects

▼ Most common: diarrhea, nausea, vomiting, constipation, gas, stomach upset or irritation, and appetite loss, especially during the first few days of treatment.

▼ Less common: stomach ulcers, GI bleeding, hepatitis, gallbladder attacks, painful urination, poor kidney function, kidney inflammation, blood and protein in the urine, dizziness, fainting, headache, drowsiness, nervousness, depression, hallucinations, confusion, disorientation, tingling in the hands or feet, light-headedness, itching, increased sweating, dry nose and mouth, heart palpitations, chest pain, ringing in the ears, breathing difficulties, and muscle cramps.

▼ Rare: severe allergic reactions including closing of the throat, fever and chills, changes in liver function, jaundice (yellowing of the skin or whites of the eyes), and kidney failure. People who experience such effects must be promptly treated in a hospital emergency room or doctor's office. NSAIDs have caused severe skin reactions; if this happens to you, see your doctor immediately.

Drug Interactions

• Nabumetone can increase the effects of oral anticoagulant (blood-thinning) drugs such as warfarin. Your anticoagulant dose may need to be reduced.

• Combining nabumetone with cyclosporine may increase the toxic kidney effects of both drugs.

• Methotrexate toxicity may be increased in people also taking nabumetone.

• Combining cholesterine with nabumetone may reduce the effectiveness of nabumetone.

• Nabumetone may reduce the blood-pressure-lowering effect of beta blockers and loop diuretics.

• Nabumetone may increase phenytoin side effects. Lithium blood levels may be increased by nabumetone.

• Nabumetone blood levels may be affected by cimetidine.

• Probenecid may increase the risk of nabumetone side effects.

• Aspirin and other salicylates should never be combined with nabumetone.

• Nabumetone may decrease the effectiveness of ACE inhibitors.

Food Interactions

Take nabumetone with food or a magnesium-aluminum antacid if it upsets your stomach.

Usual Dose

1000–2000 mg a day, taken in 1 or 2 doses.

Overdosage

People have died from NSAID overdoses. Common signs of overdose are drowsiness, nausea, vomiting, diarrhea, abdominal pain, rapid breathing, rapid heartbeat, increased sweating, ringing or buzzing in the ears, confusion, disorientation, stupor, and coma. Take the victim to a hospital emergency room at once. ALWAYS bring the prescription bottle or container.

Special Information

Take each dose with a full glass of water and do not lie down for 15 to 30 minutes afterward.

Nabumetone can make you drowsy or tired: Be careful when driving or operating hazardous equipment. Do not take any over-the-counter products containing acetaminophen or aspirin while taking nabumetone. Avoid alcohol.

Contact your doctor if you develop rash or itching, visual disturbances, weight gain, breathing difficulties, fluid retention, hallucinations, black or tarry stools, persistent headache, or any unusual or intolerable side effect.

If you forget a dose of nabumetone, take it as soon as you remember. If you take nabumetone once a day and it is within 8 hours of your next dose, or if you take several doses a day and it is within 4 hours of your next dose, skip the dose you forgot and continue with your regular schedule. Never take a double dose.

Special Populations

Pregnancy/Breast-feeding

NSAIDs may affect a fetal heart during the second half of pregnancy. Pregnant women should not take nabumetone without their doctor's approval. When this drug is considered crucial by your doctor, its potential benefits must be carefully weighed against its risks.

NSAIDs may pass into breast milk. There is a possibility that a nursing mother taking nabumetone could affect her baby's heart or cardiovascular system. Nursing mothers who must take this drug should bottle-feed.

Seniors

Seniors may be more susceptible to side effects, especially ulcer disease.

Generic Name

Naproxen/Naproxen Sodium

(nah-PROX-en) G

Brand Names

Aleve	EC-Naprosyn
Anaprox	Naprelan
Anaprox DS	Naprosyn

Type of Drug

Nonsteroidal anti-inflammatory drug (NSAID).

Prescribed For

Rheumatoid arthritis, osteoarthritis, ankylosing spondylitis, mild to moderate pain, tendinitis, bursitis, gout, fever, sunburn, toothache, migraine, and menstrual pain and headache. Only naproxen is prescribed for juvenile rheumatoid arthritis, only naproxen sodium for migraine and premenstrual syndrome (PMS).

General Information

Naproxen and other NSAIDs are used to relieve pain and inflammation. They may achieve their effects by blocking the body's production of a hormone called prostaglandin and the action of other body chemicals known as COX-1 and COX-2. Naproxen primarily blocks COX-1. Pain relief comes within 1 hour after taking the first dose of naproxen and lasts for about 7 hours, but its anti-inflammatory effect takes several days to 2 weeks to become apparent and may take a month to reach maximum effect.

Cautions and Warnings

People who are **allergic** to naproxen or any other NSAID and those with a history of **asthma** attacks brought on by an NSAID, iodides, or aspirin should not take naproxen.

Naproxen can cause **gastrointestinal (GI) bleeding, ulcers,** and **stomach perforation**. This can occur at any time, with or without warning, in people who take naproxen regularly. People with a history of active GI bleeding should be cautious about taking any NSAID. People who develop bleeding or ulcers and continue NSAID treatment should be aware of the possibility of developing more serious side effects.

Naproxen can affect platelets and **blood clotting** at high doses, and should be avoided by people with clotting problems and those taking warfarin.

People with **heart problems** who use naproxen may experience swelling in their arms, legs, or feet.

Naproxen dosage should be reduced in people with severe **liver disease**.

Naproxen can cause severe toxic effects to the **kidney**. Report any unusual side effects to your doctor, who may need to periodically test your kidney function.

Naproxen can make you **unusually sensitive to the effects of the sun**.

Possible Side Effects

▼ Most common: diarrhea, nausea, vomiting, constipation, gas, stomach upset or irritation, and appetite loss, especially during the first few days of treatment.

▼ Less common: stomach ulcers, GI bleeding, hepatitis, gallbladder attacks, painful urination, poor kidney function, kidney inflammation, blood and protein in the urine, dizziness, fainting, headache, nervousness, depression, hallucinations, confusion, disorientation, tingling in the hands or feet, light- headedness, ringing in the ears, itching, increased sweating, dry nose and mouth, heart palpitations, chest pain, difficulty breathing, and muscle cramps.

▼ Rare: severe allergic reactions including closing of the throat, fever and chills, changes in liver function, jaundice (yellowing of the skin or whites of the eyes), kidney failure, irregular breathing, hive-like swellings on the face, eyelids, mouth, lips, or tongue, wheezing, and tightening of the chest. People who experience such effects must be promptly treated in a hospital emergency room or doctor's office. NSAIDs have caused severe skin reactions; if this happens to you, see your doctor immediately.

Drug Interactions

• Naproxen can increase the effects of oral anticoagulant (blood-thinning) drugs such as warfarin. Your anticoagulant dose may need to be reduced.

• Naproxen may reduce the effect of thiazide diuretics.

• Taking naproxen with cyclosporine may increase the toxic kidney effects of both drugs.

• Methotrexate toxicity may be increased in people also taking naproxen.

• Naproxen may reduce the blood-pressure-lowering effect of beta blockers—except atenolol—and loop diuretics.

• Naproxen may increase phenytoin side effects. Lithium blood levels may be increased by naproxen.

• Naproxen blood levels may be affected by cimetidine.

• Probenecid may increase the risk of naproxen side effects.

• Aspirin and other salicylates should never be combined with naproxen.

• Naproxen may decrease the effectiveness of ACE inhibitors.

• Avoid alcohol. People who take 3 or more drinks a day are more likely to develop serious stomach problems.

Food Interactions

Take naproxen with a full glass of water. Take it with food or a magnesium-aluminum antacid if it upsets your stomach.

Usual Dose

Naproxen

Adult: starting dose—250–500 mg morning and evening; up to 1500 mg a day if needed. For mild to moderate pain, take 250–275 mg every 6–8 hours.

Child (age 2 and over): 4.5 mg per lb. of body weight divided into 2 doses a day.

Child (under age 2): not recommended.

Overdosage

People have died from NSAID overdoses. Common signs of overdose are drowsiness, heartburn, nausea, vomiting, diarrhea, abdominal pain, rapid breathing, rapid heartbeat, increased sweating, ringing or buzzing in the ears, confusion, disorientation, stupor, and coma. Take the victim to a hospital emergency room at once. ALWAYS bring the prescription bottle or container.

Special Information

Take each dose with a full glass of water and do not lie down for 15 to 30 minutes afterward.

Naproxen can make you drowsy or tired: Be careful when driving or operating hazardous equipment. Do not take any over-the-counter products containing acetaminophen or aspirin while taking naproxen. Avoid alcohol.

Contact your doctor if you develop rash or itching, visual disturbances, weight gain, breathing difficulties, fluid retention, hallucinations, black or tarry stools, persistent headache, or any unusual or intolerable side effect.

If you forget a dose of naproxen, take it as soon as you remember. If you take naproxen once a day and it is within 8 hours of your next dose, or if you take several doses a day and it is within 4 hours of your next dose, skip the dose you forgot and continue with your regular schedule. Never take a double dose.

Special Populations

Pregnancy/Breast-feeding

NSAIDs may affect fetal heart development during the second half of pregnancy. Studies in animals have shown that NSAIDs, if taken late in pregnancy, may prolong labor or cause problems during delivery. Pregnant women should not take naproxen without their doctor's approval. When the drug is considered crucial by your doctor, its potential benefits must be carefully weighed against its risks.

NSAIDs may pass into breast milk. There is a possibility that a nursing mother taking naproxen could affect her baby's heart or cardiovascular system. Nursing mothers who must take this drug should bottle-feed.

Seniors

Seniors may be more susceptible to side effects, especially ulcer disease.

Nasonex *see Corticosteroids, Nasal, page 307*

Generic Name

Nefazodone (neh-FAZ-oe-don)

Brand Name

Serzone

Type of Drug

Antidepressant.

Prescribed For

Depression.

General Information

A unique compound, nefazodone is chemically unrelated to other antidepressants. It interferes with the ability of nerve endings in the brain to absorb serotonin and norepinephrine, two key neurohormones. Nefazodone is broken down in the liver; severe liver disease may increase nefazodone blood levels by 25%. Very little of the drug is released through the kidneys.

Cautions and Warnings

Suicide is always a risk in severely depressed people, who should only be allowed to have minimal quantities of medication in their possession.

Nefazodone has been associated with potentially fatal **liver failure**. People with **liver disease** should use nefazodone with caution.

People with a history of **seizure disorders** may experience seizures while taking nefazodone.

People who have recently had a **heart attack** should use this drug with caution because it can substantially reduce heart rate.

Possible Side Effects

▼ Most common: weakness, dry mouth, nausea, headache, constipation, blurred or abnormal vision, tiredness, dizziness, constipation, light-headedness, and confusion.

▼ Common: upset stomach, increased appetite, cough, memory loss, tingling in the hands or feet, flushing or feelings of warmth, poor muscle coordination, and dizziness when rising from a lying or sitting position.

▼ Less common: low blood pressure, fever, chills, flu-like symptoms, joint pain, stiff neck, itching, rash, diarrhea, nausea, vomiting, thirst, sore throat, changes in sense of taste, ringing or buzzing in the ear, unusual dreams, poor coordination, tremors, muscle stiffness, reduced sex drive, urinary difficulties including infection, vaginitis, and breast pain.

▼ Rare: Rare side effects can affect your liver, gastrointestinal tract, joints, sexual function, and skin. Severe nefazodone allergy is rare. Contact your doctor if you experience any side effect not listed above.

Drug Interactions

• People who take nefazodone within 2 weeks of taking a monoamine oxidase inhibitor (MAOI) antidepressant may experience severe reactions including high fever, muscle rigidity or spasm, changes in mental state, and fluctuations in pulse, temperature, and breathing rate. People stopping nefazodone should wait at least 1 week before starting an MAOI.

• Combining nefazodone and sumatriptan or sibutramine may cause "serotonin syndrome"; avoid these combinations if possible.

• Combining buspirone and nefazodone may lead to increased side effects.

• Combining carbamazepine and nefazodone may raise carbamazepine and lower nefazodone blood levels.

• Nefazodone may increase blood levels of alprazolam and triazolam (benzodiazepine anti-anxiety drugs). Do not combine these drugs with nefazodone.

• Blood levels of digoxin may be substantially increased by nefazodone. People taking these drugs together should have their digoxin blood levels checked periodically.

• The clearance of haloperidol (an antipsychotic drug) may be drastically reduced by nefazodone; the implications of this are not clear.

• Combining nefazodone and propranolol may cause substantial reductions in propranolol blood levels and substantial increases in blood levels of nefazodone. Do not take these drugs together.

• Drinking alcohol or taking St. John's wort while taking nefazodone may make you very tired; avoid these combinations.

Food Interactions

Take this drug on an empty stomach at least 1 hour before or 2 hours after meals.

Usual Dose

Adult: 100 mg twice a day to start. Dosage may be increased by 100–200 mg a week to a maximum daily dose of approximately 600 mg.

Senior: Start at half the regular adult dose and increase as needed up to 600 mg a day.

Child (under age 18): Consult your physician.

Overdosage

Symptoms of overdose include nausea, vomiting, and sleepiness. Overdose victims should be taken to a hospital emergency room. ALWAYS bring the prescription bottle or container.

Special Information

Several weeks of nefazodone treatment may be necessary before you notice any effect. Continue taking the medication during this period.

Call your doctor at once if you develop hives, rash, or other allergic side effects while taking nefazodone.

Nefazodone may make you drowsy. Be careful when driving or doing any task that requires concentration. Avoid alcohol.

Check with your pharmacist or doctor before taking any over-the-counter medication because of the risk of drug interactions.

Special Populations

Pregnancy/Breast-feeding

Animal studies of nefazodone suggest decreased fertility and a risk of fetal damage. When this drug is considered crucial by your doctor, its potential benefits must be carefully weighed against its risks.

It is not known if nefazodone passes into breast milk. Nursing mothers who must take this drug should consider bottle-feeding.

Seniors

Seniors, especially women, should start treatment at half the usual dose. Dosage may be gradually increased as needed, up to the maximum recommended dosage.

Generic Name

Nelfinavir (nel-FIN-uh-vere)

Brand Name

Viracept

Type of Drug

Protease inhibitor.

Prescribed For

Human immunodeficiency virus (HIV) infection.

General Information

Part of the triple-drug cocktail responsible for the most important gains in the fight against acquired immunodeficiency syndrome (AIDS), nelfinavir belongs to a group of anti-HIV drugs called protease inhibitors. Triple-drug cocktails are considered responsible for the first overall reduction in the AIDS death rate, recorded in 1996. When the HIV virus attacks a cell, it must be converted into viral DNA. Older drugs known as reverse transcriptase inhibitors interfered with this step but are inferior to protease inhibitors. Protease inhibitors work at the end of the process of HIV reproduction, at the point when proteins are "cut" into strands of exactly the right size to duplicate HIV; these proteins are cut by protease enzymes. Protease inhibitors prevent the mature HIV virus from being formed by interfering with this cutting process. Proteins that are cut to the wrong length or remain uncut are inactive. Protease inhibitors are not a cure for HIV infection or AIDS.

Protease inhibitors are always taken with 1 or 2 nucleoside antiviral drugs such as AZT, ddI, ddC, or 3TC. Protease inhibitors revolutionized HIV treatment because, when taken in combination with other drugs, they reduce the amount of HIV virus in the bloodstream to levels that are often undetectable by current methods such as CD_4 cell counts of immune system cells and viral load (amount of virus in the blood) measurements. Multiple-drug therapy has changed the current view of HIV disease from a fatal disease to a manageable chronic (long-term) illness.

People taking a protease inhibitor may still develop infection or other conditions normally associated with HIV disease. Because of this, it is very important for you to remain under the care of a doctor or other health care provider. The long-term effects of nelfinavir are not known. You may be able to spread the HIV virus to others even if you are on triple-drug therapy.

Cautions and Warnings

Do not take nelfinavir if you are **allergic** to it. People with **liver disease** or **cirrhosis** break down nelfinavir more slowly than do those with normal liver function.

Nelfinavir may raise **blood sugar,** worsen **diabetes,** or cause new cases of diabetes to develop.

Possible Side Effects

▼ Most common: diarrhea.

▼ Common: liver inflammation, and nausea.

▼ Less common: abdominal pain, gas, weakness, and rash.

▼ Rare: Rare side effects can occur in almost any part of the body including your blood, muscles and joints, gastrointestinal tract, kidneys, and eyes, and can affect your mental state and sexual function. Contact your doctor if you experience any side effect not listed above.

Drug Interactions

• Anticonvulsant medication such as carbamazepine, phenytoin, or phenobarbital may reduce the amount of nelfinavir in the blood.

• Nelfinavir interferes with the liver's ability to break down triazolam, midazolam, statin drugs (except pravastatin and sildenafil), ergot derivatives, amiodarone, and quinidine. Do not combine nelfinavir with any of these drugs as severe side effects may result.

• Combining nelfinavir with indinavir or saquinavir, other protease inhibitors, results in large increases in the amounts of both drugs in the blood. Other drugs that increase the amount of nelfinavir in the blood are ketoconazole and ritonavir.

• Combining rifabutin with nelfinavir lowers the amount of nelfinavir in the blood and raises the amount of rifabutin. Rifabutin dosage should be cut in half when this combination is used.

• Do not combine rifampin or pimozide and nelfinavir. Combine nelfinavir and sildenafil or vardenafil with extreme caution.

• Nelfinavir reduces the amount of oral contraceptive hormones in your bloodstream (see "Special Information").

• If you combine nelfinavir, lamivudine, and zidovudine (an AIDS drug—also known as AZT), your AZT dosage may have to be increased.

• St. John's wort may decrease the effectiveness of nelfinavir. Avoid this combination.

Food Interactions

Take nelfinavir with food.

Usual Dose

Adult and Child (age 14 and over): 1250 mg twice daily or 750 mg 3 times a day.

Child (age 2–13): 9–13 mg per lb. of body weight, 3 times a day.

Overdosage

Little is known about the effects of nelfinavir overdose except that it may cause severe side effects. Take overdose victims to a hospital emergency room for treatment. ALWAYS bring the prescription bottle or container.

Special Information

It is imperative for you to take your HIV medication exactly as prescribed. Missing or skipping doses of nelfinavir increases your risk of becoming resistant to the drug and losing the benefits of nelfinavir therapy.

Nelfinavir does not cure AIDS. It will not prevent you from transmitting the HIV virus to another person; you must still practice safe sex.

Diarrhea associated with nelfinavir may be controlled by using loperamide, an over-the-counter remedy.

Do not depend on oral contraceptives while taking nelfinavir. Use another contraceptive method.

Report anything unusual to your doctor.

If you forget a dose, take it as soon as you remember. If it is almost time for your next dose, skip the dose you forgot and continue with your regular schedule. Do not take a double dose.

Special Populations

Pregnancy/Breast-feeding

The safety of using nelfinavir during pregnancy is not known. When this drug is considered crucial by your doctor, its potential benefits must be carefully weighed against its risks.

Nursing mothers with HIV should always bottle-feed, regardless of whether they take this drug, to avoid transmitting the virus.

Seniors

Seniors may take nelfinavir without special restriction.

Brand Name

Neosporin Ophthalmic

Generic Ingredients

Gramicidin + Neomycin Sulfate + Polymyxin B Sulfate G

Other Brand Names
AK-Spore

Type of Drug

Ophthalmic and antibiotic combination.

Prescribed For

Superficial eye infection.

General Information

Neosporin Ophthalmic is a combination of antibiotics that is effective against the most common types of eye infection. It is most useful when the infecting organism is known to be sensitive to any of the 3 antibiotics contained in Neosporin Ophthalmic. It may also be useful when the infecting organism is not known because of the drug's broad range of coverage. This product is also available as an eye ointment with a minor formula change—bacitracin is substituted for gramicidin. Both the eyedrops and eye ointment are used for the same kinds of eye infection.

Cautions and Warnings

Do not use Neosporin Ophthalmic if you are **allergic** or **sensitive** to any of its ingredients.

Prolonged use of any antibiotic product in the eye should be avoided because of the risk of becoming sensitive to it and because other organisms such as fungi may grow. If the infection does not clear up within a few days, call your doctor.

Possible Side Effects

▼ Less common: occasional eye irritation, itching, or burning.

Drug Interactions
None known.

Usual Dose
1 drop in the affected eye 2–4 times a day or more frequently if the infection is severe.

Overdosage
There is not enough medicine in this product to cause serious problems. Call your local poison control center or a hospital emergency room for more information. If you seek treatment, ALWAYS bring the prescription bottle or container.

Special Information
To avoid infection, do not touch the eyedropper tip to your finger, eyelid, or any other surface. Wait at least 5 minutes before using another eyedrop or eye ointment.

Call your doctor if the itching or burning does not go away after a few minutes, or if redness, irritation, swelling, visual disturbance, loss of vision, or eye pain persists.

In general, you should not wear contact lenses if you have an eye infection but your doctor may determine that the use of lenses is acceptable in your situation.

If you forget to administer a dose, do so as soon as you remember. If it is almost time for your next dose, skip the forgotten dose and continue with your regular schedule. Do not take a double dose.

Special Populations

Pregnancy/Breast-feeding
This drug has been found to be safe for use during pregnancy and breast-feeding. Remember to check with your doctor before taking any drug if you are pregnant.

Seniors

Seniors may take this drug without special restriction.

Neurontin *see Tiagabine, page 1063*

Generic Name

Nevirapine (nev-EYE-ruh-peen)

Brand Name

Viramune

Type of Drug

Antiviral.

Prescribed For

Human immunodeficiency virus (HIV) in adults whose condition has deteriorated on other anti-HIV treatments.

General Information

Nevirapine is a non-nucleoside reverse transcriptase inhibitor (NNRTI). It inhibits the reverse transcriptase (RT) enzyme, necessary for reproduction of the HIV virus in body cells, by binding directly to it. The duration of benefit from taking this drug may be limited because HIV can become resistant to nevirapine. In one study of nevirapine plus zidovudine (AZT), resistance began to develop in some people as soon as 2 weeks after treatment began. For this reason, nevirapine is generally prescribed as part of a triple therapy anti-HIV "cocktail."

Cautions and Warnings

People who are **allergic** or **sensitive** to nevirapine should avoid it.

Severe and **potentially fatal skin reactions** may develop in people taking this drug, including Stevens-Johnson syndrome (symptoms include fever, skin blisters, mouth sores, eye irritation, swelling, muscle or joint aches, and not feeling well). Call your doctor at once if any of these symptoms or any other skin reactions develop. Most rashes occur within the first 6 weeks of nevirapine treatment.

Possible Side Effects

▼ Most common: rash, fever, nausea, headache, and changes in liver function tests.

▼ Less common: abdominal pain, mouth or throat sores, tingling in the hands or feet, muscle aches, and liver inflammation.

▼ Rare: diarrhea, pain, and changes of sensation in the arms or legs.

Drug Interactions

• Rifampin and rifabutin may stimulate liver enzymes that break down nevirapine, reducing the amount of nevirapine in the blood. Neither of these drugs should be combined with nevirapine.

• Nevirapine may reduce the effectiveness of ketoconazole. This drug should not be combined with nevirapine.

• The enzyme systems that break down protease inhibitors are stimulated by nevirapine. Combining nevirapine and a protease inhibitor may reduce the amount of protease inhibitor in the blood, reducing its effectiveness and increasing the risk of protease inhibitor resistance.

• Combining nevirapine with an oral contraceptive may reduce the effectiveness of the contraceptive by lowering the amount of hormone in the blood.

Food Interactions

None known.

Usual Dose

Adult: starting dose—200 mg a day for 2 weeks. Maintenance dose—200 mg twice a day in combination with a nucleoside-type antiviral such as didanosine or AZT.

Child: (2 months–8 years): starting dose—about 2 mg per lb. of body weight a day for 2 weeks. Maintenance dose—3 mg per lb. of body weight twice a day. The total daily dose should not exceed 400 mg.

Overdosage

Little is known about the effects of nevirapine overdose. Call your local emergency room or poison control center for more information. If you seek treatment, ALWAYS bring the prescription bottle or container.

Special Information

Call your doctor at once if you develop any rash or other skin side effect (see "Cautions and Warnings").

Nevirapine does not cure AIDS. It will not prevent you from transmitting HIV to another person; you must still practice safe sex.

Take nevirapine according to your doctor's direction; this is very important in preventing the development of drug-resistant HIV. If you do forget a dose of nevirapine, take it as soon as you remember. If it almost time for your next dose, skip the dose you forgot and continue with your regular schedule. If you forget your nevirapine for a week, you will have to start the treatment program all over again, beginning with 200 mg a day for 2 weeks.

Special Populations

Pregnancy/Breast-feeding

Animal studies have shown no effect on the developing fetus but nothing is known about the safety of using nevirapine during human pregnancy. When this drug is considered crucial by your doctor, its potential benefits must be carefully weighed against its risks.

Nevirapine passes into breast milk. Nursing mothers with HIV should always bottle-feed, regardless of whether they take this drug, to avoid transmitting the virus.

Seniors

Seniors may take nevirapine without special restriction.

Nexium *see Proton-Pump Inhibitors, page 906*

Generic Name

Niacin (NYE-uh-sin) Ⓖ

Brand Names

Niacor   Nicotinex
Niaspan   Slo-Niacin
Nicolar

Type of Drug

Vitamin.

Prescribed For

Pellagra (niacin deficiency); also prescribed for high blood
levels of cholesterol and triglycerides and to dilate (widen)
blood vessels.

General Information

Niacin, also known as vitamin B3 and nicotinic acid, is essential to maintaining health through the role it plays in enzyme
activity. It is effective in lowering blood fat levels and helps to
dilate blood vessels, but we do not know exactly how it
works. The effect of niacin on blood fats is seen as early as 1
week after treatment is started.

Cautions and Warnings

Do not take niacin if you are **sensitive** or **allergic** to it or
related drugs or have **liver disease,** stomach **ulcer,** or a history of **arterial bleeding**. Niacin should be used with caution
by people with **heart disease, diabetes, gallbladder disease,**
severely **low blood pressure, gout,** or **alcoholism**.

When you are taking niacin in therapeutic dosages, your
doctor should periodically check your liver function and
blood-sugar level. People with **diabetes** may experience an
increase in blood sugar. Blood levels of uric acid may rise;
people who are prone to gout may experience an attack.

Niacin may cause postural **low blood pressure** (symptoms include dizziness or fainting when rising from a sitting or lying position).

Possible Side Effects

▼ Most common: flushing, which may occur within 2 hours of taking the first dose of niacin; itching; and gastrointestinal problems.

▼ Less common: decreased sugar tolerance in people with diabetes, nausea, vomiting, abdominal pain, diarrhea, upset stomach, jaundice (symptoms include yellowing of the skin or whites of the eyes), oily or dry skin, aggravation of skin conditions such as acne, itching, high blood levels of uric acid, low blood pressure, headache, tingling in the hands or feet, rash, abnormal heartbeats, and dizziness.

Drug Interactions

• Niacin may increase the effect of blood-pressure-lowering drugs, causing dizziness when rising quickly from a sitting or lying position.

• Niacin may interfere with sulfinpyrazone (a gout medication).

• Combining niacin and an HMG-CoA reductase inhibitor such as lovastatin may lead to the destruction of skeletal muscle.

Food Interactions

Take niacin with or after meals to reduce the risk of upset stomach.

Usual Dose

Vitamin Supplement: 15–20 mg a day.

Pellagra: not more than 500 mg a day.

High Blood-Fat Levels: 250 mg after the evening meal to start; dosage should be increased slowly, to 1500–3000 mg a day. Do not take more than 6000 mg a day. Take with a glass of cold water to help you swallow.

Overdosage

Symptoms may include drug side effects. Take the victim to a hospital emergency room. ALWAYS bring the prescription bottle or container.

Special Information

Skin reactions may occur within 2 hours of the first dose and include flushing and warmth, especially in the face, ears, or neck; tingling; itching; and headache. Call your doctor if these effects do not disappear as you continue taking niacin.

Stop taking this drug and call your doctor immediately if you experience irregular heartbeat, blurred vision, loss of appetite, flu-like symptoms, nausea, vomiting, dark-colored urine, or reduced urination.

If you forget a dose, take it as soon as you remember. If it is almost time for your next dose, skip the missed dose and continue with your regular schedule. Do not take a double dose.

Special Populations

Pregnancy/Breast-feeding

When used in normal dosages, niacin may and should be taken during pregnancy as part of a prenatal vitamin formulation. Dosages larger than 20 mg a day are not recommended during pregnancy.

Niacin passes into breast milk. Usual doses (up to 20 mg a day) will not affect a nursing infant. Larger doses used for lowering blood fats may affect a nursing infant.

Seniors

Seniors may take this drug without special restriction.

Generic Name

Nicardipine (nye-KAR-dih-pene) G

Brand Name

Cardene   Cardene SR

Type of Drug

Calcium channel blocker.

Prescribed For

Angina pectoris, high blood pressure, and congestive heart failure.

General Information

Nicardipine hydrochloride is one of many calcium channel blockers available in the U.S. These drugs block the passage of calcium, an essential factor in muscle contraction, into the heart and smooth muscles. Such blockage of calcium interferes with the contraction of these muscles, which in turn dilates (widens) the veins and vessels that supply blood to them. This dilating effect reduces blood pressure, the amount of oxygen used by the heart muscle, and the risk of blood vessel spasm. Nicardipine is therefore useful in treating not only high blood pressure but also angina pectoris (brief attacks of chest pain), a condition related to poor oxygen supply to the heart muscle.

Nicardipine affects the movement of calcium only into muscle cells; it has no effect on calcium in the blood.

Cautions and Warnings

Nicardipine can **slow your heart rate** and interfere with normal electrical conduction in heart muscle. For some people, this action can result in temporary heart stoppage, but such a reaction will not occur in people whose hearts are otherwise healthy.

You should not use nicardipine if you have had a **stroke** or bleeding in the brain or if you have advanced **hardening of the arteries**—particularly the aorta—because the drug can cause heart failure.

People who take nicardipine for congestive **heart failure** should be aware that the drug may aggravate the condition.

If you are also taking a **beta blocker,** its dosage should be reduced gradually rather than stopped abruptly when starting on nicardipine.

Nicardipine dosage should be adjusted in the presence of **kidney or liver disease**.

Nicardipine may cause **angina** when treatment is first started, when dosage is increased, or if the drug is rapidly withdrawn. This can be avoided by reducing dosage gradually.

Nicardipine may increase the risk of developing **low blood pressure,** especially if you are also taking beta blockers.

Studies of calcium channel blockers—usually those taken several times a day, not those taken only once daily—have shown that people taking them are more likely to have a **heart attack** than are people taking beta blockers or other medication for the same purposes. Discuss this with your doctor to be sure you are receiving the best possible treatment.

Possible Side Effects

▼ Most common: dizziness or light-headedness; fluid accumulation in the hands, legs, or feet; headache; weakness or fatigue; heart palpitations; angina; and facial flushing.

▼ Less common: low blood pressure; abnormal heart rhythms; fainting; increase or decrease in heart rate; heart failure; nausea; rash; nervousness; tingling in the hands or feet; hallucinations; temporary memory loss; difficulty sleeping; weakness; diarrhea; vomiting; constipation; upset stomach; itching; unusual sensitivity to the sun; painful or stiff joints; liver inflammation; increased urination, especially at night; infection; allergic reactions; sore throat; and hyperactivity.

Drug Interactions

• Combining nicardipine with a beta-blocking drug in order to treat high blood pressure is usually well tolerated but may lead to heart failure in susceptible people.

• Blood levels of cyclosporine may be increased by nicardipine, increasing the chance for cyclosporine-related kidney damage.

• The effect of quinidine (an antiarrhythmic) may be altered by nicardipine.

• Cimetidine and ranitidine may increase the amount of nicardipine in the bloodstream.

• Combining nicardipine with fentanyl or other anesthetics may cause very low blood pressure.

• Rifampin may decrease nicardipine's effectiveness.

Food Interactions

Nicardipine is best taken on an empty stomach at least 1 hour before or 2 hours after meals, but it may be taken with food or milk if it upsets your stomach. Avoid high-fat meals and grapefruit juice while on this drug.

Usual Dose

Immediate-Release: 20–40 mg 3 times a day. People with kidney disease should take 20 mg 3 times a day. People with liver disease should take 20 mg 2 times a day. Seniors should start with 20 mg 2–3 times a day and increase dosage gradually.

Sustained-Release: 30–60 mg 2 times a day. People with kidney disease should take 30 mg 2 times a day.

Overdosage

Symptoms of nicardipine overdose are very low blood pressure and reduced heart rate. Nicardipine can be removed from the victim's stomach by inducing vomiting with ipecac syrup—available at any pharmacy. This must be done within 30 minutes of the actual overdose, before the drug can be absorbed into the blood. Once symptoms develop or if more than 30 minutes have passed since the overdose, the victim must be taken to an emergency room. ALWAYS bring the prescription bottle or container.

Special Information

Call your doctor if you develop any of the following symptoms: worsening angina pain; swelling of the hands, legs, or feet; severe dizziness; constipation or nausea; or very low blood pressure.

Some people may experience a slight increase in blood pressure just before their next dose is due. You will be able to see this effect only if you use a home blood-pressure-monitoring device. If this happens, contact your doctor.

If you take nicardipine 3 times a day and forget a dose, take it as soon as you remember. If it is almost time for your next dose, take it and space the remaining doses evenly throughout the rest of the day. If you take nicardipine 2 times a day and forget a dose, take it as soon as you remember. If it is almost time for your next dose, skip the dose you forgot and continue with your regular schedule. Never take a double dose.

Special Populations

Pregnancy/Breast-feeding

In animal studies, large doses of nicardipine have been shown to harm the fetus. Nicardipine should be avoided by women who are or might be pregnant. When your doctor considers this drug crucial, its potential benefits must be carefully weighed against its risks.

Nicardipine passes into breast milk; nursing mothers who must take this drug should consider bottle-feeding.

Seniors

Seniors may be more sensitive to the side effects of nicardipine and require reduced dosage.

Generic Name

Nicotine (NIK-uh-teen) G

Brand Names

Commit	Nicorette DS
Habitrol	Nicotrol
Nicoderm	Nicotrol Inhaler
Nicoderm CQ	Nicotrol NS
Nicorette	ProStep

Type of Drug

Smoking deterrent.

Prescribed For

Addiction to cigarettes. Nicotine gum has been prescribed with haloperidol for children with Tourette's syndrome.

General Information

Nicotine replacement products are prescribed for short-term treatment and make cigarette withdrawal easier for many people. Because nicotine addiction also has a psychological component, counseling or other psychological support is necessary in order for a smoking cessation program to be successful.

The major advantage of patches over chewing gum or nasal spray is their convenience and ease of use. There are differences among the various patch products in terms of how much nicotine is absorbed into the bloodstream. All of the products are labeled according to the amount of nicotine absorbed. Obese men absorb significantly less nicotine.

Cautions and Warnings

Do not use nicotine if you are **sensitive** or **allergic** to it.

Nicotine should be used only by people addicted to nicotine. It should not be used during the period immediately following a **heart attack** or if you have severe **abnormal heart rhythms** or **angina pain**.

People with severe **temporomandibular joint (TMJ) disease** should not chew nicotine gum.

People with **heart conditions** must be evaluated by a cardiologist before starting treatment.

Nicotine should be used with caution by people with **diabetes** who take insulin and by people with an **overactive thyroid, kidney or liver disease, pheochromocytoma, hypertension** (high blood pressure), stomach **ulcer,** or chronic **dental problems** that might be worsened by nicotine chewing gum.

The nasal spray should not be used by people with **asthma, bronchospasm, allergic rhinitis, sinusitis,** or **nasal polyps.**

It is possible to become **addicted** to nicotine replacement products. Your nicotine addiction may worsen while using this product.

Possible Side Effects

Chewing Gum

▼ Most common: injury to the gums, jaw, or teeth; sore mouth or throat; stomach growling due to swallowing air while chewing.

▼ Common: nausea, vomiting, upset stomach, and hiccups.

▼ Less common: excessive salivation, dizziness, lightheadedness, irritability, headache, more frequent bowel movements, diarrhea, constipation, gas pain, dry mouth, hoarseness, flushing, sneezing, coughing, sleeplessness, swelling of the arms or legs, hypertension, heart palpitations, rapid and abnormal heartbeat, confusion,

Possible Side Effects *(continued)*

convulsions, depression, euphoria (feeling "high"), numbness, tingling in the hands or feet, ringing or buzzing in the ears, fainting, weakness, redness, itching, and rash.

Transdermal Patch

▼ Most common: feeling tired and irritation at the patch site. Transdermal systems may be more irritating to people with eczema or other skin conditions.

▼ Common: weakness, back pain, body ache, diarrhea, upset stomach, headache, sleeplessness, dizziness, nervousness, unusual dreams, increased cough or sore throat, muscle and joint pain, changes in sense of taste, and painful menstruation.

▼ Less common: chest pain, allergic reaction (symptoms include hives, breathing difficulties, and peeling skin), dry mouth, abdominal pain, vomiting, poor concentration, tingling in the hands or feet, sinus irritation or inflammation, increased sweating, and hypertension.

Nasal Spray

▼ Most common: headache, chest tightness, tingling in the hands or feet, constipation, inflammation of the mucous membranes of the mouth, and irritation of the nose, throat, or eye.

▼ Common: back pain, difficulty breathing, nausea, and joint pain.

▼ Less common: menstrual disorder, painful menstruation, heart palpitations, gas, tooth and gum problems, muscle aches, abdominal pains, confusion, acne, and itching.

Inhaler

▼ Most common: irritation of the mouth or throat, cough, runny nose, upset stomach, and headache.

▼ Common: changes in taste, flu-like symptoms, nausea, and diarrhea.

▼ Less common: pain in the neck or jaw, dental problems, sinus inflammation, back pain, numbness or tingling, gas, and fever.

Drug Interactions

• Nicotine—and cigarette smoking—reduces the effects of alcohol, benzodiazepine tranquilizers and sleeping pills, beta blockers, caffeine, clozapine, fluvoxamine, olanzapine, tacrine, theophylline, clorazepate, oral lidocaine, estradiol, imipramine, flecainide, heparin, insulin, mexiletine, opioids, and pentazocine.

Food Interactions

Do not eat or drink anything while or immediately after you chew nicotine gum. Caffeine, juice, wine, and soft drinks may interfere with its effects.

Usual Dose

Chewing Gum: 1 piece of gum whenever you feel the urge for a cigarette; do not use more than 30 pieces a day. Gradually reduce the number of pieces you chew and the time you chew each piece every 4–7 days. Substituting sugarless gum for nicotine gum may help in the process of gradual dosage reduction. Each piece contains 2–4 mg of nicotine.

Transdermal Patch: Apply the patch to the skin as soon as you remove it from the package. Nicotrol patches should be applied when you get up in the morning and removed at bedtime. Prescription nicotine patches should be left on for 16–24 hours, depending on the brand. Use a different skin site when applying a new patch. The dosage of the patch will be gradually reduced by your doctor.

Nasal Spray: 1–2 sprays in each nostril up to 5 times an hour. The spray should be used at least 8 times a day to ease symptoms of nicotine withdrawal. Do not use more than 40 doses a day.

Inhaler: Use as needed, generally 3–6 cartridges a day for the first 3–6 weeks; some people use up to 16 cartridges a day. Dosage should be gradually reduced after 12 weeks until you are able to stop.

Overdosage

Nicotine overdose may be deadly. Symptoms include excessive salivation, nausea, vomiting, diarrhea, abdominal pain, headache, cold sweats, dizziness, hearing and visual disturbances, weakness, and confusion. These symptoms may be followed by fainting; very low blood pressure; a pulse that is weak, rapid, and irregular; convulsions; and death by paralysis of the muscles that control breathing.

Nicotine stimulates the brain's vomiting center, making this reaction common but not automatic; spontaneous vomiting may be sufficient to remove the poison from the victim's system. In case of overdose, call your local poison control center or a hospital emergency room. If the victim has not already vomited, you may be told to induce vomiting with ipecac syrup—available at any pharmacy—before taking the victim to an emergency room. If you seek treatment, ALWAYS bring the nicotine package.

Special Information

When using the gum, follow the product instructions. Chew each piece slowly and intermittently for about 30 minutes. Rapid chewing releases the nicotine too quickly and may lead to side effects including nausea, hiccups, and throat irritation. Do not chew more than 30 pieces a day. The amount of gum chewed should be gradually reduced and stopped after 3 months of successful treatment.

When administering the nasal spray, tilt your head back slightly and do not sniff or inhale through your nose. A dose consists of 1 spray in each nostril. Administering fewer than 8 doses a day may not be effective. Do not exceed 40 doses a day. The spray should not be used for longer than 6 months.

Do not store nicotine patches in an area that is warmer than 86°F. Slight discoloration is not a sign of loss of potency, but do not store a patch after you have removed it from its pouch. Nicotine patches should not be used for more than 3 consecutive months.

Keep nicotine patches and nasal spray containers—used or unused—out of the reach of children or pets to avoid accidental poisoning.

Special Populations

Pregnancy/Breast-feeding
Nicotine is not safe for use during pregnancy. It is known to cause fetal harm when used during the last 3 months of pregnancy and is associated with breathing difficulties in newborns and miscarriage.

Nicotine passes into breast milk. Nursing mothers who use it should bottle-feed.

Seniors
Seniors may be more sensitive to side effects including weakness, dizziness, and body aches.

Generic Name

Nifedipine (nih-FED-ih-pene) Ⓖ

Brand Names

Adalat
Adalat CC
Nifedical XL

Nifeditab CR
Procardia
Procardia XL

The information in this profile also applies to the following drugs:

Generic Ingredient: Isradipine
DynaCirc   DynaCirc CR

Generic Ingredient: Nisoldipine
Sular

Type of Drug

Calcium channel blocker.

Prescribed For

Angina pectoris, Prinzmetal's angina, and high blood pressure; also prescribed for migraine headache prevention, asthma, heart failure, Raynaud's disease, disorders of the esophagus, gallbladder and kidney stone attacks, severe high blood pressure triggered by pregnancy, and premature labor.

General Information

Nifedipine is one of many calcium channel blockers available in the U.S. These drugs block the passage of calcium, an essential factor in muscle contractions, into the heart and smooth muscles. Such blockage of calcium interferes with the contraction of these muscles, which in turn dilates (widens) the veins and vessels that supply blood to them. This dilating effect reduces blood pressure, the amount of oxygen used by the heart muscle, and the risk of blood vessel spasm. Nifedipine is therefore useful in treating not only high blood pressure but also angina pectoris (brief attacks of chest pain), a condition related to poor oxygen supply to the heart muscle.

Nifedipine affects the movement of calcium only into muscle cells; it has no effect on calcium in the blood.

Nifedipine capsules contain liquid medication. In cases in which the drug is needed in the blood immediately, the capsules may be punctured and their content squeezed under the tongue; the medication is rapidly absorbed into the blood when taken in this manner. Thus nifedipine capsules are particularly useful when extremely high blood pressure must be lowered as quickly as possible. Some researchers assert that biting the capsule and swallowing the contents is an even faster way of absorbing the drug.

Cautions and Warnings

These drugs may cause unwanted **low blood pressure** in some people who take it for reasons other than hypertension.

Patients taking a beta-blocking drug who begin taking these drugs may develop an increase in incidences of **angina** pain. Angina may also intensify when these drugs are first started, when they are increased, or if they are stopped abruptly.

Studies have shown that people taking calcium channel blockers—usually those taken several times a day, not those that are taken only once daily—have a greater chance of having a **heart attack** than people taking beta blockers or other medications for the same purposes. Discuss this with your doctor to be sure you are receiving the best possible treatment.

Congestive **heart failure** has, on rare occasions, developed in people taking nifedipine.

Calcium channel blockers may cause **low blood pressure,** particularly if taken with beta blockers.

Do not take this drug if you have had an **allergic reaction** to it in the past.

Nifedipine may interfere with one of the mechanisms by which **blood clots** form, especially if you are also taking aspirin. Call your doctor if you develop unusual bruises, bleeding, or black-and-blue marks.

People with kidney disease or severe **liver disease** may require dosage adjustments.

Possible Side Effects

Nifedipine
Nifedipine side effects are generally mild and rarely cause people to stop taking the drug.

Possible Side Effects *(continued)*

▼ Most common: swelling of the ankles, feet, and legs; dizziness or light-headedness; flushing; a feeling of warmth; and nausea.

▼ Less common: headache; weakness, shakiness, or jitteriness; giddiness; muscle cramps, inflammation, and pain; nervousness; mood changes; heart palpitations; heart failure; heart attack; breathing difficulties; coughing; fluid in the lungs; wheezing; stuffy nose; fever and chills; and sore throat.

▼ Rare: Rare side effects can occur in your heart, stomach or intestines, urinary tract, and joints and muscles and can affect your mental and sexual function, hearing, and balance. Contact your doctor if you experience any side effect not listed above.

Isradipine

Isradipine side effects are generally mild and self-limiting.

▼ Most common: headache.

▼ Less common: low blood pressure, chest pain, abdominal pain, rapid heartbeat, dizziness, diarrhea, a feeling of warmth, nausea, light-headedness, fatigue and lethargy, itching, rash, flushing, changes in certain blood-cell components, and swelling of the legs, ankles, or feet.

▼ Rare: Rare side effects can occur in almost any part of the body. Contact your doctor if you experience any side effect not listed above.

Nisoldipine

▼ Most common: headache and swelling in the arms or legs.

▼ Common: sore throat, flushing, sinus irritation, and heart palpitations.

▼ Less common: chest pain, nausea, and rash.

▼ Rare: Rare side effects can occur in almost any part of the body. Contact your doctor if you experience any side effect not listed above.

Drug Interactions

• These drugs may interact with beta-blocking drugs to cause heart failure, very low blood pressure, or an increased incidence of angina pain. However, in many cases these drugs have been taken together with no problem.

• Nifedipine may cause unexpected blood pressure reduction in patients who also take other drugs to control their high blood pressure. Low blood pressure can also result from taking nifedipine with fentanyl and other anesthetics.

• Cimetidine, nafcillin, and ranitidine increase the amount of nifedipine in the blood and may account for a slight increase in nifedipine's effect.

• The combination of quinidine (an antiarrhythmic) and nifedipine must be used with caution because it can produce low blood pressure, very slow heart rate, abnormal heart rhythm, and swelling in the arms or legs.

• On rare occasions, nifedipine may increase the effects of oral anticoagulant (blood-thinning) drugs.

• Nifedipine may intensify the effects of cyclosporine, digoxin, and theophylline products, increasing the chances of side effects from those drugs.

• Barbiturates, melatonin, St. John's wort, and rifampin, may decrease the effectiveness of nifedipine.

• Nifedipine and diltiazem increase each other's blood levels.

• Combining isradipine with anesthetics including fentanyl can result in very low blood pressure.

• Drugs that may increase blood levels of isradipine include itraconazole, cimetidine, and ranitidine; adjust isradipine dosage if necessary.

• Rifampin may decrease the effects of isradipine, which may also require dosage adjustment.

• Isradipine may lower blood levels of lovastatin, requiring dosage adjustment.

• When nisoldipine is combined with cimetidine, blood levels of nisoldipine increase substantially.

• Quinidine reduces the amount of nisoldipine in the blood, but maximum levels remain unaffected.

Food Interactions

Avoid drinking grapefruit juice if you are taking these drugs. Avoid fatty foods when taking nisoldipine.

Usual Dose

Nifedipine
Immediate-Release: 10–30 mg 3 times a day. Do not exceed 180 mg a day.

Sustained-Release: 30–60 mg once a day.

Do not stop taking nifedipine abruptly. The dosage should be reduced gradually.

Nisoldipine
Adult: starting dose—20 mg a day. Maintenance dose—20–40 mg, as needed, up to a maximum of 50 mg.
Seniors and People with Liver Disease: starting dose—10 mg a day. Maintenance dose—20–40 mg, as needed and tolerated (maximum 60 mg).
Child: not recommended.

Isradipine
5–20 mg a day in 2 doses. Do not stop taking the drug abruptly. The dosage should be reduced gradually over a period of time.

Overdosage

Overdose of these drugs can cause low blood pressure, nausea, weakness, dizziness, drowsiness, confusion, and slurred speech. If you think you have taken an overdose of nifedipine, call your doctor or go to a hospital emergency room. ALWAYS bring the prescription bottle or container.

Special Information

Call your doctor if you develop constipation, nausea, very low blood pressure, swelling in the arms or legs, worsening angina, swelling in the hands or feet, breathing difficulties, increased heart pain, or dizziness or light-headedness, or if other side effects are particularly bothersome or persistent.

If you are taking nifedipine for high blood pressure, be sure to continue taking your medication and follow any instructions for diet restriction or other treatments. High blood pressure is a condition with few recognizable symptoms; it may seem to you that you are taking medication for no good reason. Call your doctor or pharmacist if you have any questions.

If you take Procardia XL, be sure not to break or crush the tablets. You may notice an empty tablet in your stool. This is not a cause for alarm, because the drug is normally released without actually destroying the tablet.

It is important to maintain good dental hygiene while taking nifedipine and to use extra care when using your toothbrush or dental floss: The drug may make you more susceptible to some infections.

If you forget a dose of nifedipine and you take it 3 or more times a day, take it as soon as you remember. If it is almost time for your next dose, take the dose you forgot and space the rest evenly throughout the remainder of the day. If you take nifedipine 2 times a day and forget a dose, take it as soon as you remember. If it is almost time for your next dose, skip the dose you forgot and continue with your regular schedule. Never take a double dose.

Special Populations

Pregnancy/Breast-feeding
Nifedipine crosses into the fetal blood circulation. It has been used to treat severe high blood pressure associated with pregnancy without causing any unusual effect on the fetus. Nevertheless, women who are or might be pregnant should not take nifedipine without their doctor's approval. When this drug is considered crucial by your doctor, its potential benefits must be carefully weighed against its risks.

Small amounts of nifedipine may pass into breast milk. You must consider the potential effect on the nursing infant if breast-feeding while taking this medication.

Seniors
Seniors are more sensitive to the effects of nifedipine and may require dosage adjustments.

Generic Name

Nimodipine (nih-MOE-dih-pene)

Brand Name

Nimotop

Type of Drug

Calcium channel blocker.

Prescribed For

Functional losses following a hemorrhagic stroke and migraine and cluster headaches.

General Information

Unlike other calcium channel blockers, nimodipine has a negligible effect on the heart. It is the only calcium channel blocker proven to improve neurological function after a stroke. Nimodipine has a greater effect on blood vessels in the brain than on those in other parts of the body.

Cautions and Warnings

Nimodipine should not be taken if you are **sensitive** or **allergic** to it.

People with **liver disease,** including cirrhosis, may require reduced dosage.

Possible Side Effects

▼ Most common: diarrhea, low blood pressure, rash, and headache.

▼ Less common: swelling of the arms or legs, high blood pressure, heart failure, rapid heartbeat, changes in the electrocardiogram, depression, memory loss, psychosis, paranoid feelings, hallucinations, nausea, itching, acne, anemia, bleeding or bruising, abnormal blood clotting, flushing, breathing difficulties, stomach bleeding, and muscle cramps.

▼ Rare: dizziness, heart attack, liver inflammation or jaundice, vomiting, intestinal blockage, and sexual difficulties.

Drug Interactions

• Calcium channel blockers may cause bleeding when taken alone or combined with aspirin.

• Combining nimodipine with a beta-blocking drug is usually tolerated well but may lead to heart failure in susceptible people.

- Calcium channel blockers, including nimodipine, may add to the effects of digoxin.
- Cimetidine may increase blood levels of nimodipine.

Food Interactions

Nimodipine is best taken at least 1 hour before or 2 hours after meals, but may be taken with food or milk if it upsets your stomach. Avoid drinking grapefruit juice if you are taking this drug.

Usual Dose

Stroke: 60 mg 4 times a day, beginning within 96 hours after the stroke and continuing for 21 days.

Migraine Headache: 40 mg 3 times a day.

Overdosage

Symptoms of nimodipine overdose are nausea, weakness, dizziness, drowsiness, confusion, and slurred speech. Blood pressure and heart rate may also be affected. Nimodipine can be removed from a victim's stomach by giving ipecac syrup—available at any pharmacy—to induce vomiting, but this should be done only under a doctor's supervision or direction. Once symptoms develop, the victim must be taken to a hospital emergency room for treatment. ALWAYS bring the prescription bottle or container.

Special Information

Call your doctor if you develop any of the following symptoms: swelling of the arms or legs, breathing difficulties, severe dizziness, constipation, or nausea.

Patients who are unable to swallow nimodipine capsules because of their condition may have the liquid withdrawn from the capsule with a syringe, mixed with other liquids, and given orally or through a feeding tube.

If you forget a dose of nimodipine, take it as soon as you remember. If it is almost time for your next dose, skip the dose you forgot and continue with your regular schedule. Call your doctor if you miss more than 2 consecutive doses.

Special Populations

Pregnancy/Breast-feeding

Animal studies have shown that nimodipine may cause fetal malformation. Nimodipine should be avoided by women who are or might be pregnant. When your doctor considers this drug crucial, its potential benefits must be carefully weighed against its risks.

Nimodipine passes into breast milk. Nursing mothers who must take nimodipine should bottle-feed.

Seniors

Seniors, especially those with severe liver disease, may be more sensitive to side effects.

Generic Name

Nitazoxanide (neye-tan-OX-ah-nyde)

Brand Name

Alinia

Type of Drug

Antiprotozoal.

Prescribed for

Nitazoxanide is prescribed for children ages 1–11 with diarrhea caused by the parasites *Giardia lambia* and *Cryptosporidium parvum*.

General Information

Specific enzyme reactions that occur in the body are used by the *Giardia lambia* and *Cryptosporidium parvum* microorganisms for energy production, allowing them to thrive inside the body. Nitazoxanide works by blocking these specific enzyme reactions preventing them from thriving inside people. It is broken down in the liver.

Cautions and Warnings

Do not take this drug if you are **sensitive** or **allergic** to it.

People with **liver** or **kidney** disease should take this drug with caution since it has not been studied in people with these conditions.

The safety of nitazoxanide in people with **AIDS** and those who are **HIV positive** has not been established.

Possible Side Effects

Most side effects are mild and pass with time.
▼ Most common: abdominal pain.
▼ Less common: headache, diarrhea, and vomiting.
▼ Rare: nausea, appetite changes, intestinal gas, enlarged salivary glands, fever, infections, feeling sick, itching, sweating, runny nose, dizziness, and changes in urine color.

Drug Interactions

• This drug is highly bound to proteins in the bloodstream and may interact with warfarin, digoxin, and other highly bound drugs, however, no specific interactions have been reported.

Food Interactions

Take this drug with food or meals.

Usual Dose

Child (under 12 months old): Nitazoxanide has not been studied in this age group.

Child (12 months to 47 months): 1 teaspoonful every 12 hours for 3 days.

Child (age 4 to 11): 2 teaspoons every 12 hours for 3 days.

Adult and Child (over age 11): Studies have not established the appropriate dosage for people in this age group.

Overdosage

Single doses of nitazoxanide up to 4,000 mg have been taken by adults without significant side effects. Overdose victims should be taken to a hospital emergency room for evaluation. ALWAYS bring the prescription bottle or container.

Special Information

This product contains 1.48 grams of sugar in each teaspoonful of the suspension. This information may be of importance for people with diabetes and others who must manage their sugar intake.

Special Populations

Pregnancy/Breast-feeding

Animal studies using doses about 48 times the usual dose have revealed no adverse reproductive effects. The safety of nitazoxanide during pregnancy is not known. While animal studies reveal no damage to the fetus, this drug should only be used during pregnancy after carefully weighing its potential benefits against its risks.

It is not known if nitazoxanide passes into breast milk. Nursing mothers who must take it should bottle-feed.

Seniors

This drug has not been studied in seniors.

Generic Name

Nitrofurantoin (NYE-troe-few-RAN-toe-in) G

Brand Names

Furadantin   Macrodantin
Macrobid

Type of Drug

Urinary anti-infective.

Prescribed For

Urinary tract infections (UTIs), such as pyelonephritis, pyelitis, and cystitis.

General Information

Nitrofurantoin is helpful in treating UTIs because large amounts of it pass into the urine. It works by interfering with the metabolism of carbohydrates, or sugars, in the infecting bacteria. It may also interfere with the formation of the bacterial cell wall.

Cautions and Warnings

Do not take nitrofurantoin if you are **allergic** to it or have **kidney disease**.

Rarely, severe **chest pain, breathing difficulties, cough, fever,** and **chills** may develop within a few hours to 3 weeks after taking nitrofurantoin. These symptoms usually go away within 1 to 2 days after you stop taking it. Nitrofurantoin therapy may cause **cough, breathing difficulties,** and **feelings of ill health** after 1 to 6 months. Respiratory failure and death have occurred in a few cases.

Rarely, nitrofurantoin causes **hemolytic anemia**. People with a deficiency of the enzyme G-6-PD are most susceptible to this reaction and should not take nitrofurantoin.

Rarely, nitrofurantoin causes **hepatitis,** which may lead to death. It is most likely to develop during long-term treatment.

Nitrofurantoin may cause serious or irreversible **peripheral neuropathy** (damage to the nerves in the arms and legs). People with kidney disease, anemia, diabetes, electrolyte imbalance, or vitamin B deficiency are at increased risk.

This drug is only used to treat UTIs caused by organisms susceptible to nitrofurantoin. It should not be used to treat **infections in other parts of the body.** Long-term or chronic use of nitrofurantin may lead to **secondary infection** caused by drug-resistant bacteria or fungi.

This drug may cause a false positive result in urine tests for glucose.

Possible Side Effects

Side effects are less prominent with Macrodantin than with Furadantin.

▼ Most common: loss of appetite, nausea, vomiting, stomach pain, and diarrhea. Some people develop hepatitis symptoms.

▼ Less common: fever, chills, cough, chest pain, breathing difficulties, and development of fluid in the lungs. If these reactions occur in the first week of therapy, they can generally be resolved by stopping the medication. If they develop after taking nitrofurantoin for a longer period, they are considered chronic and may be more serious.

▼ Rare: rash, itching, asthmatic attacks in people with a history of asthma, drug fever, symptoms similar to arthritis, jaundice (yellowing of the skin or whites of the eyes), effects on components of the blood, headache, dizziness, drowsiness, and temporary hair loss.

This drug is known to cause changes in white and red blood cells. It should be used only under the strict supervision of your doctor.

Drug Interactions

• Nitrofurantoin may increase other drugs' toxic effects on the liver and the risk of hemolytic anemia if you are taking another drug associated with that condition. These drugs include oral antidiabetes drugs, methyldopa, primaquine, procainamide, quinidine, quinine, and sulfa drugs.

• Nitrofurantoin interferes with nalidixic acid. Do not combine these drugs.

• Sulfinpyrazone and probenecid may reduce this drug's effectiveness and increase side effects.

• Anticholinergic drugs, including propantheline, may increase the risk of nitrofurantoin side effects.

• Magnesium, found most commonly in antacids, delays the absorption of nitrofurantoin or reduces the amount absorbed.

• Combining nitrofurantoin and metronidazole, mexiletine, ethambutol, isoniazid, lindane, lincomycin, lithium, pemoline, quinacrine, or long-term high-dose pyridoxine (vitamin B_6), may increase the risk of nervous system effects. Do not combine nitrofurantoin and any of these drugs.

Food Interactions

Nitrofurantoin should be taken with food to minimize upset stomach, loss of appetite, nausea, or other gastrointestinal symptoms. For optimal effectiveness, avoid citrus fruits while taking nitrofurantoin.

Usual Dose

Adult: 50–100 mg 4 times a day, with meals and at bedtime.
Child (over age 1 month): 2–3 mg per lb. of body weight in 4 doses.
Child (under age 1 month): not recommended.

People with chronic urinary infections may require lower-dosage, longer-term therapy.

Overdosage

Induce vomiting with ipecac syrup—available at any pharmacy—and take the victim to a hospital emergency room for treatment. If you seek treatment, ALWAYS bring the prescription bottle or container.

Special Information

Call your doctor if you develop chest pain or breathing difficulties; cough; sore throat; pale skin; unusual tiredness or
weakness; dizziness; drowsiness; headache; rash and itching; yellow skin; achy joints; fever and chills; numbness, tingling, or burning of the fingers or toes; severe diarrhea;
abdominal pain; bloody stool; or any persistent or bothersome side effect.

Continue taking this drug until your prescription is finished
even if you stop experiencing symptoms of a UTI.

Nitrofurantoin may give your urine a brownish color: This
is not a cause for concern.

The liquid form can stain your teeth if you do not swallow it
rapidly.

If you miss a dose, take it as soon as possible. If it is almost
time for your next dose and you take it 3 or more times a day,
space the missed dose and your next dose by 2 to 4 hours.

Special Populations

Pregnancy/Breast-feeding

Nitrofurantoin should never be taken by pregnant women
with G-6-PD deficiency or those who are near term because it
can interfere with the immature enzyme systems of the fetus
and cause hemolytic anemia. When this drug is considered
crucial by your doctor, its potential benefits must be carefully
weighed against its risks.

This drug passes into breast milk. Nursing mothers who
must take nitrofurantoin should consider bottle-feeding,
especially if the baby is G-6-PD deficient.

Seniors

Seniors with kidney disease may be more sensitive to nervous-system and lung effects. Seniors may also require
reduced dosage due to reduction of kidney function.

Generic Name

Nitroglycerin (nye-troe-GLIH-ser-in) Ⓖ

Brand Names

Deponit	Nitrek
Minitran	Nitro-Bid

Nitrocine	Nitrolingual
Nitro-Derm	Nitrong
Nitrodisc	NitroQuick
Nitro-Dur	Nitrostat
Nitrogard	Nitro Tab
Nitroglyn	Nitro-Time
Nitrol	Transderm-Nitro

Type of Drug

Antianginal agent.

Prescribed For

Chest pain associated with angina pectoris; prevention and management of angina; nitroglycerin injection is also used as a treatment after a heart attack, for congestive heart failure (CHF), and for high blood pressure.

General Information

Nitroglycerin and other nitrates are used to treat pain associated with heart problems. While the exact nature of their action is not fully understood, they relax vascular smooth muscle. Nitroglycerin is available in several forms: sublingual tablets, which are taken under the tongue and allowed to dissolve; capsules, which are swallowed; transmucosal tablets, which are placed between the lip or cheek and gum and allowed to dissolve; oral sprays, which are sprayed directly onto or under the tongue; transdermal patches, which deliver nitroglycerin through the skin over a 24-hour period; and ointment, which is usually spread over the chest or another area of the body. One or more forms of nitroglycerin are often used to prevent or alleviate chest pain associated with angina.

Cautions and Warnings

You should not take nitroglycerin if you are **allergic** to it or to another nitrate product, such as isosorbide. Do not use the patch form if you are allergic to adhesives.

Nitroglycerin should be taken with great caution if **head trauma** or **bleeding in the head** is present.

This drug may be inappropriate for you if you have had a recent **heart attack** or have severe **anemia, glaucoma,** severe **liver or kidney disease, overactive thyroid, glaucoma, cardiomyopathy** (loss of blood-pumping ability due to damaged heart muscle), or **low blood pressure,** especially postural low blood pressure (symptoms include dizziness or fainting when rising from a sitting or lying position).

Possible Side Effects

▼ Most common: flushing and headache, which may be severe or persistent.

▼ Less common: dizziness and weakness. Blurred vision and dry mouth may occur; if they do, stop taking the drug and call your doctor. In some people, the blood-pressure-lowering effect of nitroglycerin causes severe responses, including nausea, vomiting, weakness, restlessness, pallor (loss of facial color), increased perspiration, and collapse. Rash may also occur.

Drug Interactions

• Avoid over-the-counter drugs containing stimulants, such as cough, cold, and allergy remedies and appetite suppressants; they may aggravate heart disease.

• Do not take sildenafil, vardenafil, or taldenafil if you are taking nitroglycerin or another nitrate product. The combination can result in a rapid and potentially fatal drop in blood pressure.

• Interaction with large amounts of alcohol may rapidly lower blood pressure, resulting in weakness, dizziness, and fainting.

• Aspirin and calcium channel blockers may increase nitrate blood levels and the risk of side effects.

• Nitroglycerin may interfere with heparin (an injectable anticoagulant drug).

• Nitrates increase dihydroergotamine blood levels, which may raise blood pressure or block the effects of nitroglycerin.

Food Interactions

Do not use any oral form of nitroglycerin with food or gum in your mouth. Nitroglycerin pills intended for swallowing are best taken on an empty stomach.

Usual Dose

Use only as much as is necessary to control chest pain.

Sublingual Tablets: Since this form acts within 10–15 seconds, it should be taken only when necessary. Dissolve 1 tablet under the tongue, or between the cheek and gum. Repeat about every 5 minutes until you get relief; take no more than 3 tablets in 15 minutes.

Transmucosal Tablets: The tablets are placed between the upper lip and gum or between the cheek and gum and allowed to dissolve over a 3- to 5-hour period. The tablet releases the drug faster when touched with the tongue or when you drink a hot liquid. Insert another tablet after the previous one is dissolved. Do not sleep with a tablet in your mouth.

Sustained-Release Capsules and Tablets: Starting dose: 2.5–2.6 mg 3 or 4 times a day. Increase gradually, if needed, to a maximum of 26 mg 4 times a day.

Ointment: 1–2 in. squeezed from the tube onto a specially marked piece of paper—some people may require as much as 4–5 in. The ointment is spread on the skin every 4–8 hours as needed to control chest pain. The medication is absorbed through the skin. The application sites should be rotated to prevent skin inflammation and rash.

Transdermal Patch: The patch is placed on a hairless site on the body that is not associated with excess movement. It is applied once a day and removed after 12–14 hours. Dosages start at 0.2–0.4 mg per hour and may increase to 0.8 mg. Higher dosages are preferable for once-daily patch applications.

Aerosol: 1–2 sprays (0.4–0.8 mg) under or on your tongue; repeat as needed to relieve an angina attack, but use no more than 3 doses in a 15-minute period.

Overdosage

Overdose can result in low blood pressure; very rapid heartbeat; flushing; increased perspiration followed by cold, bluish, and clammy skin; headache; heart palpitations; blurred vision and other visual disturbances; dizziness; nausea; vomiting; slow and difficult breathing; slow pulse; confusion; moderate fever; and paralysis. Take the victim to a hospital emergency room immediately. ALWAYS bring the prescription bottle or container.

Special Information

Do not change brands of nitroglycerin without your doctor's and pharmacist's knowledge—they may not be equivalent.

Sublingual nitroglycerin should be acquired from your pharmacist only in the original, unopened bottle; the tablets must not be transferred to another bottle or container because they may lose potency. Close the bottle tightly after each use or the drug may evaporate from the tablets. Sublingual nitroglycerin should be taken while you are sitting down. This form of nitroglycerin frequently produces a burning sensation under the tongue, but this sensation does not necessarily indicate that the drug is working for you. If 1 tablet does not relieve your symptoms in 5 minutes, take another. If the second one does not work, take a third. If the pain continues or worsens, call your doctor or go to an emergency room at once.

When applying nitroglycerin ointment, do not rub or massage it into the skin. Any excess ointment should be washed from the hands after application.

People who use transdermal patches for more than 12 hours a day for an extended period can build up a tolerance to the patch and may have to use another form of nitroglycerin.

Nitroglycerin patches contain a significant amount of medication even after they have been used. They can be a hazard to children and small pets; be certain to dispose of them properly.

Orthostatic hypotension may become a problem if you take nitroglycerin over a long period of time. More blood stays in the extremities and less becomes available to the brain, resulting in light-headedness or faintness if you stand up suddenly. Avoid prolonged standing and always stand up slowly.

If you take nitroglycerin on a regular schedule and forget a dose, take it as soon as you remember. If you use immediate-release tablets and it is within 2 hours of your next dose, skip the dose you forgot and continue with your regular schedule. If you take sustained-release tablets or capsules and it is within 6 hours of your next dose, skip the dose you forgot and continue with your regular schedule.

Special Populations

Pregnancy/Breast-feeding

Nitroglycerin crosses into the fetal circulation. When this

drug is considered crucial by your doctor, its potential benefits must be carefully weighed against its risks.

Nitroglycerin passes into breast milk. Nursing mothers
who must take it should consider bottle-feeding.

Seniors

Seniors may take nitroglycerin without special restriction.
Because saliva is necessary for the absorption of sublingual
nitroglycerin, seniors with reduced saliva secretion may need
to use another form of nitroglycerin or add a saliva substitute; this also applies to younger people with dry mouth.

Generic Name

Nizatidine (nih-ZAY-tih-dene)

Brand Names

Axid   Axid AR

Type of Drug

Histamine H$_2$ antagonist.

Prescribed For

Ulcers of the stomach and duodenum (upper intestine); also
used to treat gastroesophageal reflux disease (GERD).

General Information

H$_2$ antagonists work by turning off the system that produces
stomach acid and other secretions. Nizatidine is effective in
treating the symptoms of ulcer and preventing complications
of the disease, although an ulcer that does not respond to
another histamine H$_2$ antagonist will probably not respond to
nizatidine. Histamine H$_2$ antagonists differ only in their
potency. Cimetidine is the least potent; 1000 mg are roughly
equal to 300 mg of either nizatidine or ranitidine, or 40 mg of
famotidine. All these drugs have roughly equivalent success
rates in treating ulcer disease and comparable risk of side
effects.

Cautions and Warnings

Do not take nizatidine if you have had an **allergic reaction** to it
or any histamine H$_2$ antagonist.

People with **kidney or liver disease** should take nizatidine with caution because ⅓ of each dose is broken down in the liver and the rest passes out of the body through the kidneys.

Possible Side Effects

Side effects are infrequent.
    ▼ Most common: tiredness and increased sweating.
    ▼ Rare: Rare side effects can affect the heart, liver, kidneys, stomach and intestines, blood, joints and muscles, mental status, and sexual function. Contact your doctor if you experience any side effect not listed above.

Drug Interactions

• Antacids, anticholinergics, and metoclopramide may slightly reduce the amount of nizatidine absorbed into the blood, but no precaution is needed.

• Enteric-coated tablets should not be taken with nizatidine. The change in stomach acidity produced by nizatidine causes the tablets to disintegrate prematurely in the stomach.

• Nizatidine may increase blood levels of aspirin in people taking very large doses of aspirin.

Food Interactions

You may take nizatidine without regard to food or meals.

Usual Dose

Adult: 300 mg at bedtime or 150 mg twice a day. Dosage is reduced in people with kidney disease.

Overdosage

Little is known about the effects of nizatidine overdose, but victims may experience exaggerated side effects. Your local poison control center may advise giving ipecac syrup—available at any pharmacy—to induce vomiting and remove any drug remaining in the stomach. Victims who have definite symptoms should be taken to a hospital emergency room. ALWAYS bring the prescription bottle or container.

Special Information

Take nizatidine exactly as directed and follow your doctor's instructions regarding diet and other treatments to get the maximum benefit from the drug. Antacids may be taken together with nizatidine, if needed. Cigarette smoking is associated with stomach ulcer and may reduce nizatidine's effectiveness.

Call your doctor at once if you develop any unusual side effects such as bleeding or bruising, tiredness, diarrhea, dizziness, or rash. Black or tarry stools or vomiting material that resembles coffee grounds may indicate that your ulcer is bleeding.

If you empty the nizatidine capsule and mix it with juice before taking it, you may keep it in the refrigerator. Do not store it for more than 2 days because the drug may lose potency.

If you forget a dose of nizatidine, take it as soon as you remember. If it is almost time for your next dose, skip the one you forgot and continue with your regular schedule. Do not take a double dose.

Special Populations

Pregnancy/Breast-feeding

Although animal studies revealed no damage to the fetus, nizatidine should be avoided by women who are or might be pregnant. When the drug is considered crucial by your doctor, its potential benefits must be carefully weighed against its risks.

Very small amounts of nizatidine may pass into breast milk. Nursing mothers who must take this drug should consider bottle-feeding.

Seniors

Seniors may need lower doses due to loss of kidney function and may be more susceptible to side effects.

Norvasc *see Amlodipine, page 69*

Generic Name

Olanzapine (oeh-LAN-zuh-pene)

Brand Name

Zyprexa   Zyprexa Zydis

Combination Products

Generic Ingredients: Olanzapine + Fluoxetine
Symbyax

Type of Drug

Antipsychotic.

Prescribed For

Psychotic behavior, depressive symptoms of bipolar disorder, symptoms of Alzheimer's disease, and treatment-resistant depression. Olanzapine may be prescribed both for acute and chronic conditions.

General Information

Olanzapine is a potent antipsychotic that blocks several different chemical receptors in the brain. The exact way in which olanzapine works is not known, but its antipsychotic effect may be produced by its blockage of dopamine and serotonin receptors. A small portion of each dose of olanzapine is eliminated through the kidneys, but most of it is broken down in the liver. The combination of olanzapine and fluoxetine is thought to be more effective in severe depression than either drug alone because of the combination of nervous system receptors it blocks. Specific information on fluoxetine may be found on page 965.

Cautions and Warnings

Do not take olanzapine if you are **sensitive** or **allergic** to it.

Women clear olanzapine about 30% more slowly than men, but this effect is not considered a problem. Women may respond to lower olanzapine doses than men.

Smokers clear olanzapine from their bodies about 40% faster than non-smokers, but most people do not require dosage adjustments.

People with **liver disease, heart disease,** or **breast cancer** may require dosage adjustments.

A serious set of side effects known as **neuroleptic malignant syndrome (NMS)** includes high fever, convulsions, difficult or fast breathing, rapid heartbeat, and rapid pulse. This condition has been associated with antipsychotic medicines. Other symptoms of NMS include muscle rigidity, mental changes, irregular pulse or blood pressure, and increased sweating. NMS can be fatal and requires immediate medical attention.

Tardive dyskinesia (symptoms include lip smacking or puckering, puffing of the cheeks, rapid or worm-like movements of the tongue, uncontrolled chewing motions, and uncontrolled arm or leg movements) can occur and is often considered a reason to stop taking this drug. Report any of these side effects to your doctor.

Olanzapine can cause **dizziness** or **fainting** when rising from a sitting or standing position, especially when people first start taking the drug.

Avoid being exposed to **extreme heat**. Antipsychotics can upset your body's temperature-regulating mechanism.

Swallowing problems and inhaling food intended to be swallowed, have been a problem with antipsychotics, including olanzapine.

Suicide is a danger with all psychotics. People taking this drug should be limited to no more than a 30-day supply of medication at any time to reduce the chances of possible overdose.

Seizures occur in a small number of people taking olanzapine. Olanzapine should be taken with care if you have had seizures or are at increased risk.

Olanzapine has been associated with obesity, high cholesterol, and diabetes.

Possible Side Effects

Olanzapine side effects are similar to those of placebo (sugar pill).

▼ Most common: headache, tiredness, agitation, sleeplessness, nervousness, hostility, dizziness, and runny nose.

▼ Less common: fever; abdominal, back, or chest pains; a rigid neck; dizziness or fainting when rising from a sitting or standing position; rapid heartbeat; low blood pressure; constipation; dry mouth; increased appetite; weight gain; swelling in the arms or legs; joint pain; arm or leg pain; twitching; anxiety; personality changes; restlessness or a feeling that you need to keep moving; muscle stiffness; tremors; memory loss; difficulty speaking or expressing thoughts; euphoria (feeling high); stuttering; cough; sore throat; double vision or other eye problems; and symptoms of premenstrual syndrome (PMS).

▼ Rare: Other side effects can occur in almost any part of the body. Contact your doctor if you experience any side effect not listed above.

Drug Interactions

• Your dosage of olanzapine must be adjusted when the drug is combined with carbamazepine.

• Olanzapine increases the effects of blood-pressure-lowering drugs and nervous system depressants. Dosage adjustments may be needed if you add olanzapine to another medicine.

• Do not take the combination of olanzapine and fluoxetine if you are taking an MAO inhibitor drug for depression or other mental problems or have taken one of these drugs in the past 2 weeks. Do not start taking an MAO inhibitor until at least 5 weeks after you stop taking the olanzapine-fluoxetine combination.

• Do not take the combination of olanzapine and fluoxetine if you are taking thioridazine for mental problems. Combining these drugs increases your chances of having a serious or life-threatening heart problem. Do not start taking thioridazine until at least 5 weeks after you stop taking the olanzapine-fluoxetine combination.

• Mixing the combination of olanzapine-fluoxetine with aspirin or a non-steroidal anti-inflammatory drug (NSAID) may increase your risk of bleeding.

Food Interactions

None known.

Usual Dose

Adult: starting dose—5–10 mg a day. Maintenance dose—increase gradually up to 20 mg a day if needed. Seniors should start with lower doses and increase gradually until maximum benefit is achieved.

Child (under age 18): not recommended.

Olanzapine + Fluoxetine
Adult: One 6/25 capsule every evening to start. Dosage may be increased gradually to one 12/50 capsule in the evening. Higher doses have not been studied.

Overdosage

Overdose symptoms are drowsiness and slurred speech. Overdose victims should be taken to a hospital emergency room for treatment. ALWAYS bring the prescription bottle or container.

Special Information

Sleepiness occurs in about 25% of people who take olanzapine; this effect may increase with larger doses. Take care when engaging in activities, such as driving, that require concentration or coordination.

Avoid alcohol and other nervous-system depressants while taking olanzapine.

Olanzapine can cause dry mouth. See your dentist regularly while you are taking this medication, since dental problems are more likely.

Be sure your doctor knows about all medication you are taking, including over-the-counter products.

If you forget to take a dose of olanzapine, take it as soon as you remember. If it is almost time for your next dose, skip the dose you forgot and continue with your regular schedule. Do not take a double dose.

Orally disintegrating olanzapine tablets must be used as soon as they are removed from their package. Place one in your mouth and allow it to dissolve. You may drink water or another liquid with it, but it is not needed.

Special Populations

Pregnancy/Breast-feeding

Olanzapine should only be taken by pregnant women if the potential benefits outweigh the risks. Birth defects and other problems have occurred in women taking olanzapine, but there is no definite link between the drug and these effects.

It is not known if olanzapine passes into breast milk. Nursing mothers who must take this medication should bottle-feed.

Seniors

Seniors usually need less olanzapine than younger adults.

Generic Name

Olopatadine (oe-loe-PAT-uh-dene)

Brand Name

Patanol

The information in this profile also applies to the following drugs:

Generic Ingredient: Azelastine
Optivar

Generic Ingredient: Levocabastine
Livostin

Type of Drug

Antihistamine and mast cell stabilizer.

Prescribed For

Eye itching due to allergy.

General Information

Olopatadine hydrochloride is an antihistamine eyedrop that alleviates irritation caused by conjunctivitis (pinkeye). It prevents the release of chemicals from mast cells in the eye that cause allergic symptoms and minimizes the response of nerve endings to these chemicals. Levocabastine only affects the nerve endings to minimize the allergic response.

Cautions and Warnings

Do not use olopatadine if you are **allergic** to it.

Possible Side Effects

Side effects are generally mild and subside as your body gets used to the drug.

Azelastine
▼ Common: eye stinging or burning, headache, and bitter taste in the mouth.
▼ Less common: asthma, difficulty breathing, eye pain or blurriness, fatigue, flu symptoms, itching, and sinus inflammation.

Levocabastine
▼ Most common: mild stinging or burning.
▼ Common: headache.
▼ Less common: dry mouth, visual disturbances, tiredness, sore throat, eye redness, eye tearing or discharge, eye pain or dryness, cough, nausea, skin rash or redness, eyelid swelling, and difficulty breathing.

Possible Side Effects *(continued)*

Olopatadine
  ▼ Common: headache.
  ▼ Less common: burning or stinging in the eye, dry eye, sensation that something is in your eye, eye redness, inflammation of the cornea, eyelid swelling, itching, weakness, sore throat, runny nose, common cold symptoms, sinus inflammation, and changes in sense of taste.

Drug Interactions

If you use several different eyedrops, separate them by 5 minutes.

Usual Dose

Azelastine
  Adult (age 3 and over): 1 drop in the affected eye twice a day.
  Child (under age 3): not recommended.

Levocabastine
  Adult and Child (age 12 and over): 1 drop in the affected eye 4 times a day for up to 2 weeks.
  Child (under age 12): not recommended.

Olopatadine
  Adult and Child (age 3 and over): 1–2 drops in each eye 2 times a day, 6–8 hours apart.
  Child (under age 3): not recommended.

Overdosage

Little is known about the effects of olopatadine overdose, but it is likely to increase side effects. Accidental ingestion of olopatadine is not likely to be associated with side effects because each bottle contains only small amounts of the active drug. Call your local poison control center or hospital emergency room for more information. If you seek treatment, ALWAYS bring the prescription bottle or container.

Special Information

If you wear contact lenses, wait at least 15 minutes after using olopatadine before putting in your lenses.

To avoid infection, do not touch the dropper tip to your finger, eyelid, or any other surface. Wait at least 5 minutes before using another eyedrop or eye ointment.

If you forget a dose of olopatadine, administer it as soon as you remember. If it is almost time for your next dose, skip the one you forgot and continue with your regular schedule. Do not take a double dose.

Special Populations

Pregnancy/Breast-feeding

Olopatadine can cause birth defects in laboratory animals, but there is no information on its effect in women during pregnancy. When your doctor considers this drug crucial, the potential benefits must be carefully weighed against its risks.

Olopatadine may pass into breast milk. Nursing mothers using olopatadine should consider bottle-feeding.

Seniors

Seniors may take olopatadine without special precaution.

Omnicef see Cephalosporin Antibiotics, page 210

Generic Name

Orlistat (OR-lih-stat)

Brand Name

Xenical

Type of Drug

Fat blocker.

Prescribed For

Weight reduction and maintenance.

General Information

Orlistat is the first "fat blocker" to be approved by the Food and Drug Administration (FDA). It works in the stomach and intestine by interfering with an enzyme that is key to the breakdown and absorption of one kind of fat. The unabsorbed fat, about 30% of that in your diet, passes out of the body in the stool. Since fat is the most concentrated form of calories, blocking fat absorption also reduces the number of calories you take in. People taking orlistat usually begin losing weight in a few weeks and continue to lose it for 6 months to a year. After that, weight loss is maintained. If you increase your exercise level or further reduce your caloric intake, you may lose more weight. More than 40% of people taking orlistat in clinical studies lost at least 5% of their body weight after a year of continuous treatment. About 18% lost more than 10% of body weight.

By losing weight, people taking orlistat achieved improved blood-fat profiles and lower blood pressure and blood sugar. They also reduced their waist and hip measurements—2 in. and 2.5 in., respectively—more than people taking a placebo (sugar pill) and following a weight-loss diet.

Cautions and Warnings

Do not take orlistat if you are **sensitive** or **allergic** to it. Some people may develop **kidney stones** while taking this drug, especially those prone to kidney stones.

Orlistat, like any weight-loss drug, **may be abused** or misused.

The cause of obesity must be determined before taking orlistat; it is not recommended for people who have **hyperthyroidism** or other organic causes of obesity.

A reduction in oral hypoglycemic medication or insulin may be necessary for **diabetic patients** taking orlistat.

Possible Side Effects

Most side effects are mild and temporary and tend to decrease during the second year of treatment.

▼ Most common: oily underwear spotting, gas with discharge, the feeling that you have to move your bowels, an oily or fat-laden stool, releasing an oily liquid during a bowel movement, more frequent bowel movements, abdominal pain or discomfort, flu, respiratory infections, back pain, and headache.

▼ Common: an inability to control bowel movements, nausea, infectious diarrhea, rectal pain or discomfort, arthritis, dizziness, fatigue, rash, menstrual problems, and urinary infection.

Possible Side Effects *(continued)*

▼ Less common: tooth or gum problems; vomiting; ear, nose, or throat problems; muscle pain; joint problems; tendonitis; sleep disturbances; dry skin; vaginal irritation; anxiety; depression; and swollen feet.

▼ Rare: Rare side effects can occur in almost any part of the body. Contact your doctor if you experience any side effect not listed above.

Drug Interactions

• Orlistat interferes with the absorption of fat-soluble vitamins and drugs.

• The blood-fat-lowering effect of statin cholesterol-lowering drugs is increased by orlistat.

• Orlistat may increase the effect of warfarin by interfering with the absorption of vitamin K. Warfarin dosage reduction may be needed.

Food Interactions

Take a dose with, or within an hour of, every meal.

Usual Dose

Adult: 120 mg taken 3 times a day with, or within an hour of, each meal.

Child: not recommended.

Overdosage

Symptoms are likely to include side effects, especially those related to the stomach and intestines. Take the victim to a hospital emergency room. ALWAYS bring the prescription bottle or container.

Special Information

Orlistat should be taken as part of a program of diet and exercise. Taking more than 1 capsule with each meal does not provide extra benefit.

Daily fat intake should be distributed over 3 meals to reduce the risk of developing a stomach or gastrointestinal (GI) problem.

Orlistat can interfere with the absorption of the fat-soluble vitamins A, D, and E. Take a vitamin supplement while using this drug.

If you forget to take an orlistat capsule within an hour of any meal, skip the forgotten dose and take a capsule with your next meal. Do not take a double dose.

Special Populations

Pregnancy/Breast-feeding
While animal studies of orlistat reveal no damage to the fetus, this drug is not recommended during pregnancy and should only be used after carefully weighing its potential benefits against its risks.

It is not known if orlistat passes into breast milk. Nursing mothers who must take this drug should bottle-feed.

Seniors
Orlistat has not been studied in older adults, who should use caution.

Ortho Evra 3 _see **Contraceptives**, page 291_

Ortho-Tri-Cyclen _see **Contraceptives**, page 291_

Generic Name

Oseltamivir (oe-sel-TAM-ih-veer)

Brand Name

Tamiflu

Type of Drug

Antiviral.

Prescribed For

Influenza type A and B.

General Information

Oseltamivir is the first pill approved to treat both type A and B influenza. It is thought to work by interfering with a virus enzyme called neuraminidase; this interference limits the spread of virus particles through the respiratory tract. In studies, people taking the drug for 5 days got better 1.3 days sooner than those taking a placebo (sugar pill). Oseltamivir is only prescribed for adults and children over 1 year who have had flu symptoms for no more than 2 days. It is also used to prevent the flu in adults and teens age 13 and over. This drug is broken down in the liver.

Cautions and Warnings

Do not take oseltamivir if you are **sensitive** or **allergic** to it.

People using oseltamivir to treat the flu should still get an annual **influenza vaccination**.

The effect of oseltamivir in people with chronic **heart disease, lung disease,** or any condition requiring hospitalization is not known. The safety and effectiveness of repeated oseltamivir use is not known.

Flu viruses can become resistant to oseltamivir, especially those already resistant to zanamivir (another flu medication).

People with moderate **kidney disease** require reduced dosage. People with severe kidney disease should be cautious about using oseltamivir because it has not been studied in this group.

Possible Side Effects

▼ Most common: nausea and vomiting.

▼ Common: diarrhea.

▼ Less common: bronchitis, abdominal pain, dizziness, headache, cough, sleeplessness, dizziness or fainting, fatigue, nosebleeds (occurs mainly in children), and ear disorder (occurs mainly in children).

▼ Rare: chest pain, anemia, colitis, bone fracture, pneumonia, fever, and abscesses around the tonsils.

Food and Drug Interactions

Oseltamivir may be taken with food it it upsets your stomach.

Usual Dose

Adult and Child (age 13 and over): 75 mg twice daily for 5 days. Daily dosage may be reduced to a single 75-mg capsule in people with kidney disease.

Child (age 1 and over and more than 88 lbs.): 75 mg (1$\frac{1}{4}$ tsp.) twice a day.

Child (age 1 and over and 52–88 lbs.): 60 mg (1 tsp.) twice a day.

Child (age 1 and over and 34–51 lbs.): 45 mg ($\frac{3}{4}$ tsp.) twice a day.

Child (age 1 and over and less than 34 lbs.): 30 mg ($\frac{1}{2}$ tsp.) twice a day.

Overdosage

Little is known about the effects of oseltamivir overdose, though symptoms may include nausea and vomiting. Call your local poison control center or a hospital emergency room for more information. If you seek treatment, ALWAYS bring the prescription bottle or container.

Special Information

Oseltamivir should be taken from the first appearance of flu symptoms. Taking oseltamivir is not a substitute for an annual flu shot.

If you forget a dose, take it as soon as you remember. If it is almost time for your next dose, skip the one you forgot and continue with your regular schedule. Do not take a double dose.

Special Populations

Pregnancy/Breast-feeding
Animal studies indicate that oseltamivir may cause fetal abnormalities. When this drug is considered crucial by your doctor, its potential benefits must be carefully weighed against its risks.

This drug may pass into breast milk. Nursing mothers who must take it should bottle-feed.

Seniors
Oseltamivir may be less effective in seniors.

Generic Name

Oxcarbazepine (oks-kar-BAZ-e-peen)

Brand Name

Trileptal

Type of Drug

Anticonvulsant.

Prescribed For

Partial seizures in adults, and children age 4–16 with epilepsy. Also used for panic disorder.

General Information

The exact way that oxcarbazepine works is unknown. It may stabilize sodium and calcium channels in the brain, thereby preventing the spread of seizure in the brain.

Cautions and Warnings

Do not take oxcarbazepine if you are **sensitive** or **allergic** to it. About ¼ of those who have had a reaction to carbamazepine will also react to oxcarbazepine.

People taking this drug occasionally develop **very low blood sodium levels** (symptoms include nausea, feeling sick, headache, tiredness, confusion, and reduced pain sensitivity) during the first 3 months of treatment. Your doctor will check your blood periodically and may stop the drug or lower the dose to eliminate this problem.

Possible Side Effects

▼ Most common: nausea, vomiting, abdominal pain, fatigue, headache, dizziness, tiredness, and double vision or abnormal vision.

▼ Common: poor muscle coordination, unusual eye movements, abnormal walking, memory loss, worsened convulsions, and fainting.

▼ Less common: emotional upset, reduced sensitivity to stimulation, nervousness, taste changes, earache, fever, allergy, weakness, swollen legs, weight gain, low blood pressure, speech or language problems, confusion, abnormal thinking, acne, hot flushes, rash, appetite loss, dry mouth, rectal bleeding, toothache, diarrhea, constipation, stomach irritation, thirst, runny nose, coughing, bronchitis, sore throat, nosebleed, and back pain.

▼ Rare: Rare side effects can occur in almost any part of the body. Contact your doctor if you experience any side effect not listed above.

Drug Interactions

• Carbamazepine (400–2000 mg a day), phenobarbital, and phenytoin reduce the amount of a metabolite of oxcarbazepine in the blood.

• Oxcarbazepine reduces the amount of felodipine and oral contraceptives in the blood, possibly interfering with their effectiveness. Other drugs that may be reduced in the blood by oxcarbazepine are clarithromycin, erythromycin, quinidine, benzodiazepine sedatives and tranquilizers, cyclosporine, tacrolimus, indinavir, nelfinavir, ritonavir, saquinavir, astemizole, chlorpheniramine, terfenidine, calcium channel blocker drugs, statin-type cholesterol-lowering drugs (except pravastatin), hydrocortisone, testosterone, buspirone, dapsone, codeine, dextromethorphan, finasteride, haloperidol, methadone, ondansetron, pimozide, quinine, salmeterol, sildenafil, tamoxifen, paclitaxel, terfenadine, trazodone, vincristine, zaleplon, and zolpidem.

• Oxcarbazepine may increase the amount of phenobarbital and phenytoin in the blood. It may also increase levels of amitriptyline and other tricyclic antidepressants, clomipramine, cyclophosphamide, hexobarbital, indomethacin, nilutamide, progesterone, tenoposide, lansoprozole, omeprazole, pantoprozole, and warfarin.

• Valproic acid and verapamil reduce oxcarbazepine levels in the blood.

Food Interactions

Oxcarbazepine can be taken with or without food.

Usual Dose

Adult and Child (age 16 and over): 600–2400 mg a day. People with poor kidney function should start at half the dosage and increase slowly until the desired response is reached.

Child (age 4–15): 3¾ to 4½ mg per pound up to 600 mg a day to start. Increase gradually to a maximum of 1800 mg per pound, according to body weight.

Overdosage

All overdose patients have recovered with treatment. Symptoms are likely to be exaggerated drug side effects. Overdose victims should be taken to a hospital emergency room. ALWAYS bring the prescription bottle or container.

Special Information

This drug may reduce the effectiveness of oral contraceptive pills. Use an alternate contraceptive product or method while taking oxcarbazepine.

Like all anticonvulsant medicines, oxcarbazepine must be gradually stopped to avoid experiencing sudden seizures.

Alcohol can enhance the depressive effects of this drug.

Oxcarbazepine can cause tiredness and confusion, especially when the drug is started. Driving or performing any tasks that require intense concentration should be delayed until you have taken oxcarbazepine for a while and have become used to its effects.

If you forget to take a dose of oxcarbazepine, take it as soon as you remember. If it is almost time for your next dose, skip the dose you forgot and continue with your regular schedule. Do not take a double dose. Contact your doctor if you forget 2 or more doses in a row.

Special Populations

Pregnancy/Breast-feeding

Oxcarbazepine passes into the fetus and fetal damage has been seen in animals given the drug. There is no experience with oxcarbazepine in women, but it is likely to cause fetal damage in humans. When this drug is considered crucial by your doctor, its potential benefits must be weighed against its risks.

Oxcarbazepine passes into breast milk. Nursing mothers who must take it should consider bottle-feeding.

Seniors

Older adults are likely to have 30%–60% more oxcarbazepine in their blood than younger people because of age-related differences in kidney function. Lower doses may be as effective as higher ones.

Generic Name

Oxiconazole   (ox-ih-KON-uh-zole)

Brand Name

Oxistat

Type of Drug

Antifungal.

Prescribed For

Fungal infections of the skin.

General Information

Oxiconazole nitrate is a general-purpose antifungal drug. It works by interfering with the cell membrane (outer skin) of the fungus. Little of the drug is absorbed into the bloodstream.

Cautions and Warnings

Do not use oxiconazole if you are **allergic** to it or to any other ingredient in this product.

Possible Side Effects

Oxiconazole side effects are infrequent.
 ▼ Common: itching and burning.
 ▼ Rare: stinging, irritation, rash, scaling, tingling, pain, eczema, redness and swelling, and cracked skin.

Drug Interactions

None known.

Usual Dose

Oxiconazole should be applied to affected areas 1–2 times a day for 2–4 weeks, depending on the fungus type.

Overdosage

Little is known about the effects of accidental ingestion. Victims should be taken to a hospital emergency room. ALWAYS bring the prescription bottle or container.

Special Information

Oxiconazole is meant only for application to the skin. Do not put this drug into your eyes or mouth.

Stop using the drug and call your doctor if skin irritation or redness develops.

If you forget a dose of oxiconazole, apply it as soon as you remember. If it is almost time for your next dose, skip the dose you forgot and continue with your regular schedule.

Special Populations

Pregnancy/Breast-feeding

Oxiconazole is not likely to affect your pregnancy because little is absorbed into the bloodstream. Nevertheless, you should not use this drug without your doctor's knowledge and approval.

Large amounts of oxiconazole may pass into breast milk. Nursing mothers who must use this drug should consider bottle-feeding.

Seniors

Seniors may use oxiconazole without special restriction.

Generic Name

Oxybutynin (ox-ee-BYUE-tih-nin) G

Brand Names

Ditropan   Oxytrol
Ditropan XL

Type of Drug

Antispasmodic and anticholinergic.

Prescribed For

Bladder instability including an urgent need to urinate, frequent urination, urinary leakage, and painful urination.

General Information

Oxybutynin directly affects the smooth muscle that controls the opening and closing of the bladder. It is 4 to 10 times more potent than atropine but much less likely to cause side effects.

Cautions and Warnings

Do not take oxybutynin if you are **allergic** or **sensitive** to it.

Oxybutynin should be used with caution if you have **glaucoma, urinary retention, intestinal obstruction or poor intestinal function, megacolon,** severe or ulcerative **colitis,**

myasthenia gravis, or unstable **heart disease** including abnormal heart rhythms, heart failure, or recent heart attack. **Heat prostration** may develop more easily while you are taking this drug because it makes you more sensitive to high temperatures.

Oxybutynin should be used with caution if you have **liver or kidney disease.** It may worsen symptoms of an **overactive thyroid gland, coronary heart disease, abnormal heart rhythms, rapid heartbeat, high blood pressure, prostate disease,** or **hiatal hernia.**

Possible Side Effects

▼ Most common: drowsiness, dry mouth, decreased sweating, and constipation. Transdermal patch—itching where the patch is placed.

▼ Less common: diarrhea, upset stomach, headache, difficulty urinating, blurred vision, enlarging of the pupils, worsening of glaucoma, palpitations, sleeplessness, weakness, nausea, bloating, impotence, reduced production of breast milk, rash, and itching.

Drug Interactions

• Combining oxybutynin and atenolol may increase the effect of atenolol.

• Oxybutynin may affect haloperidol blood levels, which in turn may worsen schizophrenic symptoms. Oxybutynin may increase blood levels of digoxin and nitrofurantoin, increasing the risk of side effects.

• Oxybutynin may interfere with levodopa.

• Amantadine may increase oxybutynin side effects.

• Combining oxybutynin with a phenothiazine antipsychotic drug may decrease phenothiazine blood levels.

Food Interactions

Take oxybutynin with food or milk if it upsets your stomach.

Usual Dose

Ditropan
  Adult: 10–20 mg a day in divided doses.
  Child (age 6 and over): 10–15 mg a day in divided doses.

Ditropan XL
　Adult (age 18 and over): 5–30 mg once a day.
　Child: not recommended.

Transdermal System (Oxytrol)
　Adult : Apply to dry, intact skin on the abdomen or buttock twice a week.

Overdosage

Symptoms may include restlessness, tremors, irritability, convulsions, hallucinations, flushing, fever, nausea, vomiting, rapid heartbeat, blood-pressure changes, respiratory failure, paralysis, delirium, urinary retention, and coma. Take the victim to a hospital emergency room at once. ALWAYS bring the prescription bottle or container.

Special Information

Contact your doctor if you develop severe or persistent diarrhea.

Oxybutynin may interfere with your vision and ability to concentrate. Be careful while driving or doing any task that requires concentration or clear vision. Your eyes may also become more sensitive to bright light; wearing sunglasses should help to alleviate this problem.

In warm weather, people taking oxybutynin may be at an increased risk for heatstroke due to decreased sweating.

Dry mouth may be relieved with sugarless gum, candy, or ice chips. Excessive mouth dryness may lead to tooth decay and should be brought to your dentist's attention if it lasts for more than 2 weeks.

If you forget a dose, take it as soon as you remember. If it is almost time for your next dose, skip the dose you forgot and continue with your regular schedule. Do not take a double dose.

Special Populations

Pregnancy/Breast-feeding

The safety of using oxybutynin during pregnancy is not known. When this drug is considered crucial by your doctor, its potential benefits must be carefully weighed against its risks.

It is not known if oxybutynin passes into breast milk. Nursing mothers who must take this drug should consider bottle-feeding.

Seniors

Seniors may be more susceptible to side effects and should take this drug with caution.

Generic Name

Paclitaxel (PAK-lih-tax-ul) Ⓖ

Brand Name

Onxol   Taxol

The information in this profile also applies to the following drug:

Generic Ingredient: Docetaxel
Taxotere

Type of Drug

Taxoid antineoplastic.

Prescribed For

Paclitaxel: ovarian and breast cancer, non-small-cell lung cancer, and Kaposi's sarcoma related to acquired immunodeficiency syndrome (AIDS). Also prescribed for polycystic kidney disease; cancers of the head and neck, gastrointestinal (GI) tract, pancreas, prostate, and kidney; other lung cancers; and for Hodgkin's lymphoma. Docetaxel: ovarian and breast cancer, non-small-cell lung cancer, cancers of the head and neck, melanoma, non-Hodgkin's lymphoma, soft-tissue sarcoma, and urothelial cancer.

General Information

Taxoid antineoplastic drugs interfere with cell division in cancerous cells. Generally, they are recommended only after other treatments have failed. Studies in ovarian cancer indicate that 22% to 30% of women who receive paclitaxel respond to the drug; of a total of 92 women studied, there were 6 complete and 18 partial responses. In breast cancer, response rates range from 26% and 30% to 57%. People who receive paclitaxel are premedicated with other drugs to minimize side effects.

Cautions and Warnings

Paclitaxel must be given only in adequate facilities where there is available management for the treatment of drug complications.

Severe **drug sensitivity reactions,** including breathing difficulties; low blood pressure (symptoms include dizziness and fainting); swelling of the face, hands, feet, genitals, or internal organs; and generalized itching and rash have occurred in 2–4% of people taking this drug. People who experience these reactions should not use paclitaxel.

As many as 2 out of every 100 people receiving docetaxel for breast cancer that spread to other parts of the body have died during treatment. These **deaths** have been linked to the drug treatment.

Bone-marrow suppression is the major toxic effect of paclitaxel. People with low white-blood-cell counts should not receive paclitaxel.

Fewer than 1% of people who take paclitaxel develop severe **heart problems**; these people may require cardiac therapy while continuing to receive this drug.

Paclitaxel is broken down in the liver and should be used with caution in people with severe **liver disease**.

Severe **fluid retention** has occurred in people taking docetaxel.

Possible Side Effects

In order to minimize side effects, paclitaxel should be administered before cisplatin, another antineoplastic drug.

▼ Most common: reduced blood-cell counts, anemia, infection, drug sensitivity reactions, dizziness or fainting, changes in electrocardiogram (EKG) measurements, fever, peripheral neuropathy, muscle or joint pain, nausea and vomiting, diarrhea, mouth sores, liver inflammation, kidney damage, hair loss, numbness, tingling or burning in the hands or feet, and swelling or retention of fluid.

Possible Side Effects *(continued)*

▼ Less common: bleeding, blood in the urine, bruising, black and tarry stools, severe sensitivity reactions, and slow heartbeat.

▼ Rare: severe heart problems and nail changes.

Drug Interactions

• Ketoconazole, verapamil, diazepam, quinidine, dexamethasone, cyclosporine, teniposide, etoposide, vincristine, testosterone, estradiol, and retinoic acid may increase the risk of paclitaxel side effects.

• Cyclosporine, doxorubicin, felodopine, ketoconazole, midazolam, retinoic acid, and troleandomycin may decrease the metabolism of paclitaxel.

• Paclitaxel may increase the risk of doxorubicin side effects.

Food Interactions

None known.

Usual Dose

Adult: Paclitaxel is given by intravenous injection. Dosage is individualized by condition.

Child: not recommended.

Overdosage

Little is known about the effects of paclitaxel overdose, though it is likely to cause severe side effects. Breathing difficulties, chest pain, burning eyes, sore throat, and nausea have occurred after accidental inhalation of paclitaxel. Take the overdose victim or those with symptoms of inhalation to a hospital emergency room.

Special Information

Drug therapy must be closely supervised by your doctor.

Do not receive any immunizations or vaccinations while taking paclitaxel, unless approved by your doctor.

Avoid exposure to people with bacterial or viral infections, especially when your blood counts are likely to be low.

Contact your doctor at the first sign of cold or infection. Do not touch the inside of your mouth or nose unless you have first washed your hands.

Call your doctor if you experience any unusual bleeding or bruising, black or tarry stools, blood in the urine or stool, or pinpoint red spots on the skin.

Ask your doctor about the proper way to brush and floss while using this drug, since brushing and flossing may introduce bacteria into your bloodstream. Check with your doctor before you have any dental work done and inform your dentist that you are receiving chemotherapy.

Take care to avoid accidental cuts. Avoid contact sports or other situations in which bruising or injury could occur.

Special Populations

Pregnancy/Breast-feeding

Paclitaxel can harm the fetus. Women taking this drug must be sure to use an effective contraceptive during treatment. If you are pregnant and must start taking paclitaxel or if you become pregnant while taking it, discuss the possible risks with your doctor.

It is not known if paclitaxel passes into breast milk. Nursing mothers who must use it should bottle-feed.

Seniors

Seniors may use this drug without special restriction.

Patanol see Olopatadine, page 799

Paxil see Selective Serotonin Reuptake Inhibitors (SSRIs), page 965

Paxil CR see Selective Serotonin Reuptake Inhibitors (SSRIs), page 965

Generic Name

Pemirolast (pe-MEER-oh-last)

Brand Name

Alamast

Type of Drug

Ophthalmic mast cell stabilizer.

Prescribed For

Eye allergies and redness.

General Information

Pemirolast helps relieve allergy-related itchy, red eyes by stabilizing cells in eye tissue that are responsible for releasing a number of different chemicals that cause inflammation when in the presence of an allergen.

Cautions and Warnings

Do not use pemirolast if you are **sensitive** or **allergic** to any of its ingredients.

Do not wear **contact lenses** if your eyes are red or use pemirolast for irritation caused by contact lenses because the preservative in this drug may be absorbed by soft contacts.

Do not use this drug if you have an **eye infection,** unless you are also being treated for it.

Possible Side Effects

Serious side effects are not expected with pemirolast.

▼ Most common: burning, irritation, or dryness of the eyes.

▼ Common: headache, inflammation of the mucous membranes of the nose, and flu symptoms.

Food and Drug Interactions

None known.

Usual Dose

Adult and Child (age 3 and over): 1–2 drops in each affected eye 4 times a day.

Overdosage

The amount absorbed into the blood from a dose is very small but overdose might be expected to produce ordinary drug side effects. Call your local poison control center for more information.

Special Information

To avoid infection, do not touch the dropper tip to your finger, eyelid or any other surface. Keep the bottle cap tightly closed when it is not being used.

If you wear contact lenses, remember to remove them before each dose and wait at least 10 minutes after using pemirolast before putting in your lenses.

If you forget a dose of pemirolast, administer it as soon as you remember. If it is almost time for your next dose, skip the dose you forgot and continue with your regular schedule. Do not take a double dose.

Special Populations

Pregnancy/Breast-feeding

Pemirolast causes birth defects and miscarriage in animals. Pregnant women should only use this drug if its potential benefits outweigh the possible risks.

Pemirolast passes into the breast milk of animals but no information is available for humans. Nursing mothers should consider bottle-feeding.

Seniors

Seniors may use pemirolast without special restriction.

Generic Name

Pemoline (PEM-oe-leen) Ⓖ

Brand Name

Cylert   PemADD

Type of Drug

Psychotherapeutic agent.

Prescribed For

Attention-deficit hyperactivity disorder (ADHD); may also be used to treat daytime sleepiness in adults.

General Information

This drug stimulates the central nervous system (CNS), although its exact action in children with ADHD is not known. It should be prescribed only by a doctor trained to treat ADHD, and always used as part of a total therapeutic program that includes social, psychological, and educational counseling.

Cautions and Warnings

People who are **allergic** or **sensitive** to pemoline should not use it. **Children under age 6** should not take this drug. The condition of **psychotic children** who take pemoline may get worse. Long-term treatment with pemoline may **inhibit growth** in children.

Because this drug has been linked to life-threatening **liver failure,** pemoline should only be used to treat ADHD when other treatments have failed. People taking pemoline must have blood tests to monitor liver function every 2 weeks. People with liver disease should not take pemoline.

Possible Side Effects

▼ Less common: sleeplessness, appetite loss, stomachache, rash, irritability, depression, nausea, dizziness, headache, drowsiness, hallucinations, Tourette's syndrome, and seizure.

▼ Rare: drug hypersensitivity, wandering eye, and uncontrolled movements of the lips, face, tongue, and extremities.

Drug Interactions

• Pemoline lowers the seizure threshold; anticonvulsant drug dosage may need to be increased.

• Pemoline increases the effects of other central nervous system (CNS) stimulants, which may cause nervousness, irritability, sleeplessness, and other side effects.

Food Interactions

Take this drug with food if it upsets your stomach.

Usual Dose

37.5–75 mg a day. Do not exceed 112.5 mg a day.

Overdosage

Symptoms include rapid heartbeat, hallucinations, agitation, vomiting, uncontrolled muscle movements, and restlessness. Take the victim to a hospital emergency room. ALWAYS bring the prescription bottle or container.

Special Information

Call your doctor immediately if you develop severe itching, dark-colored urine, flu-like symptoms, tiredness, appetite loss, yellowing of the skin or whites of the eyes, abdominal pain, or stomach or intestinal problems. These may be signs of liver damage.

Take your daily dose at the same time each morning. Taking pemoline too late in the day may result in trouble sleeping; call your doctor if you develop persistent insomnia.

The effects of pemoline are gradual. It may take 3–4 weeks before benefits are seen.

Your doctor may decide to stop pemoline treatment for a short period to see if symptoms return and if continued treatment is still necessary.

If you forget a dose, take it as soon as you remember. If it is almost time for your next dose, skip the dose you forgot and continue with your regular schedule. Do not take a double dose.

Special Populations

Pregnancy/Breast-feeding

Pemoline crosses into the fetal circulation. Animal studies show that large dosages of pemoline can cause stillbirth and reduce newborn survival rates. When this drug is considered crucial by your doctor, its potential benefits must be carefully weighed against its risks.

Pemoline passes into breast milk. Nursing mothers who must take this drug should consider bottle-feeding.

Seniors

Seniors should take this drug with caution.

Generic Name

Penciclovir (pen-SYE-kloe-veer)

Brand Name

Denavir

Type of Drug

Antiviral.

Prescribed For

Cold sores.

General Information

Penciclovir works against different types of herpes viruses responsible for common cold sores. Cold sores treated with penciclovir cream go away sooner and are less painful than those that are not treated. Once applied to the skin, penciclovir is converted to its active form and interferes with DNA production inside the viral particle; this inhibits the reproduction process of the herpes virus.

Cautions and Warnings

Do not use penciclovir if you are **sensitive** or **allergic** to it.

Penciclovir should **be applied only to the face or lips**. Avoid applying it near your eyes because it may be irritating. The effectiveness of penciclovir in people with **compromised immune systems** is not known.

Male animals given massive doses of penciclovir intravenously suffered damage to the testicles. This effect appears to be related to the dose of penciclovir. Men using famciclovir—the oral form of penciclovir—for 8 to 13 weeks experienced no changes in sperm count.

Drug resistance may develop with repeated use.

Possible Side Effects

Side effects are generally mild and infrequent. In studies, side effects were similar in type and frequency among people who used penciclovir and those who used an inactive cream.

▼ Common: headache, redness, and swelling.

▼ Less common: skin reactions to the cream.

▼ Rare: loss of skin sensation where the cream has been applied, changes in the sense of taste, and rash.

Drug Interactions

None known.

Usual Dose

Adult: Apply to affected areas every 2 hours, during waking hours, for 4 days.

Child: not recommended.

Overdosage

Little is known about the effects of penciclovir overdose or accidental ingestion. Call your poison control center or a hospital emergency room for more information.

Special Information

Begin cold sore treatment as early as possible. Early application of penciclovir cream will help prevent cold sores from appearing and reduce accompanying pain.

It is very important to apply penciclovir cream every 2 hours during the day for the drug to work. If you forget to apply a dose of penciclovir, apply it as soon as you remember. If you realize you forgot a dose within 30 to 45 minutes of your next dose, skip the dose you forgot and continue with your regular schedule.

Special Populations

Pregnancy/Breast-feeding

In animal studies, penciclovir had no effect on the fetus. There is no information on the effect of penciclovir in pregnant women. This drug should be used during pregnancy only if its possible benefits outweigh its risks.

It is not known if penciclovir passes into breast milk, though famciclovir—the oral form of penciclovir—passes into breast milk in concentrations larger than those found in the mother's blood. Nursing mothers who must use penciclovir should bottle-feed.

Seniors
Seniors may use this drug without special precaution.

Type of Drug

Penicillin Antibiotics (pen-ih-SIL-in)

Brand Names

Generic Ingredient: Amoxicillin G
Amoxil
Larotid
Trimox
Wymox

Generic Ingredients: Amoxicillin + Potassium Clavulanate
Augmentin
Augmentin ES-600
Augmentin XR

Generic Ingredient: Ampicillin G
Marcillin
Omnipen
Principen
Totacillin

Generic Ingredients: Ampicillin + Probenecid
Probampacin

Generic Ingredient: Bacampicillin
Spectrobid

Generic Ingredient: Carbenicillin Indanyl Sodium
Geocillin

Generic Ingredient: Cloxacillin Sodium G
Cloxapen

Generic Ingredient: Dicloxacillin Sodium G
Dycill
Dynapen
Pathocil

Generic Ingredient: Nafcillin
Unipen

Generic Ingredient: Oxacillin G
Bactocill

Generic Ingredient: Penicillin G
Pfizerpen

Generic Ingredient: Penicillin V [G]

Beepen-VK	Pen-Vee K
Betapen-VK	V-Cillin K
Ledercillin VK	Veetids
Penicillin VK	

Prescribed For

Bacterial and other infections.

General Information

Penicillin antibiotics kill bacteria and other microorganisms by destroying the cell wall of the invading organisms. Many infections respond to almost any kind of penicillin; some respond only to a specific penicillin antibiotic. Penicillin cannot cure a cold, the flu, or any other viral infection and should never be taken unless prescribed by a doctor for a specific condition. Always take penicillin exactly as prescribed, including the number of pills to take every day and number of days to take the drug, otherwise you will not get the drug's full effect.

Cautions and Warnings

Serious and sometimes **fatal allergic reactions** have occurred with penicillin. Though more common following penicillin injections, these reactions have also occurred with oral penicillin. Reactions are more common among people who have had a previous penicillin reaction and those who have had asthma, hay fever, or other allergies. Allergic symptoms include itching, rash, swelling, breathing difficulties, very low blood pressure, blood vessel collapse, peeling skin, chills, fever, muscle aches, arthritis-like pains, and feeling unwell. Sometimes, when an infection is life-threatening and can only be treated with penicillin, minor reactions may be treated with another drug while the penicillin is continued. About 1 in 20 people allergic to a penicillin antibiotic are also allergic to the cephalosporin antibiotics.

Cystic fibrosis patients are more likely to suffer from side effects of certain penicillins.

People with **kidney disease** should not take carbenicillin and will need a reduced dosage of penicillin G.

Some of these medications contain tartrazine dyes or sulfites, which may cause **allergic reactions** in certain people.

Prolonged or repeated use of penicillin may lead to a **secondary infection** that cannot be treated by the penicillin being used.

Possible Side Effects

The most common penicillin side effect, seen in up to 10% of people, is allergy. About 9% of ampicillin users develop an itchy rash, which is not a true allergic reaction.

▼ Common: upset stomach, abdominal pain, nausea, vomiting, diarrhea, colitis (symptoms include severe abdominal cramps and severe, persistent, and possibly bloody diarrhea), sore mouth, coated tongue, anemia, bleeding abnormalities, low platelet and white-blood-cell counts, and oral or rectal fungal infections.

▼ Less common: vaginal irritation, appetite loss, itchy eyes, and feelings of body warmth.

▼ Rare: yellowing of the skin or whites of the eyes.

Drug Interactions

• Penicillin should not be combined with a bacteriostatic antibiotic such as chloramphenicol, erythromycin, tetracycline, or neomycin. These drugs can interfere with each other.

• Penicillin can interfere with oral contraceptives. Use additional contraception while taking a penicillin drug. Breakthrough bleeding may occur.

• Nafcillin can interfere with cyclosporine (used to prevent rejection in people who have received an organ transplant).

• Penicillin allergies may be intensified by beta-blocking drugs.

• Combining ampicillin and allopurinol may increase the risk of rash and itching.

• Ampicillin may reduce the effect of atenolol.

• Penicillin G blood levels may be increased by aspirin, phenylbutazone, sulfa drugs, indomethacin, thiazide-type diuretics, furosemide, or ethacrynic acid.

• Nafcillin and dicloxacillin may interfere with the effects of anticoagulant (blood thinning) drugs such as warfarin.

Food Interactions

Do not take penicillin with fruit juice or carbonated beverages. The acid in these beverages may destroy the drug.

Drink a full glass of water with each glass of cloxacillin.

Most penicillins, including bacampicillin suspension, are best absorbed on an empty stomach. These medications may be taken 1 hour before or 2 hours after meals, or first thing in the morning and last thing at night with the other doses spaced evenly throughout the day.

Amoxicillin, bacampicillin tablets, and penicillin V may be taken without regard to food.

Augmentin (amoxicillin and potassium clavulanate) is best taken right before a meal for optimum effectiveness and minimum stomach upset.

Usual Dose

Amoxicillin
Adult: 250–500 mg every 8 hours.
Child: 10–20 mg per lb. a day divided into 3 doses.

Amoxicillin and Potassium Clavulanate
Adult: "250" tablet every 8 hours; "500" or "875" tablet every 12 hours. Different strengths of this product are not interchangeable. Take only the exact strength and product your doctor has prescribed.
Child: 10–20 mg per lb. a day divided into 2–3 doses.

Ampicillin
Adult: 1–12 g a day divided into 4–6 doses.
Child: 50–400 mg a day divided into 4–6 doses.
Infant: 11–23 mg per lb. a day divided into 2–4 doses.

Ampicillin with Probenecid
3.5 g of ampicillin and 1 g of probenecid as a single dose for gonorrhea.

Bacampicillin
Adult: 400–800 mg every 12 hours; 1600 mg plus 1 g of probenecid for gonorrhea.
Child: 12–25 mg per lb. a day divided into 2 doses.

Carbenicillin Indanyl Sodium
Adult: 382–764 mg 4 times a day.
Child: not recommended.

Cloxacillin Sodium
Adult and Child (45 lbs. and over): 250 mg every 6 hours.

Child (under 45 lbs.): 25 mg per lb. a day divided into 4 doses.

Dicloxacillin Sodium
  Adult and Child (90 lbs. and over): 125–250 mg every 6 hours.
  Child (under 90 lbs.): 6–12 mg per lb. a day divided into 4 doses.

Nafcillin
  Adult: 250–1000 mg every 4–6 hours.
  Child: 5–25 mg per lb. every 6–8 hours.

Oxacillin
  Adult and Child (90 lbs. and over): 500–1000 mg every 4–6 hours.
  Child (under 90 lbs.): 25–50 mg per lb. a day divided into 4 or 6 doses.

Penicillin G
  Adult (age 12 and over): 200,000–800,000 units, or 125–500 mg every 6–8 hours for 10 full days.
  Child (under age 12): 12,000–40,000 units per lb. a day divided into 3–6 doses.

Penicillin V
  Adult (age 12 and over): 125–500 mg every 6–8 hours. People with severe kidney disease should not take more than 250 mg every 6 hours.
  Child (under age 12): 12–25 mg per lb. a day divided into 3 or 4 doses.

Overdosage

Overdose is unlikely, but diarrhea or upset stomach is the primary symptom. Massive overdose may result in seizure or excitability. Call your local poison control center or a hospital emergency room for more information. ALWAYS bring the prescription bottle or container.

Special Information

Liquid penicillin should be refrigerated and must be thrown out after 14 days in the refrigerator or 7 days at room temperature.
  Call your doctor if you develop black tongue, rash, itching, hives, diarrhea, breathing difficulties, sore throat, nausea,

vomiting, fever, swollen joints, unusual bleeding or bruising, or if you are feeling unwell.

Penicillin eradicates most susceptible organisms in 7 to 10 days; be sure to take all the medication prescribed for the full period prescribed. It is best taken at evenly spaced intervals throughout the day.

If you miss a dose, take it as soon as possible. If it is almost time for your next dose, space the missed dose and your next dose by 2 to 4 hours and then continue with your regular schedule.

Special Populations

Pregnancy/Breast-feeding

Penicillin crosses into the fetal circulation but has not been known to cause birth defects and is often prescribed for pregnant women. When this drug is considered crucial by your doctor, its potential benefits must be carefully weighed against its risks.

Penicillin is generally safe during breast-feeding; however, small amounts may pass into breast milk and cause upset stomach, diarrhea, allergic reaction, or other problems in the nursing infant.

Seniors

Seniors may take penicillin without special restriction.

Generic Name

Pentosan Polysulfate Sodium

(PEN-toe-san pol-ee-SUL-fate)

Brand Name

Elmiron

Type of Drug

Kidney analgesic.

Prescribed For

Bladder pain or discomfort due to cystitis.

General Information

Interstitial cystitis is a painful, long-term infection of the bladder. Pentosan does not affect the infectious process, but it may stick to the membranes of the bladder wall, preventing irritating substances from reaching bladder cells. About ⅓ of people who take this drug for 3 months or more have less cystitis pain.

Cautions and Warnings

Do not take this product if you are **sensitive** or **allergic** to it.

Pentosan is a weak anticoagulant and can cause **black-and-blue marks, nosebleeds,** and **bleeding gums**.

People with **liver disease** should use this drug with caution because its breakdown can be reduced in people with liver problems. Pentosan may also cause mild liver toxicity.

Possible Side Effects

▼ Most common: patchy hair loss beginning within 4 weeks of treatment, diarrhea, and nausea.

▼ Common: headache, emotional upset or depression, dizziness, abdominal pain, upset stomach, and rash.

▼ Rare: Rare side effects can include sleeplessness and effects on your blood, eyes, breathing, stomach and intestines, ears, and liver. Contact your doctor if you experience any side effect not listed above.

Drug Interactions

• Aspirin, clopidogrel, warfarin, and other blood-thinning drugs should be taken with caution if you are already taking pentosan. Pentosan may increase the anticoagulant effect of these drugs.

Food Interactions

Take this drug with water on an empty stomach, at least 1 hour before or 2 hours after a meal.

Usual Dose

Adult: 100 mg 3 times a day.

Overdosage

Symptoms include bleeding, liver problems, and upset stomach. Overdose victims should be taken to a hospital emergency room at once. ALWAYS bring the prescription bottle or container.

Special Information

Pentosan has a mild anticoagulant effect. Make sure that your pharmacist, dentist, and all of your doctors know you are taking pentosan. Check with your doctor before combining aspirin or other drugs with pentosan.

Patchy hair loss, usually starting within the first 4 weeks of taking pentosan, occurs in about 4% of people who take this medication.

Pentosan should be taken exactly as directed. If you forget to take a dose of pentosan, take it as soon as you remember. If it is almost time for your next dose, skip the dose you forgot and continue with your regular schedule. Do not take a double dose.

Special Populations

Pregnancy/Breast-feeding

While animal studies of pentosan reveal no damage to the fetus, this drug should only be used during pregnancy after carefully weighing its potential benefits against its risks.

It is not known if pentosan passes into breast milk. Nursing mothers who must take it should consider bottle-feeding.

Seniors

Seniors may use this medication without special precaution.

Brand Name

Percocet

Generic Ingredients

Acetaminophen + Oxycodone Hydrochloride G

Other Brand Names

Endocet
Roxicet
Roxicet 5/500

Roxilox
Tylox

The information in this profile also applies to the following drugs:

Generic Ingredients: Acetaminophen + Codeine Phosphate G

Aceta with Codeine
Capital with Codeine
Phenaphen with Codeine No. 2
Phenaphen with Codeine No. 3
Phenaphen with Codeine No. 4
Tylenol with Codeine No. 1
Tylenol with Codeine No. 2
Tylenol with Codeine No. 3
Tylenol with Codeine No. 4

Generic Ingredients: Acetaminophen + Hydrocodone Bitartrate G

Allay	Lortab
Anexsia 5/500	Lortab 2.5/500
Anexsia 7.5/650	Lortab 5/500
Anexsia 10/660	Lortab 7.5/500
Bancap HC	Lortab 10/500
Ceta-Plus	Margesic H
Co-Gesic	Norco
Dolacet	Panacet 5/500
Duocet	Stagesic
Hydrocet	T-Gesic
Hydrogesic	Vicodin
Hy-Phen	Vicodin-ES
Lorcet-HD	Vicodin-HP
Lorcet Plus	Zydone
Lorcet 10/650	

Generic Ingredients: Acetaminophen + Pentazocine G
Talacen

Generic Ingredient: Oxycodone Hydrochloride
OxyContin   Roxicodone
Percolone

Type of Drug

Narcotic and analgesic (pain reliever) combination.

Prescribed For

Mild to moderate pain.

General Information

Percocet is generally prescribed for those who require a greater analgesic effect than acetaminophen alone can deliver or for those who cannot take aspirin. Percocet is not considered effective for arthritis or other pain caused by inflammation because it does not reduce inflammation.

Cautions and Warnings

Do not take Percocet if you are **allergic** or **sensitive** to any of its ingredients.

Use this drug with extreme caution if you suffer from **asthma or other breathing problems** or have **kidney or liver disease** or **viral infection of the liver**. This drug should be used with caution if you have **head injuries, brain disease,** a history of **seizures, inflammatory bowel disease, gallstones or gallbladder disease, enlarged prostate,** or **urinary difficulties**.

Chronic (long-term) use of Percocet may cause drug dependence or **addiction**.

Percocet may cause postural **low blood pressure** (symptoms include dizziness or fainting when rising from a sitting or lying position).

Oxycodone is a respiratory depressant and affects the central nervous system (CNS), producing **sleepiness, tiredness,** and an **inability to concentrate. Alcohol** may increase the risk of oxycodone-related drowsiness.

For additional information see "Cautions and Warnings" in Acetaminophen (p. 14).

Possible Side Effects

▼ Most common: light-headedness, dizziness, sleepiness, nausea, vomiting, appetite loss, and increased sweating. If any of these effects occur, ask your doctor to consider lowering your dosage. Most of these side effects disappear if you lie down. More serious side effects are shallow breathing or breathing difficulties.

▼ Less common: euphoria (feeling "high"), weakness, headache, agitation, uncoordinated muscle movements, minor hallucinations, disorientation, visual disturbances, dry mouth, constipation, facial flushing, rapid heartbeat, palpitations, feeling faint, urinary difficulties, reduced sex drive, impotence, rash, itching, anemia, low blood

---

Possible Side Effects *(continued)*

---

sugar, and yellowing of the skin or whites of the eyes. Narcotic pain relievers may aggravate convulsions in those who have had them.

For additional information see "Possible Side Effects" in Acetaminophen (p. 13).

Drug Interactions

• Because of its depressant effect and potential effect on breathing, Percocet should be taken with extreme care in combination with alcohol, sleeping medications, tranquilizers, antihistamines, or other drugs producing sedation.

• Combining Percocet and protease inhibitors may increase the risk of CNS depression and breathing difficulties.

For additional information see "Drug Interactions" in Acetaminophen (p. 13).

Food Interactions

Percocet is best taken with food or at least half a glass of water to prevent upset stomach.

Usual Dose

Percocet
   Adult: 1–2 tablets every 4–6 hours.
   Child: not recommended.

Acetaminophen with Codeine
   Adult and Child (age 13 and over): 1–2 tablets every 4 hours.
   Child (age 7–12): equivalent of 5–10 mg of codeine every 4–6 hours; do not exceed 60 mg in 24 hours.
   Child (age 3–6): equivalent of 2.5–5 mg of codeine every 4–6 hours; do not exceed 30 mg in 24 hours.

Acetaminophen with Hydrocodone
   Adult: 1 tablet every 4–6 hours.
   Child: not recommended.

Acetaminophen with Pentazocine
   Adult: 1 tablet every 4 hours.
   Child: not recommended.

Oxycodone
   Adult: 10–30 mg every 4 hours.
   Child: not recommended.

Overdosage

Symptoms include depressed respiration, extreme tiredness progressing to stupor and then coma, pinpointed pupils, no response to pain stimulation, cold and clammy skin, slowing of heart rate, lowering of blood pressure, yellowing of the skin or whites of the eyes, bluish discoloration of the hands or feet, fever, excitement, delirium, convulsions, cardiac arrest, and liver toxicity (symptoms include nausea, vomiting, abdominal pain, and diarrhea). Induce vomiting with ipecac syrup—available at any pharmacy—and take the victim to a hospital emergency room immediately. ALWAYS bring the prescription bottle or container.

Special Information

Percocet is a respiratory depressant that affects the CNS, producing sleepiness, tiredness, and inability to concentrate. Be careful when driving or performing any task that requires concentration.

If you have been taking this medication for more than a few weeks, do not stop taking it without your doctor's instruction. Suddenly stopping this drug may lead to withdrawal symptoms.

Call you doctor if you experience breathing difficulties or persistent nausea, vomiting, or constipation.

If you forget a dose, take it as soon as you remember. If it is almost time for your next dose, skip the dose you forgot and continue with your regular schedule. Do not take a double dose.

For additional information see "Special Information" in Acetaminophen (p. 13).

Special Populations

Pregnancy/Breast-feeding

High doses of acetaminophen, one of the ingredients in Percocet, have caused problems when taken during pregnancy. Regular use of oxycodone, the other active ingredient in Percocet, during pregnancy may cause addiction in newborns. If used during labor, it may cause breathing problems in the infant. When this drug is considered crucial by your doctor, its potential benefits must be weighed against its risks.

The ingredients in Percocet may pass into breast milk. Nursing mothers who must take this drug should wait 4 to 6 hours after their last dose before nursing or they should consider bottle-feeding.

Seniors

Seniors may be sensitive to the depressant effects of this drug and may experience dizziness, light-headedness, and fainting, particularly upon rising from a sitting or lying position.

Brand Name

Percodan

Generic Ingredients

Aspirin + Oxycodone Hydrochloride + Oxycodone Terephthalate G

Other Brand Names
Percodan-Demi   Roxiprin

The information in this profile also applies to the following drugs:

Generic Ingredients: Aspirin + Codeine Phosphate G
Empirin with Codeine No. 3
Empirin with Codeine No. 4

Generic Ingredients: Aspirin + Caffeine + Dihydrocodeine Bitartrate
Synalgos-DC

Generic Ingredients: Ibuprofen + Hydrocodone Bitartrate
Vicoprofen

Generic Ingredients: Pentazocine + Aspirin
Talwin Compound

Generic Ingredients: Pentazocine + Naloxone G
Talwin Nx

Type of Drug

Narcotic and aspirin combination.

Prescribed For

Mild to moderate pain.

General Information

Percodan is one of many combination products containing a narcotic and a non-narcotic analgesic (pain reliever). It is prescribed to relieve pain and reduce inflammation.

Cautions and Warnings

Do not take Percodan if you are **allergic** or **sensitive** to any of its ingredients.

Use this medication with extreme caution if you suffer from **asthma** or other **breathing problems**. Percodan should also be used with caution if you have **kidney or liver disease, head injuries, brain disease,** a history of **seizures, hypothyroidism** (underactive thyroid gland), **inflammatory bowel disease, gallstones or gallbladder disease, enlarged prostate,** or **urinary difficulties**.

Percodan may cause postural **low blood pressure** (symptoms include dizziness or fainting when rising from a sitting or lying position).

Chronic (long-term) use of this drug may cause drug dependence or **addiction**.

Percodan is a respiratory depressant and affects the central nervous system (CNS), producing **sleepiness, tiredness,** and an **inability to concentrate. Alcohol** may increase the CNS depression caused by this drug.

For additional information, see "Cautions and Warnings" in Aspirin (p. 111) and Ibuprofen (p. 549).

Possible Side Effects

▼ Most common: light-headedness, dizziness, sleepiness, nausea, vomiting, appetite loss, and increased sweating. If these occur, ask your doctor to consider lowering your dosage. Usually they go away if you lie down. More serious side effects are shallow breathing or other breathing difficulties.

Possible Side Effects *(continued)*

▼ Less common: euphoria (feeling "high"), weakness, headache, agitation, uncoordinated muscle movement, minor hallucinations, disorientation, visual disturbances, dry mouth, constipation, facial flushing, rapid heartbeat, palpitations, feeling faint, urinary difficulties, impotence, reduced sex drive, rash, itching, anemia, low blood sugar, and yellowing of the skin or whites of the eyes. These drugs may aggravate convulsions in those who have had them.

For additional information, see "Possible Side Effects" in Aspirin (p. 111) and Ibuprofen (p. 549).

Drug Interactions

• Combining Percodan and alcohol, tranquilizers, barbiturates, sleeping medications, antihistamines, or other drugs producing sedation increases sleepiness or an inability to concentrate and significantly increases Percodan's depressive effect.

• Combining Percodan and protease inhibitors may increase the risk of CNS depression and breathing difficulties.

For additional information, see "Drug Interactions" in Aspirin (p. 111) and Ibuprofen (p. 549).

Food Interactions

Take with food or half a glass of water to prevent upset stomach.

Usual Dose

Percodan
   Adult: 1 tablet every 4–6 hours as needed for pain relief.
   Child: Consult your doctor.

Empirin with Codeine
   Adult: 1–2 tablets 3–4 times a day.
   Child: Consult your doctor.

Synalgos-DC
   Adult: 2 capsules every 4 hours.
   Child: Consult your doctor.

Talwin Compound
   Adult: 2 tablets 3–4 times a day.
   Child: Consult your doctor.

Talwin NX
   Adult: 50 mg every 3–4 hours; increase to 100 mg if necessary. Daily dose should not exceed 600 mg.
   Child: Consult your doctor.

Vicoprofen
   Adult: 1 tablet every 4–6 hours, up to 5 tablets a day.
   Child: Consult your doctor.

Overdosage

Symptoms include breathing difficulties, extreme tiredness progressing to stupor and then coma, pinpointed pupils, no response to pain stimulation, cold and clammy skin, slowing of heartbeat, dizziness or fainting, convulsions, cardiac arrest, fever, excitement, confusion, liver or kidney failure, and bleeding. Symptoms of mild overdose include nausea, vomiting, dizziness, ringing or buzzing in the ears, flushing, increased sweating, thirst, headache, drowsiness, diarrhea, and rapid heartbeat. Take the victim to a hospital emergency room immediately. ALWAYS bring the prescription bottle or container.

Special Information

Percodan may produce sleepiness, tiredness, or an inability to concentrate. Be careful when driving or performing any tasks that require concentration.

If you have been taking this medication for more than a few weeks, do not stop taking it without your doctor's instructions. Suddenly stopping this drug may lead to withdrawal symptoms.

Call your doctor if you experience breathing difficulties or persistent nausea, vomiting, or constipation.

If you forget a dose, take it as soon as you remember. If it is almost time for your next dose, skip the one you forgot and continue with your regular schedule. Do not take a double dose.

For additional information, see "Special Information" in Aspirin (p. 111) and Ibuprofen (p. 549).

Special Populations

Pregnancy/Breast-feeding

Aspirin, one of the ingredients in Percodan, may cause bleeding problems in the fetus, particularly during the last 2 weeks of pregnancy. Taking aspirin during the last 3 months of pregnancy may lead to a low-birth-weight infant, prolong labor, and extend the duration of pregnancy; it may also cause bleeding in the mother before, during, or after delivery. Large amounts of oxycodone, the other ingredient in Percodan, may cause addiction in newborns. It may also cause breathing problems in newborns if taken just before delivery. When Percodan is considered crucial by your doctor, its potential benefits must be carefully weighed against its risks.

The ingredients in Percodan may pass into breast milk. Nursing mothers who must take this drug should consider bottle-feeding.

Seniors

Seniors may be more sensitive to the depressant effects of this drug as well as dizziness, light-headedness, and fainting, particularly upon rising suddenly from a sitting or lying position.

Generic Name

Pergolide (PER-goe-lide)

Brand Name

Permax

Type of Drug

Antiparkinsonian.

Prescribed For

Parkinson's disease.

General Information

Pergolide mesylate is combined with levodopa or carbidopa to control Parkinson's disease. It works by stimulating a specific nerve ending in the central nervous system that is normally stimulated by the hormone dopamine. Pergolide also inhibits the production of prolactin, a hormone that is involved in the production of breast milk. Pergolide affects growth-hormone levels and the reproductive hormone called luteinizing hormone (LH).

Cautions and Warnings

Do not take pergolide if you have had a reaction to it or other drugs derived from the fungus ergot.

Pergolide causes **hallucinations** in about 14% of people. If this occurs, contact your doctor at once.

People who are prone to abnormal heart rhythms should be cautious when taking pergolide because of possible **cardiac side effects**.

Possible Side Effects

In studies, about 25% of people stopped taking pergolide because of side effects.

▼ Most common: hallucinations, confusion, twisting body movements, tiredness, difficulty sleeping, anxiety, nausea, constipation, diarrhea, upset stomach, and runny nose.

▼ Less common: Other side effects can occur in almost any part of the body. Contact your doctor if you experience any side effect not listed above.

Drug Interactions

• Phenothiazines, thioxanthenes, haloperidol, droperidol, loxapine, methyldopa, molindone, papaverine, reserpine, and metoclopramide counter the effects of pergolide.

• Alcohol, tranquilizers, and other nervous-system depressants increase the depressant effects of this drug.

• Drugs that cause low blood pressure increase the blood-pressure-lowering effect of pergolide.

Food Interactions

Take pergolide with food if it upsets your stomach.

Usual Dose

Starting dosage—.05 mg a day. Dosage is increased by 0.1–0.25 mg every third day until an effect is achieved. Maximum dosage is 5 mg a day.

Overdosage

Symptoms may include nausea, vomiting, agitation, low blood pressure, hallucinations, involuntary body and muscular movements, tingling in the arms or legs, heart palpitations, abnormal heart rhythms, and nervous-system stimulation. Take the victim to a hospital emergency room. ALWAYS bring the prescription bottle or container.

Special Information

Many people taking pergolide for the first time experience dizziness and fainting caused by low blood pressure. Your doctor will need to increase your pergolide dosage gradually to reduce this effect. However, any dizziness or fainting should be reported to your doctor at once.

Contact your doctor if you experience nervous-system effects, such as confusion, uncontrolled body movements, or hallucinations; pain or burning upon urination; high blood pressure; severe headache; seizure; sudden changes in vision; severe chest pain; fainting; rapid heartbeat; severe nausea; excessive sweating; nervousness; shortness of breath; sudden weakness; or any bothersome or persistent side effect.

Do not stop taking pergolide or change your dosage without your doctor's knowledge.

This drug may make you tired, dizzy, or light-headed. Be careful when driving or doing any task that requires concentration.

Dry mouth may be relieved with sugarless gum, candy, ice, or a saliva substitute. Maintain good oral hygiene while taking pergolide because dry mouth increases the risk of oral infections.

If you forget a dose, take it as soon as you remember. If you take pergolide once a day and it is almost time for your next dose, skip the one you forgot and continue with your regular schedule. If you take pergolide 2 or 3 times a day and it is almost time for your next dose, take 1 dose as soon as you remember and another in 3 or 4 hours, then go back to your regular schedule. Never take a double dose.

Special Populations

Pregnancy/Breast-feeding

While animal studies of pergolide revealed no damage to the fetus, this drug should only be used after carefully weighing its benefits against its risks.

Pergolide may pass into breast milk and interfere with milk production. Nursing mothers who must take it should bottle-feed.

Seniors

Seniors may take pergolide without special restriction.

Generic Name

Permethrin (per-MEE-thrin) G

Brand Names

Acticin   Nix
Elimite   Rid

Type of Drug

Scabicide.

Prescribed For

Scabies and head lice.

General Information

Permethrin is a synthetic chemical that kills lice, ticks, mites, and fleas. It paralyzes the parasite by interfering with its nervous system. Only 2 or 3 in 100 people who use permethrin for head lice need to be re-treated because it kills both the parasite and its eggs. Permethrin, which remains on hair shafts after application, prevents reinfection for up to 2 weeks. Less than 2% of permethrin is absorbed through the skin into the bloodstream.

Cautions and Warnings

Do not use permethrin if you are **sensitive** or **allergic** to it or chrysanthemums. Stop using permethrin if you develop a reaction to it.

Possible Side Effects

Cream
▼ Most common: burning and stinging.
▼ Common: mild, temporary itching.

> **Possible Side Effects** *(continued)*
>
> ▼ Rare: tingling, numbness, mild swelling, and rash.
>
> *Liquid*
> ▼ Common: mild, temporary itching.
> ▼ Less common: mild, temporary burning or stinging; tingling; numbness; discomfort; mild swelling; and rash.

Drug Interactions

• Do not apply this product with any other topical medication.

Usual Dose

Cream (for scabies)*:* For adults and children age 2 months and over—Thoroughly massage the cream into the skin from the head to the soles of the feet; 1 oz. (30 g) is usually enough for a single treatment of an adult. Infants should be treated at the hairline, neck, scalp, and forehead. Leave the cream on for 8–14 hours and then remove it by washing.

Liquid (for head lice)*:* For adults and children age 2 and over—Wash your hair with regular shampoo, rinse, and towel dry. Then, apply enough permethrin liquid to saturate the hair and scalp; leave it in for 10 minutes. Rinse off with water. Repeat if lice reoccur within 7 days.

Overdosage

In case of accidental ingestion, call your local poison control center or a hospital emergency room. You may be told to induce vomiting with ipecac syrup—available at any pharmacy—before taking the victim to an emergency room. If you seek treatment, ALWAYS bring the prescription bottle or container.

Special Information

This drug should be applied only to hairy areas of the body with intact skin. It should never be swallowed.

Do not apply permethrin to areas around the eyes, nose, or mouth. Call your doctor if anything unusual develops or if irritation continues after you have stopped using the drug.

It is not necessary to comb the hair to remove parasite eggs after permethrin treatment but you may wish to do so for cosmetic reasons.

Special Populations

Pregnancy/Breast-feeding

The safety of using permethrin during pregnancy is not known. When this drug is considered crucial by your doctor, its potential benefits must be carefully weighed against its risks.

It is not known if permethrin passes into breast milk. Nursing mothers who must use it should bottle-feed.

Seniors

This drug may be used without special precaution.

Generic Name

Phenelzine (FEH-nel-zeen)

Brand Name

Nardil

The information in this profile also applies to the following drug:

Generic Ingredient: Tranylcypromine Sulfate
Parnate

Type of Drug

Monoamine oxidase inhibitor (MAOI).

Prescribed For

Atypical depression and depression that does not respond to other drugs; also prescribed for a variety of conditions including bulimia, cocaine addiction, night terrors, post-traumatic stress disorder, migraine, seasonal affective disorder, and symptoms of multiple sclerosis.

General Information

Monoamine oxidase (MAO) is a complex enzyme system found throughout the body. MAO is responsible for breaking down hormones that make the nervous system work. MAOIs such as phenelzine sulfate interfere with MAO action, causing an increase in the amount of norepinephrine and other monoamines stored throughout the nervous system. This increase is what gives phenelzine its therapeutic effect, which is long lasting and may continue for up to 2 weeks after you stop taking it.

Cautions and Warnings

Do not take phenelzine if you are **allergic** to it or have **pheochromocytoma** (adrenal-gland tumor), **heart failure, liver disease** or **abnormal liver function,** severe **kidney-function loss, heart disease,** or a history of **headaches, stroke, transient ischemic attack** (TIA)—"mini-stroke"—or **high blood pressure.** The most severe reactions to phenelzine, which can be deadly, involve very high blood pressure. **Bleeding inside the head** has occurred in people with very high blood pressure. Serious, potentially fatal reactions may occur if phenelzine and a selective serotonin reuptake inhibitor (SSRI) antidepressant are taken together (see "Drug Interactions").

Possible Side Effects

▼ Common: dizziness when rising from a sitting or lying position, dizziness, fainting, headache, tremors, muscle twitching, overly reactive reflexes, manic reactions, confusion, memory loss, sleeping difficulties, weakness, uncontrollable muscle movement, fatigue, drowsiness, restlessness, overstimulation, anxiety and agitation, constipation, nausea, diarrhea, abdominal pain, swelling, dry mouth, liver irritation, appetite loss, weight changes, and sexual difficulties.

▼ Less common: jitteriness, a need to pace the floor or change positions often, euphoria (feeling "high"), nerve irritation, chills, a need to repeat words or phrases, convulsions, tingling in the hands or feet, heart palpitations, rapid heartbeat, painful or infrequent urination, changes in blood components, glaucoma, blurred vision, uncontrolled eyeball movement, sweating, and rash.

▼ Rare: poor coordination, coma, hallucinations at high dosages, severe anxiety, schizophrenia, delirious reactions, muscle spasm, jerky movements, numbness, and yellowing of the skin or whites of the eyes.

Drug Interactions

• Do not ever combine phenelzine with meperidine, as fatal effects may occur.

• Bupropion or carbamazepine should not be combined with phenelzine.

• Phenelzine interferes with the blood-pressure-lowering effect of guanethidine. Do not combine these drugs.

• Taking an SSRI antidepressant and phenelzine at the same time or too close together may result in a serious, sometimes fatal reaction characterized by very high fever, rigidity, muscle spasms, and changes in mental state, blood pressure, pulse, and breathing rate. Two weeks should elapse between stopping phenelzine and taking an SSRI. At least 5 weeks should elapse between stopping an SSRI and taking phenelzine.

• A tricyclic antidepressant and phenelzine may be combined only under your doctor's direct supervision. If dosages are not strictly controlled, this combination can lead to seizures, sweating, coma, hyperexcitability, high fever, rapid heartbeat, rapid breathing, headache, dilated pupils, flushing, confusion, and low blood pressure. When severe, this reaction can be fatal. Generally, 2 weeks must pass between stopping phenelzine and taking a tricyclic antidepressant.

• Phenelzine increases the effects of sulfonylurea-type antidiabetic drugs, barbiturates, beta blockers, levodopa, methyldopa, rauwolfia drugs, sulfa drugs, sumatriptan, stimulants, thiazide-type diuretics, and L-tryptophan. The combination of any of these drugs and phenelzine can result in severe reactions.

• Combining dextromethorphan (a cough suppressant found in many over-the-counter products) and phenelzine may lead to a high fever and low blood pressure. Avoid this combination.

• Combining phenelzine with another MAOI or methylphenidate may lead to excessively high blood pressure.

• Combining tranylcypromine sulfate and disulfiram may lead to delirium, agitation, disorientation, and hallucinations.

Food Interactions

Avoid foods with a high dopamine, tyramine, or tryptophan level such as the following while taking phenelzine and for at least 2 weeks after stopping phenelzine as they may lead to severe high blood pressure:

Alcohol: imported beer and ale; red wine, especially Chianti; sherry; vermouth; and distilled spirits.

Cheese and Dairy: processed American cheese, blue cheese, Boursault, natural brick cheese, Brie, Camembert, cheddar, Emmenthaler, Gruyere, mozzarella, Parmesan, Romano, Roquefort, sour cream, Stilton, Swiss cheese, and yogurt.

Fruits and Vegetables: avocados, especially when overripe; yeast extracts, including marmite; canned figs; raisins; sauerkraut; soy sauce; miso soup; and bean curd.

Meat and Fish: beef or chicken liver, meats prepared with a tenderizer, summer sausage, bologna, pepperoni, salami, game, meat extracts, caviar, dried fish, anchovies, salted herring, pickled and spoiled herring, and shrimp paste.

Other: fava beans and ginseng.

Many other foods are contraindicated as well. Consult your doctor for a list of these foods.

Usual Dose

Phenelzine

Adult and Child (age 17 and over): 15 mg 3 times a day to start, increased gradually to 60–90 mg a day.

Senior: 15 mg in the morning. Dosage is increased very gradually.

Child (under age 17): not recommended.

Tranylcypromine Sulfate

Adult and Child (age 17 and over): 10–60 mg a day. Usual dosage is 30 mg a day.

Senior: starting dosage—2.5–5 mg a day.

Child (under age 17): not recommended.

Overdosage

Early symptoms may include excitement; irritability; hyperactivity; anxiety; low blood pressure; vascular system collapse; sleeplessness; restlessness; dizziness; fainting; weakness; drowsiness; hallucinations; jaw-muscle spasms; flushing; sweating; rapid breathing; rapid heartbeat; movement disorders including grimacing, rigidity, muscle tremors, and large muscle spasms; and severe headache. Death may occur.

Take the victim to a hospital emergency room at once. ALWAYS bring the prescription bottle or container.

Special Information

Serious side effects include intense headache; heart palpitations; stiff or sore neck; nausea; vomiting; sweating, sometimes accompanied by fever or cold, clammy skin; dilated pupils; and sensitivity to bright light. Report these or any bothersome or persistent side effect to your doctor.

Vivid nightmares, agitation, psychosis, and convulsions occasionally occur 1 to 3 days after phenelzine is abruptly stopped. Gradually stopping phenelzine should prevent these problems.

Phenelzine causes drowsiness and blurred vision. Be careful when driving or performing any task that requires concentration. Avoid alcohol.

People with diabetes should be cautious because this drug may lower blood-sugar readings.

Be sure your surgeon or dentist knows that you are taking phenelzine before administering any anesthetic drug.

Do not take any other prescription or over-the-counter drug without first checking with your pharmacist or the doctor who prescribed phenelzine.

If you forget a dose, take it as soon as possible. If it is less than 2 hours until your next dose, skip the dose you forgot and continue with your regular schedule. Do not take a double dose.

Special Populations

Pregnancy/Breast-feeding

Phenelzine may pass into the fetal circulation. When this drug is considered crucial by your doctor, its potential benefits must be carefully weighed against its risks.

This drug may pass into breast milk. Nursing mothers who must take it should bottle-feed.

Seniors

Seniors are more susceptible to side effects and must use caution.

Generic Name

Phenobarbital (FEEN-oe-BAR-bih-tol) Ⓖ

Brand Names

Bellatal   Solfoton

Type of Drug

Hypnotic, sedative, and anticonvulsant.

Prescribed For

Epileptic and other seizures, convulsions, daytime sedation, and sleeplessness in the short term.

General Information

Phenobarbital is a sustained-release barbiturate. It takes 30 to 60 minutes to start working and its effect lasts for 10 to 16 hours. Like other barbiturates, phenobarbital appears to act by interfering with nerve impulses to the brain. When used as an anticonvulsant, phenobarbital is not very effective by itself; when used with anticonvulsant agents such as phenytoin, the combined action is dramatic. This combination has been used very successfully to control epileptic seizure.

Cautions and Warnings

Phenobarbital may **dull your physical and mental reflexes**. Be extremely careful when driving or performing any task that requires concentration.

Phenobarbital may be **addictive** if taken for an extended period of time. It may also cause **signs of intoxication** including slurred speech, a wobbly walk, rolling of the eyes, confusion, poor judgment, irritability, and sleeplessness. Combining this drug with alcohol worsens the situation.

Barbiturates are broken down in the liver and eliminated through the kidneys; people with **liver or kidney disease** should be cautious about taking phenobarbital.

You should not take phenobarbital if you are **sensitive** or **allergic** to any barbiturate, if you have been addicted to sedatives or hypnotics, or if you have a **respiratory condition**.

People with **chronic pain** should be careful about taking this drug because it may mask symptoms or cause stimulation, though using phenobarbital after surgery and in people with cancer has proven effective.

People abruptly stopping this drug may develop **seizure**. Dosage should be reduced gradually.

Barbiturates may increase your need for **vitamin D**; take a vitamin supplement while using this drug.

Possible Side Effects

▼ Most common: drowsiness, lethargy, headache, dizziness, drug "hangover," breathing difficulties, rash, and general allergic reaction (symptoms include runny nose, watery eyes, sneezing, scratchy throat, and cough).

▼ Less common: nausea, vomiting, constipation and diarrhea, slow heartbeat, low blood pressure, and fainting. Severe adverse reactions may include anemia and yellowing of the skin or whites of the eyes.

Drug Interactions

• Alcohol, monoamine oxidase inhibitor (MAOI) antidepressants, and valproic acid increase the effects of phenobarbital.

• Charcoal, chloramphenicol, and rifampin may counteract the effects of phenobarbital.

• Phenobarbital interferes with the effects of anticoagulant (blood-thinning) drugs, beta-blocker drugs, carbamazepine, chloramphenicol, oral contraceptives ("the pill"), corticosteroids, clonazepam, digitoxin, doxorubicin, doxycycline, felodipine, fenoprofen, griseofulvin, metronidazole, phenylbutazone, quinidine, theophylline, and verapamil.

• Phenobarbital enhances the toxic effects of acetaminophen and methoxyflurane (an anesthetic).

• Phenobarbital has a variable effect on phenytoin and other antiseizure medication and on narcotic drugs. Dosage adjustments are necessary.

Food Interactions

Phenobarbital is best taken on an empty stomach but may be taken with food if it upsets your stomach.

Usual Dose

Anticonvulsant
   Adult: 60–100 mg a day.
   Child: 1.3–2.25 mg per lb. of body weight divided into 2 or 3 doses a day.

Sleeplessness
100–200 mg at bedtime.

Daytime Sedation
30–120 mg in 2–3 divided doses.

Overdosage

Severe barbiturate overdose may be fatal. Overdose symptoms include breathing difficulties, moderate reduction in pupil size, lowered body temperature progressing to fever, fluid in the lungs, and eventually coma. Take the victim to a hospital emergency room immediately. ALWAYS bring the prescription bottle or container.

Special Information

Avoid alcohol and other drugs that depress the nervous system.
   Take this medication exactly as prescribed.
   This drug causes drowsiness. Be careful when driving or doing any task that requires concentration.
   Call your doctor at once if you develop fever, sore throat, nosebleeds, mouth sores, unexplainable black-and-blue marks, or easy bruising or bleeding.
   If you forget a dose, take it as soon as you remember. If it is almost time for your next dose, skip the one you forgot and continue with your regular schedule. Do not take a double dose.

Special Populations

Pregnancy/Breast-feeding

Barbiturate use during pregnancy may increase the risk of birth defects and cause bleeding problems, brain tumors, and breathing difficulties in newborns. Regular use of a barbiturate during the last 3 months of pregnancy may cause drug dependency in newborns. However, phenobarbital may be necessary to control major episodes of seizure during pregnancy. Talk to your doctor about the potential benefits and risks of using phenobarbital.

Barbiturates pass into breast milk. They may cause drowsiness, slow heartbeat, and breathing difficulties in infants. Nursing mothers who must take phenobarbital should bottle-feed.

Seniors
Seniors are more sensitive to the effects of barbiturates and often need less medication.

Generic Name

Phenytoin (FEN-ih-toin) G

Brand Name

Dilantin   Phenytek
Dilantin Kapseals

The information in this profile also applies to the following drugs:

Generic Ingredient: Ethotoin
Peganone

Generic Ingredient: Fosphenytoin
Cerebyx

Generic Ingredient: Mephenytoin
Mesantoin

Type of Drug

Hydantoin anticonvulsant.

Prescribed For

Epileptic seizure; also prescribed for prevention of seizure following neurosurgery in nonepileptics and for abnormal heart rhythm. Phenytoin injection is used to control preeclampsia (a condition in which pregnant women experience severe increases in blood pressure during the second half of pregnancy), trigeminal neuralgia (tic douloureux), and severe skin conditions.

General Information

Phenytoin is the most widely prescribed of several hydantoin antiseizure drugs. These drugs all inhibit activity in that area of the brain responsible for grand mal seizures. People may respond to some hydantoins and not others.

Immediate-release phenytoin must be taken several times a day, while the sustained-release form can be taken either once or several times a day. Many people find the latter more convenient, but the immediate-release form allows your doctor more flexibility in designing an effective dosage schedule. Phenytoin may be used together with other anticonvulsants, such as phenobarbital.

Cautions and Warnings

Do not take phenytoin if you are **allergic** to it or any hydantoin anticonvulsant.

When discontinuing phenytoin, **dosage should be gradually reduced** over a period of about a week—otherwise, severe seizures may occur.

Phenytoin should not be used if you have **low blood pressure, myocardial insufficiency,** a very **slow heart rate,** or certain other **heart conditions.**

People with **liver disease** are more likely to experience phenytoin side effects.

Periodical blood tests are necessary to monitor **red- and white-blood-cell counts.** Sore throat, feeling unwell, fever, mucous-membrane bleeding, swollen glands, nosebleeds, black-and-blue marks, and easy bruising may be signs of blood disorders.

Rash may be a sign of a serious reaction and cause for stopping this medication. Tell your doctor at once if this happens.

If **lymph node enlargement** occurs, contact your doctor; you may be advised to substitute another anticonvulsant drug or drug combination.

Possible Side Effects

▼ Most common: drowsiness, rapid or unusual growth of the gums, slurred speech, mental confusion, nystagmus (rhythmic, uncontrolled movement of the eye), dizziness, insomnia, nervousness, uncontrollable twitching, double vision, tiredness, irritability, depression,

Possible Side Effects *(continued)*

tremors, headache. These side effects generally disappear as therapy continues and dosage is reduced.

▼ Less common: nausea, vomiting, diarrhea, constipation, fever, rash, balding, weight gain, numbness in the hands or feet, chest pain, water retention, sensitivity to bright light (especially sunlight), conjunctivitis (pinkeye), joint pain and inflammation, and high blood sugar. Phenytoin may cause coarse facial features, lip enlargement, and Peyronie's disease (in which the penis is permanently deformed or misshapen). Phenytoin rash may be accompanied by fever and may be serious or fatal. Some fatal blood-system side effects have occurred with phenytoin.

▼ Rare: liver damage (including hepatitis) and unusual body-hair growth.

Drug Interactions

• The following drugs may increase the effects of phenytoin, possibly necessitating a decrease in phenytoin dosage: alcohol in small amounts, allopurinol, amiodarone, aspirin and other salicylate drugs, benzodiazepine drugs, chloramphenicol, chlorpheniramine, cimetidine, disulfiram, fluconazole, ibuprofen, isoniazid, metronidazole, miconazole, omeprazole, phenacemide, phenothiazine antipsychotic drugs, phenylbutazone, succinimide antiseizure drugs, sulfa drugs, tricyclic antidepressants, trimethoprim, and valproic acid.

• The following drugs may interfere with the effects of phenytoin, possibly necessitating an increase in phenytoin dosage: large amounts of alcohol, antacids, anticancer drugs, barbiturates, carbamazepine, charcoal tablets, diazoxide, folic acid, influenza virus vaccine, loxapine succinate, nitrofurantoin, pyridoxine, rifampin, sucralfate, and theophylline drugs.

• Calcium supplements may slow the absorption of phenytoin

• Phenytoin may reduce the effectiveness of acetaminophen, amiodarone, carbamazepine, digitalis drugs, corticosteroids, dicumarol, disopyramide, doxycycline, estrogen drugs, haloperidol, methadone, metyrapone, mexiletine, oral contraceptives ("the pill"), quinidine, theophylline drugs, and valproic acid. Dosage increases may be necessary.

• Phenytoin may increase the risk of liver toxicity caused by acetaminophen, especially if phenytoin is taken regularly.

• Phenytoin may affect certain other drugs in an unpredictable manner. If you take phenytoin and one or more of these drugs, your doctor will have to determine if dosage adjustment is needed: cyclosporine, dopamine, furosemide, levodopa, levonorgestrel, mebendazole, phenothiazine antipsychotic drugs, and oral antidiabetes drugs.

• Combining clonazepam and phenytoin yields unpredictable results: The effect of either drug may be reduced or phenytoin side effects may occur.

• Corticosteroid drugs may mask the effects of phenytoin sensitivity reactions.

• Lithium toxicity may be increased if lithium is taken with phenytoin.

• Phenytoin may decrease meperidine's pain-relieving effects and increase the risk of meperidine side effects. This combination is not recommended.

• Long-term phenytoin therapy may result in extreme folic acid deficiency, or megaloblastic anemia. This imbalance may be corrected with folic acid supplements.

• Warfarin's effects may be increased by phenytoin; warfarin dosage must be adjusted.

Food Interactions

Take phenytoin with food to avoid stomach upset. Calcium can slow phenytoin absorption. Separate your phenytoin dose from high-calcium foods, such as milk, cheese, almonds, hazelnuts, and sesame seeds and calcium supplements, by 1 to 2 hours.

Usual Dose

Adult: starting dosage—300 mg a day. Maintenance dosage—300–400 mg a day. Dosage can be raised gradually to 600 mg a day. Sustained-release phenytoin is taken once a day; the immediate-release form must be taken throughout the day.

Child: starting dosage—2.5 mg per lb. of body weight a day, divided into 2 or 3 equal doses. Maintenance dosage—2–4 mg per lb. of body weight a day. Dosage should be adjusted according to the child's needs. Children age 6 and

over may take the adult dosage, but no child should take
more than 300 mg a day.

Overdosage

Symptoms include drug side effects. Take the victim to a hospital emergency room at once. ALWAYS bring the prescription bottle or container.

Special Information

Call your doctor at once if you feel unwell or develop a rash,
severe nausea or vomiting, swollen glands, swollen or tender
gums, yellowing of the skin or whites of the eyes, joint pain,
sore throat, fever, unusual bleeding or bruising, persistent
headache, infection, slurred speech, or poor coordination.

Do not stop taking phenytoin or change dosage without
your doctor's knowledge.

Phenytoin may cause drowsiness, dizziness, or blurred
vision, effects which are increased by alcoholic beverages. Be
careful when driving or doing any task that requires concentration.

Phenytoin sometimes produces a pink-brown color in the
urine, which is normal and not a cause for concern.

People with diabetes who take phenytoin must monitor
their urine regularly and report any changes to their doctors.

Good oral hygiene—including gum massage, frequent
brushing, and flossing—is very important because phenytoin
can cause abnormal growth of your gums.

DO NOT SWITCH PHENYTOIN BRANDS without notifying
your doctor. Different brands may not be equivalent.

If you use phenytoin suspension, be sure to shake the bottle vigorously just before a dose.

Do not use phenytoin capsules that have become discolored. Throw them away.

If you forget a dose, take it as soon as you remember. If you
take phenytoin once a day and it is almost time for your next
dose, skip the one you forgot and continue with your regular
schedule. If you take phenytoin several times a day and do
not remember it within 4 hours of your regular time, skip the
forgotten dose and go back to your regular schedule. Never
take a double dose.

Special Populations

Pregnancy/Breast-feeding

Phenytoin crosses into the fetal circulation. The great majority of mothers who take phenytoin deliver healthy babies, but some are born with cleft lip, cleft palate, or heart malformations. There is a recognized group of deformities, fetal hydantoin syndrome, which affects children of women taking phenytoin, though the drug has not been definitively established as the cause. This syndrome consists of skull and face abnormalities, reduced brain size, growth deficiency, deformed fingernails, and mental deficiency. Phenytoin increases the risk of vitamin K deficiency in newborns, which can lead to serious, life-threatening bleeding during the first 24 hours of life. Also, mothers taking phenytoin may be deficient in vitamin K, increasing the risk of bleeding during delivery.

Phenytoin passes into breast milk. Nursing mothers who must take it should bottle-feed.

Seniors

Seniors are more sensitive to side effects.

Generic Name

Pimecrolimus (pih-meh-CRO-lim-us)

Brand Name

Elidel Cream

Type of Drug

Immune system modulator.

Prescribed For

Mild to moderate eczema.

General Information

The exact way that pimecrolimus works in the management of mild to moderate dermatitis is unknown. However, it is related to drugs that are used to prevent organ rejection in transplant patients. Extremely small amounts of pimecrolimus are absorbed into the blood after application to the skin. Even after long-term use on more than half of the body, blood levels of pimecrolimus cannot be detected.

Cautions and Warnings

People who are **sensitive** or **allergic** to pimecrolimus or other related drugs should not take it.

Do not apply pimecrolimus cream to infected skin.

Possible Side Effects

▼ Most common: burning, headache, sore throat (with or without nasal pain), influenza, and cough.

▼ Less common: tonsillitis, strep throat, middle ear infection, chicken pox, fever, runny nose, worsening asthma, wheezing, nosebleeds, painful menstruation, conjunctivitis, back pain, joint pain, and earache.

▼ Rare: herpes infection, itching, toothache, constipation or loose stool, and abdominal pain.

Drug Interactions

Potential interactions between pimecrolimus and other drugs, including immunizations, have not been studied. Interactions are not expected but may still occur.

• Patients with widespread skin disease should avoid combining pimecrolimus with drugs that inhibit the liver enzyme CYP3A including calcium channel blockers, cimetidine, erythromycin, fluconazole, itraconazole, and ketoconazole.

Food Interactions

None known.

Usual Dose

Adult and Child (age 2 and over): apply a thin layer of pimecrolimus to the affected skin twice a day. Rub in gently and completely.

Child (under age 2): not recommended.

Overdosage

There have been no cases of pimecrolimus accidental ingestion. Call your local poison control center or emergency room for more information. If you seek treatment, ALWAYS bring the prescription bottle or container.

Special Information

Call your doctor if your condition does not improve after 6 weeks of using pimecrolimus cream.

Notify your doctor if you develop swollen lymph glands, or if warts, blemishes, or any other side effect worsen while using pimecrolimus.

Avoid exposure to the sun or to artificial sun lamps while using pimecrolimus.

Use pimecrolimus cream only as directed by your doctor. It is only for external application to the skin.

Wash your hands after applying pimecrolimus cream, unless your hands are the area being treated.

Do not bathe, shower, or swim immediately after applying pimecrolimus cream. This could wash off the cream.

Stop using pimecrolimus after your eczema has healed. You can begin using pimecrolimus cream again if the condition recurs.

Do not cover the skin being treated with bandages, dressings, or wraps.

Special Populations

Pregnancy/Breast-feeding

While animal studies of pimecrolimus reveal no damage to the fetus, this drug should only be used during pregnancy after carefully weighing its potential benefits against its risks.

It is not known if pimecrolimus passes into breast milk. Nursing mothers who must take it should bottle-feed.

Seniors

The effects of pimecrolimus on seniors is not known.

Generic Name

Pindolol (PIN-doe-lol) Ⓖ

Brand Name

Visken

Type of Drug

Beta-adrenergic blocking agent.

Prescribed For

High blood pressure, abnormal heart rhythms, side effects of antipsychotic drugs, and stage fright and other anxieties.

General Information

Pindolol is one of 15 beta-adrenergic blocking drugs, or beta blockers, that interfere with the action of a specific part of the nervous system. Beta receptors are found all over the body and affect many body functions. Each beta blocker has particular characteristics that make it more suitable for certain conditions or people. Pindolol is a mild heart stimulant, which is an advantage for some.

Cautions and Warnings

Do not take pindolol if you are **allergic** to beta blockers.

You should be cautious about taking pindolol if you have **asthma, severe heart failure,** a **very slow heart rate,** or **heart block** (disruption of the electrical impulses that control heart rate) because the drug may aggravate these conditions.

Do not stop taking pindolol without consulting your doctor, as the result may be **chest pain** or **heart attack.**

People with **angina** who take pindolol for high blood pressure risk aggravating their angina if they suddenly stop taking the drug. These people should have their drug dosage reduced gradually over 1 to 2 weeks.

Pindolol should be used with caution if you have **liver or kidney disease** because your ability to eliminate the drug from your body may be impaired.

Pindolol reduces the amount of blood pumped by the heart with each beat. This reduction in blood flow may aggravate the condition of people with **poor circulation** or **circulatory disease**.

Pindolol should be used with caution in people with **diabetes,** as it may affect glycemic response.

If you are undergoing **major surgery,** your doctor may want you to stop taking pindolol at least 2 days before surgery. This is a controversial practice and may not be recommended for all surgeries.

Possible Side Effects

Side effects are relatively uncommon and usually mild.

▼ Most common: impotence.

Possible Side Effects *(continued)*

▼ Less common: unusual tiredness or weakness, slow heartbeat, heart failure, dizziness, breathing difficulties, bronchospasm, depression, confusion, anxiety, nervousness, sleeplessness, disorientation, short-term memory loss, emotional instability, cold hands and feet, constipation, diarrhea, nausea, vomiting, upset stomach, increased sweating, urinary difficulties, cramps, blurred vision, rash, hair loss, stuffy nose, facial swelling, aggravation of lupus erythematosus, itching, chest pain, back or joint pain, colitis, drug allergy (symptoms include fever and sore throat), and liver toxicity.

Drug Interactions

• Pindolol may interact with surgical anesthetics to increase the risk of heart problems during surgery. Some anesthesiologists recommend gradually stopping the drug by 2 days before surgery.

• Pindolol may interfere with the normal signs of low blood sugar and with the action of oral antidiabetes drugs.

• Pindolol increases the blood-pressure-lowering effect of other blood-pressure-reducing agents, including clonidine, guanabenz, and reserpine as well as calcium channel blockers such as nifedipine.

• Aspirin, indomethacin, sulfinpyrazone, and estrogen drugs may interfere with the blood-pressure-lowering effect of pindolol.

• Cocaine may reduce the effectiveness of all beta blockers.

• Pindolol may worsen the cold hands and feet associated with taking ergot alkaloids for migraine. Gangrene is possible in people taking both ergot and pindolol.

• Pindolol counteracts thyroid hormone replacements.

• Calcium channel blockers, flecainide, hydralazine, oral contraceptives, propafenone, haloperidol, phenothiazine tranquilizers—molindone and others—quinolone antibacterials, and quinidine may increase the amount of pindolol in the bloodstream and lead to increased pindolol effects.

• Pindolol should not be taken within 2 weeks of taking a monoamine oxidase inhibitor (MAOI) antidepressant.

• Cimetidine increases the amount of pindolol absorbed into the bloodstream from oral tablets.

• Pindolol may interfere with the effectiveness of some antiasthma drugs, including theophylline and aminophylline, and especially ephedrine and isoproterenol.

• Combining pindolol and phenytoin or digitalis drugs may result in excessive slowing of the heart, possibly causing heart block.

• If you stop smoking while taking pindolol, your dose may have to be reduced because your liver will break down the drug more slowly afterward.

• Aluminum salts, barbituates, calcium salts, cholestyramine, colestipol, ampicillin, and rifampin may reduce the effectiveness of pindolol.

Food Interactions

None known.

Usual Dose

5–60 mg a day.

Overdosage

Symptoms include changes in heartbeat—unusually slow, unusually fast, or irregular; severe dizziness or fainting; breathing difficulties; bluish-colored fingernails or palms; and seizures. The victim should be taken to a hospital emergency room. ALWAYS bring the prescription bottle or container.

Special Information

Pindolol is taken continuously. When ending pindolol treatment, dosage should be reduced gradually over a period of about 2 weeks. Do not stop taking this drug unless directed to do so by your doctor: Abrupt withdrawal may cause chest pain, breathing difficulties, increased sweating, and unusually fast or irregular heartbeat.

Call your doctor at once if you develop back or joint pain, breathing difficulties, cold hands or feet, depression, rash, or changes in heartbeat. Pindolol may produce an undesirable lowering of blood pressure, leading to dizziness or fainting; call your doctor if this happens to you. Call your doctor if you experience persistent or bothersome anxiety, diarrhea, constipation, impotence, headache, itching, nausea or vomiting, nightmares or vivid dreams, upset stomach, trouble sleeping, stuffy nose, frequent urination, unusual tiredness, or weakness.

Pindolol may cause drowsiness, blurred vision, dizziness, and light-headedness. Be careful when driving or performing complex tasks.

It is best to take pindolol at the same time each day. If you forget a dose, take it as soon as you remember. If you take pindolol once a day and it is within 8 hours of your next dose, skip the dose you forgot and continue with your regular schedule. If you take it twice a day and it is within 4 hours of your next dose, skip the one you forgot and continue with your regular schedule. Never take a double dose.

Special Populations

Pregnancy/Breast-feeding
In studies, infants born to women who took a beta blocker while pregnant had lower birth weights, low blood pressure, and reduced heart rate. Pindolol should be avoided by women who are pregnant.

Pindolol passes into breast milk. Nursing mothers who must take it should bottle-feed.

Seniors
Seniors may require less of the drug to achieve results. Seniors taking pindolol may be more likely to suffer from cold hands and feet, reduced body temperature, chest pain, general feelings of ill health, sudden breathing difficulties, increased sweating, or changes in heartbeat.

Generic Name

Piroxicam (pih-ROX-ih-kam) Ⓖ

Brand Name

Feldene

Type of Drug

Nonsteroidal anti-inflammatory drug (NSAID).

Prescribed For

Rheumatoid arthritis, juvenile rheumatoid arthritis, osteoarthritis, menstrual pain, and sunburn.

General Information

Piroxicam and other NSAIDs are used to relieve pain and inflammation. We do not know exactly how NSAIDs work, but they may achieve their effects by blocking the body's production of a hormone called prostaglandin and the action of other body chemicals. Pain relief comes within 1 hour after taking the first dose of piroxicam and lasts for 2 to 3 days, but its anti-inflammatory effect takes several days to 2 weeks to become apparent and may take 3 weeks to reach maximum effect. Piroxicam is broken down in the liver and eliminated through the kidneys.

Cautions and Warnings

People who are **allergic** to piroxicam or any other NSAID and those with a history of **asthma** attacks brought on by an NSAID, iodides, or aspirin should not take piroxicam.

Piroxicam can cause **gastrointestinal (GI) bleeding, ulcers,** and **stomach perforation**. This can occur at any time, with or without warning, in people who take piroxicam regularly. People with a history of active GI bleeding should be cautious about taking any NSAID. People who develop bleeding or ulcers and continue NSAID treatment should be aware of the possibility of developing more serious drug toxicity.

Piroxicam can affect platelets and **blood clotting** at high doses and should be avoided by people with clotting problems and those taking warfarin.

People with **heart problems** who use piroxicam may experience swelling in their arms, legs, or feet.

Piroxicam can cause severe toxic effects to the **kidney**. Report any unusual side effects to your doctor, who may need to periodically test your kidney function.

Piroxicam can make you **unusually sensitive to the effects of the sun.**

Possible Side Effects

▼ Most common: diarrhea, nausea, vomiting, constipation, gas, stomach upset or irritation, and appetite loss—especially during the first few days of treatment.

▼ Less common: stomach ulcers, GI bleeding, hepatitis, gallbladder attacks, painful urination, poor kidney function, kidney inflammation, blood and protein in the

Possible Side Effects *(continued)*

urine, dizziness, fainting, nervousness, depression, hallucinations, confusion, disorientation, tingling in the hands or feet, light-headedness, itching, increased sweating, dry nose and mouth, heart palpitations, chest pain, difficulty breathing, and muscle cramps.

▼ Rare: severe allergic reactions including closing of the throat, fever and chills, changes in liver function, jaundice (yellowing of the skin or whites of the eyes), and kidney failure. People who experience such effects must be promptly treated in a hospital emergency room or doctor's office. NSAIDs have caused severe skin reactions; if this happens to you, see your doctor immediately.

Drug Interactions

• Piroxicam can increase the effects of oral anticoagulant (blood-thinning) drugs such as warfarin. Your anticoagulant dose may need to be reduced.

• Taking piroxicam with cyclosporine may increase the toxic kidney effects of both drugs.

• Methotrexate toxicity may be increased in people who are also taking piroxicam.

• Piroxicam may reduce the blood-pressure-lowering effect of beta blockers and loop diuretics.

• Piroxicam may increase phenytoin side effects. Lithium blood levels may be increased by piroxicam.

• Piroxicam blood levels may be affected by cimetidine or cholestyramine.

• Probenecid may increase the risk of piroxicam side effects.

• Aspirin and other salicylates should never be combined with piroxicam.

Food Interactions

Take piroxicam with food or a magnesium/aluminum antacid if it upsets your stomach.

Usual Dose

Adult: 20 mg a day.
Child: not recommended.

Overdosage

People have died from NSAID overdoses. Common signs of overdose are drowsiness, nausea, vomiting, diarrhea, abdominal pain, rapid breathing, rapid heartbeat, increased sweating, ringing or buzzing in the ears, confusion, disorientation, stupor, and coma. Take the victim to a hospital emergency room at once. ALWAYS bring the prescription bottle or container.

Special Information

Take each dose with a full glass of water, food, or milk and do not lie down for 15 to 30 minutes afterward.

Piroxicam can make you drowsy or tired: Be careful when driving or operating hazardous equipment. Do not take any over-the-counter products containing acetaminophen or aspirin while taking piroxicam. Avoid alcohol.

Contact your doctor if you develop rash or itching, visual disturbances, weight gain, breathing difficulties, fluid retention, hallucinations, black or tarry stools, persistent headache, or any unusual or intolerable side effect.

If you forget a dose of piroxicam, take it as soon as you remember. If you take it once a day and it is within 8 hours of your next dose, skip the missed dose and continue with your regular schedule. Do not take a double dose.

Special Populations

Pregnancy/Breast-feeding

NSAIDs may affect the fetal heart during the second half of pregnancy. When this drug is considered crucial by your doctor, its potential benefits must be carefully weighed against its risks.

NSAIDs may pass into breast milk. There is a risk that a nursing mother taking piroxicam could affect her baby's heart or cardiovascular system. Nursing mothers who must take this drug should bottle-feed.

Seniors

Seniors may be more susceptible to side effects, especially ulcer disease.

Plavix   *see Clopidogrel, page 270*

Generic Name

Podofilox (poe-DUH-fil-ox)

Brand Name

Condylox

Type of Drug

Antimitotic drug.

Prescribed For

External genital warts or warts around the anal area.

General Information

Podofilox, which can be either manufactured from chemicals or purified from natural sources, kills visible wart tissues. Exactly how it works is not known. Condylomas or genital warts are caused by the human papillomavirus and can appear in various places including the sex organs, anus, and abdomen. The risk of developing warts increases if your immune system is suppressed.

Cautions and Warnings

Do not use podofilox if you are **sensitive** or **allergic** to it.

Proper diagnosis of genital warts is necessary before you use this product: See your doctor before you start using podofilox. Do not use podofilox for any other purpose.

If you get podofilox in your **eyes,** wash it out at once with cool water and seek medical attention.

Possible Side Effects

▼ Most common: burning, pain, inflammation, skin erosion, itching, and bleeding.

▼ Common: pain during intercourse, sleeplessness, tingling, tenderness, chafing, bad odor, dizziness, scarring, small sores or ulcers, dryness, difficulty retracting the foreskin, blood in the urine, vomiting, headache, stinging, and redness.

▼ Less common: skin peeling, scabbing, skin discoloration, tenderness, crusting, skin cracks, soreness, swelling, rash, and blisters.

Drug Interactions

None known.

Usual Dose

Apply morning and night—every 12 hours—for 3 consecutive days, then apply nothing for 4 days. Repeat this cycle for up to 4 weeks in a row. Use the cotton-tipped applicator supplied with the solution, or your finger if you are using the gel. Try to limit the amount of podofilox that gets on intact skin. Thoroughly wash your hands before and after each application.

Overdosage

Swallowing podofilox may lead to nausea, vomiting, fever, diarrhea, mouth sores, tingling in the hands or feet, changes in mental state, lethargy, coma, rapid breathing, respiratory failure, blood in the urine, kidney failure, and seizures. Excess podofilox should be washed off the skin as soon as possible. In case of overdose or accidental ingestion, take the victim to a hospital emergency room. ALWAYS bring the prescription bottle or container.

Special Information

Thoroughly wash your hands before and after each application.

Call your doctor if you develop any bothersome or persistent side effect. If you do not see any improvement in 4 weeks, stop using the drug and call your doctor.

If you forget a dose, apply it as soon as you remember. If it is within 4 hours of your next dose, skip the dose you forgot and continue with your regular schedule.

Special Populations

Pregnancy/Breast-feeding

Podofilox is toxic to animal fetuses at very high dosages. When this drug is considered crucial by your doctor, its potential benefits must be carefully weighed against its risks.

It is not known if podofilox passes into breast milk. Nursing mothers who must use it should bottle-feed.

Seniors

Seniors may use podofilox without special precaution.

Brand Name

Poly-Vi-Flor

Generic Ingredients

Folic Acid + Sodium Fluoride + Vitamin A + Vitamin B_1 (Thiamine) + Vitamin B_2 (Riboflavin) + Vitamin B_3 (Niacin) + Vitamin B_6 (Pyridoxine) + Vitamin B_{12} (Cyanocobalamin) + Vitamin C + Vitamin D + Vitamin E G

Other Brand Names

Florvite*   Soluvite*
Polytabs-F   Vi-Daylin/F*

Some products in this brand-name group are alcohol- or sugar-free. Consult your pharmacist.

Type of Drug

Multivitamin supplement with fluoride.

Prescribed For

Vitamin deficiencies and prevention of dental cavities in infants and children.

General Information

Fluoride taken in small daily dosages has been effective in preventing cavities in children by strengthening the teeth. Multivitamins with fluoride are also available in preparations with iron.

Cautions and Warnings

Too much fluoride can **damage teeth**. Because of this, Poly-Vi-Flor should not be used where the fluoride content of the water supply exceeds 0.7 parts per million (ppm)—consult your pediatrician or local water company.

Possible Side Effects

▼ Common: occasional rash, itching, upset stomach, headache, and weakness.

Food and Drug Interactions

None known.

Usual Dose

1 tablet or dropperful a day.

Overdosage

Symptoms include tarry stools, bloody vomit, diarrhea, drowsiness, faintness, increased watering of the mouth or eyes, shallow breathing, stomach cramps, aching bones, rash, mouth or lip sores, or discoloration of the teeth. Check with your doctor immediately or take the victim to a hospital emergency room. ALWAYS bring the prescription bottle or container.

Special Information

If you forget to give your child a dose of Poly-Vi-Flor, do so as soon as you remember. If it is almost time for the next dose, skip the dose you forgot and continue with the regular schedule. Do not give a double dose.

Type of Drug

Potassium Replacements

Brand Names

Generic Ingredient: Potassium Chloride (Liquid) G

Cena-K S | Kay Ciel S
Kaochlor 10% | Klorvess
Kaochlor S-F S | Potasalan S
Kaon-Cl 20% S | Rum-K S

Generic Ingredient: Potassium Gluconate (Liquid) G

Kaon S | K-G Elixir
Kaylixir

Generic Ingredient: Potassium Salt Combination (Liquid) G

Kolyum | Twin-K
Tri-K

Generic Ingredient: Potassium Chloride (Powder) G

Gen-K S | K+Care

Kay Ciel $

K-Lor

Klor-Con $

Klor-Con/25 $

K-Lyte/Cl

K-Vescent

Micro-K LS

Generic Ingredient: Potassium Salt Combination (Powder) G

Klorvess $

Kolyum $

Generic Ingredient: Potassium (Effervescent Tablets) G

Effer-K

K + Care ET

Klor-Con/EF $

Klorvess $

K-Lyte

K-Lyte/Cl

K-Lyte/Cl 50

K-Lyte DS

Generic Ingredient: Potassium Chloride (Controlled-Release) G

K + 8

K + 10

Kaon-Cl-10

K-Dur 10

K-Dur 20

K-Lease

Klor-Con 8

Klor-Con 10

Klotrix

K-Norm

K-Tab

Micro-K Extencaps

Micro-K 10 Extencaps

Slow-K

Ten-K

Generic Ingredient: Potassium Gluconate (Tablets) G

Only available in generic form.

Prescribed For

Hypokalemia (low blood-potassium levels) and mild hypertension (high blood pressure).

General Information

A major component of body fluids, potassium helps to maintain electrolyte balance, kidney function, and blood pressure. Low potassium levels, which can affect the central nervous system (CNS) and heart functions, are usually caused by extended diuretic treatment, severe diarrhea, vomiting, complications of diabetes, or other medical conditions.

Potassium supplements are available in different types and forms. Potassium chloride is most often prescribed because it contains the most potassium per unit weight. Another advantage of potassium chloride is that it provides chloride ion, another important body-fluid component. Potassium gluconate provides about ⅓ as much potassium as the chloride, so you have to take 3 times as much to get an equal dose of potassium. However, it is preferable to potassium chloride in circumstances where chloride is undesirable.

Cautions and Warnings

Potassium replacement therapy should always be monitored and controlled by your doctor.

Potassium tablets have caused **ulcers of the esophagus** in some people with compression of the esophagus, who should use the liquid form. Potassium tablets have been reported to cause **small bowel ulcer,** leading to bleeding, obstruction, or perforation (formation of a hole through the bowel into the abdomen). **Seniors,** people with **diabetes, scleroderma,** and people who have had **mitral valve replacement** may be at higher risk for ulcers.

People who take potassium may develop **hyperkalemia** (high blood-potassium levels). Hyperkalemia can develop rapidly, without warning or symptoms, and is potentially fatal. It is often discovered through an EKG, but the following symptoms may also occur: tingling in the hands and feet, a feeling of heaviness or weakness in the muscles, listlessness, confusion, low blood pressure, extreme difficulty moving the arms and legs, abnormal heart rhythms, weak pulse, loss of consciousness, pallor, restlessness, and low urine output.

Do not take potassium if you are **dehydrated** or experiencing **muscle cramps** due to excessive sun exposure. Potassium should be used with caution in people with **kidney or heart disease** or untreated **Addison's disease**.

Possible Side Effects

▼ Most common: nausea, vomiting, diarrhea, gas, and abdominal discomfort.

▼ Less common: rash, tingling in hands or feet, weakness and heaviness in the legs, listlessness, mental confusion, decreased blood pressure, and heart-rhythm changes.

Drug Interactions

• Potassium supplements should not be taken with the potassium-sparing diuretics spironolactone or triamterene. Severe hyperkalemia may occur.

• Combining potassium supplements with an angiotensin-converting enzyme (ACE) inhibitor may result in hyperkalemia.

• People taking digitalis drugs must keep their blood-potassium levels within acceptable limits. Too little potassium in the blood may increase digitalis side effects and toxic reactions.

Food Interactions

Eating excess salt contributes to the problem of potassium depletion. Salt substitutes contain large amounts of potassium; do not use them while taking a potassium supplement unless directed by your doctor. If stomach upset occurs, take potassium supplements with food.

Usual Dose

16–100 milliequivalents (meq) a day.

Overdosage

Symptoms include muscle weakness, tingling in the hands or feet, a feeling of heaviness in the legs, listlessness, confusion, breathing difficulties, low blood pressure, shock, abnormal heart rhythms, and heart attack. Call your local poison control center or a hospital emergency room for more information. If you seek treatment, ALWAYS bring the prescription bottle or container.

Special Information

Directions for taking and using any potassium supplement must be followed closely. Effervescent tablets, powders, and liquids should be properly and completely dissolved, or diluted in 3 to 8 oz. of cold water or juice and drunk slowly. Noneffervescent tablets or capsules should never be chewed or crushed; they must be swallowed whole, preferably after a meal and with a full glass of water.

Many of the controlled-release potassium supplements contain potassium distributed throughout an indigestible wax core or matrix; you may notice the depleted wax matrix in your stool several hours after swallowing a tablet. This is normal and not a cause for alarm.

Call your doctor at once if you experience tingling in your hands or feet, a feeling of heaviness in the legs, unusual tiredness or weakness, nausea, vomiting, continued abdominal pain, or black stool.

If you forget a dose, take it right away if you remember within 2 hours of your regular time. If you do not remember until later, skip the dose you forgot and go back to your regular schedule. Do not take a double dose.

Special Populations

Pregnancy/Breast-feeding

The safety of using potassium salts is not known. When this medication is considered crucial by your doctor, its potential benefits must be carefully weighed against its risks.

Normal doses of potassium supplements add little to the potassium already in breast milk. Nursing mothers may take potassium supplements.

Seniors

Seniors may be at higher risk for ulcers caused by potassium supplements.

Generic Name

Pramipexole (pram-ih-PEX-ole)

Brand Name

Mirapex

Type of Drug

Antiparkinsonian.

Prescribed For

Parkinson's disease.

General Information

Pramipexole is thought to relieve symptoms of Parkinson's disease by stimulating dopamine receptors in the brain. Studies of pramipexole in people with early Parkinson's disease showed improvement after 4 weeks of treatment. People with advanced Parkinson's disease showed improvement after 6 months.

Cautions and Warnings

Do not take pramipexole if you are **sensitive** or **allergic** to it. Pramipexole may cause **low blood pressure** and make you **dizzy or faint** when rising from a sitting or lying position, especially during the early stages of treatment. About 1 in 10 to 15 people who take pramipexole experience hallucinations that may be serious enough to require stopping drug therapy.

One person taking pramipexole developed a disease in which **skeletal muscle** is destroyed.

People who stop taking other antiparkinsonians may develop **high fever** and **confusion**. Breathing difficulties caused by lung changes have also occurred with other antiparkinsonians. These symptoms have not been associated with pramipexole, but there is a risk that you may experience similar problems if you stop taking pramipexole.

Possible Side Effects

Early Parkinson's Disease

▼ Most common: sleepiness or tiredness and nausea.

▼ Common: sleeplessness, hallucinations, and constipation.

▼ Less common: dizziness, confusion, memory loss, reduced touch sensation, loss of muscle tone, a tendency to frequently change positions or pace the floor, odd thoughts, loss of sex drive, impotence, unusual muscle spasms, swelling in the arms or legs, generalized swelling, appetite loss, difficulty swallowing, weight loss, weakness, feeling unwell, fever, and abnormal vision.

Advanced Parkinson's Disease

▼ Most common: dizziness or fainting when rising from a sitting or lying position, abnormal movements, tremors, muscle rigidity, and hallucinations.

▼ Common: sleeplessness.

▼ Less common: accidental injury, weakness, generalized swelling, chest pain, feeling unwell, dizziness, abnormal dreaming, confusion, sleepiness, unusual muscle spasms, unusual walking, muscle stiffness, memory loss, a tendency to frequently change positions or pace the floor, odd thoughts, paranoid reactions, delusions, sleeping problems, frequent urination, urinary infection, loss of urinary control, swelling in the arms or

Possible Side Effects *(continued)*

legs, arthritis, twitching, bursitis, muscle weakness, breathing difficulties, runny nose, pneumonia, visual difficulties, difficulty focusing, double vision, constipation, dry mouth, and rash.

Drug Interactions

• Pramipexole increases levodopa blood levels and may worsen the uncontrolled muscle spasms that occur with levodopa. Your doctor may reduce your levodopa dosage.

• Cimetidine increases the amount of pramipexole absorbed by 50% and lengthens the time it takes for pramipexole to leave your body by 40%. Dose adjustment may be required if you take both drugs.

• Drugs that are eliminated through the kidneys—including cimetidine, ranitidine, diltiazem, triamterene, verapamil, quinidine, and quinine—reduce by 20% the ability to clear pramipexole from the body. Dosage adjustment may be required.

• Phenothiazine tranquilizers, haloperidol and similar tranquilizers, thioxanthene tranquilizers, metoclopramide, and other drugs that antagonize the effects of dopamine can reduce the effect of pramipexole.

• Pramipexole increases the sedative effect of tranquilizers, sleeping pills, and other nervous-system depressants.

Food Interactions

You may take this drug with food to prevent nausea.

Usual Dose

Adult: 0.125 mg 3 times a day to start, gradually increasing to a maximum of 4.5 mg a day. Dosage is reduced for people with kidney disease.

Overdosage

Little is known about the effects of pramipexole overdose. Symptoms are likely to include the most common side effects. Take the victim to a hospital emergency room. ALWAYS bring the prescription bottle or container.

Special Information

Take this drug exactly as prescribed.

Pramipexole causes sedation. Be careful when driving or performing any task that requires concentration. Avoid alcohol and other nervous system depressants.

Call your doctor if you develop hallucinations or any bothersome or persistent side effect.

If you forget a dose, take it as soon as you remember. Space the remaining daily dosage evenly throughout the day. Continue with your regular schedule on the next day. Do not take a double dose.

Special Populations

Pregnancy/Breast-feeding

The safety of using pramipexole during pregnancy is not known. When this drug is considered crucial by your doctor, its potential benefits must be carefully weighed against its risks.

It is not known if pramipexole passes into breast milk but this drug can interfere with milk production. Nursing mothers who must take this drug should bottle-feed.

Seniors

Seniors are more likely to experience side effects.

Pravachol *see Statin Cholesterol-Lowering Agents,*

page 987

Generic Name

Prazosin (PRAY-zoe-sin) Ⓖ

Brand Name

Minipress   Minipress XL

Combination Products

Generic Ingredients: Prazosin + Polythiazide
Minizide

Type of Drug

Antihypertensive.

Prescribed For

High blood pressure, benign prostatic hyperplasia (BPH), congestive heart failure (CHF), and Raynaud's disease. Prasozin combined with the diuretic polythiazide is used to treat high blood pressure.

General Information

Prazosin hydrochloride and other alpha-adrenergic blocking agents, or alpha blockers, reduce blood pressure by dilating (widening) blood vessels. They achieve this effect by blocking nerve endings known as alpha$_1$ receptors. The maximum blood-pressure-lowering effect of prazosin is seen between 2 and 6 hours after taking a dose. Prazosin's effect in CHF is seen within 1 hour of taking the drug. In BPH treatment, prazosin works by relaxing smooth muscles in the prostate and neck of the bladder. Despite the fact that prazosin reduces the symptoms of BPH, the drug's long-term effect on complications of BPH or the need for urinary surgery is not known. Prazosin's effect lasts between 6 and 10 hours. It is broken down in the liver.

Cautions and Warnings

Prazosin may cause **dizziness** and **fainting,** especially the first few doses. This is known as the first-dose effect, which can be minimized by limiting the first dose to 1 mg at bedtime. First-dose effects occur in about 1% of people taking an alpha blocker and may recur if the drug is stopped for a few days and then restarted.

People who are **allergic** or **sensitive** to any alpha blocker should avoid prazosin.

Prazosin may slightly reduce cholesterol levels and improve the ratio of high-density lipoprotein (HDL)—"good" cholesterol—and low-density lipoprotein (LDL), a positive step for people with a blood-cholesterol problem.

Possible Side Effects

Side effects occur less often with prazosin than with other alpha blockers.

▼ Most common: dizziness, drowsiness, weakness, nausea, headache, and heart palpitations.

Possible Side Effects *(continued)*

▼ Less common: low blood pressure, dizziness when rising from a sitting or lying position, rapid heartbeat, vomiting, dry mouth, diarrhea, constipation, abdominal pain or discomfort, breathing difficulties, stuffy nose, nosebleed, joint or muscle pain, blurred vision, conjunctivitis (pinkeye), ringing or buzzing in the ears, depression, nervousness, tingling in the hands or feet, frequent urination, impotence, poor urinary control, painful erection, itching, sweating, rash, hair loss, fluid retention, and fever.

Drug Interactions

• Prazosin may interact with beta blockers to increase the risk of dizziness or fainting after the first dose of prazosin.

• The blood-pressure-lowering effect of prazosin may be reduced by indomethacin.

• When taken with verapamil, prazosin produces an exaggerated reduction of blood pressure.

• The blood-pressure-lowering effect of clonidine may be reduced by prazosin.

• People taking this drug for high blood pressure should avoid over-the-counter cough medicine, cold and allergy remedies, and appetite suppressants. These products often contain stimulant ingredients that can increase blood pressure.

• People taking prazosin should avoid alcohol, which may increase the risk of low blood pressure.

Food Interactions

None known.

Usual Dose

1 mg 2–3 times a day to start; may be increased to a total daily dose of 20 mg although 40 mg a day has been used in some cases.

Overdosage

Overdose may produce drowsiness, poor reflexes, and very low blood pressure. Overdose victims should be taken to a hospital emergency room immediately. ALWAYS bring the prescription bottle or container.

Special Information

Take prazosin exactly as prescribed. Do not stop taking prazosin unless directed to do so by your doctor.

Prazosin may cause dizziness, headache, and drowsiness, especially 2 to 6 hours after you take your first dose, although these effects can persist after the first few doses. Use caution when getting up from a sitting or lying position.

Call your doctor if you develop severe dizziness, heart palpitations, or any bothersome or persistent side effect.

Wait 12 to 24 hours after taking your first dose of prazosin before driving or doing anything that requires intense concentration. Take your dose at bedtime to minimize this problem.

If you forget a dose, take it as soon as you remember. If it is almost time for your next dose, skip the dose you forgot and continue with your regular schedule. Do not take a double dose.

Special Populations

Pregnancy/Breast-feeding

The safety of using prazosin during pregnancy is not known, although animal studies have shown that alpha blockers may affect fetal development. When this drug is considered crucial by your doctor, its potential benefits must be carefully weighed against its risks.

Small amounts of prazosin pass into breast milk. Nursing mothers who must take this drug should bottle-feed.

Seniors

Seniors, especially those with CHF or kidney disease, may be more sensitive to the side effects of prazosin.

Premarin   see **Estrogens,** page 445

Prempro   see **Estrogens,** page 445

Prevacid   see **Proton-Pump Inhibitors,** page 906

Prilosec *see Proton-Pump Inhibitors, page 906*

Generic Name

Procainamide (proe-KAY-nuh-mide) Ⓖ

Brand Names

Procan-SR
Procanbid
Promine

Pronestyl
Pronestyl-SR

Type of Drug

Antiarrhythmic.

Prescribed For

Abnormal heart rhythms.

General Information

Procainamide hydrochloride works by slowing the response of heart muscle to nervous-system stimulation. It also slows the rate at which nervous-system impulses are carried through the heart. Procainamide begins working 30 minutes after you take it and continues working for 3 or more hours. As with other antiarrhythmic drugs, studies have not proven that people who take procainamide live longer than people who do not take it.

Sustained-release or long-acting forms of generic procainamide may not be equivalent to each other and should not be interchanged without your doctor's knowledge.

Cautions and Warnings

About 1 in 200 people taking procainamide in the usual dosage range develop bone marrow depression, a drastic drop in white-blood-cell count, low platelet count, or other **abnormalities of blood components**. Because these abnormalities happen most often during the first 3 months of taking procainamide, you should be checked with weekly blood counts during your first 3 months on this drug.

Procainamide and other antiarrhythmic agents should be taken only by patients with **life-threatening ventricular arrhythmias.**

Procainamide should not be taken by people who have complete **heart block** or the arrhythmia called **"torsade de pointes."** Long-term use may cause up to 30% of people taking procainamide to test positive for **lupus erythematosus** (long-term condition affecting the body's connective tissues). If you already have this condition, you should not take procainamide.

If you have **myasthenia gravis,** tell your doctor when procainamide is first prescribed; you should be taking a drug other than procainamide. You should also tell your doctor if you are **allergic** to procainamide or to the local anesthetic **procaine**.

Procainamide may aggravate congestive **heart failure**.

This drug is eliminated from the body through the kidney and liver. If you have either **kidney or liver disease,** your dosage of procainamide may have to be adjusted.

Possible Side Effects

▼ Common: appetite loss; nausea; itching; symptoms resembling the disease lupus erythematosus (fever and chills, nausea, vomiting, muscle aches, skin lesions, arthritis, and abdominal pains); enlargement of the liver or changes in blood tests that indicate a change in the liver; soreness of the mouth or throat; unusual bleeding; rash; and fever. If any of these symptoms occur while you are taking procainamide, tell your doctor immediately.

▼ Less common: bitter taste in the mouth, vomiting, diarrhea, weakness, dizziness, mental depression, giddiness, hallucinations, and drug allergy (symptoms include rash, itching, and fever).

Drug Interactions

• Procainamide blood levels and the risk of side effects are increased by propranolol and other beta blockers; cimetidine, ranitidine, and other H_2 antagonists; quinidine; and trimethoprim.

• Procainamide may increase the action of lidocaine, producing dangerous side effects. Procainamide may also increase the effects of succinylcholine.

• Do not take procainamide with other antiarrhythmic drugs unless specifically instructed by your doctor. These combinations can depress heart function.

• The interaction between alcohol and procainamide is variable and may alter the effects of procainamide.

• Avoid over-the-counter (OTC) cough, cold, or allergy remedies containing drugs that have a stimulating effect on the heart. Ask your pharmacist about the ingredients in OTC remedies.

Food Interactions

This medication is best taken on an empty stomach, but you may take it with food if it upsets your stomach.

Usual Dose

Starting dosage—1000 mg in divided doses. Maintenance dosage—23 mg a day per lb. of body weight, in doses every 3 hours around the clock, adjusted according to individual needs. Taking a sustained-release product allows doses to be spaced 6 hours apart. Seniors and people with kidney or liver disease are treated with lower dosages or given the medication less often.

Overdosage

Symptoms include abnormal heart rhythms, slow heart rate, low blood pressure, tremors, and nervous-system depression. Overdose victims should be taken to an emergency room immediately. ALWAYS bring the prescription bottle or container.

Special Information

Call your doctor at once if you develop any sign of infection, including fever, chills, sore throat, or mouth sores, or if you develop any of the following: joint or muscle pain, dark urine, wheezing, weakness, chest or abdominal pains, heart palpitations, nausea, vomiting, diarrhea, appetite loss, dizziness, depression, hallucinations, or unusual bruising or bleeding.

Be sure you discuss with your doctor any drug sensitivity or reaction, especially to procaine or other local anesthetics or to aspirin. Also, be sure your doctor knows if you have heart failure, lupus erythematosus, liver or kidney disease, or myasthenia gravis.

Because procainamide is taken so frequently during the day, it is essential that you follow your doctor's directions about taking your medicine. Taking more medicine will not necessarily help you, and skipping doses or taking them less often than directed may lead to a loss of control over your heart problem.

If you forget to take a dose of procainamide and remember within 2 hours, or within 4 hours if you are taking long-acting procainamide, take it right away. If it is almost time for your next dose, skip the one you forgot and continue with your regular schedule. Do not take a double dose.

Special Populations

Pregnancy/Breast-feeding

Procainamide passes into the fetal circulation. When this drug is considered crucial by your doctor, its potential benefits must be carefully weighed against its risks.

This drug passes into breast milk. Nursing mothers who must take it should bottle-feed.

Seniors

Seniors are more sensitive to procainamide.

Generic Name

Prochlorperazine (proe-klor-PER-uh-zeen) Ⓖ

Brand Name

Compazine
Compazine Spansule

Compro

Type of Drug

Antinauseant and phenothiazine antipsychotic.

Prescribed For

Severe nausea and vomiting; also prescribed for psychotic disorders such as excessive anxiety, tension, and agitation.

General Information

Prochlorperazine and other phenothiazine drugs act on a portion of the brain called the hypothalamus. They affect areas of the hypothalamus that control metabolism, body temperature, alertness, muscle tone, hormone balance, and vomiting. How phenothiazines work is not completely understood.

Cautions and Warnings

Prochlorperazine may depress the **gag (cough) reflex**. Some people who have taken this drug have accidentally choked to death because the gag reflex failed to respond. Because it can prevent vomiting, prochlorperazine **may obscure symptoms of disease or toxicity** due to drug overdose.

Do not take prochlorperazine if you are **allergic** to it or any phenothiazine drug or have **very high or low blood pressure, Parkinson's disease,** or **blood, lung, liver, kidney, or heart disease**. If you have **glaucoma, epilepsy, ulcers, intestinal obstruction,** or **difficulty passing urine,** prochlorperazine should be used with caution and under the strict supervision of your doctor.

Because this drug may both increase the risk of **Reye's syndrome** and mask its symptoms, it should not be used to treat vomiting in children when the underlying cause is unknown. It should be used with caution in children with acute illnesses such as **chickenpox, measles, central nervous system (CNS) infections, gastroenteritis,** or any illness that causes **dehydration**.

Some people taking prochlorperazine develop **tardive dyskinesia** (symptoms include lip smacking or puckering, puffing of the cheeks, rapid or worm like tongue movements, uncontrolled chewing motions, and uncontrolled arm and leg movements). This risk increases with long-term use of the medication.

Avoid **extreme heat** because prochlorperazine can upset your body's temperature-control mechanism.

Possible Side Effects

▼ Most common: drowsiness, especially during the first or second week of therapy. If the drowsiness becomes troublesome, call your doctor. Prochlorperazine can cause jaundice (symptoms include yellowing of the skin or whites of the eyes), typically within the first 4 weeks of treatment. It usually goes away when the drug is discontinued. If you notice this effect or feel feverish or unwell, call your doctor immediately.

Possible Side Effects *(continued)*

▼ Less common: changes in blood components including anemia (condition characterized by a reduction in the number of red blood cells or amount of hemoglobin or blood), raised or lowered blood pressure, abnormal heart rate, heart attack, feeling faint, and dizziness. Phenothiazines may produce extrapyramidal effects such as spasm of the neck muscles, rolling back of the eyes, convulsions, difficulty swallowing, and symptoms associated with Parkinson's disease. These effects look very serious but disappear after the drug is withdrawn; however, face, tongue, and jaw symptoms may persist for several years, especially in seniors with a history of brain damage. If you experience extrapyramidal effects, contact your doctor immediately.

▼ Rare: Prochlorperazine may cause an increase in psychotic symptoms or cause paranoid reactions. Other rare side effects can occur in almost any part of the body. Contact your doctor if you experience any side effect not listed above.

Drug Interactions

• Be cautious about combining prochlorperazine and barbiturates, sleeping pills, narcotics, tranquilizers, other phenothiazines, or other drugs that produce a depressive effect. Avoid alcohol.

• Aluminum antacids may reduce the effectiveness of prochlorperazine. Anticholinergic drugs may reduce the effectiveness of prochlorperazine and increase the risk of side effects.

• Prochlorperazine may reduce the effects of bromocriptine and appetite suppressants. The blood-pressure-lowering effect of guanethidine may be counteracted by this drug.

• Combining lithium and prochlorperazine may lead to disorientation, loss of consciousness, and uncontrolled muscle movements. Combining propranolol and prochlorperazine may lead to unusually low blood pressure.

• Combining phenytoin and prochlorperazine may either increase or decrease phenytoin levels in the blood.

• Prochlorperazine may increase blood levels of tricyclic antidepressant and the risk or their side effects.

Food Interactions

Prochlorperazine's effectiveness as an antipsychotic may be counteracted by beverages or foods containing caffeine.

Usual Dose

Adult: by mouth for nausea and vomiting—15–40 mg a day; rectal suppositories—25 mg twice a day; psychosis—15–150 mg a day.

Child (40–85 lbs.): 2.5 mg 3 times a day or 5 mg 2 times a day. The syrup form contains 5 mg of prochlorperazine per tsp.

Child (30–39 lbs.): 2.5 mg 2–3 times a day.

Child (20–29 lbs.): 2.5 mg 1–2 times a day.

Child (under age 2 or 20 lbs.): not recommended unless considered to be life-saving. Usually only 1–2 days of therapy are needed to relieve nausea and vomiting.

Overdosage

Symptoms include depression, extreme weakness, tiredness or a desire to sleep, lowered blood pressure, uncontrolled muscle spasms, agitation, restlessness, convulsions, fever, dry mouth, abnormal heart rhythms, and coma. Take the victim to a hospital emergency room immediately. ALWAYS bring the prescription bottle or container.

Special Information

Prochlorperazine is a tranquilizer and may have a depressive effect, especially during the first few days of therapy. Be careful when driving or performing any task that requires concentration.

Call your doctor if you develop sore throat, fever, rash, weakness, tremors, visual disturbances, or yellowing of the skin or whites of the eyes.

Do not take any over-the-counter medications without first consulting your doctor.

Prochlorperazine may cause increased sensitivity to the sun. It may also turn your urine reddish-brown to pink; this is not a cause for concern.

If dizziness occurs, avoid sudden changes in posture and climbing stairs. Use caution in hot weather because this medication may make you more prone to heatstroke.

The liquid form of prochlorperazine may cause skin irritation or rash; do not get it on your skin. Liquid prochlorperazine must be protected from light. Do not remove it from its opaque bottle.

If you miss a dose, take it as soon as you remember. If it is almost time for your next dose, skip the dose you forgot and go back to your regular schedule. Do not take a double dose.

Special Populations

Pregnancy/Breast-feeding

Taking prochlorperazine during pregnancy may cause jaundice and CNS effects in newborns. When this drug is considered crucial by your doctor, its potential benefits must be carefully weighed against its risks.

Prochlorperazine may pass into breast milk. Nursing mothers who must take it should consider bottle-feeding.

Seniors

Seniors are more sensitive to prochlorperazine's effects and usually require lower dosages to achieve desired results. Some experts feel that they should be treated with 25% to 50% of the usual adult dosage.

Generic Name

Promethazine (proe-METH-uh-zeen) G

Brand Name

Phenergan
Prometh Plain

Promethacon
Promethegen

Combination Products

Generic Ingredients: Promethazine + Codeine Phosphate G
Pentazine VC with Codeine Liquid A
Phenergan with Codeine Syrup
Pherazine with Codeine Syrup
Prometh with Codeine Syrup

Generic Ingredients: Promethazine + Dextromethorphan Hydrobromide G
Phenergan with Dextromethorphan Syrup
Phenameth DM Syrup A
Pherazine DM Syrup
Prometh with Dextromethorphan Syrup

Generic Ingredients: Promethazine + Phenylephrine Hydrochloride G
Phenergan VC Syrup
Promethazine VC Plain Syrup
Prometh VC Plain Liquid A

Generic Ingredients: Promethazine + Codeine Phosphate + Phenylephrine Hydrochloride G
Phenergan VC with Codeine Syrup
Pherazine VC with Codeine Syrup
Prometh VC with Codeine Liquid A
Promethist with Codeine Syrup A

Type of Drug

Antihistamine.

Prescribed For

Allergy, motion sickness, nausea, vomiting, nighttime seda-tion, and pain relief. Combination products are used to treat cough and stuffy/runny nose due to allergy or cold.

General Information

Promethazine hydrochloride, one of the older members of the phenothiazine antihistamine group, is used alone and in combination with cough suppressants and decongestants.

Cautions and Warnings

Do not use promethazine if you are **allergic** to it or if you can-not tolerate any other phenothiazine drug such as chlorpro-mazine and prochlorperazine.

Promethazine should be used with caution if you have **very low blood pressure; sleep apnea; Parkinson's disease; intesti-nal obstruction; or heart, blood, respiratory, liver, or kidney disease**. This drug should be used under your doctor's strict supervision if you have an **ulcer,** a **seizure disorder, bone-marrow depression, glaucoma,** or **urinary difficulties,** includ-ing an enlarged prostate.

Children with **liver disease,** any illness that causes **dehydra-tion,** a history of **sleep apnea,** a family history of **sudden infant death syndrome** (SIDS), or **Reye's syndrome** should not take promethazine.

This medication is not recommended for any child under age 2.

Possible Side Effects

The suppositories can cause rectal burning or stinging.

▼ Most common: drowsiness, thick mucus, and sedation.

▼ Less common: sore throat and fever; unusual bleeding or bruising; tiredness; weakness; dizziness; feeling faint; clumsiness; unsteadiness; dry mouth, nose, or throat; facial redness; breathing difficulties; hallucinations; confusion; seizure; muscle spasm, especially in the back and neck; restlessness; a shuffling walk; jerky movements of the head and face; shaking and trembling of the hands; blurred vision or other changes in vision; urinary difficulties; rapid heartbeat; sensitivity to the sun; increased sweating; and appetite loss. Children and older adults are more likely to develop difficulty sleeping, excitability, nervousness, restlessness, or irritability.

Drug Interactions

• This drug should not be taken with a monoamine oxidase inhibitor (MAOI) antidepressant.

• The sedating effects of promethazine are increased by central nervous system (CNS) depressants including tranquilizers, alcohol, hypnotics, sedatives, antianxiety drugs, and narcotics. These combinations should be used with extreme caution.

• Promethazine will antagonize the effects of amphetamines and other appetite suppressants such as diet pills.

• The combination of promethazine and an oral antithyroid drug may increase the risk of agranulocytosis (condition characterized by a reduction in the number of white blood cells).

• The combination of quinidine and promethazine may increase the cardiac effects of both drugs.

• Increasing the dosage of anticonvulsant medication, bromocriptine, guanadrel, guanethidine, or levodopa may be necessary when any of these drugs are taken with promethazine.

• Riboflavin requirements are increased in people taking promethazine.

• Promethazine may interfere with blood-sugar tests and home pregnancy tests.

Food Interactions

Take promethazine with food if it upsets your stomach.

Usual Dose

Allergy
    Adult: 12.5 mg before meals and 12.5–25 mg at bedtime.
    Child (age 2 and over): 6.25–12.5 mg 3 times a day or 25 mg at bedtime.

Motion Sickness
    Adult: 12.5–25 mg half an hour before travel; repeat in 8–12 hours if needed. Then take 1 dose upon arising and another before dinner.
    Child (age 2 and over): 12.5–25 mg 2 times a day.

Nausea and Vomiting
    Adult: 12.5–25 mg when needed, up to 6 times a day if necessary.
    Child (age 2 and over): 10–25 mg when needed, or 0.5 mg per lb. of body weight; 10–25 mg every 4–6 hours if necessary.

Nighttime Sedation
    Adult: 25–50 mg at bedtime.
    Child (age 2 and over): 12.5–25 mg at bedtime.

Overdosage

Symptoms include drowsiness; confusion; clumsiness; dry mouth, nose, or throat; hallucinations; seizure; and other promethazine side effects. Overdose victims should be taken to a hospital emergency room for treatment. ALWAYS bring the prescription bottle or container.

Special Information

Be careful when performing tasks requiring concentration and coordination, such as driving, because the drug may cause tiredness, dizziness, or light-headedness. Avoid alcohol.

Call your doctor if you develop sore throat; dry mouth, nose, or throat; fever; chills; unusual bleeding or bruising; tiredness; weakness; clumsiness; unsteadiness; hallucinations; seizure; sleeping problems; feeling faint; flushing; breathing difficulties; or any bothersome or persistent side effect.

Maintain good dental hygiene while taking promethazine because dry mouth may cause you to be more susceptible to oral infections. If the dry mouth caused by promethazine is not eased by gum or hard candy or lasts more than 2 weeks, call your doctor or dentist. Any dental work should be completed prior to starting on this drug.

If you forget a dose of promethazine, take it as soon as you remember. If you take it twice a day and it is almost time for your next dose, take 1 dose right away and another in 5 or 6 hours, then continue with your regular schedule. If you take promethazine 3 or more times a day and forget a dose, take it as soon as you remember. If it is almost time for your next dose, take 1 dose right away and another in 3 or 4 hours, then continue with your regular schedule. Never take a double dose.

Special Populations

Pregnancy/Breast-feeding

Babies born to women who took phenothiazines have suffered side effects at birth such as yellowing of the skin and whites of the eyes, CNS effects, and blood-clotting problems. Do not take any antihistamine without your doctor's knowledge if you are or might be pregnant—especially during the last 3 months of pregnancy—because newborns may have severe reactions to antihistamines.

Nursing mothers who must take promethazine should bottle-feed.

Seniors

Seniors are more sensitive to side effects and may require lower dosages.

Generic Name

Propoxyphene Hydrochloride

(proe-POK-sih-fene hye-droe-KLOR-ide) G

Brand Names

Darvon Pulvules	Dolene
Darvon	Kesso-Gesic

Combination Products

Generic Ingredients: Propoxyphene Hydrochloride +
Aspirin + Caffeine Ⓖ
Darvon Compound

Generic Ingredients: Propoxyphene Hydrochloride +
Acetaminophen Ⓖ
Wygesic

The information in this profile also applies to the following
drugs:

Generic Ingredient: Propoxyphene Napsylate
Darvon-N

Generic Ingredients: Propoxyphene Napsylate +
Acetaminophen Ⓖ
Darvocet-N 50   Propacet 100
Darvocet-N 100

Type of Drug

Analgesic.

Prescribed For

Mild to moderate pain.

General Information

A chemical derivative of methadone (a narcotic pain reliever),
propoxyphene hydrochloride is widely used for mild pain. It
is estimated that propoxyphene hydrochloride is about ½ to
⅔ as strong a pain reliever as codeine and about as equally
effective as aspirin. Propoxyphene hydrochloride is more
effective when combined with aspirin or acetaminophen than
when used alone. Propoxyphene hydrochloride is about 30%
more potent than propoxyphene napsylate.

Cautions and Warnings

Do not take propoxyphene hydrochloride if you are **allergic** to
it or to similar drugs. This medication should be used with
caution if you have **liver or kidney disease**.

Psychological or physical **drug dependence** (addiction)
may result when propoxyphene hydrochloride is taken in
doses larger than those needed for pain relief for long periods of time. The major sign of psychological dependence is

anxiety when the drug is suddenly stopped. People may also become physically addicted to propoxyphene hydrochloride; it can be abused to the same degree as codeine.

Never take more of this medication than is prescribed by your doctor. Use this medication with extreme caution if you also take **tranquilizers** or **antidepressants**.

Propoxyphene hydrochloride should be considered a **potentially dangerous drug,** especially in the hands of anyone with a history of addiction or severe depression. Excessive doses of propoxyphene hydrochloride, either by itself or together with alcohol or other central nervous system (CNS) depressants, are a major cause of **drug-related deaths**. Many of these deaths have occurred in people with a history of emotional disturbances, suicidal ideas or suicide attempts, and misuse of tranquilizers, alcohol, and other CNS depressants.

Propoxyphene hydrochloride should not be taken by **children**.

For Combination Products, see "Cautions and Warnings" in Acetaminophen (p. 13) for additional information.

Possible Side Effects

▼ Common: dizziness, sedation, nausea, and vomiting. These effects usually disappear if you lie down and relax for a few moments.

▼ Less common: constipation, stomach pain, rash, light-headedness, headache, weakness, euphoria (feeling "high"), dysphoria (feeling sad), hallucinations, and minor visual disturbances.

▼ Rare: jaundice.

Taking propoxyphene hydrochloride over long periods of time and in very high doses has caused subacute painful myopathy (muscle disease).

For Combination Products, see "Possible Side Effects" in Acetaminophen (p. 13) for additional information.

Drug Interactions

• Propoxyphene hydrochloride may cause drowsiness when taken with other drugs that cause drowsiness, such as tranquilizers, sedatives, hypnotics, narcotics, alcohol, and possibly antihistamines.

• Carbamazepine levels may be increased by propoxyphene hydrochloride, resulting in dizziness, nausea, and poor coordination.

• Charcoal tablets decrease the absorption of propoxyphene hydrochloride into the bloodstream.

• Cigarette smoking increases the rate at which this drug is broken down in the liver. Heavy smokers may need more propoxyphene hydrochloride to obtain pain relief but will have to take less of the drug if they stop smoking.

• Propoxyphene hydrochloride may increase the anticoagulant (blood-thinning) effect of warfarin.

• Combining propoxyphene hydrochloride and protease inhibitors is not recommended.

For Combination Products, see "Drug Interactions" in Acetaminophen (p. 13) for additional information.

Food Interactions

Take propoxyphene hydrochloride with a full glass of water or with food if it upsets your stomach.

Usual Dose

Propoxyphene Hydrochloride: 65 mg every 4 hours as needed.

Propoxyphene Napsylate: 100 mg every 4 hours as needed. Seniors and people with poor liver or kidney function may need to take the medication less often.

Overdosage

Symptoms include a decrease in respiratory rate, changes in breathing pattern, pinpointed pupils, convulsions, extreme sleepiness leading to stupor or coma, and abnormal heart rhythms. The overdose victim should be taken to a hospital emergency room immediately. ALWAYS bring the prescription bottle or container.

Special Information

Use caution while driving or performing any tasks that require you to be awake and alert. Avoid alcohol and other CNS depressants.

Call your doctor if you develop nausea or vomiting while taking this drug, or if you develop breathing difficulties.

If you forget a dose, take it as soon as you remember. If it is almost time for your next dose, skip the one you forgot and continue with your regular schedule. Do not take a double dose.

For Combination Products see "Special Information" in Acetaminophen (p. 13) for additional information.

Special Populations

Pregnancy/Breast-feeding
No clinical studies of this medication have been conducted in pregnant women, but a survey of almost 3,000 pregnant women who took propoxyphene hydrochloride found that 46—1.6%—had infants with birth defects. Animal studies show that high doses of the drug can cause problems in a fetus. Pregnant women who must take propoxyphene hydrochloride should talk to their doctor about the risks of this drug.

Small amounts of propoxyphene hydrochloride pass into breast milk. Nursing mothers who must take this drug should consider bottle-feeding.

Seniors
Seniors, especially those with reduced kidney or liver function, are more likely to be sensitive to the effects of this drug and should be treated with smaller dosages.

Generic Name

Propranolol (proe-PRAN-oe-lol) Ⓖ

Brand Name

Inderal   Innopran XL
Inderal LA

Combination Products

Generic Ingredients: Propranolol + Hydrochlorothiazide Ⓖ
Inderide   Inderide LA

Type of Drug

Beta-adrenergic blocking agent.

Prescribed For

High blood pressure, angina pectoris, abnormal heart rhythm, prevention of second heart attack or migraine, tremors, aggressive behavior, side effects of antipsychotic drugs, acute panic, stage fright and other anxieties, and schizophrenia; also used to treat bleeding from the stomach or esophagus, and symptoms of hyperthyroidism (overactive thyroid gland).

General Information

Propranolol hydrochloride is one of 15 beta-adrenergic blocking drugs, or beta blockers, that interfere with the action of a specific part of the nervous system. Beta receptors are found all over the body and affect many body functions. Each beta blocker has particular characteristics that make it more suitable for certain conditions or people.

Cautions and Warnings

Do not take propanolol if you are allergic to beta blockers.

You should be cautious about taking propranolol if you have **asthma, severe heart failure,** a very **slow heart rate,** or **heart block** (disruption of the electrical impulses that control heart rate) because the drug may aggravate these conditions.

People with **angina** who take propranolol for high blood pressure risk aggravating their angina if they suddenly stop taking the drug. These people should have their drug dosage reduced gradually over 1 to 2 weeks.

Propranolol should be used with caution if you have **liver or kidney disease** because your ability to eliminate this drug from your body may be impaired.

Propranolol reduces the amount of blood pumped by the heart with each beat. This reduction in blood flow may aggravate the condition of people with **poor circulation** or **circulatory disease.**

If you are undergoing **major surgery,** your doctor may want you to stop taking propranolol at least 2 days before surgery.

Possible Side Effects

Side effects are relatively uncommon and usually mild.

▼ Most common: impotence.

▼ Less common: tiredness or weakness, slow heartbeat, heart failure, dizziness, breathing difficulties,

Possible Side Effects *(continued)*

bronchospasm, depression, confusion, anxiety, nervousness, sleeplessness, disorientation, short-term memory loss, emotional instability, cold hands and feet, constipation, diarrhea, nausea, vomiting, upset stomach, increased sweating, urinary difficulties, cramps, blurred vision, rash, hair loss, stuffy nose, facial swelling, aggravation of lupus erythematosus, itching, chest pain, back or joint pain, colitis, drug allergy (symptoms include fever and sore throat), and liver toxicity.

Drug Interactions

- Propranolol may interact with surgical anesthetics to increase the risk of heart problems during surgery. Some anesthesiologists recommend gradually stopping the drug by 2 days before surgery.

- Propranolol may interfere with the normal signs of low blood sugar and with the action of oral antidiabetes medications.

- Propranolol increases the blood-pressure-lowering effect of other blood-pressure-reducing agents including clonidine, guanabenz, and reserpine, as well as calcium channel blockers such as nifedipine.

- Aspirin-containing drugs, indomethacin, sulfinpyrazone, and estrogen drugs may interfere with the blood-pressure-lowering effect of propranolol.

- Cocaine may reduce the effectiveness of all beta blockers.

- Propranolol may worsen the problem of cold hands and feet associated with ergot alkaloids, used to treat migraine. Gangrene is a possibility in people taking both ergot and propranolol.

- The effect of benzodiazepine antianxiety drugs may be increased by propranolol.

- Propranolol will counteract thyroid hormone replacements.

- Calcium channel blockers, flecainide, hydralazine, oral contraceptives, propafenone, haloperidol, phenothiazine tranquilizers—molindone and others—quinolone antibacterials, and quinidine may increase the amount of propranolol in the bloodstream and lead to increased propranolol effects.

• Propranolol should not be taken within 2 weeks of taking a monoamine oxidase inhibitor (MAOI) antidepressant.

• Cimetidine increases the amount of propranolol absorbed into the bloodstream from oral tablets.

• Propranolol may interfere with the effectiveness of some antiasthma medications including theophylline and aminophylline, and especially ephedrine and isoproterenol.

• Combining propranolol and phenytoin or digitalis drugs may result in excessive slowing of the heart, possibly causing heart block.

• Your propranolol dose may have to be reduced if you stop smoking because your liver will break down the drug more slowly after you stop.

• Aluminum salts, barbituates, calcium salts, cholestyramine, colestipol, ampicillin and rifampin may reduce the effectiveness of propranolol.

• Propanolol may increase the anticoagulant effect of warfarin.

Food Interactions

Although it is best to take propranolol without food or on an empty stomach, it is more important to be consistent about taking it with or without food in order to maintain consistent effects.

Usual Dose

30–700 mg a day.

Overdosage

Symptoms include changes in heartbeat—unusually slow, fast, or irregular; severe dizziness or fainting; breathing difficulties; bluish-colored fingernails or palms; and seizures. The victim should be taken to a hospital emergency room. ALWAYS bring the prescription bottle or container.

Special Information

Propranolol is for continuous use. Do not stop taking this drug unless directed to do so by your doctor: Abrupt withdrawal may cause chest pain, breathing difficulties, increased sweating, and unusually fast or irregular heartbeat. When ending propranolol treatment, dosage should be reduced gradually over a period of about 2 weeks.

Call your doctor at once if you develop back or joint pain, breathing difficulties, cold hands or feet, depression, rash, or

changes in heartbeat. Propranolol may produce an undesirable lowering of blood pressure, leading to dizziness or fainting; call your doctor if this happens to you. Call your doctor if you experience persistent or bothersome anxiety, diarrhea, constipation, impotence, headache, itching, nausea or vomiting, nightmares or vivid dreams, upset stomach, trouble sleeping, stuffy nose, frequent urination, unusual tiredness, or weakness.

Propranolol may cause drowsiness, light-headedness, dizziness, or blurred vision. Be careful when driving or performing complex tasks.

It is best to take propranolol at the same time each day. If you forget a dose, take it as soon as you remember. If you take propranolol once a day and it is within 8 hours of your next dose, skip the dose you forgot and continue with your regular schedule. If you take it twice a day and it is within 4 hours of your next dose, skip the dose you forgot and continue with your regular schedule. Never take a double dose.

Special Populations

Pregnancy/Breast-feeding

In studies, infants born to women who took a beta blocker while pregnant had lower birth weights, low blood pressure, and reduced heart rates. Propranolol should be avoided by pregnant women.

Propranolol passes into breast milk in concentrations too small to have any effect.

Seniors

Seniors may require less of the drug to achieve results. Seniors taking propranolol may be more likely to suffer from cold hands and feet, reduced body temperature, chest pain, general feelings of ill health, sudden breathing difficulties, increased sweating, or changes in heartbeat.

Type of Drug

Prostaglandin Agonists

Brand Names

Generic Ingredient: Bimatoprost
Lumigan

Generic Ingredient: Travoprost
Travatan

Generic Ingredient: Latanoprost
Xalatan

Generic Ingredient: Unoprostone
Rescula

Prescribed For

Open-angle glaucoma and ocular hypertension (high pressure inside the eye).

General Information

Prostaglandin agonists are believed to reduce pressure inside the eye by combining with prostaglandin receptors to increase the outflow of eye fluid. They are absorbed through the cornea, where all but bimatoprost are transformed into their active forms. Pressure is lowered within 2 hours and lasts up to 12 hours.

Cautions and Warnings

Do not use these medicines if you are **allergic** or **sensitive** to them. Sensitivity to one member of this group may not indicate sensitivity to all.

Prostaglandin agonists may change your **eye color** because they increase the number of pigment granules in the cornea, which in turn increases brown pigment in the iris. This color change occurs gradually over a period of months or years. Typically, the brown color around the pupil spreads slowly to the outer part of the iris. This change is more noticeable in people with green-brown, blue/gray-brown or yellow-brown eye color. The long-term effect of these medicines on eye pigment granules is not known; your doctor may tell you to stop using these eyedrops if the color change persists or is especially noticeable. They can also increase eyelash color and length, as well as the number of eyelashes.

The effect of prostaglandin agonists on the cornea is not known.

Possible Side Effects

▼ Most common: blurred vision; stinging, burning, itching and redness of the eyes; and brownish eye coloration.

Possible Side Effects *(continued)*

▼ Common: abnormal vision, eyelid problems, excessive tearing, and a sensation of something in the eye.

▼ Less common: dry eye, swelling or redness of the eyelid, eyelid discomfort, inflammation or pain, and increased sensitivity to bright light.

▼ Rare: blood clot in the artery supplying the retina, bleeding inside the eye, detachment of the retina, increased eye pressure, color blindness, corneal deposits, corneal swelling, droopy eyelid, and irritation of the iris.

Systemic side effects from traces of these drugs passing into the blood:

▼ Common: cold, flu, or other respiratory infections.

▼ Less common: muscle, joint, or back pain, accidental injury, chest pain, angina pain, bronchitis, cough, diabetes, dizziness, headache, high blood pressure, sleeplessness, sore throat, runny nose, sinus irritation, and rash or allergic reactions.

Drug Interactions

• If you use other eyedrops that contain a thimerosal preservative, separate the administration of each eyedrop by at least 5 minutes.

Usual Dose

Bimatoprost, Latanoprost, and Travoprost
   Adult: 1 drop in the affected eye every evening.
   Child: not recommended.

Unoprostone
   Adult: 1 drop in the affected eye 2 times a day.
   Child: not recommended.

Overdosage

Overdose symptoms include eye irritation and redness. Severe overdosage may also cause abdominal pain, dizziness, fatigue, flushing, nausea, and sweating. Call your doctor, local poison control center, or a hospital emergency room for more information. If you go to a hospital emergency room ALWAYS bring the prescription bottle or container.

Special Information

Call your doctor if you develop eye irritation or any other side effect.

If you use any other eye medication, wait 5 minutes between each application.

To prevent infection, keep the eyedropper from touching your fingers, eyelids, or any surface.

Contact your doctor immediately if you are having eye surgery, you experience an eye injury, or you develop an eye infection to determine if you should continue to use the eyedrops.

If you wear contact lenses, take them out before using these eyedrops. They contain a benzalkonium preservative that can be absorbed by the contacts.

Store unopened bottles of latanoprost in the refrigerator. Once opened, the eyedrops can be kept at room temperature—up to 77°F—for 6 weeks. All other products can be stored at room temperature and should be discarded 6–8 weeks after opening.

Do not take more medication than your doctor has prescribed. Taking it more often may actually reduce its effectiveness. If you forget to administer a dose, do so as soon as you remember. If it is almost time for your next dose, skip the one you forgot and continue with your regular schedule. Do not take a double dose.

Special Populations

Pregnancy/Breast-feeding

Animal studies have shown that prostaglandin agonists may be harmful to the fetus at extremely high dosages. When your doctor considers this drug crucial, its potential benefits must be carefully weighed against its risks.

It is not known if these medications pass into breast milk. Nursing mothers who must use a prostaglandin agonist should consider bottle-feeding.

Seniors

Seniors may use these medicines without special precaution.

Protonix *see Proton-Pump Inhibitors, page 906*

Type of Drug

Proton-Pump Inhibitors

Brand Names

Generic Ingredient: Esomeporazole Magnesium
Nexium

Generic Ingredient: Lansoprazole
Prevacid

Generic Ingredients: Lansoprazole + Amoxicillin + Clarithromycin
Prevpac

Generic Ingredient: Omeprazole
Prilosec

Generic Ingredient: Pantoprozole
Protonix

Generic Ingredient: Rabeprazole
Aciphex

Prescribed For

Stomach or duodenal (upper intestinal) ulcers, gastroesophageal reflux disease (GERD), and conditions in which there is an excess of stomach acid; also used to treat and maintain healing of ulcers of the esophagus.

General Information

Proton pump inhibitors (PPIs) stop the production of stomach acid by interfering with the "proton pump" in the mucous lining of the stomach at the last stage of acid production. PPIs can turn off stomach acid production within 1 hour. These drugs are useful in treating conditions in which stomach acid plays a key role, as with ulcers and GERD. It is prescribed together with amoxicillin and clarithromycin for people with ulcers caused by Heliobacter pylori infections.

Cautions and Warnings

Do not take PPIs if you are **allergic** to them.

PPIs should not be taken as maintenance treatment for duodenal ulcers and are not recommended for treatment of GERD beyond 8 to16 weeks.

People with **liver disease** may need to take a lower dose of PPIs.

Possible Side Effects

Generally, PPIs cause few side effects. Those that may occur include headache, diarrhea, abdominal pain, nausea, sore throat, upper respiratory infection, fever, vomiting, dizziness, rash, constipation, muscle pain, unusual tiredness, cough, and back pain.

▼ Rare: Rare side effects can occur in almost any part of the body. Contact your doctor if you experience any side effect not listed above.

Drug Interactions

• PPIs may increase the effects of diazepam, phenytoin, and warfarin. They may also interact with other drugs broken down by the liver.

• Combining PPIs and clarithromycin may increase blood levels of both drugs.

• PPIs may interfere with the absorption of iron, ampicillin, and ketoconazole.

• PPIs may increase the effects of drugs that reduce the production of blood cells by bone marrow.

• Lansoprazole may reduce the amount of theophylline drugs in the blood.

Food Interactions

PPIs should be taken immediately before a meal, preferably breakfast. Esomeprazole must taken at least 1 hour before a meal.

Usual Dose

Esomeprazole

Adult: 20–40 mg a day, 1 hour before a meal. Capsules may be opened and mixed with a tablespoon of cool applesauce for people having difficulty swallowing. Eat the mixture right away and do not chew the pellets.

Child (under age 18): not recommended.

Lansoprazole

Adult: 30 mg 2 or 3 times a day. Capsules may be opened and mixed with a tablespoon of cool applesauce for people having difficulty swallowing. Dosage may be increased up to 120 mg a day. People with liver disease need a lower dosage.
Child: (under age 18): not recommended.

Omeprazole

Adult: 40 mg once a day for days 1–14, then 20 mg once a day for days 15–28. Antacids may be taken with omeprazole.
Child: (age 3 months–13 years): 20–60 mg a day.
Child: (under age 3 months): 0.22 mg per lb. of body weight a day.

Pantoprazole

Adult: 40 mg once a day, preferably in the morning, for 4–8 weeks. A second 8-week course of treatment may be prescribed.

Prevpac

2 amoxicillin (Trimox) capsules, 1 clarithromycin (Biaxin) tablet, and 1 lansoprazole (Prevacid) capsule before breakfast and dinner for 14 days.

Rabeprazole

Adult: 20 mg a day.
Child (under 18): not recommended.

Overdosage

Little is known about the effects of PPI overdose. Symptoms are likely to resemble side effects. Call your local poison control center or a hospital emergency room for more information. If you seek treatment, ALWAYS bring the prescription bottle or container.

Special Information

Call your doctor if you are unusually tired or weak, or if you develop a sore throat, fever, sores in the mouth that do not heal, unusual bleeding or bruising, bloody or cloudy urine, urinary difficulties, or any persistent or bothersome side effect.

Take the full course of treatment prescribed, even if your symptoms improve after 1 or 2 weeks.

Do not open, crush, or chew the capsule; swallow it whole.

If you forget a dose, take it as soon as you remember. If it is almost time for your next dose, skip the one you forgot and

continue with your regular schedule. Do not take a double dose.

Special Populations

Pregnancy/Breast-feeding

PPIs may be toxic to pregnant animals. When your doctor considers this drug crucial, its potential benefits must be carefully weighed against its risks.

It is not known if PPIs pass into breast milk. Nursing mothers who use this drug should consider bottle-feeding.

Seniors

Seniors report the same side effects as younger adults.

Generic Name

Quetiapine (kwe-TYE-uh-pene)

Brand Name

Seroquel

Type of Drug

Antipsychotic.

Prescribed For

Psychotic disorders and schizophrenia.

General Information

Quetiapine fumarate is effective against a wide variety of symptoms. It may work by antagonizing a number of different types of brain receptors. This means that the drug decreases levels of certain neurotransmitters including serotonin, dopamine, and histamine, by preventing them from binding to cell receptors. Quetiapine is broken down by the liver.

Cautions and Warnings

People who are **sensitive** or **allergic** to quetiapine should avoid it.

A potentially fatal condition called **neuroleptic malignant syndrome** (symptoms include convulsions, breathing difficulties, and back, neck, or leg pain) may occur with some antipsychotic drugs. People who have experienced this syndrome with another antipsychotic drug should be cautious when taking quetiapine.

Antipsychotic drugs are often associated with **involuntary, uncoordinated, and uncontrolled movements**. This reaction is most common among older adults, especially women. Call your doctor if you develop any unusual movements while taking quetiapine.

Quetiapine may make you **dizzy** or cause you to **faint** if you rise suddenly from a sitting or lying position. It should be used with caution if you have a history of **heart disease** including heart attack, angina pains, and abnormal heart rhythms. Take this drug with caution if you have a condition or take any drug that can cause **low blood pressure**.

People taking this drug for a long period have developed cataracts, but they have not been directly related to the drug. People taking quetiapine should have an eye exam when they start the drug and every 6 months thereafter to detect any cataract formation.

Quetiapine should be used with caution if you have had a **seizure,** or have a seizure disorder or other condition that may make you more susceptible to seizures, such as Alzheimer's disease.

Quetiapine treatment has been associated with low levels of **thyroid hormone** in the blood. This is usually not a problem, although a small percentage of people taking this drug may need a thyroid supplement.

Quetiapine may cause increases in **blood cholesterol** and **triglyceride** levels.

Quetiapine has caused **liver inflammation** without any symptoms, as measured by increases in enzymes produced by the liver. These enzymes generally return to normal with continued treatment.

The possibility of **suicide** exists in any person with schizophrenia. People at risk of suicide should keep only small amounts of medication at any time.

Quetiapine has been associated with **obesity, high cholesterol**, and **diabetes**.

Possible Side Effects

▼ Most common: dizziness, headache, upset stomach, tiredness, dizziness or fainting when rising from a sitting

Possible Side Effects

or lying position, abdominal pain, weight gain, and dry mouth.

▼ Common: swelling in the arms or legs, heart palpitations, spastic movements, difficulty talking, sore throat, runny nose, increased coughing, breathing difficulties, flu symptoms, appetite loss, sweating, and low white-blood-cell counts.

▼ Less common: other side effects can occur in almost any part of the body. Contact your doctor if you experience any side effect not listed above.

Drug Interactions

• Drinking alcohol while taking quetiapine can cause drowsiness.

• Quetiapine may antagonize the effects of levodopa and other drugs used to treat Parkinson's disease.

• Combining quetiapine with phenytoin increases the rate at which quetiapine is released from the body by 5 times. You may require an increase in quetiapine dosage to achieve the same effect. Once dosage has been adjusted, special caution should be taken if phenytoin is replaced by another anti-seizure drug that does not stimulate the body's breakdown of quetiapine. Other drugs that have a similar effect on quetiapine are thioridazine, carbamazepine, barbiturates, rifampin, and oral corticosteroids.

• Ketoconazole, itraconazole, fluconazole, and erythromycin may affect quetiapine. Caution should be exercised when combining these drugs with quetiapine.

• Quetiapine may reduce the rate at which the body clears lorazepam.

Food Interactions

Taking quetiapine with food increases the amount of drug absorbed by a small amount. This is not likely to change its effect on your body.

Usual Dose

Adult: 150–750 mg a day. Seniors may obtain maximum benefit with smaller doses.

Overdosage

Overdose victims should be taken to a hospital emergency room at once. ALWAYS bring the prescription bottle or container.

Special Information

Quetiapine may make you drowsy. Take care while driving or performing any task that requires concentration.

Antipsychotic drugs may increase your sensitivity to hot weather and your susceptibility to dehydration by interfering with temperature-control mechanisms.

Special Populations

Pregnancy/Breast-feeding

Quetiapine should only be taken during pregnancy if the possible benefits outweigh the risks. Talk to your doctor if you become pregnant or are trying to become pregnant while taking this drug.

Quetiapine passes into breast milk. Nursing mothers who must take quetiapine should bottle-feed.

Seniors

Seniors may be more sensitive to side effects, especially dizziness, fainting, and tiredness.

Generic Name

Quinapril (QUIN-uh-pril)

Brand Name

Accupril

Combination Products

Generic Ingredients: Quinapril + Hydrochlorothiazide
Accuretic 10/12.5   Accuretic 20/12.5

The information in this profile also applies to the following drugs:

Generic Ingredient: Perindopril
Aceon

Generic Ingredient: Ramipril
Altace

Type of Drug

Angiotensin-converting enzyme (ACE) inhibitor.

Prescribed For

High blood pressure and congestive heart failure.

General Information

Quinapril and other ACE inhibitors work by preventing the conversion of a hormone called angiotensin I to another hormone called angiotensin II, a potent blood-vessel constrictor. Preventing this conversion relaxes blood vessels, thus reducing blood pressure and relieving the symptoms of heart failure. Quinapril also affects the production of other hormones and enzymes that participate in the regulation of blood-vessel dilation. Quinapril begins working about 1 hour after you take it and lasts for 24 hours.

Some people who start taking an ACE inhibitor after they are already on a diuretic (an agent that increases urination) experience a rapid blood-pressure drop after their first doses or when the dosage is increased. To prevent this from happening, you may be told to stop taking the diuretic 2 or 3 days before starting the ACE inhibitor or to increase your salt intake during that time. The diuretic may then be restarted gradually.

Cautions and Warnings

Do not take quinapril if you have had an **allergic reaction** to it.

Quinapril occasionally causes **very low blood pressure**. Quinapril can affect your **kidneys,** especially if you have congestive **heart failure**. It is advisable for your doctor to check your urine for changes during the first few months of treatment. Dosage adjustment is necessary if you have reduced kidney function.

Rarely, quinapril affects white-blood-cell count, possibly increasing your susceptibility to **infection**. Blood counts should be monitored periodically.

Quinapril can cause fetal injury or death; do not take quinapril if you are **pregnant.**

Possible Side Effects

▼ Most common: dizziness, tiredness, headache, and chronic cough. The cough usually goes away a few days after you stop taking the medication.

▼ Less common: nausea, vomiting, and abdominal pain.

▼ Rare: Rare side effects can occur in almost any part of the body. Contact your doctor if you experience any side effect not listed above.

Drug Interactions

• The blood-pressure-lowering effect of quinapril is additive with diuretic drugs and beta blockers. Any other drug that causes a rapid drop in blood pressure should be used with caution if you are taking an ACE inhibitor.

• Quinapril may increase potassium levels in your blood, especially when taken with dyazide or other potassium-sparing diuretics.

• Quinapril may increase the effects of lithium; this combination should be used with caution.

• Antacids and quinapril should be taken at least 2 hours apart.

• Quinapril decreases the absorption of tetracycline by about ⅓, possibly because of the high magnesium content of quinapril tablets.

• Quinapril may increase blood levels of digoxin, possibly increasing the chance of digoxin-related side effects.

• Capsaicin may trigger or aggravate the cough associated with quinapril therapy.

• Indomethacin may reduce the blood-pressure-lowering effect of quinapril.

• Phenothiazine tranquilizers and antiemetics may increase the effects of quinapril.

• Combining allopurinol and quinapril increases the risk of side effects.

Food Interactions

Quinapril is affected by high-fat food and should be taken on an empty stomach, at least 1 hour before or 2 hours after a meal.

Usual Dose

Perindopril: Adult dosage is 4–8 mg a day. Seniors and people with kidney disease may require a lower dosage.

Quinapril: Adult dosage is 10–80 mg a day in 1 or 2 doses. Seniors and people with kidney disease may require a lower dosage.

Accuretic: 1 tablet a day.

Ramipril: Adult dosage is 2.5–20 mg a day. Seniors and people with moderate to severe kidney disease should begin with 1.25 mg a day; dosage may then be increased up to 5 mg a day.

Overdosage

The principal effect of quinapril overdose is a rapid drop in blood pressure, as evidenced by dizziness and fainting. Take the overdose victim to a hospital emergency room at once. ALWAYS bring the prescription bottle or container.

Special Information

ACE inhibitors may cause unexplained swelling of the face, lips, hands, and feet. This swelling can also affect the larynx (throat) and tongue and interfere with breathing. If this happens, go to a hospital emergency room for treatment immediately. Call your doctor if you develop a sore throat, mouth sores, abnormal heartbeat, chest pain, a persistent rash, or loss of taste perception.

You may get dizzy if you rise too quickly from a sitting or lying position.

Avoid strenuous exercise and very hot weather because heavy sweating or dehydration can cause a rapid drop in blood pressure.

Avoid over-the-counter diet pills, decongestants, and other stimulants that can raise blood pressure.

If you forget a dose, take it as soon as you remember. If it is within 8 hours of your next dose, skip the one you forgot and continue with your regular schedule. Do not take a double dose.

Special Populations

Pregnancy/Breast-feeding

ACE inhibitors can cause fetal injury or death. They are not considered safe for use during pregnancy.

Small amounts of quinapril pass into breast milk. Nursing mothers who must take this drug should consider bottle-feeding.

Seniors

Seniors may be more sensitive to the effects of quinapril due to age-related kidney impairment; the starting dosage for seniors is 10 mg daily.

Generic Name

Quinidine (QUIN-ih-dene) Ⓖ

Brand Names

Cardioquin	Quinidex Extentabs
Quinaglute Dura-Tabs	Quinora
Quinalan	Quin-Release

Type of Drug

Antiarrhythmic.

Prescribed For

Abnormal heart rhythms.

General Information

Derived from the bark of the cinchona tree, which also gives us quinine, quinidine works by affecting the flow of potassium into and out of heart muscle cells. This helps quinidine slow the flow of nerve impulses throughout the heart muscle, which allows control mechanisms in the heart to take over and keep the heart beating at a normal, even rate. The 3 kinds of quinidine—gluconate, polygalacturonate, and sulfate—provide different amounts of active drug and cannot be interchanged without dosage adjustments.

Cautions and Warnings

Do not take quinidine if you are **allergic** to it, to quinine, or to a related drug. Quinidine sensitivity may be masked if you have **asthma, muscle weakness,** or an **infection** when you start taking the drug.

Liver toxicity related to quinidine sensitivity occurs rarely. Unexplained fever or liver inflammation may indicate this effect. Your doctor should monitor your liver function during the first 4–8 weeks of therapy. People with **kidney or liver disease** may require lower dosages.

Quinidine can also cause **abnormal heart rhythms**.

People taking quinidine for long periods may experience sudden **fainting** or an abnormal heart rhythm. Occasionally, these episodes may be fatal.

Possible Side Effects

▼ Most common: nausea, vomiting, abdominal pain, diarrhea, and appetite loss. These may be accompanied by fever.

▼ Less common: unusual heart rhythms, altering of blood components; irritation of the esophagus, headache, dizziness, feelings of apprehension or excitement, confusion, delirium, muscle ache or joint pain, ringing or buzzing in the ears, mild hearing loss, blurred vision, changes in color perception, sensitivity to bright light, double vision, difficulty seeing at night, flushing of the skin, itching, sensitivity to the sun, cramps, an unusual urge to defecate or urinate, and cold sweat.

▼ Rare: collapse of blood vessels; asthma; swelling of the face, hands, and feet; respiratory collapse; and liver problems.

High dosages of quinidine may cause rash, hearing loss, dizziness, ringing in the ears, headache, nausea, or disturbed vision. This group of symptoms, called cinchonism, is usually related to taking a large amount of quinidine but may appear after a single dose of the medication. Cinchonism is not necessarily a toxic reaction, but you should immediately report any sign of it to your doctor. Do not stop taking this drug unless instructed to do so by your doctor.

Drug Interactions

• Quinidine increases the effect of warfarin and other oral anticoagulants (blood thinners).

• Quinidine may increase the effects of metoprolol, procainamide, propafenone, propranolol, and other beta blockers; succinylcholine; benztropine, oxybutynin, atropine, trihexyphenidyl, and other anticholinergic drugs; and tricyclic antidepressants.

• The effect of quinidine may be decreased by the following medicines: phenobarbital and other barbiturates, phenytoin and other hydantoins, nifedipine, rifampin, sucralfate, and cholinergic drugs such as bethanechol.

• The effectiveness and side effects of quinidine may be increased by taking amiodarone, some antacids, cimetidine, anything that decreases urine acid levels, and verapamil.

• Quinidine may dramatically increase the amount of digoxin in the blood, causing possible digoxin toxicity. This combination should be monitored closely by your doctor.

• The combination of disopyramide and quinidine may result in increased disopyramide levels and possible side effects; reduced quinidine activity may also result.

• Avoid over-the-counter cough, cold, allergy, and diet preparations. These medications may contain drugs that stimulate the heart and may be dangerous in combination with quinidine.

Food Interactions

You may take quinidine with food if it upsets your stomach. Some forms of quinidine are less irritating to the stomach.

Usual Dose

Immediate-Release: extremely variable; generally, 600–1200 mg a day.

Sustained-Release: generally, 600–1800 mg a day.

Overdosage

Overdose produces depressed mental function, including lethargy, decreased breathing, seizures, and coma. Other symptoms are abdominal pain and diarrhea, abnormal heart rhythms, and symptoms of cinchonism (see "Possible Side

Effects"). The victim should be taken to a hospital emergency room. ALWAYS bring the prescription bottle or container.

Special Information

Call your doctor if you develop ringing or buzzing in the ears, hearing or visual disturbances, dizziness, headache, nausea, rash, breathing difficulties, or any intolerable side effect.

Do not crush or chew the sustained-release products.

Some side effects of quinidine may lead to oral discomfort including dry mouth, cavities, periodontal disease, and oral *Candida* infections. See your dentist regularly while taking this drug.

If you forget to take a dose of quinidine and you remember within 2 hours of your regular time, take it right away. If you do not remember until later, skip the dose you forgot and continue your regular schedule. Do not take a double dose.

Special Populations

Pregnancy/Breast-feeding

Quinidine may cause birth defects. When this drug is considered crucial by your doctor, its potential benefits must be carefully weighed against its risks.

Quinidine passes into breast milk but is considered acceptable for use while breast-feeding. Consult your doctor.

Seniors

Seniors may be more sensitive to the effects of this medication due to decreased kidney function.

Generic Name

Raloxifene (rah-LOX-ih-feen)

Brand Name

Evista

Type of Drug

Selective Estrogen Receptor Modulator (SERM).

Prescribed For

Osteoporosis prevention and treatment. Also used for breast cancer prevention.

General Information

The female hormone estrogen plays an important role in maintaining bone strength in women by regulating the body's use of calcium. When the ovaries stop producing estrogen after menopause, a woman's risk of developing osteoporosis increases significantly. Raloxifene hydrochloride, which belongs to the SERM class of drugs, is used to increase bone density and prevent broken bones in postmenopausal women by mimicking the protective effect that estrogen has on bone. This drug also lowers cholesterol levels by acting like estrogen therapy in the cardiovascular system. Raloxifene has a potential advantage over estrogen therapy in the treatment of osteoporosis because it does not appear to have an estrogen-like effect in the breast or uterus, where the hormone may increase cancer risk. Raloxifene is broken down in the liver.

Cautions and Warnings

Do not take raloxifene if you are **sensitive** or **allergic** to it, are **pregnant,** or have had **blood-clotting problems** or clots in the lung, leg, eye, or another part of the body.

Only postmenopausal women should use raloxifene.

People with **liver disease** should use this drug with caution.

Possible Side Effects

▼ Most common: infections, flu-like symptoms, hot flashes, joint pain, and sinus irritation.

▼ Common: depression, sleeplessness, rash, nausea, headaches, upset stomach, weight gain, muscle aches, leg cramps, sore throat, and cough.

▼ Less common: chest pain, fever, migraine, sweating, vomiting, gas, stomach and intestinal problems, vaginal irritation, vaginal discharge, urinary infection, cystitis, endometrial problems, swelling in the arms or legs, arthritis, pneumonia, and laryngitis.

▼ Rare: coughing up of blood; loss of or changes in speech, coordination, or vision; pain or numbness in the chest, arm, or leg; and shortness of breath. Rare side effects can occur in almost any part of the body. Contact your doctor if you experience any side effect not listed above.

> **Possible Side Effects** *(continued)*
>
> Raloxifene is more likely to cause hot flashes, infection, and chest pain than estrogen therapy but is much less likely to cause abdominal pain, vaginal bleeding, breast pain, and gas.

Drug Interactions

- Taking raloxifene and estrogen therapy is not recommended because the effects of this combination are unknown.
- Raloxifene can increase blood levels of clofibrate, indomethacin, naproxen, ibuprofen, diazepam, and diazoxide.
- Ampicillin can reduce the absorption of raloxifene, but this interaction is not considered important.
- Cholestyramine can reduce the amount of raloxifene absorbed by 60%. Separate doses of these drugs by 2 hours or more.
- Raloxifene can reduce the effect of warfarin (a blood thinner). Your warfarin dosage may need adjustment.
- Raloxifene interferes with the absorption of levothyroxine, interfering with its effectiveness. Separate these two medicines by 12 hours.

Food Interactions

Raloxifene can be taken with or without food.

Usual Dose

Adult: 60 mg once a day.
Child: not recommended.

Overdosage

Little is known about the effects of raloxifene overdose. Call your local poison control center or a hospital emergency room for information. If you seek treatment, ALWAYS bring the prescription bottle or container.

Special Information

Raloxifene can increase your risk of developing a blood clot in the lung, leg, or another part of the body during any extended period of inactivity. Stop taking raloxifene 3 days before surgery, a long period of bed rest, or lengthy plane or car trips.

It is very important for all postmenopausal women and women age 51 and over to get 1200 mg of calcium and 10 mcg (400 IU) of vitamin D every day, either from food or a dietary supplement. Women age 70 and over require 1200 mg of calcium and 15 mcg (600 IU) of vitamin D daily.

Regular exercise is recommended for all postmenopausal women because it helps build strong bones.

Raloxifene does not reduce the hot flashes or flushes associated with menopause. Call your doctor if you experience hot flashes or flushes while taking raloxifene.

If you forget a dose, take it as soon as you remember. If a whole day has passed without taking your medication, skip the forgotten dose and continue with your regular schedule. Do not take a double dose.

Special Populations

Pregnancy/Breast-feeding

Raloxifene can harm the fetus. It is not considered safe for use during pregnancy.

It is not known if raloxifene passes into breast milk. Nursing mothers who must take it should bottle-feed.

Seniors

Seniors can use raloxifene without special precaution.

Generic Name

Ranitidine (rah-NIT-ih-deen) G

Brand Names

Zantac   Zantac EFFERdose
Zantac 75

Type of Drug

Antiulcer and histamine H_2 antagonist.

Prescribed For

Duodenal (intestinal) and gastric (stomach) ulcers; also prescribed for gastroesophageal reflux disease (GERD), other conditions characterized by the secretion of large amounts of gastric fluids, and to prevent bleeding in the stomach and upper intestines, stress ulcers, stomach damage caused by nonsteroidal anti-inflammatory drugs (NSAIDs), and the production of stomach acid during surgery.

General Information

Ranitidine hydrochloride and other H_2 antagonists work by turning off the system that produces stomach acid and other secretions. Ranitidine starts working within 1 hour and reaches its peak effect in 1 to 3 hours. Its effect lasts for up to 15 hours. Ranitidine is effective in treating ulcer symptoms and preventing complications of the disease. It is prescribed for short-term and maintenance therapy. Since all H_2 antagonists work in the same way, ulcers that do not respond to one will probably not respond to another. The only difference among H_2 antagonists is their potency. Cimetidine is the least potent, with 1000 mg roughly equal to 300 mg of ranitidine and nizatidine or 40 mg of famotidine. The ulcer-healing rates of all of these drugs are roughly equivalent, as is the risk of side effects.

Cautions and Warnings

Do not take ranitidine if you have had an **allergic reaction** to it or another H_2 antagonist. Caution must be exercised by people with **kidney or liver disease** who take ranitidine because the drug is partly broken down in the liver and passes out of the body through the kidneys. Occasionally, reversible **hepatitis or other liver abnormality** may occur, with or without jaundice (symptoms include yellowing of the skin or whites of the eyes). Reducing stomach acid levels in a person with **compromised immune function** may increase the risk of intestinal worm infection.

Possible Side Effects

Side effects with ranitidine are rare.

▼ Most common: dizziness, confusion, hallucinations, depression, sleeplessness, hair loss, inflammation of the pancreas, joint pain, and drug reactions.

▼ Less common: headache, blurred vision, agitation or anxiety, nausea, vomiting, constipation, diarrhea, abdominal discomfort, painful breast swelling, impotence, loss of sex drive, and rash.

Possible Side Effects *(continued)*

▼ Rare: rapid or irregular heartbeat, reversible reduction in white-blood-cell or blood-platelet count, and hepatitis.

Drug Interactions

• Antacids slightly reduce the effects of ranitidine. To avoid this interaction, separate doses of these drugs by about 2 to 3 hours.

• Ranitidine may interfere with the absorption of diazepam tablets. This interaction is considered minor and is unlikely to affect most people.

• Ranitidine may increase blood concentrations of glipizide, glyburide, theophylline drugs, and procainamide, increasing the risk of side effects. Interactions between ranitidine and glyburide or a theophylline drug are rare.

• Ranitidine may interact with warfarin, an anticoagulant (blood thinner). Your warfarin dosage may need an adjustment.

Food Interactions

You may take ranitidine with or without food.

Usual Dose

150–300 mg a day. People with severe conditions may require up to 600 mg a day. People with severe kidney disease need less medication.

Overdosage

Little is known about the effects of ranitidine overdose, though symptoms are likely to include severe side effects. Induce vomiting with ipecac syrup—available at any pharmacy. Call your doctor or a local poison control center before doing this. If you seek treatment, ALWAYS bring the prescription bottle or container.

Special Information

It may take several days for ranitidine to begin to relieve stomach pain. You must take this drug exactly as directed and follow your doctor's instructions for diet and other treatments to get the maximum benefit from it.

Call your doctor at once if any unusual side effects develop. Especially important are unusual bleeding or bruising, unusual tiredness, diarrhea, dizziness, rash, or hallucinations. Black, tarry stools or vomiting "coffee-ground"-like material may indicate that your ulcer is bleeding.

If you forget a dose, take it as soon as you remember. If it is almost time for your next dose, skip the one you forgot and continue with your regular schedule. Do not take a double dose.

Special Populations

Pregnancy/Breast-feeding

While animal studies of ranitidine reveal no damage to the fetus, this drug should only be used during pregnancy after carefully weighing its potential benefits against its risks.

Large amounts of ranitidine pass into breast milk. Nursing mothers who must take this drug should consider bottle-feeding.

Seniors

Seniors may obtain maximum benefit with smaller dosages. They also may be more susceptible to side effects, especially confusion.

Generic Name

Ranitidine Bismuth Citrate

(rah-NIT-ih-deen BIZ-muth SIH-trate)

Brand Name

Tritec

Type of Drug

Antibacterial and antiulcer combination.

Prescribed For

Duodenal (upper intestinal) ulcer.

General Information

Research into the causes of ulcer disease has shown that the microorganism *Heliobacter pylori* is almost always present.

Drugs that combine an acid blocker with an antibiotic are used to treat the ulcer and the infection that may be causing it. Ranitidine bismuth citrate, which is prescribed in conjunction with the antibiotic clarithromycin, is a combination of ranitidine and bismuth. Ranitidine turns off the system that produces stomach acid, providing relief from ulcer symptoms. Bismuth works against *H. pylori* by disrupting the bacterial cell wall. It may also prevent bacteria from sticking to cells in the stomach lining and from becoming resistant to antibiotics.

Cautions and Warnings

Ranitidine bismuth citrate should **not be used alone** for active duodenal ulcers. Active ulcer treatment also requires the use of clarithromycin.

If you have taken clarithromycin for *H. pylori* and your **ulcer symptoms persist,** it is likely that you have a resistant form of the bacterium. A different antibiotic may be needed.

Do not take this drug if you are **sensitive** or **allergic** to it.

People with **porphyria** should not take ranitidine bismuth citrate and clarithromycin.

People with **kidney disease** should take ranitidine bismuth citrate and clarithromycin with caution. Some people with kidney disease may require lower dosages.

Ranitidine may interfere with the **Multistix urine test**.

Possible Side Effects

Ranitidine Bismuth Citrate
Side effects can be expected to be minimal. In studies, they are approximately equal to those reported with a placebo (sugar pill). For more information, see "Ranitidine," p. 922.

Ranitidine Bismuth Citrate in Conjunction with Clarithromycin

▼ Most common: diarrhea and changes in sense of taste.

▼ Less common: headache, nausea, vomiting, and gynecological problems.

▼ Rare: tremors, abdominal discomfort, stomach pain, rash, transient changes in liver enzymes, and drug reactions.

Drug Interactions

• Combining clarithromycin, ranitidine, and bismuth increases blood levels of all 3 drugs. This interaction is beneficial to people taking the combination.

• High-dose antacids may reduce ranitidine and bismuth blood levels.

Food Interactions

This drug may be taken with food if it upsets your stomach.

Usual Dose

Adult: 400 mg 2 times a day for 4 weeks; 500 mg of clarithromycin is taken 3 times a day for the first 2 weeks.

Child: not recommended.

Overdosage

Bismuth overdose may lead to kidney and nervous system toxicity, but this has not been seen with ranitidine bismuth citrate, only with other bismuth products. Ranitidine overdose may cause dizziness, confusion, hallucinations, depression, sleeplessness, hair loss, inflammation of the pancreas, and joint pain; these effects usually are not permanent. Take the victim to a hospital emergency room. ALWAYS bring the prescription bottle or container.

Special Information

Bismuth may cause a temporary darkening of your tongue or stool. This is a harmless effect. Darkening of the stool should not be confused with blood in the stool, which turns it black.

If you forget a dose, take it as soon as you remember. If it is almost time for your next dose, skip the dose you forgot and continue with your regular schedule. Do not take a double dose.

Special Populations

Pregnancy/Breast-feeding

While animal studies of ranitidine bismuth citrate reveal no damage to the fetus, this drug should only be used during pregnancy after carefully weighing its potential benefits against its risks. Information in humans is limited. Of the 4 known cases in which ranitidine bismuth citrate was used in the course of a full-term pregnancy, 1 child was born with birth defects, which doctors considered unrelated to the medication.

It is not known if ranitidine bismuth citrate passes into breast milk, though both ingredients pass into rat breast milk. Nursing mothers who must take this drug should consider bottle-feeding.

Seniors

Seniors may take this drug without special restriction.

Brand Name

Rebetron

Generic Ingredients

Interferon Alfa-2b + Ribavirin

Type of Drug

Antiviral combination.

Prescribed For

Hepatitis C.

General Information

This combination should be used only when interferon alpha, the only other approved treatment for hepatitis C, has failed. Ribavirin is not effective against hepatitis C by itself. The way that this combination works against hepatitis C is not known.

Cautions and Warnings

All people taking this combination must be closely **monitored by their doctors,** including periodic **blood and liver and thyroid function** tests.

People with **kidney disease** or **heart disease** should use this medication with caution. If heart disease worsens during treatment, the drug should be discontinued.

Rebetron can affect both sperm and egg. Men and women taking Rebetron must **use effective contraception** during treatment and for 6 months after treatment is completed. Call your doctor if pregnancy occurs.

People who develop **severe side effects** or become **depressed** while taking this medication should have their interferon dosage temporarily lowered. The medication should be stopped if severe depression develops.

Children as young as age 1 have been treated with interferon alpha, but the combination product has not been studied in **children** of any age.

Possible Side Effects

Some people experience no side effects while taking Rebetron, and most feel well enough to work and travel during treatment.

▼ Most common: depression, fever, tiredness, headache, muscle aches, chills, flu-like symptoms, irritability, nausea, diarrhea, appetite loss, abdominal pain, weakness, joint pain, muscle pain, and feeling unwell.

▼ Common: dry mouth, thirst, dizziness, tingling in the hands or feet, sleep disturbances, vomiting, upset stomach, weight loss, and hemolytic anemia (red-blood-cell destruction).

▼ Less common: loss of concentration, nervousness, constipation, loose stools, changes in sense of taste, sore throat, breathing difficulties, sinus irritation, inflamed injection site (interferon only), chest pain, and sweating.

▼ Rare: confusion, loss of sex drive, stuffy nose, coughing, facial swelling, and cold sores. Other rare side effects can occur in almost any part of the body. Contact your doctor if you experience any side effect not listed above.

Drug Interactions

• Antacids may reduce the amount of ribavirin absorbed.

• Interferon alfa-2b can significantly increase the level of theophyline in the blood.

• Combining interferon alfa-2b with zidoudine may result in serious side effects. If taking this combination, your white blood cell count must be monitored carefully.

Food Interactions

High-fat meals can increase the amount of ribavirin absorbed, though the importance of this is not known. These drugs may be taken with or without food.

Usual Dose

Adult (under 166 lbs.): Ribavirin—400 mg in the morning and 600 mg at night. Interferon alfa—3 million units 3 times a week by injection under the skin.

Adult (166 lbs. and over): Ribavirin—600 mg morning and night. Interferon alfa—3 million units 3 times a week by injection under the skin.

Child: not recommended.

Overdosage

Little is known about the effects of Rebetron overdose. Take the victim to a hospital emergency room. ALWAYS bring the prescription bottle or container.

Special Information

This medication can make you drowsy. Be careful when driving or performing any task that requires concentration.

Drink lots of water while using Rebetron to make sure you are well hydrated.

Call your doctor at once if hives, itching, chest tightness, coughing, breathing difficulties, visual difficulties, wheezing, low blood pressure, or light-headedness develop. These can be signs of drug allergy.

Rebetron can make you more sensitive to the sun. Avoid spending a lot of time in the sun while taking it.

If you forget to take a dose of interferon, take it as soon as you remember. If it is almost time for your next dose, space your remaining weekly doses throughout the rest of the week. If you forget a dose of ribavirin, take it as soon as you remember. If it is almost time for your next dose, skip the dose you forgot and continue with your regular schedule. Do not take a double dose. Call your doctor if you forget 2 or more doses in a row.

Do not change brands of interferon without your doctor's knowledge—they may not be equivalent.

Special Populations

Pregnancy/Breast-feeding

Rebetron should not be taken by pregnant women or their male partners because of its effect on the sperm, egg, and fetus. Women must be tested monthly to be sure they are not pregnant.

It is not known if the ingredients in Rebetron pass into breast milk. Nursing mothers who must take this medication should bottle-feed.

Seniors

Seniors may use Rebetron without special restriction.

Generic Name

Repaglinide (reh-PAG-lih-nide)

Brand Name

Prandin

The information in this profile also applies to the following drug:

Generic Ingredient: Nateglinide
Starlix

Type of Drug

Antidiabetic.

Prescribed For

Type II diabetes.

General Information

In people with type II diabetes, the pancreas does not make enough insulin, or the hormone fails to work. Because insulin regulates the amount of sugar in the blood, lack of this hormone causes blood sugar to rise to unhealthy levels. Repaglinide is the first in a new group of drugs designed to control diabetes by increasing insulin production. When taken with meals, this drug temporarily stimulates the pancreas to release more insulin when it is needed to help process dietary sugar. This helps to stabilize blood sugar.

Repaglinide may be used alone or combined with metformin or other antidiabetes drugs. Repaglinide works only if beta cells in the pancreas are functioning.

Cautions and Warnings

Because repaglinide is broken down in the liver, people with **liver problems** may require reduced dosage or more time between doses.

Any antidiabetes drug can excessively **lower blood sugar**. Low blood sugar can develop when you do not consume enough calories, overexert yourself physically, drink alcohol, or combine blood-sugar-lowering drugs (see "Overdosage" for low blood sugar symptoms).

You may need to temporarily switch to insulin therapy if you have **surgery** or experience **fever, infection,** or **trauma**.

Possible Side Effects

Netaglinide
▼ Most common: respiratory infection.
▼ Less common: bronchitis, cough, back pain, flu symptoms, dizziness, joint disease, diarrhea, accidents, and low blood sugar.

Repaglinide
▼ Most common: low blood sugar, headache, and respiratory infection.
▼ Common: sinus irritation, runny nose, bronchitis, nausea, diarrhea, and back or joint pain.
▼ Less common: constipation, vomiting, upset stomach, tingling in the hands or feet, chest pain, urinary infection, and tooth problems.
▼ Rare: allergy.

Drug Interactions

• Combining repaglinide and ketoconazole, miconazole, or erythromycin may result in low blood sugar.
• Combining repaglinide and rifampin, barbiturates, gemfibrozil or carbamazepine may result in high blood sugar.
• The blood sugar-lowering effect of all antidiabetes drugs may be increased by sulfa drugs; aspirin, ibuprofen, and other nonsteroidal anti-inflammatory drugs (NSAIDs); chloramphenicol; coumadin-type anticoagulants (blood thinners);

probenecid; monoamine oxidase inhibitor (MAOI) drugs; and beta blockers.

• Thiazides and other diuretics, corticosteroid anti-inflammatory drugs, phenothiazines, thyroid drugs, estrogens, oral contraceptives ("the pill"), phenytoin, nicotinic acid, stimulants, calcium channel blockers, and isoniazid may increase blood sugar levels. Your dosage of repaglinide may need to be increased if you combine it with any of these drugs.

Food Interactions

Repaglinide should be taken before meals because food interferes with its absorption in the blood.

Usual Dose

Nateglinide
    Adult: 60–120 mg 1–30 minutes before each meal, 3 times a day.
    Child: not recommended.

Repaglinide
    Adult: 0.5–4 mg 15–30 minutes before each meal, up to 4 times a day.
    Child: not recommended.

Overdosage

People taking up to 80 mg a day of repaglinide for 2 weeks had few problems other than low blood sugar. Up to 720 mg a day of nateglinide has been taken for 7 days with no adverse effect, but low blood sugar may occur. Symptoms of low blood sugar are cold sweats, anxiety, cool and pale skin, difficulty concentrating, drowsiness, excessive hunger, headache, nausea, nervousness, rapid pulse, shakiness, unusual tiredness or weakness, and vision changes. Take the overdose victim to a hospital emergency room. ALWAYS bring the prescription bottle or container.

Special Information

Measurements of blood sugar and glycosylated hemoglobin (hemoglobin A1$_c$) are essential to your doctor's evaluation of your progress. See your doctor regularly.

    Repaglinide must be taken before you eat. If you skip a meal, do not take this drug. If you have an extra meal, take an extra dose of repaglinide before that meal.

The timing of each repaglinide dose is key to its effectiveness. If you forget to take repaglinide before a meal, take it during the meal. If you have already eaten and forgotten your medication, skip the forgotten dose. If you cannot remember to take repaglinide before each meal, talk to your doctor about changing drugs.

Special Populations

Pregnancy/Breast-feeding

Repaglinide should not be taken during pregnancy. Animal studies indicate that it may affect the skeletal development of the fetus. Most experts recommend that diabetes be controlled with insulin during pregnancy.

It is not known if repaglinide passes into breast milk. Nursing mothers who must take it should bottle-feed.

Seniors

Some seniors may be more sensitive to the effects of this drug.

Rhinocort Aqua *see Corticosteroids, Nasal,*

page 306

Generic Name

Rifampin (rih-FAM-pin) Ⓖ

Brand Names

Rifadin   Rimactane

Combination Products

Generic Ingredients: Rifampin + Isoniazid
Rifamate

Generic Ingredients: Rifampin + Isoniazid + Pyrazinamide
Rifater

Type of Drug

Antitubercular.

Prescribed For

Tuberculosis, meningitis carriers, and other infections.

General Information

Rifampin, an important agent in the treatment of tuberculosis, is always used with at least one other tuberculosis drug. It is also prescribed to eradicate the organism that causes meningitis in carriers—people who are not infected themselves but carry the organism and can spread it to others. Rifampin can be used to treat strep throat; staphylococcal infections of the skin, bones, or prostate; legionnaires' disease; leprosy; and to prevent meningitis caused by *Haemophilus influenzae*.

Cautions and Warnings

Do not take this drug if you are **allergic** to it or rifabutin, prescribed for *Mycobacterium avium* complex (an infection associated with advanced cases of AIDS).

Liver damage and death have been reported in people taking rifabutin, a drug that is very similar to rifampin. People taking other drugs that may cause liver damage should avoid rifampin. If you have **liver disease,** your liver function should be monitored by your doctor.

Bacterial resistance develops very quickly if rifampin is used for active meningococcus infection. It should not be used for this purpose.

A few cases of accelerated **lung cancer growth** have been reported, but a link to rifampin use is not established. Rifampin has the potential to **suppress the immune system**.

Possible Side Effects

▼ Most common: flu-like symptoms, heartburn, upset stomach, appetite loss, nausea, vomiting, gas, cramps, diarrhea, headache, drowsiness, tiredness, menstrual disturbances, dizziness, fever, pain in the arms and legs, confusion, visual disturbances, numbness, and hypersensitivity to the drug.

▼ Less common: effects on the blood, kidneys, or liver.

Drug Interactions

- Severe and sometimes fatal hepatitis has also occurred in people taking izoniazid, another antitubercular drug often combined with rifampin. This combination produces more liver damage than either drug taken alone. People with liver disease should be carefully monitored by their doctors and receive reduced dosage.
- Severe liver damage may develop when rifampin is combined with other drugs that cause liver toxicity.
- Rifampin may increase your need for oral anticoagulant (blood-thinning) drugs and may also affect angiotensin-converting enzyme (ACE) inhibitors, especially enalapril; acetaminophen; oral antidiabetes drugs; barbiturates; benzodiazepine tranquilizers; beta blockers; buspirone, clarithromycin; erythromycin and other macrolide antibiotics; chloramphenicol; corticosteroids; cyclosporine; dapsone; digoxin; disopyramide; doxycycline; estrogens; fluroquinolone anti-infectives; haloperidol; inamrinone; itraconazole; ketoconazole; losartan; narcotics; ondansetron; phenytoin; methadone; mexiletine; quinine drugs; quinidine; sulfa drugs; tacrolimus; theophylline drugs; tocainide; tricyclic antidepressants; thyroid hormones; verapamil; and zolpidem.
- Drugs that can interfere with rifampin include aminosalicylic acid, itraconazole, and ketoconazole.
- Women taking birth control pills should use another contraceptive method while taking rifampin.
- Rifampin increases the breakdown of AIDS antiviral drugs and may reduce their effectiveness. Rifampin is not recommended for people taking these drugs.
- Liver toxicity has developed when people taking rifampin were given halothane, a general anesthetic, prior to surgery.

Food Interactions

Take rifampin 1 hour before or 2 hours after a meal, at the same time every day.

Usual Dose

Adult: 4.5 mg per lb., up to 600 mg a day.
Child: 4.5–9 mg per lb. of body weight, up to 600 mg a day.

Overdosage

Symptoms include nausea, vomiting, and tiredness. Unconsciousness is possible in cases of severe liver damage.

Brown-red or orange skin discoloration may also develop. Take the victim to a hospital emergency room at once. ALWAYS bring the prescription bottle or container.

Special Information

Rifampin may cause a red-brown or orange discoloration of the urine, stool, saliva, sweat, and tears; this is not harmful. Soft contact lenses may become permanently stained.

Call your doctor if you develop flu-like symptoms, fever, chills, muscle pain, headache, tiredness or weakness, appetite loss, nausea, vomiting, sore throat, unusual bleeding or bruising, yellowing of the skin or whites of the eyes, rash, or itching.

If you take rifampin once a day and miss a dose, take it as soon as you remember. If it is almost time for your next dose, skip the dose you forgot and continue with your regular schedule. Do not take a double dose. Regularly missing doses of rifampin increases the risk of side effects.

Special Populations

Pregnancy/Breast-feeding

Animal studies indicate that rifampin may cause cleft palate and spina bifida (birth defect in which bones of the lower spinal column do not form properly, leaving the spinal canal partially exposed) in the fetus. Pregnant women should use this drug only if absolutely necessary.

This drug may pass into breast milk. Nursing mothers who must take it should bottle-feed.

Seniors

Seniors with liver disease may be more sensitive to the effects of this drug.

Generic Name

Riluzole (RIL-ue-zole)

Brand Name

Rilutek

Type of Drug

Glutamate-release blocker.

Prescribed For

Amyotrophic lateral sclerosis (ALS), also known as Lou Gehrig's disease.

General Information

ALS is a chronic disease of the nervous system. Riluzole, the only drug proven to affect ALS, has a number of different actions, though nobody knows exactly how it works. The drug slows the release of glutamate, which is thought to damage important nerve centers in the brains of people with ALS, and protects other aspects of nerve function. Riluzole extended survival in people with ALS during 18 months of treatment, though muscle strength and nerve function did not improve. Overall, death rates at the end of the studies were the same whether people took riluzole or not. In one study, the average life extension for people taking riluzole was 60 days. Riluzole is broken down in the liver.

Cautions and Warnings

Do not take riluzole if you are **allergic** to it.

Riluzole causes **liver inflammation;** people with severe liver disease should use this drug with caution. Liver function should be evaluated regularly. People with **kidney disease** should also use riluzole with caution.

Women and people of Japanese descent may eliminate riluzole from their bodies twice as slowly as do male Caucasians. The drug may be eliminated more slowly due to genetic factors or because of differences in diet such as decreased use of alcohol, nicotine, and caffeine.

Cigarette smoking is likely to increase the rate at which riluzole is broken down by the liver. The drug may break down more quickly in women than in men. There is no indication that either of these factors is important in determining riluzole dosage.

Taking more than 100 mg a day of riluzole increases side effects and is not more effective.

Possible Side Effects

About 14% of people stop taking riluzole because of side effects.

▼ Most common: weakness, nausea, dizziness (twice as common in women), diarrhea, a tingling sensation

Possible Side Effects *(continued)*

around the mouth, appetite loss, fainting, and tiredness. These effects increase with dosage.

▼ Common: poor lung function, abdominal pain, pneumonia, and vomiting.

▼ Less common: back pain, headache, upset stomach at high dosages, gas, stuffy nose, runny nose, cough, high blood pressure, joint aches, and swelling in the arms and legs. At high dosages—urinary infection and painful urination, and dizziness when rising from a lying or sitting position.

▼ Rare: aggravation, feeling unwell, mouth infection, eczema, rapid heartbeat, and vein irritation. Other rare side effects can occur in almost any part of the body. Contact your doctor if you experience any side effects not listed above.

Drug Interactions

• Allopurinol, methyldopa, sulfasalazine, and other drugs that are toxic to the liver may interact with riluzole. Combinations of liver-toxic drugs should be taken with caution.

• Caffeine, theophylline, phenacetin, amitriptyline, and quinolone antibacterials may slow the elimination of riluzole, increasing the risk of drug side effects.

• Rifampin and omeprazole may quicken the elimination of riluzole.

• Riluzole can accelerate the breakdown of caffeine, theophylline, and tacrine, but these effects have not actually been seen in people.

Food Interactions

Take riluzole on an empty stomach, at least 1 hour before or 2 hours after meals. Avoid charcoal-broiled foods, which may speed the elimination of riluzole. Avoid high-fat meals, which decrease the absorption of riluzole.

Usual Dose

Adult: 50 mg every 12 hours.
Child: not recommended.

Overdosage

Little is known about the effects of riluzole overdose. Take the victim to a hospital emergency room at once. ALWAYS bring the prescription bottle or container.

Special Information

Taking more than 50 mg twice a day will not improve your condition and may increase drug side effects.

Call your doctor at once if you become feverish or ill. This could be a sign of a very low white-blood-cell count.

Riluzole should be taken at the same time each day—morning and evening—to achieve maximum benefit.

Riluzole can make you dizzy, tired, or faint. Be careful when driving or doing any task that requires concentration.

People taking riluzole should not drink to excess.

Store riluzole tablets between 68°F and 77°F and protect them from bright light.

If you forget a dose, take it as soon as you remember. If it is almost time for your next dose, skip the dose you forgot and continue with your regular schedule.

Special Populations

Pregnancy/Breast-feeding

Riluzole is toxic to pregnant lab animals at high dosages. When this drug is considered crucial by your doctor, its potential benefits must be carefully weighed against its risks.

It is not known if riluzole passes into breast milk. Nursing mothers who must take it should bottle-feed.

Seniors

Seniors with kidney or liver disease should use riluzole with caution.

Generic Name

Rimantadine (rih-MAN-tuh-dene)

Brand Name

Flumadine

Type of Drug

Antiviral.

Prescribed For

Influenza A viral infection (type A flu).

General Information

Rimantadine hydrochloride is a synthetic antiviral agent that appears to interfere with the reproduction of various strains of the influenza A virus, a common cause of viral infection. Rimantadine is used both to treat and to prevent type A flu. Annual vaccination against the virus is the best way of preventing the flu, but immunity takes 2 to 4 weeks to develop. In the meantime, rimantadine may be taken to prevent viral infection in high-risk people or people who may experience greater exposure to the virus.

Cautions and Warnings

Do not take rimantadine if you are **allergic** to it or to **amantadine**.

People with severe **liver or kidney disease** clear this drug from their bodies only half as fast as those with normal organ function; they will need to have their dosage adjusted appropriately.

People with a history of **seizures** are likely to suffer another one while taking rimantadine. Call your doctor if this happens to you.

The influenza virus may become **resistant** to rimantadine in up to 30% of people taking the drug. When this happens, the resistant virus can infect people who are not protected by the vaccine.

Possible Side Effects

▼ Most common: sleeplessness, nervousness, loss of concentration, headache, fatigue, weakness, nausea, vomiting, appetite loss, dry mouth, and abdominal pains.

▼ Less common: diarrhea, upset stomach, dizziness, depression, euphoria (feeling "high"), changes in gait or walk, tremors, hallucinations, convulsions, fainting,

Possible Side Effects *(continued)*

ringing or buzzing in the ears, changes in or loss of the senses of taste or smell, breathing difficulties, pallor, rash, heart palpitations, rapid heartbeat, high blood pressure, heart failure, swelling of the ankles or feet, and heart block.

▼ Rare: constipation, swallowing difficulties, mouth sores, agitation, sweating, diminished sense of touch, eye pain or tearing, cough, bronchospasm, increased urination, fever, and fluid oozing from the nipples in women.

Drug Interactions

The importance of rimantadine's drug interactions is not known because there is no established relationship between the amount of drug in the blood and its antiviral effect.

• Aspirin and acetaminophen may reduce the amount of rimantadine in the blood by about 10%.

• Cimetidine decreases the rate at which rimantadine is broken down by the liver.

Food Interactions

Rimantadine is best taken on an empty stomach, or at least 1 hour before or 2 hours after meals. You may take it with food if it upsets your stomach.

Usual Dose

Adult and Child (age 10 and over): 100 mg twice a day. People with severe liver or kidney disease—no more than 100 mg a day.

Child (under age 10): 2.25 mg per lb. of body weight, up to 150 mg, taken once a day.

Overdosage

Symptoms include agitation, hallucination, and abnormal heart rhythm. Overdose victims should be made to vomit with ipecac syrup—available at any pharmacy—as soon as possible. Call your local poison control center or a hospital emergency room before giving ipecac. Take overdose victims to a hospital emergency room. ALWAYS bring the prescription bottle or container.

Special Information

Rimantadine may be given to children to prevent influenza infection, but it is not recommended for treatment of their flu symptoms.

Call your doctor if you develop seizures, convulsions, or any other serious or unusual side effects.

If you forget a dose, take it as soon as you remember. If it is almost time for your next dose, skip the dose you forgot and continue with your regular schedule. Do not take a double dose.

Special Populations

Pregnancy/Breast-feeding

In animal studies, rimantadine is toxic to fetuses. When this drug is considered crucial by your doctor, its potential benefits must be carefully weighed against its risks.

Rimantadine passes into breast milk. Nursing mothers who must take it should bottle-feed.

Seniors

Seniors are more likely to suffer from rimantadine side effects of the nervous system, stomach, and intestine and may require reduced dosage due to liver or kidney dysfunction.

Risperdal   *see* **Risperidone,** *below*

Generic Name

Risperidone   (ris-PER-ih-done)

Brand Name

Risperdal   Risperdal M-TAB

Type of Drug

Antipsychotic.

Prescribed For

Psychotic disorders and schizophrenia; also prescribed for bipolar disorders, symptoms of Alzheimer's disease, and treatment-resistant depression.

General Information

Risperidone affects brain receptors for serotonin and dopamine, two important neurohormones. It is broken down in the liver. Between 6% and 8% of Caucasians and a very small number of Asians have little of the liver enzyme that breaks down risperidone and are considered to be "poor metabolizers" of the drug. Because these people break risperidone down very slowly, the drug takes about 5 days to reach a steady level in their blood. People with normal amounts of the enzyme reach a steady level in about 1 day. People with kidney or liver disease require reduced dosage.

Cautions and Warnings

Do not take this drug if you are **sensitive** or **allergic** to it. People taking it for longer than 6 to 8 weeks must be reevaluated at least every 2 months.

A serious set of side effects known as **neuroleptic malignant syndrome (NMS)** has been associated with some antipsychotic drugs. The symptoms that constitute NMS include high fever, muscle rigidity, mental changes, irregular pulse or blood pressure, sweating, and abnormal heart rhythm. NMS is potentially fatal and requires **immediate medical attention**.

Risperidone can produce **uncontrolled movements,** including tremor, spasm of the neck muscles, rolling back of the eyes, convulsions, difficulty swallowing, and symptoms associated with Parkinson's disease. These effects usually disappear after the drug has been discontinued. Face, tongue, and jaw symptoms may persist, especially in older women. Contact your doctor immediately if you experience any of these symptoms.

Risperidone can cause a life-threatening abnormal heart rhythm called **torsade de pointes**. The drug should therefore be used with caution in people with **heart disease**. Slow heart rate, electrolyte imbalance, and taking other drugs that carry a risk of torsade de pointes may increase the chances of developing this abnormality.

Risperidone raises levels of a hormone called prolactin. Increased prolactin has been associated with **tumors of the pituitary gland, breast, and pancreas,** but no problems have been noted with risperidone specifically.

Risperidone has been associated with **obesity, high cholesterol,** and **diabetes**.

Possible Side Effects

▼ Most common: sleepiness, sleeplessness, agitation, anxiety, uncontrolled movements, headache, and nasal stuffiness and irritation.

▼ Less common: dizziness, constipation, nausea, vomiting, upset stomach, abdominal pain, weight gain, absence of menstrual periods, increased sleep duration, coughing, upper respiratory infection, sinus infection, sore throat, breathing difficulties, rapid heartbeat, joint or back pain, chest pain, fever, abnormal vision, rash, dry skin, and dandruff.

Other side effects can occur in almost any part of the body. Contact your doctor if you experience any side effect not listed above.

Drug Interactions

• Risperidone may decrease the effects of levodopa and other dopamine agonists.

• Carbamazepine and clozapine may reduce the effect of this drug.

• Risperidone increases the effects of blood-pressure-lowering drugs and central nervous system (CNS) depressants.

Food Interactions

None known.

Usual Dose

Adult: starting dosage—1 mg 2 times a day. Maintenance dosage—increase gradually up to 8 mg a day if needed.

Senior: starting dosage—0.5 mg 2 times a day. Increase gradually if needed.

Child: not recommended.

Overdosage

Symptoms include drowsiness, rapid heartbeat, low blood pressure, and abnormal and uncontrolled muscle movements. Overdose victims should be taken to a hospital emergency room. ALWAYS bring the prescription bottle or container.

Special Information

Risperidone can make you tired and affect your judgment, an effect that increases with dosage. Be careful when driving or performing any task that requires concentration. Avoid alcohol.

Some antipsychotic drugs can interfere with the body's temperature-regulating mechanism. Avoid extreme heat while you are taking risperidone.

Some people develop a rapid heartbeat and become dizzy or faint when first taking risperidone. This risk can be minimized by starting at a low dose, such as 2 mg a day in adults, or 1 mg in seniors or those with kidney or liver disease.

Risperidone can make you unusually sensitive to the sun. Wear protective clothes and use sunscreen.

If you forget a dose, take it as soon as you remember. If it is almost time for your next dose, skip the dose you forgot and continue with your regular schedule. Call your doctor if you forget 2 doses in a row.

Special Populations

Pregnancy/Breast-feeding

Studies of risperidone in animals show an increase in birth defects and stillbirth. There is also a report of an infant who was born with an abnormally developed brain after the mother took risperidone. Risperidone should not be taken by pregnant women unless the potential benefits are carefully weighed against the risks.

It is not known if risperidone passes into breast milk. Nursing mothers who must take this medication should bottle-feed.

Seniors

Seniors with reduced kidney function require lower dosage. Seniors may also be more sensitive to side effects.

Generic Name

Ritonavir (rih-TON-uh-vere)

Brand Name

Norvir

Combination Products

Generic Ingredients: Ritonavir + Lopinavir
Kaletra

Type of Drug

Protease inhibitor.

Prescribed For

Human immunodeficiency virus (HIV) infection.

General Information

Part of the multidrug cocktail responsible for the most important gains in the fight against acquired immunodeficiency syndrome (AIDS), ritonavir and lopinavir belong to a group of anti-HIV drugs called protease inhibitors. Triple-drug cocktails are considered responsible for the first overall reduction in the AIDS death rate, recorded in 1996. Protease inhibitors work in a unique way but are not a cure for HIV infection or AIDS. When the HIV virus attacks a cell, it must be converted into viral DNA. Older drugs, known as reverse transcriptase inhibitors, interfere with this step, but they need help in fighting HIV. Protease inhibitors work at the end of the HIV reproduction process, when proteins are "cut" into strands of exactly the right size to duplicate HIV. The protein is cut by a protease enzyme. Protease inhibitors prevent the mature HIV virus from being formed by interfering with this cutting process. Proteins that are cut to the wrong length or that remain uncut are inactive.

Protease inhibitors are always taken with 1 or 2 nucleoside antiviral drugs such as AZT, ddl, ddC, or 3TC. Protease inhibitors revolutionized HIV treatment because when taken in combination, they reduce the amount of HIV virus in the bloodstream to levels that are often undetectable by current methods—CD_4 cell counts (immune system cells) and viral load (amount of virus in the blood) measurements. Multiple-drug therapy has changed the current view of HIV from a fatal disease to a manageable chronic illness.

People taking a protease inhibitor may still develop infections or other conditions associated with HIV disease. Because of this, it is very important for you to remain under the care of a doctor or other health care provider. The long-term effects of ritonavir are not known at this time. You may be able to pass the HIV virus to others even if you are on triple-drug therapy.

Cautions and Warnings

Do not take ritonavir if you are **allergic** to it. People with mild or moderate **liver disease** and **cirrhosis** break down ritonavir more slowly than those with normal liver function and may be more likely to develop side effects. People with cirrhosis should receive a reduced dose of ritonavir.

Ritonavir may raise your blood sugar, worsen your **diabetes,** or bring out latent diabetes. Diabetics who take ritonavir may have to have the dosage of their antidiabetes medication adjusted.

Some of ritonavir's drug interactions may be dangerous (see "Drug Interactions").

Ritonavir can affect a wide variety of **blood tests,** including those for triglycerides, liver function, and blood sugar.

Possible Side Effects

▼ Most common: weakness, tiredness, nausea, abnormal stools, diarrhea, vomiting, appetite loss, abdominal pains, taste changes, and tingling around the mouth and in the hands or feet.

▼ Less common: increased levels of cholesterol and other blood fats, diabetes and high blood sugar, and increased fat deposits in some areas of the body, including the back of the neck.

▼ Rare: Rare side effects can occur in almost any part of the body, including muscles and joints, blood components, and the mouth, stomach and intestines, nervous system, skin, kidneys, liver, and urinary and respiratory tracts. Changes in mental state and sexual function may also occur.

Drug Interactions

• Combining ritonavir and lopinavir with statin-type cholesterol-lowering drugs can result in serious reactions.

• The following drugs should not be combined with ritonavir: amiodarone, astemizole, bepridil, bupropion, clozapine, encainide, flecainide, meperidine, piroxicam, propafenone, propoxyphene, quinidine, and rifabutin. Ritonavir can be expected to substantially raise the blood levels of all these drugs, which may cause serious abnormal heart rhythms, blood problems, seizures, and other serious side effects.

• Combining ritonavir with any of the following drugs may cause excessive sedation and breathing difficulties: alprazolam, clorazepate, diazepam, estazolam, flurazepam, midazolam, triazolam, and zolpidem. The effectiveness of other sedative-hypnotics is likely to be reduced by ritonavir. Ritonavir may interact with narcotic pain relievers, but the exact interaction is not predictable.

• Combining rifampin with ritonavir decreases the amount of ritonavir absorbed by about 35% and should be avoided.

• Ritonavir and lopinavir should not be combined with pimozide.

• Combining ritonavir with clarithromycin raises the amount of clarithromycin in the blood. Mixing ritonavir with isoniazid increases the amount of isoniazid in the blood.

• Combining ritonavir with didanosine (ddI) may reduce the amount of ddI in the blood by about 15%. Take ddI 1 hour before of 2 hours after taking ritonavir.

• Combining fluconazole or fluoxetine with ritonavir increases the amount of ritonavir in the blood.

• Combining ritonavir with desipramine or trazodone substantially increases the amount of these drugs in the blood. Dosage adjustment may be required.

• Do not combine ritonavir oral solution and disulfiram or metronidazole.

• Combining ritonavir with oral contraceptives containing ethinyl estradiol can lower blood hormone levels, possibly reducing their effectiveness.

• Combining ritonavir with saquinavir, another protease inhibitor, slows the breakdown of saquinavir and increases its blood levels.

• Ritonavir lowers the amount of sulfamethoxazole absorbed into the blood by about 20% and raises trimethoprim by about 20%.

• Combining ritonavir with theophylline reduces the amount of theophylline absorbed by about 40%.

- Taking ritonavir with AZT reduces the amount of AZT in the blood by about 10%.
- Ritonavir is likely to increase the absorption of these drugs into the blood: alpha blockers, antiarrhythmics, anticancer drugs, antidepressants, antiemetics, antifungals, antimalarials, beta blockers, blood-fat reducers, calcium entry blockers, cimetidine, corticosteroids, erythromycin, immunosuppressants, methylphenidate, pentoxifylline, phenothiazines, and warfarin.
- Ritonavir is likely to reduce the amount of these drugs absorbed into the blood: atovaquone, clofibrate, daunorubicin, diphenoxylate, theophylline, and metoclopramide.
- St. John's wort significantly reduces blood levels of ritonavir and should not be used together.

Food Interactions

To increase the effectiveness of ritonavir capsules, take them with meals. Ritonavir oral solution should be taken on an empty stomach, 1 hour before or 2 hours after meals. The taste of the oral liquid may be improved by mixing it with chocolate milk, Ensure, or Advera. Do not mix earlier than 1 hour before you take your dose.

Usual Dose

Adult: 600 mg 2 times a day. You may start with a lower dosage and increase gradually to avoid upset stomach. Kaletra—3 capsules 2 times a day.

Child: consult your doctor.

Overdosage

Little is known about the effects of ritonavir overdose. Take the victim to a hospital emergency room at once. ALWAYS bring the prescription bottle or container.

Special Information

It is imperative to take your HIV medication exactly as prescribed. Missing doses of ritonavir makes you more likely to become resistant to the drug and to lose the benefits of therapy.

Ritonavir does not cure AIDS. It will not prevent you from transmitting the HIV virus to another person; you must still practice safe sex.

Stay in close touch with your doctor while taking ritonavir and report unusual symptoms. Abdominal pain, nausea, and vomiting may be signs of pancreatitis (inflammation of the pancreas), which can be fatal.

Ritonavir and Kaletra capsules should be stored in the refrigerator. The ritonavir liquid may be kept at room temperature, but only for 30 days; Kaletra liquid may be kept at room temperature for 2 months.

If you forget a dose of ritonavir, take it as soon as you remember. If it is almost time for your next dose, skip the dose you forgot and continue with your regular schedule. Do not take a double dose.

Special Populations

Pregnancy/Breast-feeding

Animal studies indicate that ritonavir may affect the fetus. When this drug is considered crucial by your doctor, its potential benefits must be carefully weighed against its risks.

It is not known if ritonavir passes into breast milk. Nursing mothers who must take ritonavir should bottle-feed.

Seniors

Seniors may take ritonavir without special restriction.

Generic Name

Rofecoxib (roe-feh-KOX-ib)

Brand Name

Vioxx

Type of Drug

Cyclooxygenase-2 (COX-2) inhibitor and nonsteroidal anti-inflammatory drug (NSAID).

Prescribed For

Osteoarthritis, painful menstruation, and acute pain.

General Information

Traditional NSAIDs works primarily by blocking the effects of COX-2, a body enzyme that plays an important role in regulating pain and inflammation. But these NSAIDs also have an unwanted effect: They interfere with cyclooxygenase-1 (COX-

1), a related enzyme that helps to maintain the stomach's protective lining. NSAIDs that block the effects of this enzyme may produce side effects such as stomach irritation, gas, and stomach ulcers.

COX-2 inhibitors such as rofecoxib are a new class of NSAIDs that interfere primarily with COX-2, leaving the stomach-protecting COX-1 relatively unaffected. This means that COX-2 inhibitor NSAIDs can relieve pain and inflammation just like traditional NSAIDs but are less likely to cause gastrointestinal (GI) side effects. Another potential advantage of rofecoxib is that it does not cause thinning of the blood or affect blood platelets like older NSAIDs do. Rofecoxib is broken down in the liver.

African Americans and Hispanics absorb 10% to 15% more rofecoxib than Caucasians. The importance of this fact is unclear.

Cautions and Warnings

Do not take rofecoxib if you are **sensitive** or **allergic** to it or to sulfa drugs. NSAIDs should not be taken by people with **asthma** or by those who have had an **allergic reaction to aspirin or another NSAID**. People who have experienced a group of symptoms (runny nose with or without nasal polyps and severe bronchial spasm) known as the aspirin triad after taking aspirin or another NSAID are at greatest risk.

NSAIDs can cause **gastrointestinal (GI) bleeding and ulcers** and **stomach perforation**. This can occur at any time, with or without warning, in people who take NSAIDs regularly. Minor **upper GI problems,** such as upset stomach, are common and may occur at any time during NSAID therapy. People who develop bleeding or ulcers and continue NSAID treatment should be aware of the risk of developing more serious side effects.

Rofecoxib should be used with caution by people who have had **stomach ulcers** or **GI bleeding**. It should also be used with caution in people with other **bleeding problems, anemia, high blood pressure, heart disease,** or **fluid retention**.

Rofecoxib should not be used by people with severe **kidney disease**.

Rofecoxib can cause **liver irritation** and should be used with caution by people with **hepatitis** or **cirrhosis**. People with moderate liver disease require reduced dosages. The effect of rofecoxib in people with severe liver failure is not known.

Possible Side Effects

Side effects are similar to those of traditional NSAIDs. Stomach and intestinal effects are about half as common.

▼ Common: respiratory infection, diarrhea, and nausea.

▼ Less common: abdominal pain, weakness, fatigue, dizziness, flu-like symptoms, swollen legs, high blood pressure, upset stomach, heartburn, sinus irritation, back pain, headache, and urinary infection.

▼ Rare: Rare side effects can occur in almost any part of the body. Contact your doctor if you experience any side effect not listed above.

Drug Interactions

• Alcohol may increase the risk of serious GI-related side effects. Avoid alcohol while taking this medication.

• Combining rofecoxib and an aluminum and magnesium antacid slightly reduces the amount of drug absorbed. Separate doses of these antacids and rofecoxib by 1 to 2 hours.

• Rofecoxib may raise lithium blood levels and increase the risk of side effects.

• While rofecoxib may be combined with low dosages of aspirin, taking these two drugs together can increase the risk of stomach or intestinal ulcers or other complications. Speak with your doctor before taking aspirin or any other NSAID while you are taking rofecoxib.

• Rofecoxib can reduce the blood-pressure-lowering effect of angiotensin-converting enzyme (ACE) inhibitor and diuretic drugs. This combination can also increase the risk of kidney damage after chronic rofecoxib use.

• High dosages of cimetidine (800 mg twice a day) can increase the amount of rofecoxib in the blood, but no dosage adjustment is necessary.

• NSAIDs can reduce the effect of furosemide and thiazide-type diuretics in some people.

• Rofecoxib can elevate methotrexate blood levels by about 25% and increase the risk of methotrexate side effects.

• Rifampin reduces the amount of rofecoxib in the blood by 50%. People taking rifampin may need a higher starting dosage of rofecoxib.

• Rofecoxib may increase the blood-thinning effect of warfarin. Your doctor should check your blood if you are combining these drugs.

Food Interactions

Rofecoxib may be taken without regard to food or meals. For optimal effectiveness, avoid taking this drug with high-fat meals.

Usual Dose

Adult (age 18 and over): 12.5–50 mg once a day.
Child (under age 18): consult your doctor.

Overdosage

Overdose symptoms are usually limited to lethargy, drowsiness, nausea, vomiting, and stomach pain. Stomach or intestinal bleeding may occur. High blood pressure, kidney failure, breathing difficulty, and coma can occur but are rare. Severe allergic reactions may occur following an overdose. In case of overdose, call your local poison control center or a hospital emergency room. You may be told to induce vomiting with ipecac syrup—available at any pharmacy—before taking the victim to an emergency room. If you seek treatment, ALWAYS bring the prescription bottle or container.

Special Information

This medication can cause a serious allergic reaction in some people. If you experience irregular breathing or other breathing difficulties, irregular and rapid heartbeat, hives, swelling around the eyes, or changes in skin color, call an ambulance or have someone bring you to the nearest emergency room.

Call your doctor if you develop rash, itching, unexplained weight gain, nausea, fatigue, yellowing of the skin or whites of the eyes, flu-like symptoms, lethargy, swelling, black stools, severe stomach pain, persistent headache, or any bothersome or persistent side effect.

If you forget a dose, take it as soon as you remember. If it is almost time for your next dose, skip the forgotten dose and continue with your regular schedule.

Special Populations

Pregnancy/Breast-feeding

Any NSAID may affect fetal heart development during the second half of pregnancy. Pregnant women should not take rofecoxib without their doctor's approval. When this drug is considered crucial by your doctor, its potential benefits must be carefully weighed against its risks.

NSAIDs may pass into breast milk. There is a possibility that a nursing mother taking rofecoxib could affect her baby's heart or cardiovascular system. Nursing mothers who take this drug should bottle-feed.

Seniors
Generally, seniors can take this drug without special precaution. They should use the lowest effective dosage.

Generic Name

Ropinirole (roe-PIN-ih-role)

Brand Name

Requip

Type of Drug

Antiparkinsonian.

Prescribed For

Parkinson's disease.

General Information

Ropinirole relieves symptoms of Parkinson's disease by stimulating dopamine receptors in the brain. A study of people with early Parkinson's disease showed improvement in about 70% of people taking the drug for 10 to 12 weeks, compared to 40% of people taking a placebo (sugar pill). In another study, 28% of people with advanced Parkinson's disease who received ropinirole for 6 months showed improvement compared to 11% of people in the placebo group. Ropinirole is broken down in the liver.

Cautions and Warnings

Do not take ropinirole if you are **sensitive** or **allergic** to it. Ropinirole may cause **low blood pressure** and make you **dizzy or faint** when rising from a sitting or lying position, especially during the early stages of treatment. About 1 in 10 to 15 people who take ropinirole experience **hallucinations** that may be serious enough to require stopping drug therapy.

People stopping other treatments for Parkinson's disease have developed **high fever** and **confusion**. **Breathing difficulties** caused by lung changes have occurred with the use of other antiparkinsonians. These problems have not been associated with ropinirole but there is a risk that you may experience similar problems if you stop taking ropinirole.

Possible Side Effects

Early Parkinson's Disease

▼ Most common: sleepiness or tiredness, nausea, dizziness, fainting, upset stomach, vomiting, and virus infection.

▼ Common: general pain, sweating, weakness, fainting, abdominal pain, sore throat, and changes in vision.

▼ Less common: dry mouth, flushing, chest pain, feeling unwell, blood-pressure changes, heart palpitations, rapid heartbeat, hallucinations, confusion, memory loss, very sensitive reflexes, yawning, unusual movements, difficulty concentrating, appetite loss, gas, swollen arms or legs, runny nose, sinus irritation, bronchitis, breathing difficulties, eye problems, urinary infection, impotence, and poor blood supply to the hands, legs, and feet.

Advanced Parkinson's Disease

▼ Most common: abnormal movements, tremor, muscle rigidity, hallucinations, and urinary infection.

▼ Common: confusion, constipation, pneumonia, sweating, abdominal pain, and twitching.

▼ Less common: dizziness or fainting when rising from a sitting or lying position, unusual dreaming, changes in the way you walk, poor muscle coordination, memory loss, nervousness, tingling in the hands or feet, temporary paralysis, diarrhea, difficulty swallowing, gas, increased salivation, poor urinary control, pus in the urine, arthritis, breathing difficulties, dry mouth, anemia, and weight loss.

Drug Interactions

• Ropinirole increases levodopa blood levels and may worsen uncontrolled muscle spasm that occurs with levodopa. Your doctor may reduce your levodopa dosage.

• Ciprofloxacin, diltiazem, enoxacin, erythromycin, estrogen, fluvoxamine, mexilitene, norfloxacin, tacrine, cimetidine, and cigarette smoking increase ropinirole's effects.

• Phenothiazine tranquilizers, haloperidol and similar tranquilizers, thioxanthene tranquilizers, and metoclopramide and other drugs that antagonize the effects of dopamine may reduce the effect of ropinirole.

• Ropinirole increases the sedative effect of tranquilizers, sleeping pills, and other nervous system depressants.

Food Interactions

You may take this drug with food to prevent nausea.

Usual Dose

Adult: 0.25 mg 3 times a day to start, gradually increasing, if needed, in intervals of .75 mg a week, to a maximum of 24 mg a day. Dosage is reduced for people with kidney disease.

Overdosage

Little is known about the effects of ropinirole overdose. Symptoms are likely to include the most common side effects. Take the victim to a hospital emergency room. ALWAYS bring the prescription bottle or container.

Special Information

Take this drug exactly as prescribed.

Ropinirole causes sedation. Be careful when driving or performing any task that requires concentration. Avoid alcohol and other nervous system depressants.

Hallucinations may occur with this drug, especially among seniors. Call your doctor if you develop hallucinations or bothersome or persistent side effects.

If you forget a dose, take it as soon as you remember. Space the remaining daily dosage evenly throughout the day. Go back to your regular schedule the next day. Do not take a double dose.

Special Populations

Pregnancy/Breast-feeding

In animal studies, ropinirole causes birth defects and damages the fetus. When this drug is considered crucial by your doctor, its potential benefits must be carefully weighed against its risks.

Animal studies show that ropinirole passes into breast milk, but it is not known if this occurs in humans. Ropinirole may interfere with milk production. Nursing mothers who must take this drug should bottle-feed.

Seniors

Hallucinations are more likely in seniors.

Generic Name

Salmeterol (sal-METE-er-ol)

Brand Name

Serevent   Severent Diskus

The information in this profile also applies to the following drug:

Generic Ingredients: Salmeterol + Fluticasone
Advair Diskus

Type of Drug

Bronchodilator.

Prescribed For

Asthma and bronchospasm.

General Information

Salmeterol xinafoate differs from other bronchodilators in that it does not provide immediate symptom relief but is instead prescribed for long-term prevention. When you start salmeterol treatment, you may need to continue your other asthma inhalers for symptom relief. After a while, however, you should have less need for the other drugs. Salmeterol works like other bronchodilator drugs, such as albuterol, terbutaline, and metaproterenol, but it has a weaker effect on nerve receptors in the heart and blood vessels; for this reason, it is somewhat safer for people with heart conditions. Still, very large doses of salmeterol may lead to abnormal heart rhythms. Salmeterol begins working within 20 minutes after a dose and continues for 12 hours. Salmeterol and fluticasone, a corticosteriod, have been combined into a single product for inhalation because both drugs are prescribed in the long-term prevention of asthma.

Cautions and Warnings

Salmeterol should be used with caution by people with a history of **angina pectoris** (condition characterized by brief attacks of chest pain), **heart disease, high blood pressure, stroke** or **seizure, thyroid disease, prostate disease,** or **glaucoma**.

Used in excess, salmeterol can actually lead to more **breathing difficulties,** rather than breathing relief. In the most extreme cases, people have had **heart attacks** after using excessive amounts of inhalant bronchodilators.

Long-term use of salmeterol, and related drugs, can lead to increases in certain **ovarian tumors**.

Salmeterol should not be used in patients with acutely deteriorating asthma, which can lead to **serious respiratory events**.

Possible Side Effects

▼ Most common: heart palpitations, rapid heartbeat, tremors, cough, dizziness and fainting, shakiness, nervousness, tension, headache, diarrhea, heartburn or upset stomach, dry or sore and irritated throat, respiratory infections, and nasal or sinus conditions.

▼ Less common: nausea and vomiting, joint or back pain, muscle cramps, muscle soreness, muscle ache or pain, giddiness, viral stomach infections, itching, dental pain, not feeling well, rash, and menstrual irregularity.

Drug Interactions

• Monoamine oxidase inhibitors (MAOIs), tricyclic antidepressants, thyroid drugs, other bronchodilator drugs, and some antihistamines may increase the effects of salmeterol.

• The risk of cardiotoxicity may be increased in people taking both salmeterol and theophylline.

• Salmeterol may decrease the effects of blood-pressure-lowering drugs, especially reserpine, methyldopa, and guanethidine.

Food Interactions

None known.

Usual Dose

Salmeterol (aerosol)
  Adult and Child (age 12 and over): 2 inhalations every 12 hours.
  Child (under age 12): not recommended.

Salmeterol (powder)
  Adult and Child (age 4 and over): 1 inhalation every 12 hours.
  Child (under age 4): not recommended.

Salmeterol and Fluticasone
  Adult and Child (age 12 and over): 1 inhalation every 12 hours.
  Child (under age 12): not recommended.

Overdosage

Overdose of salmeterol inhalation usually results in exaggerated side effects, including chest pain and high blood pressure, although blood pressure may drop to a low level after a short period of elevation. People who inhale too much salmeterol should see a doctor. ALWAYS bring the prescription bottle or container.

Special Information

Be sure to follow the inhalation instructions that come with the product. Wait at least 1 minute between puffs. Do not inhale salmeterol if you have food or anything else in your mouth. Rinse mouth with water after each use.

Call your doctor immediately if you develop chest pain, palpitations, rapid heartbeat, muscle tremors, dizziness, headache, facial flushing, or urinary difficulty, or if you continue to experience difficulty in breathing after using salmeterol.

If you forget a dose of salmeterol, take it as soon as you remember. If it is almost time for your next dose, skip the one you forgot and go back to your regular schedule. Do not take a double dose.

If your doctor is switching you from an inhaled corticosteroid to the salmeterol with fluticasone combination, it is important for you to report any changes in symptoms as soon as they occur.

Special Populations

Pregnancy/Breast-feeding
When used during childbirth, salmeterol may slow or delay natural labor. It can cause rapid heartbeat and high blood sugar in the mother and rapid heartbeat and low blood sugar in the baby. It is not known whether salmeterol causes birth defects in humans, but it has caused defects in animals. When your doctor considers this drug crucial, its potential benefits must be carefully weighed against its risks.

Salmeterol may pass into breast milk. Nursing mothers who must take this drug should consider bottle-feeding.

Seniors
Seniors should use the same dosage of salmeterol as younger adults.

Generic Name

Saquinavir Mesylate

(suh-QUIN-uh-vere MES-uh-late)

Brand Names

Invirase   Fortovase

Type of Drug

Protease inhibitor.

Prescribed For

Advanced human immunodeficiency virus (HIV) infection.

General Information

Part of the multidrug cocktail responsible for important gains in the fight against acquired immunodeficiency syndrome (AIDS), saquinavir is a member of a group of anti-HIV drugs called protease inhibitors. These drugs work at the end of the HIV reproduction process, when proteins are "cut" into strands of exactly the correct size to duplicate HIV. The protein is cut by an enzyme known as protease. Protease inhibitors prevent the mature HIV virus from being formed by inhibiting this cutting process. Proteins that are cut to the wrong length or that remain uncut are inactive.

Protease inhibitors are always taken with 1 or 2 nucleoside antiviral drugs such as AZT, ddI, ddC, or 3TC. They revolutionized HIV treatment because, when taken in combination, they reduce the amount of HIV virus in the bloodstream to levels that are often undetectable by current methods—CD$_4$ cell (immune system cell) counts and viral load (amount of virus in the blood) measurements. Multiple-drug therapy has changed the current view of HIV from a fatal disease to a manageable chronic illness.

Cautions and Warnings

Saquinivir mesylate capsules (Invirase) and saquinavir soft gelatin capsules (Fortovase) **should not be used interchangeably**. Fortovase is recommended when using saquinavir as part of an antiviral regimen. Invirase may be considered in rare circumstances if it is combined with antiretrovirals that significantly inhibit saquinavir's metabolism.

Do not take this drug if you are **sensitive** or **allergic** to it.

If a serious **toxic reaction** occurs while taking saquinavir, you should stop the drug until your doctor can determine the cause or until the reaction resolves itself. Then treatment can be resumed.

Use caution if you have moderate to severe **liver disease**.

Saquinavir may raise your **blood sugar,** worsen your **diabetes,** or bring out latent diabetes. People with diabetes who take saquinavir may need the dosage of their antidiabetes medication adjusted.

HIV virus may become **resistant** to saquinavir or other protease inhibitors. For this reason it is essential that you take saquinavir exactly according to your doctor's directions.

Possible Side Effects

Most side effects are mild. Other side effects become more prominent when saquinavir is taken together with antiretroviral drugs; these include weakness, muscle pain, and mouth ulcers.

▼ Most common: diarrhea, dyspepsia, nausea, and abdominal discomfort.

Possible Side Effects (continued)

▼ Less common: upset stomach, abdominal pain, headache, tingling or numbness in the hands or feet, dizziness, nerve damage, changes in appetite, and rash.

▼ Rare: Rare side effects can occur in almost any part of the body. Contact your doctor if you experience any side effect not listed above.

Drug Interactions

• Rifampin and rifabutin reduce saquinavir blood levels by 80% and 40%, respectively. Do not combine these drugs with saquinavir. Other drugs that can reduce saquinavir blood levels are phenobarbital, phenytoin, carbamazepine, and dexamethasone.

• Blood levels of saquinavir may be elevated by terfenidine, astemizole, ketoconazole, and itraconazole. Other drugs that may elevate saquinavir levels and lead to serious side effects are calcium channel blockers, clindamycin, dapsone, delavirdine, clarithomycin, ergot derivatives, quinidine, and triazolam.

• Ritonavir increases blood levels of saquinavir and increases the risk of side effects.

• St. John's wort decreases the effectiveness of saquinavir. Do not combine.

• Protease inhibitors may drastically increase sildenafil blood levels, increasing the risk of sildenafil, vardenafil, and tadalafil side effects including low blood pressure, visual changes, and persistent, painful erection.

• Phenobarbital, phenytoin, dexamethasone, carbomazepine, and nevirapine may reduce blood levels of saquinavir.

Food Interactions

Take saquinavir within 2 hours after a full meal. The amount of saquinavir absorbed into the blood is vastly reduced when it is taken on an empty stomach, thus negating its antiviral effects.

Usual Dose

Invirase

Adult (age 16 and over): 600 mg 3 times a day, within 2 hours after a full meal.

Child (under age 16): consult your doctor.

Fortovase

Adult (age 16 and over): 1200 mg 3 times a day, within 2 hours after a meal.

Child (under age 16): consult your doctor.

Overdosage

Little is known about the effects of saquinavir overdose. Take the victim to a hospital emergency room. ALWAYS bring the prescription bottle or container.

Special Information

Saquinavir does not cure HIV infection or AIDS. It will not prevent you from transmitting the HIV virus to another person; you must still practice safe sex. You may still develop opportunistic infections or other illnesses associated with advanced HIV disease. The long-term effects of this drug are not known.

It is imperative for you to take this medication exactly according to your doctor's instructions. Missing doses of saquinavir increases the risk that you will become resistant to the drug. It should be taken after meals with your nucleoside antiviral drug. If you forget a dose of saquinavir, take it as soon as you remember. Do not take a double dose.

Special Populations

Pregnancy/Breast-feeding

While animal studies of saquinavir reveal no damage to the fetus, this drug should only be used during pregnancy after carefully weighing its potential benefits against its risks.

It is not known if saquinavir passes into breast milk. Nursing mothers with HIV should always bottle-feed, regardless of whether they take this drug, to avoid transmitting the virus.

Seniors

Seniors can take this drug without special precaution.

Type of Drug

Selective Serotonin Reuptake Inhibitors (SSRIs)

Brand Name

Generic Ingredient: Citalopram
Celexa

Generic Ingredient: Escitalopram
Lexapro

Generic Ingredient: Fluoxetine G
Prozac   Sarafem
Prozac Weekly

Generic Ingredient: Fluvoxamine G
Luvox

Generic Ingredient: Paroxetine
Paxil   Paxil CR

Generic Ingredient: Sertraline
Zoloft

Prescribed For

Depression, bulimic binge-eating and vomiting, obsessive-compulsive disorder (OCD), obesity, alcoholism, anorexia, attention-deficit hyperactivity disorder (ADHD), bipolar affective disorder, borderline personality disorder, cataplexy and narcolepsy, generalized anxiety disorder, kleptomania, migraine, chronic daily headaches, tension headaches, post-traumatic stress disorder (PTSD), schizophrenia, Tourette's syndrome, dyskinetic side effects of levodopa, and social phobias.

General Information

SSRIs, which are chemically unrelated to other antidepressant drugs, prevent the movement of the neurotransmitter serotonin into nerve endings. This forces serotonin to remain in the spaces surrounding nerve endings, increasing its action. Abnormal serotonin function may be involved in depression, and the SSRIs are effective in treating the common symptoms of depression. They can help improve mood and mental alertness, increase physical activity, and improve sleep patterns. There are some differences in the time it takes for the different SSRIs to start working and how they are eliminated from the body.

Drug	Time to start working	Mode of elimination
Citalopram	About 7 days	35% kidney, 65% liver
Escitalopram	About 7 days	18% kidney, 82% liver
Fluoxetine	About 28 days	100% liver
Fluvoxamine	About 7 days	About 94% kidney
Paroxetine	About 10 days	64% kidney, 36% liver
Paroxetine CR	14 days	64% kidney, 36% liver
Sertraline	7 days	40–45% kidney, 40–45% liver

Cautions and Warnings

Do not take these drugs if you are **allergic** to them. Some people have experienced serious **drug reactions** to SSRIs.

Serious, **potentially fatal reactions** may occur if SSRIs and a **monoamine oxidase inhibitor (MAOI)** antidepressant are taken within 2 weeks of one another (see "Drug Interactions").

About 7% of people taking fluoxetine develop an **itching rash,** 1/3 of whom have to stop taking the medication. Other symptoms associated with the rash are fever, joint pain, swelling, wrist and hand pain, breathing difficulties, swollen lymph glands, and laboratory abnormalities. In most people, these symptoms go away when they stop taking fluoxetine and receive antihistamines or corticosteroids.

As many as 1/3 of people taking an SSRI experience **anxiety, sleeplessness,** and **nervousness.**

Underweight depressed people who take fluoxetine may lose more weight. About 9% of people taking fluoxetine experience appetite loss, while 13% lose more than 5% of their body weight.

SSRIs may affect **blood platelets,** though their exact effect is not known. Some people have had **abnormal bleeding** while taking these drugs.

SSRIs are significantly broken down in the liver. People with **liver disease** should use these drugs with caution and may require lower doses than people without liver disease. People with severe **kidney disease** should begin with smaller doses of citalopram, paroxetine, and sertraline.

People taking citalopram may experience a severe drop in their blood sodium level.

Manic depressive people taking escitalopram may experience a worsening of their condition.

SSRIs should be used with caution by people with **seizure disorders**.

A few people with **mania or hypomania** may experience an activation of their condition when taking SSRIs.

Fluoxetine may alter **glycemic control** in people with diabetes.

The possibility of **suicide** exists in severely depressed patients and may be present until the condition is significantly improved. Severely depressed people should be allowed to carry only small quantities of SSRIs to limit the risk of overdose.

Possible Side Effects

▼ Most common: headache, anxiety, nervousness, sleeplessness, drowsiness, tiredness, weakness, changes in sex drive, tremors, sweating, dizziness, light-headedness, dry mouth, upset or irritated stomach, appetite loss, nausea, vomiting, diarrhea, gas, rash, and itching.

▼ Less common: abnormal ejaculation, impotence, abnormal dreams, difficulty concentrating, increased appetite, acne, hair loss, dry skin, chest pain, allergy, runny nose, bronchitis, abnormal heart rhythms, bleeding, blood pressure changes, dizziness or fainting when rising suddenly from a sitting position, bone pain, bursitis, twitching, breast pain, fibrocystic disease of the breast, cystitis, urinary pain, double vision, eye or ear pain, conjunctivitis (pinkeye), anemia, swelling, low blood sugar, weight loss or gain, and low thyroid activity.

▼ Rare: Rare side effects can affect almost any part of the body. Contact your doctor if you experience any side effect not listed above.

Drug Interactions

• Five weeks should elapse between stopping fluoxetine and starting an MAOI antidepressant. At least 2 weeks should elapse between stopping other SSRIs and starting an MAOI.

Two weeks should elapse between stopping an MAOI and starting an SSRI. Taking these drugs too close together or at the same time may cause serious, life-threatening reactions.

• Combining an SSRI and NSAIDs substantially increases the risk of gastrointestinal side effects. This combination should be avoided over the long term.

• Fluoxetine blood levels may increase if the drug is taken with a tricyclic antidepressant. SSRIs may increase tricyclic antidepressant blood levels.

• SSRIs affect lithium blood levels. Your lithium dosage may need to be adjusted.

• People taking warfarin and SSRIs may experience increased bleeding or increased warfarin side effects.

• Combining sertraline and pimozide can significantly increase the amount of pimozide in the blood. Do not combine these drugs.

• Cyproheptadine (an antihistamine) may reverse the effects of fluoxetine and paroxetine.

• Hallucinations have occurred after combining fluoxetine with dextromethorphan (the most common cough suppressant in over-the-counter products).

• Combining fluoxetine, paroxetine, or sertraline with phenytoin can lead to increased phenytoin side effects and reduce blood levels of paroxetine.

• Fluoxetine, fluvoxamine, and sertraline can raise the blood level of the antipsychotic drug clozapine.

• People who combine l-tryptophan and SSRIs may become agitated and restless, and may experience an upset stomach.

• Alcohol may increase tiredness and other depressant effects of SSRIs.

• Fluoxetine and fluvoxamine may reduce the effectiveness of buspirone, which can lead to a worsening of OCD in people taking this combination to treat OCD.

• Fluoxetine and fluvoxamine may increase the risk of carbamazepine side effects and increase haloperidol levels.

• Fluoxetine, fluvoxamine, and sertraline may increase the effect of benzodiazepine antianxiety drugs.

• Cimetidine can increase paroxetine and citalopram levels in the blood.

• Smoking increases the metabolism of fluvoxamine.

• Fluvoxamine and citalopram may increase the effects of beta blockers.

• Paroxetine may affect the effectiveness of digoxin, and may increase phenothiazine tranquilizer levels and the effects of procyclidine.

• Fluvoxamine may increase methadone and tacrine blood levels, and may increase the effects of diltiazem.

• Paroxetine and fluvoxamine may increase the effects of sumatriptan and affect theophylline blood levels.

• Fluoxetine can raise the blood levels of pimozide and cyclosporine (an immune suppressant).

Food Interactions

These drugs may be taken without regard to food or meals.

Usual Dose

Citalopram

Adult: 20–40 mg a day. Seniors and people with liver disease should take no more than 20 mg a day. People with kidney disease may need a lower dose.

Child: not recommended.

Escitalopram

Adult: 10–20 mg once a day. Seniors and people with liver disease should take no more than 10 mg.

Child: consult your doctor.

Fluoxetine

Adult: 20–80 mg a day, taken in the morning, or a single 90 mg capsule weekly. Seniors, people with kidney or liver disease, and people taking several different drugs may need a lower dose.

Child (age 8–18): 10–20 mg a day.

Fluvoxamine

Adult: 50–300 mg a day at bedtime. Seniors and people with liver disease may need a lower dose.

Child (age 8–17): 25–200 mg a day. Doses larger than 50 mg should be divided in two and given morning and night. If the 2 divided doses are not equal, give the larger dose at bedtime.

Child (up to age 8): not recommended.

Paroxetine

Adult: 20–60 mg a day, or 25–62.5 mg a day for the controlled-release form. Seniors and people with liver disease

should start at 10 mg a day and take no more than 40 mg a day. People with kidney disease may need a lower dose.
    Child: not recommended.

Sertraline
    Adult: 50–200 mg a day. Lower doses may be used to start, but most adults take at least 50 mg a day. Seniors and people with liver disease should take a lower dose.
    Child (age 6–17 years): 25–50 mg to start. Maximum dose is 200 mg a day.

Overdosage

Overdose symptoms may include seizures, nausea, vomiting, agitation, restlessness, and nervous system excitation. Any person suspected of having taken an SSRI overdose should be taken to a hospital emergency room at once. ALWAYS bring the prescription bottle or container.

Special Information

SSRIs can make you dizzy or drowsy. Take care when driving or performing other tasks that require alertness and concentration, especially when you first start the drug or increase your dose. Avoid alcohol.

Be sure your doctor knows if you are pregnant, breast-feeding, or taking other drugs, including over- the-counter drugs, while taking an SSRI.

Call your doctor if you develop a rash or hives, become excessively nervous or anxious, lose your appetite—especially if you are already underweight—or experience any unusual side effects.

If you forget a dose, take it as soon as you remember. If it is almost time for your next dose, skip the dose you forgot and continue with your regular schedule. Do not take a double dose.

Special Populations

Pregnancy/Breast-feeding

In one study, about 5% of pregnant women who took fluoxetine during the first 3 months had babies with major abnormalities. Animal studies with the other SSRIs show similar results. In addition, women taking this drug were more likely to deliver prematurely. Do not take an SSRI if you are or might be pregnant without first weighing the potential benefits and risks with your doctor.

The SSRIs pass into breast milk. There are 2 reports of nursing infants whose mothers were taking an SSRI. The infants became sleepy, ate less, and lost weight. Nursing mothers who must take an SSRI should consider bottle-feeding.

Seniors

Seniors generally start with lower doses and may need less of the drug to achieve the desired results.

Generic Name

Selegiline (seh-LEG-uh-leen) G

Brand Names

Atapryl	Eldepryl
Carbex	

Type of Drug

Antiparkinsonian and selective monoamine oxidase inhibitor (MAOI).

Prescribed For

Parkinson's disease.

General Information

Selegiline hydrochloride is often combined with levodopa or carbidopa to control Parkinson's disease. Selegiline blocks the effects of the enzyme monoamine oxidase (MAO); it interferes with a form of it found almost exclusively in the brain. Selegiline also stimulates dopamine receptors. In order for any drug to work in Parkinson's disease, it must increase the activity of dopamine in the brain.

Cautions and Warnings

Be cautious about using selegiline if you have had a **reaction** to it.

If you take **Sinemet**—which contains levodopa and carbidopa—and start taking selegiline, you may experience an increase in levodopa side effects. Your Sinemet dosage may need to be reduced.

Taking more than 10 mg of selegiline a day may cause **severe reactions,** including possibly fatal high blood pressure.

Selegiline should not be used with **meperidine or other narcotic drugs** because of the risk of severe, possibly fatal reactions.

Possible Side Effects

Some of selegiline's side effects may be caused by methamphetamine and amphetamine; these potent stimulants are products of the body's breakdown of selegiline. When selegiline dosage is less than 10 mg per day, most side effects are not caused by the drug itself; rather, selegiline increases the side effects of levodopa. It is important for your doctor to reduce your levodopa dosage as much as possible.

▼ Most common: nausea, vomiting, dizziness, light-headedness or fainting, and abdominal pain.

▼ Less common: tremors or uncontrolled muscle movements, loss of balance, inability to move, increasingly slow movements associated with Parkinson's disease, facial grimacing, falling due to loss of balance, stiff neck, muscle cramps, hallucinations, overstimulation, confusion, anxiety, depression, drowsiness, changes in mood or behavior, nightmares or unusual dreams, tiredness, delusions, disorientation, feeling unwell, apathy, sleep disturbances, restlessness, weakness, irritability-generalized aches and pains, migraine or other headaches, muscle pains in the back or legs, ringing or buzzing in the ears, eye pain, finger or toe numbness, changes in sense of taste, dizziness when rising from a sitting or lying position, blood-pressure changes, abnormal heart rhythm, heart palpitations, chest pain, rapid heartbeat, swelling in the arms or legs, constipation, appetite loss, weight loss, difficulty swallowing, diarrhea, heartburn, rectal bleeding, urinary difficulties, impotence, swelling of the prostate, increased sweating, increased facial hair, hair loss, rash, increased sensitivity to the sun, bruising or black-and-blue marks, asthma, blurred or double vision, shortness of breath, speech problems, and dry mouth.

At dosages above 10 mg a day, selegiline may cause muscle twitching or spasms, memory loss, increased

---

Possible Side Effects *(continued)*

energy, transient euphoria (feeling "high"), grinding of
the teeth, decreased sensation in the penis, and inability
to achieve orgasm in men.

Drug Interactions

• Selegiline should not be used with meperidine or other
narcotics because of the risk of severe, possibly fatal reactions (see "Cautions and Warnings").

• Combining fluoxetine with MAOIs other than selegiline
has been deadly. This effect has not been seen with selegiline, but the combination should be avoided. Allow 5 weeks
between stopping fluoxetine and starting on any MAOI. If you
are already taking an MAOI, allow at least 2 weeks between
stopping that drug and starting on selegiline.

Food Interactions

Take selegiline with food to avoid nausea or stomach upset,
but avoid the following: Chianti and red wine, vermouth,
unpasteurized or imported beer, beef or chicken liver, fermented sausages, tenderized or prepared meats, caviar,
dried fish, pickled herring, cheese (American, Brie, cheddar,
Camembert, Emmentaler, Boursault, Stilton, and others),
avocados, yeast extracts, bananas, figs, raisins, soy sauce,
miso soup, bean curd, fava beans, caffeine, and chocolate.
These foods may cause severe, sudden high blood pressure
in people taking selegiline.

Usual Dose

5 mg with breakfast and lunch.

Overdosage

Symptoms may include excitement, irritability, anxiety, low
blood pressure, sleeplessness, restlessness, dizziness, weakness, drowsiness, flushing, sweating, heart palpitations, and
unusual movements, including grimacing and muscle twitching. Serious overdoses may lead to convulsions, incoherence
or confusion, severe headache, high fever, heart attack, shock,
and coma. Take the victim to a hospital emergency room.
ALWAYS bring the prescription bottle or container.

Special Information

After you have taken selegiline for 2 or 3 days, your doctor will probably reduce your carbidopa or levodopa dosage by 10% to 30%. If the disease is still under control, your dosage may be reduced further.

Contact your doctor if you develop headache, unusual body movements or muscle spasms, mood changes, or any bothersome or persistent side effects. Do not stop taking selegiline or change your dosage without your doctor's knowledge.

Selegiline reduces saliva flow in the mouth and may increase the risk of cavities, gum disease, and oral infections. Use candy, ice, sugarless gum, or a saliva substitute to avoid dry mouth.

If you forget a dose, take it as soon as you remember. If it is almost time for your next dose, take 1 dose right away and another in 5 or 6 hours, then go back to your regular schedule. Do not take a double dose.

Special Populations

Pregnancy/Breast-feeding

The safety of using selegiline during pregnancy is not known. When this drug is considered crucial by your doctor, its potential benefits must be carefully weighed against its risks.

It is not known if selegiline passes into breast milk. Nursing mothers who must take it should consider bottle-feeding.

Seniors

Seniors should receive the lowest effective dosage to minimize side effects.

Brand Name

Septra

Generic Ingredients

Sulfamethoxazole + Trimethoprim G

Other Brand Names

Bactrim
Bactrim DS
Bactrim Pediatric
Cotrim
Cotrim DS
Cotrim Pediatric

Septra
Septra DS
Sulfamethoprim
Sulfamethoprim DS
Sulfatrim
TMP-SMZ

Type of Drug

Anti-infective.

Prescribed For

A wide variety of infections, including urinary tract infection, bronchitis, and ear infection in children; also prescribed for traveler's diarrhea, pneumocystis carinii pneumonia (PCP), prostate infection, cholera, nocardiosis (lung infection), and *Salmonella* infection.

General Information

Septra is effective in many situations where other drugs are not. It is unique because it interferes with the infecting microorganism's normal use of folic acid in two ways, making it more efficient than other antibacterial drugs.

Cautions and Warnings

Do not take Septra if you have a **folic acid deficiency** or are **allergic** to either ingredient or to any sulfa drug, antidiabetes drug, or thiazide-type diuretic. Septra should be used with caution by people with **liver or kidney disease. Infants under 2 months of age** should not be given this combination product.

Symptoms such as unusual bleeding or bruising, extreme tiredness, rash, sore throat, fever, pallor, or yellowing of the skin or eyes may be early indications of a serious **blood disorder**. If any of these effects occur, contact your doctor immediately and stop taking the drug. **People taking Septra for PCP** also have compromised immune function. They may not respond to Septra and are more likely to develop the less common side effects.

Septra should not be used for **strep throat** because of a greater chance of treatment failure than with penicillin.

Possible Side Effects

▼ Most common: nausea, vomiting, upset stomach, loss of appetite, and rash or itching.

▼ Less common: reduced levels of red and white blood cells and platelets, allergic reaction (symptoms include rash, itching, hives, and breathing difficulties), swelling around the eyes, arthritis-like pain, diarrhea, coating of the tongue, headache, tingling in the arms or

> **Possible Side Effects** *(continued)*
>
> legs, depression, convulsions, hallucinations, ringing in the ears, dizziness, difficulty sleeping, apathy, tiredness, weakness, and nervousness. Septra may also affect your kidneys and cause you to produce less urine.

Drug Interactions

• Septra may prolong the effects of anticoagulant (blood-thinning) agents—such as warfarin—and oral antidiabetes drugs.

• The trimethoprim in Septra may reduce the effectiveness of cyclosporine and increase its toxic effect on the kidney.

• The sulfamethoxazole in Septra can increase the amount of phenytoin and methotrexate in the bloodstream, increasing the chance of side effects. Dosage reduction of phenytoin or methotrexate may be needed to adjust for the presence of Septra.

• Older adults taking a thiazide diuretic with Septra are more likely to develop reduced levels of blood platelets and an increased chance of bleeding under the skin.

• Taking Septra together with dapsone can result in increased blood levels of both drugs. Septra can interfere with the elimination of zidovudine (AZT) through the kidneys, increasing the amount of AZT in the blood.

Food Interactions

Take each dose with a full glass of water. Continue to drink plenty of fluids throughout the day to decrease the risk of kidney-stone formation.

Usual Dose

Adult: 2 regular tablets or 1 Septra DS tablet every 12 hours for 5–14 days, depending on the condition being treated.

Child (67–88 lbs.): 4 tsp. (or 2 tablets) every 12 hours.

Child (45–66 lbs.): 3 tsp. (or 1½ tablets) every 12 hours.

Child (23–44 lbs.): 2 tsp. (or 1 tablet) every 12 hours.

Child (under 22 lbs.): 1 tsp. every 12 hours.

Child (under age 2 months): not recommended.

Overdosage

Large overdoses can cause exaggerated side effects. Call your local poison control center or emergency room for more information. If you go to the hospital for treatment, ALWAYS bring the prescription bottle or container.

Special Information

Take Septra exactly as prescribed for the full length of the prescription. Do not stop taking it just because you are beginning to feel better. Take each dose with a full glass of water and drink plenty of fluids all day to lower the risk of kidney-stone formation.

Call your doctor if you develop sore throat, rash, unusual bleeding or bruising, or any other persistent or intolerable side effect.

You may develop unusual sensitivity to bright light, particularly sunlight. If you have a history of light sensitivity or if you have sensitive skin, avoid prolonged exposure to sunlight while using Septra.

If you miss a dose of Septra, take it as soon as possible. If you take it twice a day and it is almost time for your next dose, take 1 dose as soon as you remember and another in 5 to 6 hours, then go back to your regular schedule. If you take Septra 3 or more times a day and it is almost time for your next dose, take 1 dose as soon as you remember and another in 2 to 4 hours, then continue with your regular schedule. Never take a double dose.

Special Populations

Pregnancy/Breast-feeding
Septra may affect folic acid in the fetus throughout pregnancy and should be used with caution. It should never be taken near term because of the effects of sulfamethoxazole on the newborn, including yellowing of the skin or eyes. Talk to your doctor about Septra's risks versus its benefits if the drug is to be used during pregnancy.

Septra is not recommended for use if you are nursing because of possible effects on the newborn infant.

Seniors
Seniors are more likely to be sensitive to the effects of this drug, especially if they have liver or kidney problems; dosage adjustments may be required.

Seroquel   *see Quetiapine, page 909*

Generic Name

Sevelamer (seh-VEL-ah-mer)

Brand Name

Renagel

Type of Drug

Phosphate binder.

Prescribed For

High blood-phosphate levels in people with end-stage renal disease (ESRD).

General Information

People with ESRD, a form of kidney disease, tend to retain phosphorous. High phosphate levels, in turn, can effect calcium balance in the body and cause deposits of this mineral to build up in the wrong places. Sevelamer hydrochloride helps to reduce phosphate levels by limiting the amount of phosphorous absorbed from food. Sevelamer also lowers levels of total and low-density lipoprotein (LDL) cholesterol.

Cautions and Warnings

Do not take sevelamer if you are **sensitive** or **allergic** to it or have a **low phosphate level** or a **bowel obstruction**.

Use this drug with caution if you have had **gastrointestinal (GI) surgery** or have **difficulty swallowing** or severe **stomach or intestinal problems**.

Possible Side Effects

▼ Most common: headache, infection, pain, blood pressure changes, blood clotting problems, diarrhea, upset stomach, and vomiting.

▼ Common: nausea.

▼ Less common: cough, gas, and constipation.

▼ Rare: Rare side effects can occur in almost any part of the body. Contact your doctor if you experience any side effect not listed above.

Drug Interactions

• Sevelamer may interfere with other drugs taken at the same time. Take sevelamer either 1 hour before or 3 hours after other medications.

Food Interactions

Sevelamer should be taken with meals.

Usual Dose

Adult: 1–4 capsules with each meal; maximum dosage is 30 capsules a day.

Child: There is no information on the use of this drug in children. Those receiving it must be closely monitored by their doctors.

Overdosage

Symptoms may include drug side effects. Call your local poison control center or a hospital emergency room for more information. If you seek treatment, ALWAYS bring the prescription bottle or container.

Special Information

Sevelamer can interfere with the absorption of vitamins from food. Take a supplemental multivitamin while using this drug.

It is important to take sevelamer with each meal. If you forget a dose, skip it and continue to take the drug with subsequent meals.

Do not chew or dismantle the capsules before swallowing them.

Special Populations

Pregnancy/Breast-feeding

In animal studies, sevelamer interfered with fetal bone development. It also interferes with the absorption of vitamins and nutrients, which are essential for a healthy pregnancy. When this drug is considered crucial by your doctor, its potential benefits must be carefully weighed against its risks.

It is not known if sevelamer passes into breast milk. Nursing mothers who must take it should consider bottle-feeding.

Seniors

Seniors may take this drug without special precaution.

Generic Name

Sibutramine (sih-BYUE-trah-meen)

Brand Name

Meridia

Type of Drug

Appetite suppressant.

Prescribed For

Weight loss.

General Information

Sibutramine works by increasing levels of norepinephrine, serotonin, and dopamine in the brain. By preventing the re-uptake of these chemicals into nerve endings, sibutramine stimulates areas of the brain associated with appetite control. About 6 in 10 people who take sibutramine in conjunction with a diet and exercise program lose 4 lbs. or more during the first 4 weeks of treatment and are likely to lose about 5% of their total body weight in 6 to 12 months.

Cautions and Warnings

Do not take sibutramine if you are **allergic** to it.

People taking sibutramine may develop **drug dependency**.

People taking sibutramine may eventually become resistant to the drug, requiring increased dosage to achieve the same effect.

People who have had a **stroke** or who have **heart disease** should not take sibutramine.

People with **narrow-angle glaucoma** should take this drug with caution because it can dilate pupils.

Sibutramine should not be taken by people with severe **liver or kidney disease**.

Sibutramine can **raise blood pressure and pulse rate,** especially if you already have high blood pressure. Check your blood pressure and pulse regularly.

Rarely, people taking sibutramine develop a group of symptoms called **serotonin syndrome,** consisting of one or more of the following symptoms: excitement, a mild manic reaction, restlessness, loss of consciousness, confusion, disorientation, anxiety, agitation, muscle weakness, muscle spasms, tremors, involuntary muscle movements on one side of the body, shivering and dilated pupils, sweating, vomiting, and rapid heartbeat. Serotonin syndrome requires immediate medical treatment.

Other weight loss drugs that act on the nervous system like sibutramine does can cause a rare condition called pulmonary hypertension. This has not been reported with sibutramine.

Rapid weight loss can cause or worsen **gallstones**.

Possible Side Effects

▼ Most common: headache, dry mouth, sleeplessness, appetite loss, constipation, runny nose, and sore throat.

▼ Common: back pain, flu-like symptoms, injuries, weakness, dizziness, nervousness, increased appetite, nausea, joint pain, and sinus irritation.

▼ Less common: abdominal pain, chest pain, neck pain, allergy, rapid heartbeat, flushing, migraine, high blood pressure, heart palpitations, anxiety, depression, tingling in the hands or feet, tiredness, stimulation, emotional instability, rash, sweating, herpes infections, acne, upset stomach, stomach irritation, vomiting, rectal problems, painful menstruation, urinary or vaginal infections, excessive menstrual flow, thirst, swelling, muscle aches, tendon inflammation, joint problems, increased cough, laryngitis, changes in sense of taste, and ear problems.

▼ Rare: seizures, agitation, leg cramps, gas, tooth problems, abnormal thinking, bronchitis, breathing difficulties, bleeding problems, and kidney problems.

Drug Interactions

• Cimetidine, erythromycin, and ketoconazole can mildly increase sibutramine blood levels, but this effect is not considered important.

• Do not drink alcohol to excess while taking sibutramine.

• Do not combine monoamine oxidase inhibitor (MAOI) drugs and sibutramine. This combination could lead to serotonin syndrome (see "Cautions and Warnings").

• Do not combine sibutramine and other weight loss pills that act on the nervous system (usually these are prescription-only diet pills), triptan-type migraine drugs, dihydroergotamine, antidepressants, decongestants, cough medications, lithium, or L-tryptophan.

• Stimulants found in some over-the-counter medications—such as decongestants, weight loss pills, or cough, cold, or allergy drugs—can raise blood pressure or heart rate when combined with sibutramine.

Food Interactions

Sibutramine can be taken with or without food.

Usual Dose

Adult and Child (age 16 and over): 5–15 mg once a day.
Child (under age 16): not recommended.

Overdosage

Little is known about the effects of sibutramine overdose, though symptoms may include rapid heartbeat. Take the victim to a hospital emergency room. ALWAYS bring the prescription bottle or container.

Special Information

Call your doctor if you develop an allergic reaction such as rash or hives or experience any bothersome or persistent side effect.

This drug can cause an inability to concentrate. Be careful when driving or performing any task that requires concentration or good judgment.

If you forget a dose, take it as soon as you remember. If it is almost time for your next dose, skip the forgotten dose and continue with your regular schedule. Do not take a double dose.

Special Populations

Pregnancy/Breast-feeding
Pregnant women should not take sibutramine under any circumstances. Women of childbearing age should be sure to use effective contraception while taking this medication.

It is not known if sibutramine passes into breast milk. Nursing mothers who must take it should consider bottle-feeding.

Seniors
Seniors with reduced kidney or liver function should receive the lowest effective dosage.

Brand Name

Sinemet

Generic Ingredients

Carbidopa + Levodopa G

Other Brand Names

Sinemet CR

The information in this profile also applies to the following drug:

Generic Ingredient: Carbidopa

Lodosyn

Type of Drug

Antiparkinsonian.

Prescribed For

Parkinson's disease.

General Information

In Sinemet, levodopa is the active ingredient that affects Parkinson's disease; carbidopa slows the breakdown of levodopa, making more available to the brain. This combination is so effective that your dosage of levodopa may be reduced by about 75%, which results in fewer side effects. Unfortunately, people eventually develop a resistance to levodopa in any form. Carbidopa is sold under the brand name Lodosyn for people who need individual doses of both carbidopa and levodopa.

Cautions and Warnings

Do not take Sinemet if you are **allergic** to either of its ingredients. If you are switching from levodopa to Sinemet, you should stop taking levodopa 8 hours before your first dose of Sinemet. The sustained-release form of Sinemet has a lesser incidence of **nervous-system side effects;** the immediate-release version may produce such effects even at lower dosages.

Possible Side Effects

▼ Common: uncontrolled muscle movements, appetite loss, nausea, vomiting, stomach pain, dry mouth, difficulty swallowing, drooling, shaky hands, headache, dizziness, numbness, weakness, feeling faint, grinding of the teeth, confusion, sleeplessness, nightmares, hallucinations, anxiety, agitation, tiredness, feeling unwell, and euphoria (feeling "high").

▼ Less common: heart palpitations; dizziness when rising quickly from a sitting or lying position; sudden extreme slowness of movement ("on-off" phenomenon); changes in mental state, including paranoia, psychosis, depression, and a slowdown of mental functioning; difficulty urinating; muscle twitching; eyelid spasms; lockjaw; burning sensation on the tongue; bitter taste; diarrhea; constipation; gas; flushing; rash; sweating; unusual breathing; blurred or double vision; pupil dilation; hot flashes; weight changes; and darkening of urine or sweat.

▼ Rare: Rare side effects can occur in almost any part of the body. Contact your doctor if you experience any side effect not listed above.

Drug Interactions

• Sinemet's effectiveness may be increased by anticholinergic drugs such as trihexyphenidyl.

• Methyldopa (an antihypertensive drug) may increase the amount of levodopa available in the central nervous system and may have a slight effect on Sinemet as well.

• People taking guanethidine or a diuretic to treat high blood pressure may need less of either if they start taking Sinemet.

• Reserpine, benzodiazepine tranquilizers, antipsychotic drugs, phenytoin, and papaverine may interfere with Sinemet. Vitamin B_6 interferes with levodopa but not with Sinemet.

• Combining Sinemet and a monoamine oxidase inhibitor (MAOI) may cause a rapid increase in blood pressure. MAOIs should be stopped 2 weeks before starting on Sinemet.

• Sinemet may increase the effects of ephedrine, amphetamines, epinephrine, and isoproterenol. This interaction, which may also occur with antidepressant drugs, can result in adverse effects on the heart.

Food Interactions

Immediate-release Sinemet may be taken with food to reduce upset stomach. Sinemet CR, the sustained-release form, should be taken on an empty stomach.

Usual Dose

Three Sinemet strengths are available: 10/100, 25/100, and 25/250. The first number represents carbidopa content, the second the levodopa content, in mg. Dosage must be individualized based on previous drug treatment. Dosage adjustments are made by adding or omitting ½–1 tablet a day. Maximum daily dosage is eight 25/250-tablets. Sinemet CR is started at dosages roughly equal to 10% more levodopa a day than was being taken previously.

If extra carbidopa is needed, your doctor may prescribe Lodosyn to be taken together with Sinemet. Lodosyn is added in steps of no more than 25 mg a day until the desired effect is achieved.

Overdosage

Symptoms include exaggerated side effects. Take the victim to a hospital emergency room. ALWAYS bring the prescription bottle or container.

Special Information

Sinemet can cause tiredness or an inability to concentrate: Be careful when driving or doing any task that requires concentration.

Call your doctor if you experience dizziness; light-headedness or fainting spells; changes in mood or mental state; abnormal heart rhythm or heart palpitations; difficulty urinating; persistent nausea, vomiting, or other stomach complaints; or uncontrollable movements of the face, eyelids, mouth, tongue, neck, arms, hands, or legs.

This drug may cause darkening of urine or sweat. This effect is not harmful, but may interfere with urine tests for diabetes. Make sure all your doctors know you are taking this medication.

Take Sinemet exactly as prescribed.

If you forget a dose, take it as soon as you remember. If it is within 2 hours of your next dose, skip the one you forgot and

continue with your regular schedule. Do not take a double dose.

Special Populations

Pregnancy/Breast-feeding
Both of the ingredients in Sinemet cause birth defects in animals. When this drug is considered crucial by your doctor, its potential benefits must be carefully weighed against its risks.

The ingredients in Sinemet may pass into breast milk and are considered unsafe for infants. Nursing mothers who must take this drug should bottle-feed.

Seniors
Seniors may require reduced dosage. They are also more likely to develop abnormal heart rhythms or other cardiac side effects, especially if they have heart disease.

Singulair *see Leukotriene Antagonists/Inhibitors,* page 617

Skelaxin *see Metaxalone,* page 682

Type of Drug
Statin Cholesterol-Lowering Agents

Brand Names

Generic Ingredient: Atorvastatin
Lipitor

Generic Ingredient: Fluvastatin
Lescol   Lescol XL

Generic Ingredient: Lovastatin G
Altocor   Mevacor

Generic Ingredients: Lovastatin + Niacin
Advicor

Generic Ingredient: Pravastatin
Pravachol

Generic Ingredients: Pravastatin + Aspirin
Pravigard PAC

Generic Ingredient: Rosuvastatin [G]
Crestor

Generic Ingredient: Simvastatin
Zocor

Prescribed For

High blood levels of cholesterol, low-density lipoprotein (LDL) cholesterol, and triglycerides; also prescribed for atherosclerosis (hardening of the arteries), diabetes-related blood-fat problems, preventing heart attacks and strokes, and reducing the risk of cardiac bypass surgery. Some of these drugs may also be used for blood-fat disorders related to kidney disease and inherited blood-fat problems.

General Information

High blood-fat levels are believed to play a role in the development of cardiovascular disease. Statin drugs help to lower blood-fat levels by blocking the effects of the enzyme HMG-CoA reductase, which in turn interferes with the production of cholesterol in the body. They also increase levels of high-density lipoprotein (HDL) cholesterol, the "good" cholesterol considered to have a beneficial effect on heart health. Statin drugs are proven to slow the progression of atherosclerosis, help prevent heart attacks, and reduce the risk of dying from heart disease. Other related benefits have been discovered. Atorvastatin, for example, has been found to improve the ability of people with intermittent claudication (a blood vessel disease) to walk. Advicor combines lovastatin with niacin, a nutrient that helps raise levels of "good" cholesterol. One product combines pravastatin with a small dose (81 mg) of aspirin in an effort to combine two drugs commonly taken at the same time for heart-attack prevention.

These drugs begin working quickly. Blood-fat levels are significantly improved after 1 to 2 weeks of treatment. Maximum effect occurs in 4 to 6 weeks, persists for the remainder of drug therapy, and continues for 4 to 6 weeks after you stop taking these drugs. These drugs are generally not recommended for people under age 30, though they may be prescribed for teenagers under certain circumstances. Only a small amount of these drugs enters the bloodstream. They are largely broken down in the liver.

Cautions and Warnings

Do not take any of these drugs if you are **allergic** to them. It is possible to be allergic to one of these drugs and tolerate another.

People with a history of **liver disease** and those who drink **large amounts of alcohol** should avoid these drugs because they may aggravate or cause liver disease. About 1 in 100 people who take these drugs develops high liver-enzyme counts; the risk of this effect is highest with lovastatin and lowest with atorvastatin and cerivastatin. Your doctor should take a blood sample to test your liver function every month or so during the first year of treatment.

People taking these drugs may develop severe **muscle aches** or **weakness,** which can be a sign of a more serious condition. This is usually a rare problem but is more common at higher drug doses.

People with **kidney disease** who take pravastatin, rosuvastatin, or simvastatin must be closely monitored by their doctors.

People in early studies of lovastatin developed **cloudy vision,** due to an effect on the lens of the eye, but this effect has not been seen in further studies. Statins have also been reported to cause degeneration of the optic nerve and cataracts at doses 30 to 60 times the average dose. Report any changes in vision to your doctor.

Possible Side Effects

Side effects are usually mild and temporary. Rare side effects associated with these drugs can occur in almost any part of the body. Contact your doctor if you experience any side effect not listed below.

Atorvastatin
▼ Most common: headache, diarrhea, joint pain, sinusitis, infection, and flu-like symptoms.

Possible Side Effects *(continued)*

▼ Common: muscle aches and weakness.

▼ Less common: gas, upset stomach, itching, rash, and allergy.

Fluvastatin

▼ Most common: upper respiratory infection, headache, upset stomach, and diarrhea.

▼ Common: muscle aches, abdominal pain or cramps, changes in sense of taste, flu-like symptoms, allergy, and back pain.

▼ Less common: dizziness, sleeplessness, nausea, vomiting, constipation, gas, tooth problems, arthritis, joint pain, runny nose, cough, sore throat, sinus irritation, itching, rash, and fatigue.

Lovastatin

▼ Common: stomach pain, cramps, gas, constipation, diarrhea, and headache.

▼ Less common: dizziness, heartburn, upset stomach, itching, rash, allergy, infection, nausea, vomiting, muscle aches or pain, joint pain, blurred vision, and eye irritation.

Lovastatin and Niacin

▼ Most common: flushing, which may occur within 2 hours of the first dose.

▼ Common: stomach pain, cramps, gas, and constipation.

▼ Less common: headache, dizziness, heartburn, upset stomach, itching, rash, allergy, infection, nausea, vomiting, diarrhea, muscle aches or pain, joint pain, blurred vision, eye irritation, decreased sugar tolerance in diabetics, stomach ulcer activation, jaundice (yellowing of the skin or eyes), oily or dry skin, aggravation of skin conditions such as acne, low blood pressure, tingling in the hands or feet, and abnormal heartbeats.

Pravastatin

▼ Most common: localized pain.

▼ Common: headache, nausea, vomiting, diarrhea, abdominal pain or cramps, and common cold symptoms.

Possible Side Effects *(continued)*

▼ Less common: dizziness, constipation, heartburn, upset stomach, muscle aches, cough, runny nose, chest pain, itching, rash, flu-like symptoms, fatigue, and urinary difficulties.

Rosuvastatin
▼ Common: sore throat and headache.
▼ Less common: diarrhea, upset stomach, stomach pain, muscle aches, constipation, nausea, back pain, flu-like symptoms, weakness, accidental injury, chest pain, infection, pain, high blood pressure, swelling in the arms or legs, arthritis, joint pains, dizziness, sleeplessness, depression, tingling in the hands or feet, extreme muscle tension, coughing, bronchitis, and rash.
▼ Rare: severe muscle pain and muscle weakness resulting in kidney damage.

Simvastatin
▼ Less common: headache, weakness, nausea, vomiting, diarrhea, abdominal pain or cramps, constipation, gas, upset stomach, and respiratory infection.

Drug Interactions

• Antioxidant supplements, including vitamins E and C and beta-carotene, may reverse the effects of statin drugs. These combinations should be avoided.
• Drinking alcohol regularly increases the amount of fluvastatin in the blood by 30%.
• Antacids reduce statin blood levels, though their actual cholesterol lowering may not change. Separate doses of these drugs by at least 1 hour.
• Itraconazole and ketoconazole can increase lovastatin blood levels by 20 times. Avoid this combination by temporarily stopping your cholesterol medication if you take itraconazole.
• Other drugs that interfere with the breakdown of statin drugs (except pravastatin) are delavirdine, indinavir, nelfinavir, ritonavir, saquinavir, amiodarone, ciprofloxacin, clarithromycin, diltiazem, erythromycin, fluconazole, fluvoxamine, mifepristone, nefazodone, norfloxacin, mibefradil, and troleandomycin.

• Carbamazepine, phenobarbital, phenytoin, pioglitazone, rosiglitazone, and rifampin may reduce statin drug blood levels by stimulating the liver to break it down faster than normal.

• The cholesterol-lowering effects of these drugs and cholestyramine are additive. Take a statin drug 1 hour before or 4 hours after cholestyramine. Colestipol reduces atorvastatin blood levels, but this combination more effectively lowers blood-fat levels than either drug used alone.

• Combining these drugs and cyclosporine, erythromycin, niacin, or gemfibrozil can lead to severe muscle aches or degeneration or other muscle problems. Generally, these combinations should be avoided.

• Digoxin can reduce fluvastatin blood levels. Statin drugs can increase the amount of digoxin in the blood by about 20%.

• Isradipine may speed the elimination of lovastatin from the body.

• Statins increase blood levels of oral contraceptives ("the pill"), which can lead to side effects. If you must take both drugs, talk to your doctor about lowering your contraceptive dosage to the lowest effective dose.

• These drugs may increase the effects of warfarin. People taking these drugs together should be periodically examined by their doctors. Warfarin dosage adjustment may be necessary.

• Propranolol can reduce the effectiveness of these drugs.

Food Interactions

Grapefruit juice can slow the breakdown of statin drugs (except pravastatin) in the liver, increasing the risk of drug side effects. Lovastatin must be taken with meals. Other statin drugs may be taken with or without food.

Usual Dose

Atorvastatin
   Adult: 10–80 mg a day.
   Senior: 10–20 mg a day. Dosage should be adjusted monthly based on how well the drug is working.

Fluvastatin
   Adult: 20–80 mg a day, taken in the evening. Dosage may be adjusted up to 80 mg based on how well the drug is working.

Lovastatin
Adult: 10–80 mg a day, usually taken with your evening meal. Dosage should be adjusted monthly based on how well the drug is working.

Lovastatin and Niacin
Adult: 1 tablet, taken at bedtime. Dosage should be adjusted monthly based on how well the drug is working.

Pravastatin
Adult: 10–40 mg, taken at bedtime.
Senior: 10–20 mg, taken at bedtime. Dosage should be adjusted monthly based on how well the drug is working.

Rosuvastatin
Adult: 5–20 mg a day. Dosage may be increased to a maximum of 40 mg a day.

Simvastatin
Adults: 5–80 mg, taken in the evening.
Senior: 5–20 mg, taken in the evening. Dosage may be adjusted monthly based on how well the drug is working.

Overdosage

People taking overdoses of these drugs have experienced no specific symptoms and have recovered without a problem after the drug was removed from their stomachs by making them vomit. Overdose victims should be taken to a hospital emergency room for evaluation and treatment. ALWAYS bring the prescription bottle or container.

Special Information

Call your doctor if you develop blurred vision or muscle aches, pain, tenderness, or weakness, especially if you are also feverish or don't feel well.

Statin drugs are prescribed in combination with a low-fat diet. Following your doctor's dietary instructions will help reduce your blood fats and keep them low. Do not take more cholesterol-lowering medication than your doctor has prescribed. Do not stop taking it without your doctor's knowledge.

These drugs may cause increased sensitivity to the sun. Use sunscreen and wear protective clothing.

If you forget a dose, take it as soon as you remember. If it is almost time for your next dose, skip the one you forgot and

continue with your regular schedule. Do not take a double dose.

Special Populations

Pregnancy/Breast-feeding

Pregnant women and those who might become pregnant must not take any of these drugs.

These drugs may pass into breast milk. Nursing mothers who must take them should bottle-feed.

Seniors

Seniors are more sensitive to the effects of some statin drugs and may require reduced dosage.

Generic Name

Stavudine (STAV-ue-dene)

Brand Name

Zerit   Zerit XR

Type of Drug

Antiviral.

Prescribed For

Advanced human immunodeficiency virus (HIV) infection.

General Information

Stavudine is a synthetic nucleoside antiviral drug that inhibits the reproduction of the HIV virus by interfering with viral DNA duplication. Stavudine can also interfere with DNA in human cells and may affect the duplication of some body cells. The drug is eliminated primarily through the kidneys.

Cautions and Warnings

Stavudine should be taken only by adults with **advanced HIV infection** who cannot take or tolerate other AIDS treatments, or whose disease has progressed despite treatment with other antiviral drugs. There is no proof that stavudine prolongs the lives of people with AIDS.

People taking stavudine or any other anti-HIV drug may continue to develop **opportunistic infections** and other complications of the disease, and should remain under the direct care of a doctor.

In some cases, **lactic acidosis** (a potentially fatal metabolic imbalance) and severe **liver enlargement** has occurred with the use of stavudine. Patients with **liver disease** should use this drug with caution.

Pancreatic inflammation occurs in 1% of people taking stavudine and has been associated with 14 deaths in people taking this drug.

Peripheral neuropathy is the most common side effect of stavudine (see "Special Information"). People who have had these symptoms before are more likely to have this problem while taking stavudine.

Possible Side Effects

▼ Most common: peripheral neuropathy, which can produce tingling, burning, numbness, or pain in the hands, arms, feet, or legs; diarrhea; nausea; vomiting; headache; fever; chills; weakness; abdominal pain; back pain; muscle or joint ache; generalized pain; not feeling well; sleeplessness; anxiety; depression; nervousness; breathing difficulties; appetite and weight loss; rash; itching; and sweating.

▼ Common: allergic reactions; flu-like symptoms; swollen lymph glands, usually felt under the arms or in the neck; chest pain; constipation; upset stomach; and dizziness.

▼ Less common: pelvic pain, tumors, hypertension (high blood pressure), swelling, flushing, stomach ulcers, confusion, migraine headache, sleepiness, tremors, nerve pain, asthma, pneumonia, skin tumors, conjunctivitis, visual disturbances, painful urination, genital pain, painful menstruation, and vaginitis.

▼ Rare: frequent urination, blood in the urine, impotence, fainting, inflammation of the pancreas, nerve pain, and peeling skin.

Drug Interactions

• Combining stavudine with didanosine or hydroxyurea may increase the risk of lactic acidosis, peripheral neuropathy, inflamed pancreas, or liver toxicity.

• Methadone may reduce blood levels of stavudine by more than 25%.

• Doxorubicin and ribavirin may affect stavudine; use with caution.

Usual Dose

Adult and Child (66 lbs. and over): 30–40 mg every 12 hours. Dosage reduction may be needed in seniors.

Child (under 66 lbs.): 0.5 mg per lb. every 12 hours.

Overdosage

Chronic overdose can produce peripheral neuropathy (see "Special Information") and liver toxicity. Call your local poison control center for more information. Overdose victims should be taken to a hospital emergency room for treatment. ALWAYS bring the prescription bottle or container.

Special Information

Peripheral neuropathy (symptoms include tingling, pain, or numbness in the hands, arms, legs, or feet) occurs in 15% to 20% of people who take stavudine. If the drug is stopped, symptoms may disappear, although they can actually worsen for a time after you stop taking stavudine. If the symptoms do go away, your doctor may restart stavudine treatment at a lower daily dosage.

Your stavudine dosage will be reduced if you develop symptoms of neuropathy or if you have reduced kidney function.

Stavudine does not cure AIDS. It will not prevent you from transmitting the virus to another person; you must still practice safe sex. Stavudine may not prevent some illnesses associated with AIDS from developing. The long-term effects of stavudine are not known.

It is very important to take stavudine according to your doctor's directions. If you forget a dose, take it as soon as you remember. If it is almost time for your next dose, take the dose you forgot, take the next 2 doses 8 hours apart, and then go back to your regular schedule. Do not take a double dose. Call your doctor if you skip more than 2 consecutive doses.

Special Populations

Pregnancy/Breast-feeding

Animal studies show that stavudine passes to the fetus and causes birth defects, but there is no direct information on what happens in humans. Stavudine should be taken during pregnancy only if it is absolutely necessary.

Animal studies show that stavudine passes into breast milk, but it is not known if this occurs in humans. In any case, mothers who are HIV positive should bottle-feed their babies to avoid transmitting the virus through their milk.

Seniors

Older adults are likely to have reduced kidney function and may need to have their daily dose adjusted accordingly.

Generic Name

Sucralfate (sue-KRAL-fate) G

Brand Name

Carafate

Type of Drug

Antiulcer.

Prescribed For

Short-term (less than 8-week) treatment of duodenal (intestinal) ulcer; also used for stomach ulcer, irritation, and bleeding; gastroesophageal reflux disease (GERD); irritation of the esophagus and mouth; throat ulcer; and prevention of stress ulcer and stomach bleeding.

General Information

Sucralfate works within the gastrointestinal (GI) tract by exerting a soothing local effect on ulcer tissue; very little of the drug is absorbed into the bloodstream. After the drug binds to proteins in the damaged mucous tissue within the ulcer, it forms a barrier to the normal acids and enzymes of the GI tract. This barrier protects ulcer tissue from further damage, allowing it to heal naturally. Sucralfate is not an antacid and works differently than cimetidine, omeprazole, and other antiulcer drugs, but it is as effective in treating duodenal ulcer disease as these drugs.

Cautions and Warnings

Duodenal ulcer is a chronic disease. Short-term treatments like sucralfate can completely heal an ulcer, but this does not reduce the risk of having another ulcer.

Small amounts of aluminum are absorbed while you take sucralfate. This can be a problem for people with chronic **kidney failure** and for those on **dialysis**.

Possible Side Effects

Side effects are usually minimal.

▼ Most common: constipation.

▼ Less common: diarrhea, nausea, upset stomach, indigestion, dry mouth, rash, itching, back pain, dizziness, and sleepiness.

Drug Interactions

• Sucralfate may decrease the effects of digoxin, ketoconazole, phenytoin, quinidine, tetracycline, warfarin, and ciprofloxacin, norfloxacin, and other quinolone antibacterials. Separate these drugs and sucralfate by 2 hours to avoid this effect.

• Do not take antacids 30 minutes before or after taking sucralfate.

• Do not take aluminum-containing antacids at all while you are taking sucralfate. This combination increases aluminum absorption into the bloodstream and may lead to aluminum toxicity.

Food Interactions

Take each dose on an empty stomach, at least 1 hour before or 2 hours after meals.

Usual Dose

Adult: starting dosage—1 tablet 4 times a day for active ulcers. Maintenance dosage—1 tablet 2 times a day.

Child: not recommended.

Overdosage

Little is known about the effects of sucralfate overdose, though the risk associated with it is thought to be minimal. Call your local poison control center or a hospital emergency room for more information. If you seek treatment, ALWAYS bring the prescription bottle or container.

Special Information

Complete the full course of drug therapy.

Notify your doctor if you develop constipation, diarrhea, or other GI side effects.

If you forget a dose, take it as soon as you remember. If it is almost time for your next dose, skip the one you forgot and continue with your regular schedule. Do not take a double dose.

Special Populations

Pregnancy/Breast-feeding

While animal studies of sucralfate reveal no damage to the fetus, this drug should only be used during pregnancy after carefully weighing its potential benefits against its risks.

It is not known if sucralfate passes into breast milk. Nursing mothers who must take it should consider bottle-feeding.

Seniors

Seniors may take sucralfate without special restriction.

Type of Drug

Sulfa Drugs

Brand Names

Generic Ingredient: Sulfadiazine G
Only available in generic form.

Generic Ingredient: Sulfadoxine + Pyrimethamine
Fansidar

Generic Ingredient: Sulfamethizole
Thiosulfil Forte

Generic Ingredient: Sulfamethoxazole G
Gantanol

Generic Ingredient: Sulfasalazine G
Azulfidine   Azulfidine EN-Tabs

Generic Ingredient: Sulfisoxazole G
Gantrisin   Sosol

Generic Ingredients: Triple Sulfa (Sulfathiazole +
Sulfacetamide + Sulfabenzamide) Ⓖ

Dayto Sulf	Trysul
Gyne-Sulf	V.V.S.
Sultrin	

Prescribed For

Urinary and other infections; may also be prescribed for rheumatoid, juvenile, and psoriatic arthritis; ulcerative and other forms of colitis; Crohn's disease; ankylosing spondylitis; and psoriasis. Sulfisoxazole has also been used to prevent middle ear infection. Triple sulfa is used only to treat vaginal infection. Fansidar (sufladoxine and pyrimethamine) is prescribed for the treatment and prevention of malaria.

General Information

In use for many years, sulfa drugs are prescribed for infections in various parts of the body but are particularly helpful for urinary tract infections. They kill bacteria and some fungi by interfering with the metabolic processes of these organisms. Some organisms may become resistant to the effects of sulfa drugs.

Sulfasalazine is different from the other sulfa drugs in that only about ⅓ of it is absorbed into the bloodstream; the rest remains in the intestines. Because of its specific anti-inflammatory and immune system effects, sulfasalazine is effective against colitis, intestinal irritation, and arthritis and other inflammatory conditions.

Cautions and Warnings

Do not take sulfa drugs if you are **allergic** to them or any drug chemically related to the sulfa drugs including thiazide and loop diuretics, carbonic anhydrase inhibitors, and sulfonylurea-type oral antidiabetes drugs—which do not include metformin. Do not use any sulfa drug if you are allergic to PABA-containing sunscreens or local anesthetics, or if you have **porphyria**.

Fansidar has been associated with **fatal rash** and **skin tissue decay**. Stop taking this medication if you develop a skin rash or bacterial or fungal infection.

Sulfa drugs can cause **increased sensitivity to the sun or bright light**. Use sunscreen and wear protective clothing.

Sulfa drugs should be taken by people with severe **kidney or liver disease** only after a doctor has evaluated their condition and need for the drug.

Sulfasalazine should not be used by people with aspirin allergy or by **children under age 2**.

Men taking sulfasalazine may have **low sperm count** or become **infertile**. This effect reverses when the drug is stopped.

Deaths in people taking sulfasalazine have been related to a variety of effects on the blood, liver damage, and nervous system changes. **Deaths** in people taking fansidar have occured due to toxic skin reactions. Call your doctor if a rash or anything unusual develops while taking a sulfa drug.

Possible Side Effects

▼ Most common: headache, itching, rash, skin sensitivity to strong sunlight, nausea, vomiting, abdominal or stomach cramps or pain, feeling unwell, hallucinations, diarrhea, dizziness, ringing or buzzing in the ears, and chills.

▼ Less common: blood diseases or changes in blood composition, arthritic pain, appetite loss, drowsiness, hearing loss, itchy eyes, fever, hair loss, and yellowing of the skin or whites of the eyes. Sulfasalazine may reduce sperm count.

Drug Interactions

• Sulfa drugs may increase the effects of sulfonylurea-type oral antidiabetes drugs, methotrexate, warfarin, and phenytoin and other hydantoin antiseizure drugs. Dosages of these drugs may have to be reduced by your doctor.

• Cyclosporine blood levels may be reduced by sulfa drugs, possibly increasing kidney toxicity.

• Sulfa drugs may increase blood levels of indomethacin, probenecid, and aspirin and other salicylates, increasing the risks of side effects.

• When methenamine and a sulfa drug are taken together, an insoluble substance may form in acid urine. Avoid this combination.

• Erythromycin increases the effect of sulfa drugs against infections caused by *Haemophilus influenzae,* a common cause of middle-ear infections.

• The effects of folic acid and digoxin may be diminished by sulfasalazine; dosage increases may be needed.

• Sulfa drugs may increase the effects of barbiturate anesthetics.

• Combining diuretics and sulfa drugs may lead to a decrease in blood platelets.

Food Interactions

Sulfa drugs should be taken on an empty stomach with a full glass of water. Sulfasalazine and fansidar may be taken with food if they upset your stomach.

Usual Dose

Sulfadiazine

Adult: 2–4 g a day.

Child (age 2 months and over): 34–68 mg per lb. of body weight a day.

Child (under age 2 months): not recommended, except to treat certain infections present at birth. In these cases, dosage is 11.3 mg per lb. of body weight, 4 times a day.

Fansidar (sulfadoxine and pyrimethamine)

Adult: 2–3 tablets for an acute attack of malaria; for prevention, first dose prior to departure, then 1–2 tablets every week or every other week.

Child: ½–2 tablets for an acute attack of malaria; for prevention, first dose prior to departure, then ¼–1½ tablets every week or every other week.

Sulfamethizole

Adult: 1.5–4 g a day.

Child (age 2 months and over): 13–20 mg per lb. of body weight a day, in divided doses.

Sulfamethoxazole

Adult: 2–6 g a day.

Child (age 2 months and over): 23–27 mg per lb. of body weight a day.

Sulfasalazine

Adult: 1–4 g a day in evenly divided doses.

Child (age 2 and over): 18–27 mg per lb. of body weight a day, in evenly divided doses.

Child (under age 2): not recommended.

Sulfisoxazole

Adult: 4–8 g a day, in 4–6 divided doses.

Child (age 2 months and over): 34–68 mg per lb. of body weight a day, in 4–6 divided doses.

Triple Sulfa
    Adult: 1 applicator's worth twice a day for 4–6 days, then ¼–½ applicator's worth twice a day; or 1 intravaginal tablet morning and evening for 10 days.

Overdosage

Symptoms include appetite loss, nausea, vomiting and colic, dizziness, headache, drowsiness, unconsciousness, high fever, severe bleeding or bruising, and irritation or soreness of the tongue. Take the victim to a hospital emergency room at once. ALWAYS take the prescription bottle or container.

Special Information

Sulfa drugs often cause increased sensitivity to the sun. Use sunscreen or wear protective clothing.

Sore throat, fever, chills, unusual bleeding or bruising, rash, and drowsiness are signs of serious blood disorders and should be reported to your doctor at once. Also contact your doctor if you experience ringing in the ears, blood in the urine, or breathing difficulties.

Be sure to take the full course of medication as prescribed, even if you notice an improvement in your symptoms.

Sulfasalazine may turn your urine orange-yellow. This is a harmless reaction. Skin discoloration has also occurred. This drug may permanently stain soft contact lenses.

Maintain adequate fluid intake to reduce the chance of kidney stone formation when taking sulfasalazine.

Sulfa drugs may interfere with some tests for sugar in the urine.

If you forget a dose, take it as soon as you remember. If you take the drug twice a day and it is almost time for your next dose, take 1 dose right away, another after 5 to 6 hours, and then go back to your regular schedule. If you take the drug 3 or more times a day and it is almost time for your next dose, take 1 dose right away, another after 2 to 4 hours, and then go back to your regular schedule. Never take a double dose.

Special Populations

Pregnancy/Breast-feeding
Sulfa drugs pass into the fetal circulation and may affect the fetus. Malformations have been seen in animal studies. Sulfa

drugs are not recommended during pregnancy. When a sulfa drug is considered crucial by your doctor, its potential benefits must be carefully weighed against its risks.

Small amounts of sulfa drugs pass into breast milk. Nursing mothers who must take them should consider bottle-feeding, especially if their babies are premature, deficient in the enzyme G-6-PD, or have hyperbilirubinemia (condition in which there is too much bilirubin in the blood). Mothers taking sulfadoxine should not breast-feed.

Seniors
Seniors with kidney or liver problems should take sulfa drugs with caution.

Type of Drug
Sulfonylurea Antidiabetes Drugs

Brand Names

Generic Ingredient: Acetohexamide G
Dymelor

Generic Ingredient: Chlorpropamide G
Diabinese

Generic Ingredient: Glimepiride
Amaryl

Generic Ingredient: Glipizide G
Glucotrol   Glucotrol XL

Generic Ingredient: Glyburide G
DiaBeta   Micronase
Glynase PresTab

Generic Ingredient: Tolazamide G
Tolinase

Generic Ingredient: Tolbutamide G
Orinase

Combination Products

Generic Ingredients: Glipizide + Metformin
Metaglip

Prescribed For

Type 2 diabetes mellitus. Chlorpropamide may also be used to treat diabetes insipidus (a hormonal condition unrelated to blood sugar).

General Information

These medicines work by stimulating the production and release of insulin from the pancreas. They differ from each other in how long they take to start working, the duration of their effectiveness, and the amount of each required to produce a roughly equivalent antidiabetic effect (see table). These drugs do not lower blood sugar directly; they require some working pancreas cells. The "second-generation" antidiabetes drugs (glimepiride, glipizide, and glyburide) belong to the same chemical class as the older "first generation" ones, but lower doses of the second-generation agents are required to accomplish the same effect.

Drug	Equivalent dose (mg)	Hours to start working	Hours of effectiveness
Acetohexamide	500–750	1–2	12 to 24
Chlorpropamide	250–375	1	Up to 60
Glimepiride	NA	2–3	24
Glipizide	10	1 to 3	10 to 24
Glyburide (DiaBeta, Micronase)	5	2 to 4	16 to 24
Glyburide (Glynase PresTab)	3	1	12 to 24
Tolazamide	250–375	4 to 6	12 to 24
Tolbutamide	1000–1500	1	6 to 12

NA = not applicable

Cautions and Warnings

Mild stress, such as **infection, minor surgery,** or **emotional upset,** reduces the effectiveness of these drugs. You must be under your doctor's continuous care while taking any of these drugs.

These drugs are **not a form of oral insulin** or a substitute for insulin. They do not lower blood sugar by themselves.

Studies conducted in the 1960s and confirmed in 1999 found that people taking oral sulfonylurea antidiabetes drugs are more likely to have **fatal heart trouble** than those who can control their diabetes with diet alone or diet plus insulin.

These drugs can cause **low blood sugar** (see "Overdosage") that may require medical attention.

These drugs should be used with caution if you have serious **liver, kidney, or endocrine disease;** monitor your blood sugar very closely.

Possible Side Effects

▼ Most common: loss of appetite, nausea, vomiting, and stomach upset. At times you may experience weakness or tingling in the hands and feet.

▼ Less common: Oral sulfonylurea antidiabetes drugs may produce abnormally low blood sugar levels when too much is taken for your immediate requirements.

▼ Rare: yellowing of the skin or whites of the eyes, itching, and rash. Usually these reactions will disappear in time. If they persist, contact your doctor.

For additional side effects for Metaglip, see Metformin, page 685.

Drug Interactions

• The following drugs may increase your need for oral sulfonylurea antidiabetes drugs: beta blockers, calcium channel blockers, cholestyramine, corticosteroids, diazoxide, estrogens, isoniazid, nicotinic acid, oral contraceptives, phenothiazines, phenytoin and other hydantoin drugs, rifampin, stimulants, thiazide diuretics, thyroid replacement drugs, charcoal tablets, and anything that makes your urine less acidic.

• The following drugs may decrease your need for oral sulfonylurea antidiabetes drugs and some of these drugs can cause drastic drops in blood sugar levels: androgens (male hormones), anticoagulants, sulfa drugs, aspirin and other salicylates, bishydroxycoumarin, chloramphenicol, cimetidine, clarithromycin, clofibrate, dicumarol, famotidine, fenfluramine, fluconazole, gemfibrozil, itraconazole, ketoconazole, ranitidine, magnesium-containing products, methyldopa, miconazole, monoamine oxidase inhibitor (MAOI) drugs, nizatidine, oxyphenbutazone, phenylbutazone, probenecid, warfarin, phenyramidol, sulfinpyrazone, tricyclic antidepressants, large doses of vitamin C, and citrus fruits and other foods that make your urine more acidic.

• Mixing insulin with one of these medicines may lead to severely low blood sugar, though it can be successfully used by some people with type 2 diabetes. This combination must be used only under a doctor's supervision.

• Mixing these drugs with alcohol can cause flushing and breathlessness. Other possible effects are throbbing pain in the head and neck, breathing difficulties, nausea, vomiting, increased sweating, excessive thirst, chest pains, palpitations, lowered blood pressure, weakness, dizziness, blurred vision, and confusion. If you experience any of these reactions, contact your doctor immediately.

• Combining a fluoroquinolone antibiotic, such as ciprofloxacin or gatifloxacin, with glyburide can increase its blood-sugar-lowering effect.

• Chlorpropamide may increase the effects of barbiturates.

• Glyburide may alter the effectiveness of oral anticoagulant (blood-thinning) drugs. Dosage may have to be adjusted by your doctor.

• These drugs may increase the effects of digitalis drugs.

• The stimulants in many over-the-counter cough, cold, and allergy remedies may affect your blood sugar; avoid them unless your doctor advises otherwise.

For additional drug interactions for Metaglip, see Metformin, page 685.

Food Interactions

All these drugs except glipizide may be taken with food. Glipizide should be taken 30 minutes before a meal for best results.

Usual Dose

Acetohexamide: 250–1500 mg a day.

Chlorpropamide: starting dose—100–250 mg a day. Your doctor will then raise or lower your dose according to your response. Maintenance dose—100–250 mg a day; rarely, 750 mg a day may be prescribed.

Glimepiride: 1–8 mg once a day.

Glipizide: 5 mg once a day. Seniors may be started on 2.5 mg a day. Doses up to 40 mg a day divided into 2 doses may be needed to control more severe diabetes.

Glyburide: DiaBeta/Micronase—2.5–20 mg once a day, usually with breakfast or the first main meal. Seniors may start with 1.25 mg a day. Glynase PresTab—1.5–12 mg a day, usually with breakfast or the first main meal. Seniors may start with 0.75 mg a day. Glynase PresTab is not equivalent to DiaBeta or Micronase and may not be substituted for either of them. DiaBeta and Micronase are interchangeable.

Metaglip: 2.5 mg/250 mg–10 mg/2000 mg once a day with a meal.

Tolazamide: moderate diabetes—100–250 mg a day. Severe diabetes—500–1000 mg a day.

Tolbutamide: starting dose—1–2 g a day. Your doctor will then raise or lower your dosage based on your response. Maintenance dose—0.25–2 g a day; rarely, 3 g a day may be prescribed.

Overdosage

A mild overdose causes low blood sugar (symptoms include tingling of the lips and tongue, nausea, lethargy, yawning, confusion, agitation, nervousness, rapid heartbeat, increased sweating, tremors, and hunger). This can be treated by consuming sugar in such forms as candy, orange juice, or glucose tablets. Ultimately, low blood sugar may lead to convulsions, stupor, and coma. Call your doctor, local poison control center, or hospital emergency room to find out if the overdose victim should be taken to a hospital emergency room. ALWAYS bring the prescription bottle or container.

Special Information

Treating diabetes is your responsibility. Follow your doctor's instructions about diet, body weight, exercise, personal hygiene, and all measures to avoid infection.

Call your doctor if you develop low blood sugar (see "Overdosage") or high blood sugar (symptoms include excessive thirst or urination and sugar or ketones in the urine), if you are not feeling well, or if you have symptoms such as itching, rash, yellowing of the whites of the eyes, abnormally light-colored stools, a low-grade fever, sore throat, diarrhea, or unusual bruising or bleeding.

Do not stop taking these drugs, except under your doctor's supervision. If you forget a dose, take it as soon as you remember. If it is almost time for your next dose, skip the one you forgot and continue with your regular schedule. Do not take a double dose.

Special Populations

Pregnancy/Breast-feeding

Animal studies have shown that all these drugs except glyburide cause birth defects or interfere with fetal development. Check with your doctor before taking an oral sulfonylurea antidiabetes drug if you are or might be pregnant. Pregnant women are best treated with insulin because oral sulfonylurea antidiabetes drugs generally will not control their blood sugar, and high blood sugar increases the risk of birth defects.

These drugs pass into breast milk. They may lower blood-sugar levels in an infant. Nursing mothers taking one of these medications should bottle-feed.

Seniors

Seniors, especially those with reduced kidney function, are very sensitive to the blood-sugar-lowering effects and side effects of these drugs. Low blood sugar, the major sign of drug overdose, may be more difficult to identify in seniors and is more likely to cause nervous-system side effects. Seniors taking these drugs must keep in close contact with their doctors and follow their directions.

Synthroid   see *Thyroid Hormone Replacements, page*

1058

Generic Name

Tacrolimus (tak-ROE-lim-us)

Brand Name

Prograf   Protopic

Generic Ingredient: Sirolimus
Rapamune

Type of Drug

Immunosuppressant.

Prescribed For

Organ transplant rejection, autoimmune disease, and severe psoriasis, and atopic dermatitis.

General Information

Formerly known as FK506, tacrolimus is derived from a bacterium and is used to prevent the rejection of transplanted organs. The drug is used in liver transplants and has been studied in kidney, bone marrow, heart, pancreas, and small bowel transplants, among others. Tacrolimus works by blocking the activity of T-cells, which protect the body against invading microorganisms or foreign substances, producing immune-system suppression. Tacrolimus may be used with corticosteroids and cyclosporine for further transplant protection.

Cautions and Warnings

Transplant patients who are **sensitive** or **allergic** to tacrolimus should be given another drug. Some people may also be allergic to chemically modified castor oil, which is used in tacrolimus injection.

Between 10% and 20% of transplant patients treated with tacrolimus develop **post-transplant diabetes mellitus (PTDM),** though the condition is sometimes reversible.

Tacrolimus may be **toxic to the nerves and the kidneys;** the latter has been found in more than 50% of kidney transplant patients and about 40% of liver transplant patients. **Neurotoxicity** (including tremor and headache) has been found in about 55% of liver transplant recipients.

About 10% to 44% of liver transplant patients who take tacrolimus develop mild **elevations of blood potassium**.

Tremors, headaches, muscle function changes, changes in mental state and sense perception, or other nervous system problems occur in about half of the people receiving liver transplants. Seizure has also occurred. In some cases, these side effects may be associated with large amounts of tacrolimus in the blood.

As with other immune suppressants, people taking tacrolimus have an increased risk of developing a **lymphoma**

or other malignancy. The risk increases with the degree of immune suppression and the length of time that the drug is taken. A disorder related to **Epstein-Barr virus** (EBV) infection has also been reported.

People with **kidney disease** should receive lower dosages. People who experience post-transplant reduction in liver function may develop kidney damage. Mild to moderate **high blood pressure** is a common side effect of tacrolimus and may be a sign of kidney damage. People taking this drug should measure their blood pressure regularly.

Sirolimus can cause increases in **cholesterol and triglyceride levels** that may require treatment with diet or lipid-lowering drugs.

Possible Side Effects

Sirolimus
Drug side effects increase as drug dosage increases.

▼ Most common: sore throat; difficulty breathing; upper respiratory infection; abdominal pain; weakness; back pain; chest pain; fever; headache; joint pain; urinary infection; high blood pressure; high blood lipids; tremors; acne; rash; constipation; diarrhea; nausea; vomiting; upset stomach; anemia; low blood platelet levels; swollen legs, ankles, or arms; kidney damage; high blood potassium; low blood phosphate; and weight gain.

▼ Common: sleeplessness, low white blood cell counts, and nosebleeds.

▼ Rare: Rare side effects can occur in almost any part of the body. Contact your doctor if you experience any side effect not listed above.

Tacrolimus
▼ Most common: headache, tremors, sleeplessness, tingling in the hands or feet, diarrhea, nausea, constipation, appetite loss, vomiting, liver or kidney abnormalities, high blood pressure, urinary infection, infrequent urination, anemia, increased white-blood-cell counts, reduced blood-platelet counts, changes in blood-potassium level, reduced blood magnesium, high blood sugar, fluid in the lungs and other lung problems, breathing difficulties, itching, rash, abdominal pain, generalized pain, fever, weakness, back pain, abdominal-fluid buildup, and retention of fluid.

Possible Side Effects *(continued)*

▼ Less common: abnormal dreaming, anxiety, confusion, depression, dizziness, instability, hallucination, poor coordination, muscle spasms, psychosis, tiredness, unusual thoughts, double vision or other visual disturbances, ringing or buzzing in the ears, upset stomach, yellowing of the skin or whites of the eyes, difficulty swallowing, gas, stomach bleeding, fungal infection of the mouth, blood in the urine, chest pain, rapid heartbeat, low blood pressure, diabetes, black-and-blue marks, muscle and joint aches, leg cramps, muscle weakness, asthma, bronchitis, coughing, sore throat, pneumonia, stuffy and runny nose, sinus irritation, voice changes, sweating, and herpes infection.

Protopic

▼ Most common: burning or itching skin, redness or infection of the skin, headache, and flu-like symptoms.

▼ Less common: herpes simplex, rash, acne, allergic reaction, asthma, sinusitis, sleeplessness, and painful menstruation.

Drug Interactions

• Tacrolimus should not be taken at the same time as other immune suppressants so as to avoid excessive suppression of the immune system.

• Combining tacrolimus with cyclosporine (another organ transplant drug) can worsen kidney disease. Administration of these drugs should be separated by at least 24 hours.

• Tacrolimus may cause more kidney damage when combined with other drugs that also cause kidney problems including aminoglycoside antibiotics, amphotericin B, cisplatin, and cyclosporine.

• Antifungal drugs such as ketoconazole and itraconazole, bromocriptine, calcium channel blockers, cimetidine, clarithromycin, danazol, diltiazem, erythromycin, methylprednisolone, protease inhibitors, and metoclopramide may increase tacrolimus blood levels and side effects.

• Carbamazepine, phenobarbital, phenytoin, rifampin, St. John's wort, and rifampicin may reduce tacrolimus blood levels.

• Vaccination may be less effective during tacrolimus use. Live vaccines such as those for measles, mumps, rubella, oral polio, and BCG should be avoided.

Food Interactions

Do not drink grapefruit juice while taking tacrolimus, since it interferes with the breakdown of the drug. Take tacrolimus at least 1 hour before or 2 hours after meals. Sirolimus should be taken consistently before or after meals.

Usual Dose

Sirolimus

   Adult and Child (age 13 and over): Dosage is individualized based on height and weight, and is usually in the range of 2–6 mg a day. Dosing is usually started at the high end of the recommended amount and then reduced to the lowest effective level. Mix the solution with only 2 or more ounces of water or orange juice.

Tacrolimus

   Adult and Child: 0.075–0.15 mg per lb. of body weight a day divided into 2 doses. Children may require more than adults. Dosing is usually started at the high end of the recommended amount and then reduced to the lowest effective level.

Protopic

   Adult and Child: Rub ointment into affected areas twice a day and continue for 1 week after symptoms go away.

Overdosage

Sirolimus overdose has produced abnormal heart rhythms.

   Tacrolimus overdose produces expected drug side effects. Take the victim to a hospital emergency room. ALWAYS bring the prescription bottle or container.

Special Information

It is extremely important to take this drug exactly as prescribed. If you forget a dose, take it as soon as you remember. If it is almost time for your next dose, skip the forgotten dose and continue with your regular schedule. Do not take a double dose. Call your doctor if you forget 2 or more doses in a row.

   Sirolimus solution must be stored in the refrigerator. If the solution becomes cloudy in the refrigerator, let it stand at room temperature until the cloudiness disappears. The cloudiness does not affect the quality of the drug.

People taking tacrolimus require regular testing to monitor their progress.

Call your doctor at the first sign of fever; sore throat; tiredness; weakness; nervousness; unusual bleeding or bruising; tender or swollen gums; convulsions; irregular heartbeat; confusion; numbness or tingling of your hands, feet, or lips; breathing difficulties; severe stomach pain with nausea; or blood in the urine. Other side effects should be brought to your doctor's attention.

Maintain good dental hygiene while taking tacrolimus and use extra care when brushing and flossing because the drug increases your risk of oral infection. See your dentist regularly.

Tacrolimus should be continued as long as prescribed by your doctor. Do not stop taking it because of side effects or other problems. If you cannot tolerate the oral form, this drug may be given by injection, though the oral capsules are preferable.

Special Populations

Pregnancy/Breast-feeding

Tacrolimus passes into the fetal circulation, and in animals causes miscarriage and reduced fertility. In humans, babies born to mothers taking this drug have had high blood potassium and poor kidney function. When this drug is considered crucial by your doctor, its potential benefits must be carefully weighed against its risks. Contraception should begin before starting tacrolimus and continue 12 weeks after treatment has stopped.

Tacrolimus passes into breast milk. Nursing mothers who must take tacrolimus should bottle-feed.

Seniors

Seniors may require reduced dosage due to loss of kidney function.

Generic Name

Tamoxifen Citrate (tuh-MOX-ih-fen SYE-trate) Ⓖ

Brand Name

Nolvadex

The information in this profile also applies to the following drug:

Generic Ingredient: Toremifene Citrate
Fareston

Type of Drug

Anti-estrogen.

Prescribed For

Breast cancer. Tamoxifen is also used for painful breasts in women; swollen or painful breasts and breast cancer in men; and pancreatic, endometrial, and liver cell cancer.

General Information

Tamoxifen is effective in treating estrogen-positive breast cancer in women. It works by blocking the effects of estrogen in breast tissue. When used together with chemotherapy after mastectomy, tamoxifen can prevent or delay the recurrence of breast cancer. It is used to treat metastatic breast cancer (that which has spread) and to prevent breast cancer in women at high risk. Up to 60% of women whose breast cancer has metastasized may benefit from taking tamoxifen. Toremifene is used only to treat breast cancer, not to prevent it.

Cautions and Warnings

Women taking tamoxifen for **ductal carcinoma,** or those at **high risk for breast cancer,** have an increased risk of uterine cancer, stroke, or pulmonary embolism.

Visual difficulties have occurred in people taking tamoxifen for 1 year or more in dosages at least 4 times above the maximum recommended dosage. A few cases of decreased visual clarity and other vision problems have been reported at normal dosages.

People taking tamoxifen have experienced **liver inflammation** and, rarely, more serious liver abnormalities. Very high dosages of this drug (15 mg per lb. of body weight) may cause **liver cancer.**

Women taking tamoxifen may have an increased risk of **thromboembolic events** such as deep vein thrombosis and pulmonary embolism.

Women undergoing coumarin-type anticoagulant therapy or with a history of heart disease should not take tamoxifen.

Possible Side Effects

Side effects are generally mild. Lowering drug dosage can sometimes control severe reactions.

▼ Most common: hot flashes, weight changes, fluid retention, vaginal discharge, menstrual changes, and nausea. Increased bone and tumor pain sometimes occur shortly after starting tamoxifen. These may be a sign of a good response to the drug and usually decline rapidly.

▼ Less common: vomiting, vaginal bleeding, skin changes, and kidney problems.

▼ Rare: high blood-calcium levels, swelling of the arms or legs, changes in sense of taste, vaginal itching, depression, dizziness, light-headedness, headache, visual difficulties, and reduced white-blood-cell or platelet count. Ovarian cysts have occurred in premenopausal women with advanced breast cancer who took tamoxifen.

Drug Interactions

• The effects of warfarin and other anticoagulant (blood-thinning) drugs may be increased by tamoxifen. Tamoxifen may increase blood-calcium levels.

• Bromocriptine may increase tamoxifen blood levels.

• The use of tamovifen and cytotoxic agents may increase the risk of blood cots.

Food Interactions

Tamoxifen may be taken with food or milk if it upsets your stomach.

Usual Dose

Tamoxifen: 20–40 a day. Doses higher than 20 mg should be divided and taken morning and evening.

Toremifene: 60 mg once a day.

Overdosage

Symptoms may include breathing difficulties, convulsions, tremors, overactive reflexes, dizziness, and unsteadiness. Take the victim to a hospital emergency room. ALWAYS bring the prescription bottle or container.

Special Information

Take this medication according to your doctor's directions. Inform your doctor if you become very weak or sleepy or if you experience confusion, pain, swelling of the legs, breathing difficulties, blurred vision, bone pain, hot flashes, nausea or vomiting, weight gain, irregular periods, dizziness, headache, or appetite loss. Call your doctor if you vomit shortly after taking a dose of tamoxifen. Your doctor may tell you to take another dose immediately or wait until the next dose.

Women taking tamoxifen should use a condom, diaphragm, or other non-hormonal contraceptive during sexual intercourse until treatment is complete.

If you forget a dose, call your doctor. If you cannot reach your doctor, skip the forgotten dose and continue your regular schedule. Do not take a double dose.

Special Populations

Pregnancy/Breast-feeding

Tamoxifen can harm the fetus and cause vaginal bleeding and spontaneous abortion. It should not be taken by any pregnant women. Women of childbearing age taking tamoxifen must use barrier contraception to prevent pregnancy. Contact your doctor at once if you think you may be pregnant.

It is not known if tamoxifen passes into breast milk. Nursing mothers who must take it should bottle-feed.

Seniors

Seniors may take tamoxifen without special restriction.

Generic Name

Tamsulosin (tam-SUE-loe-sin)

Brand Name

Flomax

Type of Drug

Alpha blocker.

Prescribed For

Benign prostatic hyperplasia (BPH).

General Information

Tamsulosin hydrochloride and similar drugs block nerve endings known as alpha₁ receptors. In BPH, tamsulosin works by relaxing smooth muscles in the prostate and neck of the bladder. This effect is produced by blocking alpha₁ receptors in the affected muscles. Despite the fact that tamsulosin alleviates the urinary symptoms of BPH, the drug's long-term effect on complications of BPH or the need for urinary surgery is not known. Alpha blockers are broken down in the liver.

Cautions and Warnings

Tamsulosin may cause **dizziness and fainting,** especially after the first few doses. This is known as the first-dose effect and may be minimized by limiting the first dose to 1 mg at bedtime. The first-dose effect occurs in about 1% of people and may recur if the drug is stopped for a few days and then restarted.

Do not take this drug if you are **allergic** or **sensitive** to any alpha blocker.

Tamsulosin may slightly reduce **cholesterol levels** and improve the high-density lipoprotein (HDL)/low-density lipoprotein (LDL) ratio, a positive step for people with blood-cholesterol problems.

Red- and white-blood-cell counts may be slightly reduced by other alpha blockers. This effect should be monitored in people taking tamsulosin.

Possible Side Effects

▼ Most common: dizziness, weakness, and headache.

▼ Less common: low blood pressure; rapid heartbeat; abnormal heart rhythms; chest pain; flushing in the face, arms, or legs; fainting; vomiting; dry mouth; diarrhea; constipation; abdominal pain or discomfort; gas; breathing difficulties; stuffy nose; sinus inflammation; cold or flu-like symptoms; cough; bronchitis; worsening of asthma; nosebleed; sore throat; runny nose; shoulder, neck, or back pain; pain in the arms or legs; joint pain; arthritis; muscle pain; blurred vision or other visual disturbances; conjunctivitis (pinkeye); eye pain; nervousness; tingling in the hands or feet; tiredness; anxiety; difficulty sleeping; frequent urination; urinary infection; itching; rash; sweating; swelling of the face, arms, or legs; and fever.

Possible Side Effects *(continued)*

▼ Rare: depression, reduced sex drive or abnormal sexual function (including priapism), fluid retention, and weight gain.

Drug Interactions

• Tamsulosin may interact with beta-blocking drugs to produce a higher rate of dizziness or fainting after taking the first dose of tamsulosin.

• Cimetidine increases blood levels of tamsulosin and should be used with caution.

• The blood-pressure-lowering effect of tamsulosin may be reduced by indomethacin.

• When taken with blood-pressure-lowering drugs, tamsulosin produces severe reduction of blood pressure.

• The blood-pressure-lowering effect of clonidine may be reduced by tamsulosin.

Food Interactions

None known.

Usual Dose

Starting dosage—0.4 mg a half hour after the same meal each day. Dosage may be increased by 0.8 mg a day if there has been no response after 2 weeks.

Overdosage

Symptoms may include severe side effects. Take the victim to a hospital emergency room at once. ALWAYS bring the prescription bottle or container.

Special Information

Take tamsulosin exactly as prescribed and do not stop taking it unless directed to do so by your doctor. Avoid over-the-counter drugs that contain stimulants because they may increase your blood pressure.

Tamsulosin may cause dizziness, headache, and drowsiness, especially 2 to 6 hours after you take your first dose, though these effects may persist after the first few doses. Wait 12 to 24 hours after taking the first dose before driving or doing any task that requires concentration. You should take it at bedtime to minimize this problem.

Call your doctor if you develop severe dizziness, heart palpitations, or any bothersome or persistent side effect.

If you forget a dose, take it as soon as you remember. If it is almost time for your next dose, skip the forgotten dose and continue with your regular schedule. If you forget your medication for several days in a row, you will have to begin again at the lower dosage of 0.4 mg a day regardless of the dosage you were taking before.

Special Populations

Pregnancy/Breast-feeding
Tamsulosin is intended only for men. The safety of using tamsulosin during pregnancy and breast-feeding is not known.

Seniors
Seniors may be more sensitive to the action and side effects of tamsulosin.

Generic Name

Tazarotene (tuh-ZAR-oe-tene)

Brand Name

Avage   Tazorac

Type of Drug

Anti-acne.

Prescribed For

Mild to moderate acne, and psoriasis. Also, prescribed for actinic keratosis.

General Information

Tazarotene is converted to its active form after it is applied to the skin. A retinoid related to vitamin A, tazarotene is in the same family as retinoic acid—the active ingredient in Retin-A anti-acne products.

Cautions and Warnings

Women who are or might be **pregnant** should not use this drug.

Tazarotene may cause a temporary **burning** or **stinging** sensation. It may cause severe burning if applied to eczema. Other skin medications and makeup can make the skin very dry and should be avoided while you are using tazarotene. It may also be advisable to "rest" your skin between using other drugs or makeup and starting tazarotene.

Tazarotene can cause **rash, allergy,** or a severe **toxic reaction,** especially if used together with another drug that sensitizes the skin such as a tetracycline antibiotic, a fluoroquinolone, or a phenothiazine tranquilizer.

Possible Side Effects

▼ Most common: peeling skin, a burning or stinging sensation, dry skin, redness, and itching.

▼ Common: irritation, skin pain, cracking, swelling, and skin discoloration.

Drug Interactions

None known.

Usual Dose

Adult: Gently clean your face and apply a thin layer of tazarotene to the affected area every evening.

Overdosage

Accidental ingestion of tazarotene may cause symptoms similar to vitamin A overdose. Call your local poison control center for information about what to do in the case of tazarotene ingestion.

Special Information

If skin irritation, redness, itching, or peeling is excessive, stop using tazarotene until your skin is completely healed. Extreme wind or cold may worsen skin irritation.

Applying excessive amounts of tazarotene to your skin can cause redness, peeling skin, or other discomfort.

Special Populations

Pregnancy/Breast-feeding
Tazarotene caused birth defects in lab animals. Women who are or might be pregnant should not use this drug.

It is not known if tazarotene passes into breast milk. Nursing mothers should be aware when using this drug that some may be passed on to their babies.

Seniors
Seniors may use this drug without special restriction.

Generic Name

Tegaserod (te-GAS-er-odd)

Brand Name
Zelnorm

Type of Drug
Serotonin receptor agonist.

Prescribed For
Women with irritable bowel syndrome (IBS) whose primary bowel symptom is constipation and who have not responded to other treatments.

General Information
Tegaserod stimulates one type of serotonin ($5HT_4$) receptor. Serotonin—95% of which is found in the gastrointestinal tract—is thought to be a key element in all aspects of bowel function. Tegaserod triggers the release of neurotransmitters from sensory neurons in the gastrointestinal tract. This stimulates normal bowel movement and intestinal secretion. Tegaserod studies indicate that it improves muscle and nerve activity in the GI tract and normalizes movement throughout the gastrointestinal tract that is impaired because of IBS. In addition, animal studies show that tegaserod moderates visceral sensitivity during colorectal distension in animals, making them less sensitive to the effects of experimental IBS.

Cautions and Warnings
Do not take tegaserod if you are **sensitive** or **allergic** to it.

Do not take tegaserod if you currently have **diarrhea** or if you frequently have attacks of diarrhea.

People with severe **kidney disease,** moderate to severe **liver disease,** or a history of **bowel obstruction, dysfunction, or gallbladder disease** should not use tegaserod.

Possible Side Effects

▼ Most common: abdominal pain, diarrhea, and headache.

▼ Common: nausea, intestinal gas, and leg pain.

▼ Less common: dizziness, migraine, and back or joint pain.

▼ Rare: Rare side effects can occur in almost any part of the body. Contact your doctor if you experience any side effect not listed above.

Drug Interactions

Tegaserod has been studied with a variety of different medicines and few drug interactions are likely to occur. However, some may appear as the drug is more widely adopted.

• Tegaserod reduces blood levels of digoxin, but dose adjustment is unlikely.

Food Interactions

Food interferes with the absorption of tegaserod. Take this drug 30 to 60 minutes before a meal.

Usual Dose

Adults: 6 mg twice a day for 4 to 6 weeks. If the drug works, it may be prescribed for a second 4 to 6 week period.
Child: not recommended.

Overdosage

Symptoms include diarrhea and headache. Other possible overdose symptoms include intermittent abdominal pain, dizziness or fainting when rising from a seated or lying position, intestinal gas, nausea, and vomiting. Call your local poison control center or a hospital emergency room for more information. If you seek treatment, ALWAYS bring the prescription bottle or container.

Special Information

Stop taking tegaserod immediately if you have new or sudden worsening of abdominal pain.

You may develop diarrhea during tegaserod therapy. Most people have one episode within the first week of treatment.

Typically, diarrhea does not reoccur with continued treatment.

Call your doctor if you have severe diarrhea, or if severe cramping, abdominal pain, or dizziness accompanies the diarrhea.

If you forget to take a dose of tegaserod, take it as soon as you remember. If it is almost time for your next dose, skip the one you forgot and continue with your regular schedule. Do not take a double dose.

Special Populations

Pregnancy/Breast-feeding
While animal studies of tegaserod reveal no damage to the fetus, this drug should only be used during pregnancy after carefully weighing its potential benefits against its risks.

Tegaserod passes into breast milk. Nursing mothers who must take it should bottle-feed.

Seniors
Blood levels of tegaserod are usually higher in older women, but dosage adjustments are not required.

Generic Name

Temozolomide (tem-oh-ZOHL-oh-mide)

Brand Name

Temodar

Type of Drug

Antineoplastic.

Prescribed For

Brain cancer.

General Information

Temozolomide is used to treat astrocytoma, a specific type of cancer of the brain, in adults whose tumors have returned after other chemotherapy. Once absorbed, it seems to interfere with the growth of cancer cells, which are then eventually destroyed by the body.

Cautions and Warnings

Do not take this medicine if you are **sensitive** or **allergic** to it or dacarbazine, another antineoplastic drug.

People taking temozolomide may experience **reduced white blood cell and platelet counts**. These generally occur late in the first treatment cycle and may increase your risk of infection.

People with **impaired liver function** should use temozolomide with caution.

Temozolomide may cause **infertility** in men.

Possible Side Effects

▼ Most common: headache, fatigue, diarrhea, nausea, constipation, and vomiting.

▼ Common: convulsions, weakness on one side of the body, dizziness, poor muscle coordination, memory loss, sleeplessness, viral infection, leg or arm swelling, fever, and general weakness.

▼ Less common: partial paralysis, anxiety, difficulty swallowing, jerking movements of the face, trunk, arms, or legs, depression, walking unusually, confusion, itching, rash, increased urination, loss of urinary control, urinary infection, appetite loss, abdominal pain, double vision and other visual abnormalities, muscle aches, breast pain (women), weight gain, and back pain.

Drug Interactions

• Valproic acid reduces the amount of temozolomide cleared through the kidney. The importance of this interaction is not known.

Food Interactions

Food interferes with the absorption of this drug into the blood. Take it on an empty stomach to reduce nausea and vomiting.

Usual Dose

Adult: 100–200 mg at bedtime. Dosage is adjusted according to body weight and white blood cell and platelet counts.
Child: not recommended.

Overdosage

Temozolomide overdose causes drastic reductions in platelets and white blood cells. Overdose victims must be taken to a hospital emergency room at once. ALWAYS bring the prescription bottle or container.

Special Information

Nausea and vomiting usually decline with time and are readily controlled with antinauseant drugs. Antinauseant medication may be taken before or after your temozolomide dose.

Women clear temozolomide from the body more slowly than men and are more likely experience low white blood cell and platelet counts in the first cycle of temozolomide treatment.

Exposure to temozolomide powder causes malignant tumors in animals. Be sure that you and others do not inhale the contents of any capsule or get any of the drug on your skin or mucous membranes from a capsule that has been damaged or opened.

Do not open or chew temozolomide capsules. Swallow them whole with a glass of water.

Keep this drug away from children and pets.

If you forget to take a dose of temozolomide, be sure to tell your doctor and continue with your regular schedule on the next day. Do not take a double dose.

Special Populations

Pregnancy/Breast-feeding

Temozolomide will damage a developing fetus. Women who must take it should use an effective contraceptive method and wait 6 months after the treatment is finished before becoming pregnant. Men should not father a child up to 6 months after treatment.

Women who must take temozolomide should bottle-feed because temozolomide may pass into breast milk and cause severe reactions in the nursing infant.

Seniors

Seniors are more likely to experience reduced white blood cell and platelet counts.

Generic Name

Tenofovir (te-NOE-foh-veer)

Brand Name

Viread

Type of Drug

Antiviral.

Prescribed For

Human immunodeficiency virus (HIV) infection.

General Information

Tenofovir is a nucleotide reverse transcriptase inhibitor (NRTI). It inhibits the reverse transcriptase (RT) enzyme, necessary for reproduction of HIV in body cells, by binding directly to it. Unlike many other HIV antivirals, tenofovir is not broken down in the liver. Most of the tenofovir taken in a typical dose passes out of the body in the urine. The HIV virus can become resistant to tenofovir. For this reason, tenofovir is always prescribed as part of a multi-drug anti-HIV "cocktail." Tenofovir can also help control cytomegalovirus.

Cautions and Warnings

Do not take this drug if you are **allergic** or **sensitive** to it.

HIV becomes **resistant** to tenofovir if it is used alone. Treatment must always include at least 1 other anti-HIV drug.

Tenofovir can be toxic to the **liver** and may cause **lactic acidosis,** which can be fatal. People with a history of hepatitis should have their liver function evaluated periodically and probably should use an alternate drug.

Tenofovir is eliminated through the kidneys. People with severe **kidney disease** should not take this medication until more is known about how this drug affects the kidneys.

Bone and kidney toxicity, problems associated with other antiretroviral medicines, have not been seen with tenofovir, but may become a problem in people taking this drug for more than 1 year.

Patients taking anti-retroviral drugs for HIV have experienced **fat redistribution** and **weight gain, loss of fat from the**

arms, legs, and face, breast enlargement, and a **moon-shaped face**. The origins and long-term consequences of these developments are not known.

Possible Side Effects

▼ Most common: nausea, diarrhea, weakness, and headache.

▼ Common: vomiting, stomach gas, abdominal pain, and loss of appetite.

Drug Interactions

• Tenofovir may reduce the breakdown of amitriptyline, caffeine, clomipramine, clozapine, cyclobenzaprine, estradiol, fluvoxamine, haloperidol, imipramine, mexiletine, naproxen, acetaminophen, propranolol, riluzole, ropivacaine, tacrine, theophylline, verapamil, waerfarin, zileuton, and zolmitriptan, modestly increasing the amount of these drugs in the blood.

• Tenofovir increases blood levels of didanosine, which increases the risk of side effects. People taking both of these drugs must take tenofovir either 2 hours before or 1 hour after taking didanosine.

• Tenofovir decreases the amount of ritonavir and lopinavir (with higher tenofovir doses) absorbed into the bloodstream.

• At higher tenofovir doses, the blood concentration of lamivudine may be reduced.

• The effect of tenofovir on oral contraceptives ("the pill") is not known, but it can increase the amount of estradiol (a contraceptive hormone) in the blood. People combining these drugs should use an additional contraceptive method because "the pill" may not be effective.

• Tenofovir may decrease blood levels of atazanavir.

Food Interactions

None known.

Usual Dose

Adult (age 18 and over): 300 mg once a day.
Child: not recommended.

Overdosage

Little is known about tenofovir overdose. Take the overdose victim to a hospital emergency room. ALWAYS bring the prescription bottle or container.

Special Information

It is imperative that you take your HIV medication exactly as prescribed. Missing or skipping doses of tenofovir increases your risk of becoming resistant to the drug and losing the benefits of tenofovir therapy.

If you are also taking didanosine, take your tenofovir 2 hours before or 1 hour after taking didanosine.

Tenofovir does not cure acquired immunodeficiency syndrome (AIDS). It does not prevent you from transmitting the HIV virus to another person; you must still practice safe sex.

If you forget a dose, take it as soon as you remember. If it is almost time for your next dose, skip the dose you forgot and continue with your regular schedule. Do not take a double dose. Skipping doses of this drug increases the risk that your HIV will become resistant to its effects.

Special Populations

Pregnancy/Breast-feeding

Animal studies of tenofovir using up to 19 times the human dose have revealed no birth defects. There are no studies in women. Pregnant women should take tenofovir only after discussing its potential benefits and risks with their doctor.

Tenofovir passes into breast milk. Nursing mothers with HIV should always bottle-feed to avoid transmitting the virus to their babies.

Seniors

It is not known if seniors respond differently to tenofovir than younger adults. Kidney function declines with age and the lowest possible tenofovir dose is recommended.

Generic Name

Terbinafine (ter-BIN-uh-feen)

Brand Name

Desenex Max   Lamisil AT
Lamisil

Type of Drug

Antifungal.

Prescribed For

Fungus infections of the skin, fingernails, or toenails.

General Information

Terbinafine hydrochloride is a general-purpose antifungal. It can cure common athlete's foot, jock itch, and ringworm faster than other drugs of this type. It is also effective against *Candida* and other fungal infections of the skin. Terbinafine is unique because it accumulates in the skin and continues to kill fungus organisms even after you stop using it. Most other antifungals do not kill the fungus; they only stop it from growing.

Cautions and Warnings

Do not take this product if you are **allergic** to terbinafine or any other ingredient in the product. **Kidney or liver disease** can increase the amount of terbinafine in your blood by 50%. Rare cases of liver failure have been reported in people without a preexisting liver condition.

   Terbinafine cream is only meant to be applied to the skin. Do not put it into your eyes or use it for a vaginal infection. **Do not swallow** terbinafine cream. Only the capsules are meant for oral use.

   Terbinafine should be used only for specific fungal infections and only as prescribed. Rarely, people taking terbinafine have experienced severe eyesight changes or a severe drop in **white-blood-cell count,** leading to serious **infection** and fever. Serious skin reactions to terbinafine have been reported; if skin rash occurs, contact your doctor immediately. Call your doctor if anything unusual develops.

Possible Side Effects

Cream
   ▼ Most common: itching and irritation of the skin immediately after application.
   ▼ Less common: burning, irritation, and dryness of the skin.

Possible Side Effects *(continued)*

Tablets
▼ Most common: headache.
▼ Common: diarrhea and rash.
▼ Less common: upset stomach, abdominal pain, nausea, gas, itching, liver irritation, taste changes, and temporary eyesight changes.
▼ Rare: aching joints and muscle, yellowing of the skin or eyes, loss of appetite, severe reactions of the liver or skin, low white-blood-cell count, and allergic reactions.

Drug Interactions

• Cimetidine and terfenadine increase the amount of terbinafine in the blood.
• Do not combine terbinafine and rifampin.
• Terbinafine may reduce the effect of cyclosporine.
• Terbinafine may increase the effect of caffeine.
• Terbinafine may raise blood levels of dextromethorphan, a common ingredient in cough syrups.

Food Interactions

Take terbinafine tablets 1 hour before or 2 hours after eating.

Usual Dose

Cream: Apply to affected areas morning and night for 1–4 weeks.

Spray: Once or twice a day for 1 week.

Tablets: 250 mg a day for 6 or 12 weeks, depending on condition being treated.

Overdosage

Terbinafine overdose may lead to nausea, vomiting, abdominal pain, dizziness, rash, frequent urination, and headache. Overdose victims should be taken to a hospital emergency room. ALWAYS bring the prescription bottle or container.

Special Information

Do not put terbinafine cream in contact with your eyes, nose, mouth, or any other mucous membrane tissues.

Do not stop using terbinafine before your prescription is complete, even if your rash clears up. The full prescription may be necessary to eliminate the offending fungus.

Do not cover the cream with plastic wrap or anything else that restricts ventilation unless so instructed by your doctor.

Call your doctor if your skin becomes red, burns, itches, blisters, swells, or if oozing develops.

If you forget to administer a dose, do so as soon as you remember. If it is almost time for your next dose, skip the one you forgot and continue with your regular schedule.

Special Populations

Pregnancy/Breast-feeding

The effect of terbinafine during pregnancy is not known. Women who are pregnant should not use terbinafine because the treatment of toenail or fingernail fungus infections can be postponed until after pregnancy.

Terbinafine passes into breast milk. Nursing mothers who must use this drug should bottle-feed.

Seniors

Seniors may use terbinafine without special restriction.

Generic Name

Terbutaline (ter-BUE-tuh-leen) G

Brand Names

Brethaire   Bricanyl
Brethine

Type of Drug

Bronchodilator.

Prescribed For

Asthma, bronchospasm, and premature labor.

General Information

Terbutaline sulfate is similar to other bronchodilator drugs, such as metaproterenol and isoetharine, but it has a weaker effect on nerve receptors in the heart and blood vessels. For this reason, it is somewhat safer for people with heart conditions.

Terbutaline tablets begin to work within 30 minutes and continue working for 4 to 8 hours. Terbutaline inhalation begins working in 5 to 30 minutes and continues for 3 to 6 hours. Terbutaline injection starts working in 5 to 15 minutes and lasts for 1½ to 4 hours.

Cautions and Warnings

Terbutaline should be used with caution by people with a history of **angina pectoris** (condition characterized by brief attacks of chest pain), **heart disease, high blood pressure, cardiac arrythmia, stroke, seizure, diabetes, thyroid disease, prostate disease,** or **glaucoma**.

Using excessive amounts of terbutaline can lead to **increased difficulty breathing** rather than relief. In the most extreme cases, people have had heart attacks after using excessive amounts of inhalant.

Possible Side Effects

▼ Most common: heart palpitations, abnormal heart rhythm, tremors, dizziness and fainting, shakiness, nervousness, tension, drowsiness, headache, nausea and vomiting, and heartburn or upset stomach.

▼ Less common: rapid heartbeat, chest pain and discomfort, angina, weakness, sleeplessness, wheezing, bronchial spasms and difficulty breathing, dry throat, sore or irritated throat, flushing, sweating, and changes in sense of smell and taste.

Drug Interactions

• Terbutaline's effects may be increased by monoamine oxidase inhibitors (MAOIs), tricyclic antidepressants, thyroid drugs, other bronchodilator drugs, and some antihistamines.

• The risk of cardiac toxicity may be increased in people taking both terbutaline and theophylline.

• Terbutaline's effectiveness is reduced by beta-blocking drugs such as propranolol.

• Terbutaline may reduce the effects of blood-pressure-lowering drugs, especially reserpine, methyldopa, and guanethidine.

Food Interactions

Terbutaline tablets are more effective when taken on an empty stomach—1 hour before or 2 hours after meals—but can be taken with food if they upset your stomach.

Usual Dose

Inhaler

Adult and Child (age 12 and over): 1 or 2 puffs every 4–6 hours. Asthma triggered by exercise may be prevented by taking 2 puffs 15 minutes before exercising.

Tablets

Adult and Child (age 15 and over): 2.5–5 mg every 6 hours, 3 times a day. Do not take more than 15 mg a day.

Child (age 12–14): 2.5 mg 3 times a day. Do not take more than 7.5 mg a day.

Child (under age 12): not recommended.

Overdosage

Overdose of terbutaline inhalation usually results in exaggerated side effects, including chest pain and high blood pressure, although blood pressure may drop to a low level after a short period of elevation. People who inhale too much terbutaline should see a doctor.

Overdose of terbutaline tablets is more likely to trigger changes in heart rate, palpitations, unusual heart rhythms, chest pain, high blood pressure, fever, chills, cold sweats, nausea, vomiting, and dilation of the pupils. Convulsions, sleeplessness, anxiety, and tremors may also develop, and the victim may collapse.

If the overdose was taken within the past 30 minutes, give the victim ipecac syrup—available at any pharmacy—to induce vomiting and to remove any remaining medication from the stomach. DO NOT GIVE IPECAC SYRUP IF THE VICTIM IS UNCONSCIOUS OR CONVULSING. If symptoms have already begun to develop, the victim should be taken to a hospital emergency room. ALWAYS bring the prescription bottle or container.

Special Information

If you are inhaling terbutaline, be sure to follow the inhalation instructions that come with the product. The drug should be inhaled during the second half of your inward breath, since this will allow it to reach deeper into your lungs. Wait at least 1 minute between puffs if you use more than 1 puff per dose. Do not inhale terbutaline if you have food or anything else in your mouth.

Do not take more terbutaline than your doctor prescribes. Taking more than you need could actually worsen your symptoms. If your condition worsens rather than improves after taking terbutaline, stop taking it and call your doctor.

Call your doctor immediately if you develop chest pain, palpitations, rapid heartbeat, muscle tremors, dizziness, headache, facial flushing, or urinary difficulty, or if you continue to experience difficulty in breathing after using the medication.

If you forget a dose of terbutaline, take it as soon as you remember. If it is almost time for your next dose, skip the one you forgot and return to your regular schedule. Do not take a double dose.

Special Populations

Pregnancy/Breast-feeding

When used during childbirth, terbutaline can slow or delay labor. Generally, terbutaline should not be taken after the first 3 months of pregnancy: It can cause rapid heartbeat and high blood sugar in the mother, and rapid heartbeat and low blood sugar in the fetus. It is not known if terbutaline causes birth defects in humans, but it has caused defects in pregnant animals. When your doctor considers this drug crucial, its potential benefits must be carefully weighed against its risks.

Terbutaline passes into breast milk. Nursing mothers who must take this drug should consider bottle-feeding.

Seniors

Seniors are more sensitive to the effects of terbutaline. Follow your doctor's directions closely and report any side effects at once.

Generic Name

Terconazole (ter-KON-uh-zole)

Brand Names

Terazol 3   Terazol 7

Type of Drug

Antifungal.

Prescribed For

Fungal infections of the vagina.

General Information

Terconazole is available as a vaginal cream or suppository. It may also be applied to the skin to treat common fungal infections. Exactly how it works is unknown.

Cautions and Warnings

Do not use terconazole if you are **allergic** to it. Proper diagnosis is essential for effective treatment. Do not use this product without first consulting your doctor.

Notify your physician if fever, chills, or flu-like symptoms occur during use.

Possible Side Effects

▼ Most common: headache, which affects 1 in 4 women who use it.

▼ Rare: painful menstruation, genital pain, body pain, abdominal pain, fever, chills, vaginal burning or irritation, and itching. Application of terconazole cream to the skin can cause unusual sensitivity to the sun.

Food and Drug Interactions

None known.

Usual Dose

Vaginal Suppositories or Cream: 1 applicator's worth or 1 suppository into the vagina at bedtime for 3 or 7 days, depending on formulation.

Topical: Apply to affected areas of skin twice a day for up to 1 month.

Overdosage

Terconazole overdose may cause irritation and accidental ingestion may cause upset stomach. Call your local poison control center or hospital emergency room for more information.

Special Information

When using the vaginal cream, insert the whole applicatorful of cream high into the vagina. Be sure to complete the full course of treatment prescribed. Call your doctor if you develop burning or itching.

Refrain from sexual intercourse or use a condom to avoid reinfection while using this product. Using sanitary napkins may keep terconazole from staining your clothing.

If you forget a dose, administer it as soon as you remember. If it is almost time for your next dose, skip the dose you forgot and continue with your regular schedule. Do not administer a double dose.

Special Populations

Pregnancy/Breast-feeding

Pregnant women should avoid using the vaginal cream during the first 3 months of pregnancy; during the last 6 months, it should be used only if absolutely necessary.

Terconazole may cause problems in breast-fed infants. Nursing mothers who must use this drug should bottle-feed.

Seniors

Seniors may take this medication without special restriction.

Generic Name

Teriparatide (terr-ih-PAR-a-tide)

Brand Name

Forteo

Type of Drug

Parathyroid hormone.

Prescribed For

Post-menopausal osteoporosis; also used to treat osteopenia (low bone mass) in men.

General Information

Teriparatide is a synthetic form of the human parathyroid hormone, which is involved in maintaining calcium balance in the body. This treatment is the first proven to actually build new bone and improve bone structure in women suffering from osteoporosis. All other osteoporosis drugs change the rate at which calcium is lost from bone, so they slow the rate of bone loss. Studies of teriparatide have shown that people taking it experience significant increases in bone mineral density and suffer fewer bone fractures while they are taking teriparatide as well as after they stop it. Typically, people take teriparatide for one to two years to build bone mass and prevent additional fractures.

Cautions and Warnings

Do not take teriparatide if you are **sensitive** or **allergic** to it.

When teriparatide was given to rats, it increased their risk for developing **osteosarcoma,** a rare but very serious cancer of the bone. This effect has not appeared in humans. People with a **bone disease,** such as **Paget's Disease,** a history or risk of **bone cancer,** or **cancer that has spread to the bone** should not take teriparatide.

People who have had **radiation therapy** should not take this drug.

The long-term safety of teriparatide has not been studied past 2 years.

People who have or have had **kidney stones** should use teriparatide with caution because of the risk that it could worsen this condition.

Possible Side Effects

In most cases, studies of teriparatide found that its side effects were similar to people who took an inactive placebo.

▼ Most common: generalized pain and joint pain.

▼ Common: headache, weakness, high blood pressure, nausea, constipation, diarrhea, upset stomach, dizziness, runny nose, coughing, and sore throat.

Possible Side Effects *(continued)*

▼ Less common: neck pain, angina pain, fainting, vomiting, stomach problems, dental problems, leg cramps, depression, sleeplessness, a sense of spinning or whirling, shortness of breath, pneumonia, rash, and sweating.

▼ Rare: Rare side effects can occur in almost any part of the body. Contact your doctor if you experience any side effect not listed above.

Drug Interactions

• Teriparatide increases blood levels of calcium and should be used cautiously when combining with digoxin.

• Bisphosphonates reduce the ability of teriparatide to build new bone. Teriparatide alone produces better improvements in bone density than either a bisphosphonate alone or taking the two drugs together.

Food Interactions

You may take this drug without regard to food or meals.

Usual Dose

Adult: 20 mcg a day by subcutaneous injection (under the skin) in the thigh or abdomen (lower stomach area). Teriparatide comes in a 'pen' containing 28-days worth of medicine. Teriparatide is a clear and colorless liquid. Do not use if there are particles in it or if the solution is cloudy or colored. *Child:* not recommended.

Overdosage

Little is known about the effects of teriparatide overdose. Likely symptoms include high blood calcium, dizziness or fainting, low blood pressure, hypotension, nausea, vomiting, and headache. Take the victim to a hospital emergency room. ALWAYS bring the prescription bottle or container.

Special Information

Take teriparatide at the same time every day. If you forget to take a dose, take it as soon as you remember. Do not take a double dose and do not take more than one dose a day.

Teriparatide must be injected under the skin. If you cannot inject yourself, you must have someone else do it for you every day.

When you first start taking teriparatide, you should be in a place where you can sit or lie down if you get dizzy. Contact your doctor if dizziness continues.

You must continue taking calcium and/or vitamin D supplements as prescribed by your doctor. Also, regular weight bearing exercise, reducing alcohol consumption, and stopping smoking will help improve your osteoporosis.

Do not use teriparatide after the expiration date printed on the pen and pen packaging. Throw away your teriparatide pen 28 days after you start using it, even if it still contains medicine.

Store this product in the refrigerator. Teriparatide should be injected shortly after you take the pen out of the refrigerator. Replace the cap and put it back into the refrigerator immediately after use.

Special Populations

Pregnancy/Breast-feeding
Teriparatide enters fetal circulation. Pregnant women should not take this drug.

Teriparatide passes into breast milk. Nursing mothers who must take it should bottle feed.

Seniors
Seniors may use this drug without special precaution.

Generic Name

Testosterone (tes-TOS-ter-one)

Brand Names

Androderm Transdermal System	Testin Testoderm
Androgel	Transdermal System
Striant	Testopel

The information in this profile also applies to the following drug:

Generic Ingredient: Methyltestosterone ☐G

Android   Testred
Oreton Methyl   Virilon

Type of Drug

Hormone replacement.

Prescribed For

Impotence due to hormone deficiency and testosterone replacement in men who have lost their testicle function or have low blood levels of testosterone. Androgen may be prescribed for boys before they reach puberty to maintain secondary sex characteristics if testosterone is lacking or if puberty is delayed. In women, testosterone may be used to treat metastatic cancer (cancer that has spread from one part of the body to another) and breast enlargement or pain in women who have just given birth.

General Information

Testosterone is the principal androgen (male hormone). In men, testosterone is produced in the testicles. Women make small amounts of testosterone in their ovaries and in the adrenal gland. Testosterone is responsible for the growth and development of male sex organs as well as secondary sex characteristics such as beard, pubic, chest, and underarm hair; vocal cord thickening, which lowers the voice; and muscle and fat distribution. Androgens are also responsible for the adolescent growth spurt.

Weekly testosterone injection of 200 mg, for up to 1 year, has been studied as a reversible male contraceptive.

Cautions and Warnings

The following people should avoid testosterone: **pregnant women, men with breast or prostate cancer,** those who are **allergic** to it, and people with **heart or kidney disease,** who may respond to the drug by retaining fluid.

Some athletes have taken testosterone in order to improve performance, but this is unsafe and ineffective. Male hormones may cause very **high blood calcium levels** in women with breast cancer and in people who are immobilized; these groups should avoid taking testosterone. Continuous use of high dosages of male hormones may cause life-threatening **liver problems**. Taking male hormones for an extended period of time causes **reduced sperm count and semen volume**.

Men taking testosterone as hormone replacement may develop **enlarged breasts**.

Sometimes, people taking male hormones develop a condition called **acute intermittent porphyria** (symptoms include abdominal pain, nausea and vomiting, constipation, neurotic or psychotic behavior, and nerve irritation).

Blood **cholesterol** may rise while you are taking testosterone. People with heart disease; those who have had a stroke or transient ischemic attack (TIA)—"mini-stroke;" and those who have blood vessel disease, such as claudication, should be cautious about taking a male hormone.

A man using a **scrotal testosterone patch** may transfer some hormone to his sexual partner, which may result in unwanted changes in the partner's secondary sex characteristics.

Testosterone may affect glycemic control in people with **diabetes**.

Testosterone must be used with caution in **children**. They should be treated only by specialists who are experienced with testosterone and understand its effects on children's bone development.

Possible Side Effects

▼ Most common: women—menstrual irregularities, a deepening voice, hairiness, acne, and enlargement of the clitoris. Men—breast soreness or enlargement, excessive erections, and skin reactions at the site of application.

▼ Common: men and women—swelling of the feet or lower legs, rapid weight gain, water retention, dizziness, headache, tiredness, flushing or redness, bleeding, nausea, vomiting, yellowing of the skin or whites of the eyes, confusion, depression, increased or decreased libido, thirst, increased urination, and constipation. Men—chills, pain in the scrotum or groin, prostate cancer, and difficult urination.

▼ Less common: men and women—mild acne, diarrhea, increased pubic hair, and difficulty sleeping. Men—impotence, irritation or infection of the skin of the scrotum, and decreased testicle size.

▼ Rare: men and women—male pattern baldness, oily skin, jaundice, and changes in liver function tests.

Drug Interactions

• Testosterone may increase the effects of anticoagulants (blood thinners) such as warfarin.

• Combining testosterone and imipramine (an antidepressant) may lead to a paranoid reaction.

• Testosterone may interfere with laboratory tests of thyroid function; it does not affect the thyroid gland or normal thyroid function.

Food Interactions

You may take this drug with food if it upsets your stomach. Food does not interfere with testosterone skin patches or gel.

Usual Dose

Oral Tablets
  Men: 10–50 mg a day.
  Women: 50–200 mg a day.

Skin Patches
Apply nightly. Testoderm patches should be placed on clean dry skin of the scrotum. Androderm is applied to clean dry skin on your back, abdomen, upper arm, or thigh. Androderm dosage starts at one 5 mg or two 2.5 mg patches a night. Dosage may be adjusted to 1 or 3 patches nightly.

Topical Gel
Apply to shoulders, upper arms, and/or abdomen once daily.

Striant
Apply to the gums every 12 hours.

Overdosage

Symptoms resemble drug side effects. Call your local poison control center or a hospital emergency room for more information. If you seek treatment, ALWAYS bring the prescription package or container.

Special Information

If you are using a testosterone skin patch, apply it as directed by your doctor. The site of Androderm application should be rotated, with an interval of 7 days between application to the same site. The patch should not be applied to oily or irritated skin.

Take this drug exactly as prescribed. If you forget a dose, take it as soon as possible. If it is almost time for your next dose, skip the dose you forgot and continue with your regular schedule. Do not take a double dose.

Special Populations

Pregnancy/Breast-feeding

Testosterone is not safe for use during pregnancy. Taking this drug during pregnancy, especially during the first 3 months, results in excessive masculinization of the fetus.

It is not known if testosterone passes into breast milk. Nursing mothers who must take it should bottle-feed.

Seniors

Seniors who take testosterone may have an increased risk of developing prostate disease, including cancer. A marked increase in sex drive may also develop.

Type of Drug

Tetracycline Antibiotics (teh-tra-SIKE-lene)

Brand Names

Generic Ingredient: Demeclocycline
Declomycin

Generic Ingredient: Doxycycline G

Adoxa	Doxychel Hyclate
Atridox	Monodox
Bio-Tab	Periostat
Doryx	Vibramycin
Doxy Caps	Vibra-Tabs

Generic Ingredient: Meclocycline Sulfosalicylate
Meclan

Generic Ingredient: Minocycline Hydrochloride G

Arestin	Minocin
Dynacin	Vectrin

Generic Ingredient: Oxytetracycline G

Terramycin	Uri-Tet

Generic Ingredient: Tetracycline Hydrochloride G

Achromycin V	Sumycin
Ala-Tet	Tetracap
Bristacycline	Tetracyn
Nor-Tet	Tetralan
Panmycin	Topicycline

Prescribed For

Infection including gonorrhea; infection of the mouth, gums, and teeth; Rocky Mountain spotted fever and other types of fever caused by ticks and lice including Lyme disease; urinary tract infection; and respiratory infection such as pneumonia or bronchitis. Doxycycline has been prescribed to treat and prevent traveler's diarrhea. Tetracycline hydrochloride has been used to treat amebic dysentery.

General Information

Tetracycline antibiotics are effective against a variety of bacterial infections. They work by interfering with the normal growth cycle of the invading bacteria. This allows the body's normal defenses to fight off the infection. Tetracycline may be substituted for penicillin in people who are allergic to penicillin.

Tetracyclines have been used to treat skin infection but are not considered the first-choice antibiotic. Tetracycline hydrochloride and meclocycline have been used successfully in the treatment of adolescent acne, in low dosages over a long period of time.

Cautions and Warnings

Tetracycline should not be given to people with **liver disease** or **kidney or certain urinary problems**.

If the antibiotic that your doctor has prescribed does not work, a number of things may have happened. You may not have taken the drug long enough. You may be the victim of a superinfection, in which another organism—usually a fungus—unaffected by the tetracycline antibiotic begins to grow in the same area as the bacteria being treated. If this happens, it may seem like a relapse or new infection. Only your doctor can determine which drug to take for it.

Avoid prolonged **exposure to the sun** if you are taking high dosages of tetracycline, especially demeclocycline, because these antibiotics may interfere with your body's normal sun-screening mechanism, making you more prone to severe sunburn.

If you are **allergic** to any tetracycline antibiotic, you are probably allergic to them all. Do not use tetracycline if you are allergic to it.

Tetracyclines should not be used by **children under age 8** because they have been shown to interfere with the development of the long bones and may retard growth. Permanent tooth discoloration may also result.

People taking demeclocycline may experience **diabetes insipidus syndrome** (symptoms include excessive thirst, urination, and weakness). The severity of this condition depends on the amount of drug taken and is reversible when the drug is withdrawn.

Minocycline may cause **light-headedness, dizziness,** or **fainting**.

Tetracycline has been associated with **pseudotumor cerebri** (condition characterized by increased pressure in the brain—symptoms include headache and blurred vision).

Treatment with antibacterial medications such as tetracycline may cause **diarrhea** or, more seriously, **colitis**. Contact your doctor if you develop diarrhea while taking tetracycline.

Possible Side Effects

▼ Most common: upset stomach, nausea, vomiting, diarrhea, sensitivity of the skin to the sun, and rash.

▼ Less common: hairy tongue and itching and irritation of the anal or vaginal region. If these symptoms appear, call your doctor immediately. Periodic physical examinations and laboratory tests should be given to those who are on long-term tetracycline therapy.

▼ Rare: appetite loss, peeling skin, fever, chills, anemia, brown spotting of the skin, reduced kidney function, and liver damage.

Drug Interactions

• Tetracycline may interfere with bactericidal (bacteria-killing) agents such as penicillin. You should not take both kinds of antibiotics for the same infection.

• Do not combine tetracycline with isotretinoin or methoxyflurane.

• Antacids, mineral supplements, and multivitamins containing bismuth, calcium, zinc, magnesium, or iron may reduce the effectiveness of tetracycline—with the exception of doxycycline and minocycline. Sodium bicarbonate powder may also be a problem if used as an antacid. Separate doses of an antacid, mineral supplement, vitamin with minerals, or sodium bicarbonate and a tetracycline antibiotic by at least 2 hours.

• Tetracycline may increase the effect of anticoagulant (blood-thinning) drugs such as warfarin. Your anticoagulant dosage may need an adjustment.

• Barbiturates, carbamazepine, and hydantoin antiseizure drugs may reduce doxycycline's effectiveness. More doxycycline or a different antibiotic may be required.

• Cimetidine, ranitidine, and other H_2-antagonists may reduce the effectiveness of tetracycline.

• Tetracycline may increase digoxin side effects in a small number of people. This effect may last for months after the tetracycline has been withdrawn. If you are taking this combination, be vigilant for the appearance of digoxin side effects; call your doctor if they develop.

• Tetracycline may reduce insulin requirements for diabetics. If you are using this combination, be sure to carefully monitor your blood-sugar level.

• Tetracycline may increase or decrease blood-lithium levels.

• These drugs may reduce the effectiveness of oral contraceptives ("the pill"). Breakthrough bleeding or pregnancy is possible; you should use another method of contraception in addition to an oral contraceptive while taking one of these antibiotics.

Food Interactions

Take all tetracycline antibiotics, except for doxycycline and minocycline, on an empty stomach, 1 hour before or 2 hours after meals and with 8 oz. of water. The antibacterial effect of these antibiotics may be neutralized when they are taken with food, dairy products such as milk or cheese, or antacids. Doxycycline and minocycline may be taken with food or milk.

Usual Dose

Demeclocycline
    Adult: 600 mg a day.

Child (age 9 and over): 3–6 mg per lb. of body weight a day.
Child (under age 9): not recommended.

Doxycycline Hydrochloride

Adult and Child (age 9 and over, and over 100 lbs.): starting dosage—200 mg in 2 doses of 100 mg given 12 hours apart. Maintenance dosage—100 mg a day in 1 or 2 doses. For gonorrhea, take 300 mg in 1 dose and then a second 300-mg dose in 1 hour, or 100 mg twice daily for at least 7 days; for syphilis, 100–300 mg for 10 days to 4 weeks.

Child (age 9 and over, but under 100 lbs.): starting dosage—2 mg per lb. of body weight divided into 2 doses. Maintenance dosage—1 mg per lb. of body weight as a single daily dose.

Your doctor may double the maintenance dosage for severe infection. An increased incidence of side effects is observed with dosages over 200 mg a day.

Meclocycline Sulfosalicylate
Apply to affected area morning and night.

Minocycline Hydrochloride

Adult: starting dosage—200 mg. Maintenance dosage—100 mg every 12 hours. Alternate dosage: starting dosage—100-200 mg. Maintenance dosage—50 mg 4 times a day.

Child (age 9 and over): starting dosage—2 mg per lb. of body weight. Maintenance dosage—1 mg per lb. every 12 hours.

Child (under age 9): not recommended.

Oxytetracycline and Oral Tetracycline Hydrochloride

Adult: 250–500 mg 4 times a day.

Child (age 9 and over): 10–20 mg per lb. of body weight a day in 4 equal doses.

Child (under age 9): not recommended.

Tetracycline Hydrochloride Ointment and Solution
Apply to affected area morning and night.

Overdosage

Overdose is most likely to affect the stomach and digestive system. Call your local poison control center or a hospital emergency room for more information. ALWAYS bring the prescription bottle or container if you go for treatment.

Special Information

Do not take any antibiotic after the expiration date on the label. Decomposed tetracycline may cause serious kidney damage.

Since the action of tetracycline depends on its concentration within the invading bacteria, it is imperative that you completely follow the doctor's directions and complete the full course of treatment prescribed.

Call your doctor if you develop excessive thirst, urination, and weakness; blue-gray discoloration of the skin or mucous membranes (with minocycline); appetite loss; headache; vomiting; changes in vision; abdominal pain with nausea and vomiting; yellowing of the skin or whites of the eyes; or any persistent or intolerable side effect including dizziness, light-headedness, or unsteadiness; burning or cramps in the stomach; diarrhea with nausea and vomiting; or itching of the mouth, rectal, or vaginal areas (may indicate the presence of a superinfection). Call your doctor if your child develops tooth discoloration.

Avoid excessive exposure to the sun while taking tetracycline, especially demeclocycline, because these drugs may cause susceptibility to sunburn.

Tetracycline may cause dizziness, light-headedness, or fainting. Be careful when driving or performing any task that requires concentration.

If you are using tetracycline hydrochloride topical solution or meclocycline sulfosalicylate for acne, apply the product generously to your skin until the area to be treated is completely wet. Stinging or burning may occur but this lasts only a few minutes. Tetracycline hydrochloride solution may stain your skin yellow but the stain usually washes away. Do not apply the solution or cream inside your eyes, nose, or mouth.

If you miss a dose of oral tetracycline, take it as soon as possible. If you take the drug once a day and it is almost time for your next dose, space the missed dose and your next dose 10 to 12 hours apart, then go back to your regular schedule. If you take tetracycline twice a day and it is almost time for your next dose, space the missed dose and your next dose by 5 to 6 hours, then go back to your regular schedule. If you take the drug 3 or more times a day and it is almost time for your next dose, space the missed dose and your next dose by 2 to 4 hours, then go back to your regular schedule. Never take a double dose.

Special Populations

Pregnancy/Breast-feeding

Tetracycline should not be taken if you are pregnant, especially during the last 5 months of pregnancy. It interferes with the formation of skull and bone structures in the fetus.

Tetracycline passes into breast milk. It interferes with the development of a child's skull, bones, and teeth. Nursing mothers who must take tetracycline should bottle-feed.

Seniors

Seniors, especially those with poor kidney function, are more likely to suffer from less common side effects.

Generic Name

Thalidomide (thal-IH-doe-mide)

Brand Name

Thalomid

Type of Drug

Immune-system modulator.

Prescribed For

Erythema nodosum leprosum (ENL)—a painful skin condition associated with leprosy.

General Information

Thalidomide was approved by the Food and Drug Administration (FDA) in 1998 for ENL under a very strict distribution system called S.T.E.P.S. (System for Thalidomide Education and Prescribing Safety), as this drug causes serious birth defects. Only doctors who are registered with the S.T.E.P.S. program can prescribe thalidomide. The exact way that thalidomide works is not known, but it appears to suppress excessive amounts of tumor necrosis factor (TFN) and also affects the movement of white blood cells. Thalidomide is also prescribed for leprosy, scleroderma and other skin conditions, and is being studied for prostate and other cancers.

Cautions and Warnings

As little as 1 dose of thalidomide can cause **birth defects**. It should not be taken by pregnant women under any circumstances. Women must take a pregnancy test before the drug will be prescribed. Women who might become pregnant should consider taking thalidomide only if other treatments have failed. Men taking thalidomide can also transmit the drug to the fetus. To protect the health of the fetus, these men should use a condom during intercourse with a pregnant partner; using 2 methods of barrier contraception is preferred.

A **drug sensitivity or allergic reaction** to thalidomide (symptoms include rash, fever, rapid heartbeat, and low blood pressure) may be cause to temporarily stop your treatment.

Thalidomide should not be used as the sole treatment for ENL by people with **neuritis** (nerve irritation).

Thalidomide frequently causes **nerve damage** (symptoms include numbness, tingling, or pain in the hands or feet) that may be permanent. It generally occurs after a few months of regular treatment but can also develop after taking thalidomide for a short time.

Thalidomide can cause a rapid drop in white-blood-cell count, increasing the risk of **infection**.

Thalidomide can increase the level of HIV RNA in people with AIDS, but the importance of this finding is unclear.

Thalidomide is generally not recommended for **children under age 18,** though a small number of children have been safely treated with the drug.

Possible Side Effects

▼ Most common: drowsiness, rash, dizziness, impotence, fainting, headache, and stomach pain.

▼ Common: muscle weakness; tingling, burning, numbness, or pain in the hands, arms, feet, or legs; tremors; constipation; diarrhea; nausea; mouth infections; sinus irritation; back pain; fever, alone or with chills and sore throat; infections; and feeling unwell.

▼ Less common: dry mouth, liver inflammation, gas, dry skin, mood change, leg swelling, acne, fungal skin infections, nail problems, itching, sweating, loss of

Possible Side Effects *(continued)*

appetite, tooth pain, anemia, low white-blood-cell count, swollen lymph glands, runny nose, abdominal pain, accidental injuries, and a rigid or painful neck.

▼ Rare: blood in the urine, decreased urination, irregular heartbeat, low blood pressure, and agitation. Other rare side effects can occur in almost any part of the body. Contact your doctor if you experience any side effect not listed above.

Drug Interactions

• Combining thalidomide with alcohol, barbiturates, chlorpromazine, reserpine, sedatives, tricyclic antidepressants, tranquilizers, or other nervous system depressants can cause extreme tiredness. Avoid this combination.

• Combining thalidomide and chloramphenicol, cisplatin, dapsone, didanosine, ethambutol, ethionamide, hydralazine, isoniazid, lithium, metronidazole, nitrofurantoin, nitrous oxide, phenytoin, stavudine, vincristine, or zalcitabine may worsen peripheral neuropathy (symptoms include tingling, burning, numbness, or pain in the hands or feet) or increase your risk of developing it.

• Medications that interfere with oral contraceptives ("the pill") must be avoided if you are taking thalidomide because they increase the risk of an unwanted pregnancy. These drugs include protease inhibitors—used in the treatment of human immunodeficiency virus (HIV) infection; griseofulvin; rifampin; rifabutin; phenytoin; and carbamazepine.

Food Interactions

For optimal effectiveness, do not take thalidomide with a high-fat meal.

Usual Dose

Adult: 100–400 mg a day at bedtime.

Overdosage

Symptoms are likely to be common side effects. Take the victim to a hospital emergency room. ALWAYS bring the prescription bottle or container.

Special Information

Women of childbearing age who take thalidomide should have weekly pregnancy tests. Women with irregular periods may have to be tested every 2 weeks. Stop taking the drug at once if you are or think you may be pregnant.

Drowsiness is common with thalidomide. Be careful when driving or performing any task that requires concentration.

Thalidomide can make you dizzy or faint if you rise suddenly from a lying position. Sitting up for a few minutes before attempting to stand may help prevent this problem.

Thalidomide can increase your sensitivity to the sun. Use sunscreen and wear protective clothing while taking this drug.

Take this drug exactly as prescribed. Do not stop taking it without your doctor's knowledge.

If you forget a dose, take it as soon as you remember. If it is almost time for your next dose, skip the one you forgot and continue with your regular schedule. Do not take a double dose.

Special Populations

Pregnancy/Breast-feeding

Women who are or might be pregnant should never take thalidomide, especially during the first 2 months of pregnancy. Women of childbearing age who take thalidomide should use 2 reliable methods of contraception (for example, an oral contraceptive and a condom). Contraception must be used for at least 1 month before treatment is begun, during treatment, and for 1 month after treatment has been completed.

It is not known if thalidomide passes into breast milk but it could cause serious reactions in a nursing infant. Nursing mothers who must take thalidomide should bottle-feed.

Seniors

Seniors may take this drug without special restriction.

Type of Drug

Thiazide Diuretics (THYE-uh-zide dye-ur-RET-iks)

Brand Names

Generic Ingredient: Bendroflumethiazide
Naturetin

Generic Ingredient: Chlorothiazide G
Diurigen   Diuril

Generic Ingredient: Chlorthalidone G
Hygroton   Thalitone

Generic Ingredient: Hydrochlorothiazide G
Esidrix   Hydro-Par
Ezide   Microzide
HydroDIURIL   Oretic

Generic Ingredient: Hydroflumethiazide G
Diucardin   Saluron

Generic Ingredient: Indapamide G
Lozol

Generic Ingredient: Methyclothiazide G
Aquatensen   Enduron

Generic Ingredient: Metolazone
Mykrox   Zaroxolyn

Generic Ingredient: Polythiazide
Renese

Generic Ingredient: Quinethazone
Hydromox

Generic Ingredient: Trichlormethiazide G
Diurese   Naqua
Metahydrin

Prescribed For

Congestive heart failure (CHF), cirrhosis of the liver, kidney malfunction, hypertension (high blood pressure), and other conditions where it is necessary to rid the body of excess water.

General Information

Thiazide diuretics increase urine production by affecting the movement of sodium and chloride in the kidney. Thiazide diuretics reduce sodium, magnesium, bicarbonate, chloride, and potassium-ion levels. Calcium elimination is moderated and uric acid is retained as a result of thiazide treatment. Thiazide diuretics may also raise blood sugar. These drugs are used in the treatment of any disease where it is desirable to eliminate large quantities of water. Thiazide diuretics are often taken with other drugs to treat high blood pressure and other conditions. The exact way in which they reduce blood pressure is not known; sodium elimination is of primary importance. These diuretics begin to work within 2 hours and produce their effect in 2 to 6 hours. The differences between thiazide diuretic drugs lie in duration of effect—6 to 12 hours for some and as long as 48 to 72 hours for others—and quantity of drug absorbed.

Cautions and Warnings

Do not take a thiazide diuretic if you are **allergic** or **sensitive** to any drugs in this group or to sulfa drugs. If you have a history of allergy or bronchial asthma, you may also have a sensitivity or allergy to thiazide diuretics. Thiazide diuretics may aggravate **lupus erythematosus** (chronic condition affecting the body's connective tissue).

Thiazides may raise total **cholesterol,** low-density lipoprotein (LDL) cholesterol, and total triglyceride levels. They should be used with caution by people with moderate to high blood-cholesterol or triglyceride levels. Thiazides should be used with caution if you have severe **kidney disease** because they may precipitate kidney failure; only metolazone and indapamide may be safely given in this group. People with severe **liver disease** should be treated carefully with diuretics because minor changes in electrolyte (body-fluid) balance may cause hepatic coma.

Switching between brands of metolazone is not recommended. They are not equivalent.

Possible Side Effects

▼ Most common: Thiazide diuretics cause loss of body potassium. Symptoms of low potassium include dry mouth, thirst, weakness, lethargy, drowsiness, restlessness, muscle pain or cramp, muscular tiredness, low blood pressure, decreased frequency of urination and decreased urine production, abnormal heart rate, and upset stomach including nausea and vomiting. Potassium supplements are given to prevent this problem—or you may eat high-potassium foods such as bananas, citrus fruits, melons, and tomatoes.

Possible Side Effects *(continued)*

▼ Less common: appetite loss, abdominal pain, bloating, diarrhea, constipation, dizziness, yellowing of the skin or whites of the eyes, headache, tingling of the toes and fingers, restlessness, changes in blood composition, increased sensitivity to the sun, rash, itching, fever, breathing difficulties, allergic reaction, dizziness when rising quickly from a sitting or lying position, muscle spasm, impotence and reduced sex drive, weakness, and blurred vision.

Drug Interactions

• Thiazide diuretics increase the action of other blood-pressure-lowering drugs. Consequently, people with high blood pressure often take more than 1 drug.

• The risk of developing imbalances in electrolytes is increased if you take medications such as digitalis drugs, amphotericin B, and adrenal corticosteroids while taking a thiazide diuretic.

• If you begin taking a thiazide diuretic, your insulin or antidiabetic dosage may have to be modified.

• Thiazide diuretics may increase the risk of allopurinol side effects.

• Thiazide diuretics may decrease the effects of oral anticoagulant (blood-thinning) drugs.

• Antigout drug dosage may have to be modified since thiazide diuretics raise blood uric-acid levels.

• Thiazide diuretics may prolong the white-blood-cell-reducing effects of chemotherapy drugs.

• Thiazide diuretics may increase the effects of diazoxide, leading to symptoms of diabetes.

• Combining thiazide diuretics and loop diuretics may lead to an extreme diuretic effect and extreme effect on blood-electrolyte levels.

• Thiazide diuretics may increase the action of vitamin D, possibly leading to high blood-calcium levels.

• Propantheline and other anticholinergics may increase the effects of thiazide diuretics.

• Thiazide diuretics increase the risk of lithium side effects.

- Cholestyramine and colestipol block the absorption of thiazide diuretics. Thiazide diuretics should be taken more than 2 hours before cholestyramine or colestipol.
- Methenamine and other urinary agents may reduce the effect of thiazide diuretics.
- Certain nonsteroidal anti-inflammatory drugs (NSAIDs), particularly indomethacin, may reduce the effectiveness of thiazide diuretics. Sulindac, another NSAID, may increase the effect of thiazide diuretics.

Food Interactions

Thiazide diuretics may be taken with food if they upset your stomach. Your doctor may recommend high-potassium foods like bananas and orange juice to offset the potassium-lowering effect of these drugs.

Usual Dose

Bendroflumethiazide
Starting dosage—5–20 mg a day, either in 1 dose or divided into 2 doses. Maintenance dosage—2.5–5 mg a day.

Chlorothiazide
Adult: 0.5–1 g 1–2 times a day. Often people respond to intermittent therapy, that is, taking the drug on alternate days or 3–5 days a week. This reduces side effects.

Child (age 6 months and over): 10 mg per lb. of body weight a day in 2 equal doses.

Child (under age 6 months): not more than 15 mg per lb. of body weight a day in 2 equal doses.

Chlorthalidone
50–100 mg (Thalitone, 30–60 mg) a day, or 100 mg (Thalitone, 60 mg) on alternate days. Some patients may need 150–200 mg (Thalitone, 90–120 mg) at these intervals, or 120 mg Thalitone daily.
Hypertension: 25 mg (Thalitone, 15 mg) daily, increased if necessary to 50–100 mg (Thalitone, 30–50 mg) once a day.

Hydrochlorothiazide
Adult: 25–200 mg a day depending on the condition being treated. Maintenance dosage—25–100 mg a day. 200 mg a day is sometimes required.

Child (age 6 months and over): 1 mg per lb. of body weight a day in 2 doses.

Child (under age 6 months): 1.5 mg per lb. of body weight a day in 2 doses.

Hydroflumethiazide
Starting dosage—50 mg 1–2 times a day. Maintenance dosage—25–200 mg a day. Daily dosages of more than 100 mg should be divided into separate doses.

Indapamide
1.25–5 mg every morning. Dosage may be increased to 5 mg a day.

Methyclothiazide
2.5–10 mg a day.

Metolazone
Dosage is individualized. Zaroxolyn—2.5–20 mg once a day. Mykrox—0.5 mg once a day, in the morning. Dosage may be increased to 1 mg a day.

Polythiazide
1–4 mg a day.

Quinethazone
50–100 mg a day. Occasionally, dosages of 100 mg are divided into 2 doses. 150–200 mg a day is sometimes required.

Trichlormethiazide
2–4 mg a day.

Overdosage

Symptoms include tingling in the arms or legs, weakness, fatigue, fainting, dizziness, changes in heartbeat, feeling unwell, dry mouth, restlessness, muscle pain or cramp, urinary difficulties, nausea, and vomiting. Take the victim to a hospital emergency room at once. ALWAYS bring the prescription bottle or container.

Special Information

Ordinarily, diuretics are prescribed early in the day to prevent excessive nighttime urination from interfering with sleep.

Thiazide diuretics cause excess urination at first but it subsides after several weeks.

Contact your doctor if you develop muscle pain, sudden joint pain, weakness, cramps, nausea, vomiting, restlessness, excessive thirst, tiredness, drowsiness, increased heart or pulse rate, diarrhea, or dizziness. People with diabetes may experience increased blood-sugar levels and need dosage adjustments of their antidiabetic medication.

Avoid alcohol and other medications while taking a thiazide diuretic, unless directed by your doctor.

Avoid over-the-counter medications for the treatment of coughs, colds, and allergy if you have hypertension or CHF because such medication may contain stimulants.

If you forget a dose, take it as soon as you remember. If it is almost time for your next dose, skip the one you forgot and continue with your regular schedule. Do not take a double dose.

Special Populations

Pregnancy/Breast-feeding

Thiazide diuretics enter the fetal circulation and may cause side effects in the newborn such as jaundice, blood problems, and low potassium levels. Diuretics are used to treat specific medical conditions during pregnancy but their routine use during a normal pregnancy is improper. When any of these drugs is considered crucial by your doctor, its potential benefits must be carefully weighed against its risks.

Thiazide diuretics pass into breast milk. Nursing mothers who must take diuretics should bottle-feed.

Seniors

Seniors are more sensitive to side effects, especially dizziness.

Type of Drug

Thyroid Hormone Replacements

Brand Names

Generic Ingredient: Levothyroxine Sodium G
Levotabs   Synthroid
Levothroid   Thyro-Tabs
Levoxyl   Unithyroid

Generic Ingredient: Liothyronine Sodium G
Cytomel   Triostat

Generic Ingredient: Liotrix G
Thyrolar

Generic Ingredient: Thyroglobulin
Only available in generic form.

Generic Ingredient: Thyroid Hormone Ⓖ

Armour Thyroid	Thyroid Strong
S-P-T	Thyrar

Prescribed For

Hypothyroidism (underactive thyroid gland).

General Information

The major differences between these drugs are their sources and hormone content. Thyroid hormone is made from beef and pork thyroid. It is effective but lacks standardization, making it difficult for doctors to control dosage. Synthetic drugs are more desirable because their content is easily standardized, ensuring that you receive the correct amount of hormone.

Basically, there are 2 important thyroid hormones: levothyroxine and liothyronine. Levothyroxine is converted to liothyronine in the body. This process slows the absorption of levothyroxine and lowers the risk of side effects. Liothyronine's potency and its potential for side effects make it less desirable for older adults. Thyroglobulin and liotrix contain both levothyroxine and liothyronine; since levothyroxine is converted naturally to liothyronine, there is usually no advantage in taking both hormones. These considerations tend to make levothyroxine the treatment of choice for thyroid hormone replacement.

Cautions and Warnings

If you have **hyperthyroid disease** (symptoms include headache, nervousness, sweating, rapid heartbeat, chest pain, and other signs of central nervous system [CNS] stimulation) or **high output of thyroid hormone,** you should not use these drugs.

If you have **heart disease** or **hypertension** (high blood pressure), thyroid hormone replacement therapy should not be used unless it is clearly indicated and supervised by your doctor, as it can aggravate the condition. If you develop chest pain or other signs of heart disease while taking this drug, call your doctor immediately.

These drugs should not be used to treat **infertility** unless the person also has hypothyroidism.

Thyroid hormone replacements have been prescribed for **weight loss**. Thyroid treatments do not work in people with a normal thyroid status unless large dosages are used—these dosages may produce serious or fatal side effects, especially when taken with appetite-suppressing drugs.

Thyroid hormone replacement therapy increases metabolism and may worsen the symptoms of other endocrine system—hormone-related—diseases including **diabetes** and **Addison's disease**. Adjustments in the levels of treatment for these diseases may be needed when you begin using these drugs.

Possible Side Effects

Side effects are rare except during the start of therapy or when dosage is adjusted.

▼ Most common: heart palpitations, rapid heartbeat, abnormal heart rhythms, weight loss, chest pain, hand tremor, headache, diarrhea, nervousness, menstrual irregularity, inability to sleep, sweating, and intolerance to heat. These symptoms may be controlled by adjusting dosage.

Drug Interactions

• Antacids, simethicone, sucralfate, colestipol, and cholestyramine may reduce the effect of these drugs. Take your thyroid hormone replacement and these drugs 4 to 6 hours apart.

• Estrogen drugs may increase your need for thyroid hormone replacement therapy.

• Raloxifene interferes with the absorption of levothyroxine. Separate these medicines by 12 hours.

• Avoid taking over-the-counter drugs that contain stimulants—such as many of the products used to treat cough, cold, or allergy—which affect the heart and may cause symptoms of overdose.

• People with diabetes may need to have their doctors increase their insulin or oral antidiabetic drug dosages when they start taking a thyroid hormone replacement.

• These drugs may reduce the effectiveness of beta blockers. Beta-blocker dosage may need to be increased.

• Dosage reduction of theophylline may be required if you take a thyroid hormone replacement.

• Blood levels of digitalis drugs, and their effectiveness, may be reduced by thyroid hormone replacements.

• Use of carbamazapine, phenobarbital, and SSRIs may result in a need for increased dosages of levothyroxine.

• Combining tricyclic antidepressants and levothyroxine may increase the risk of toxic effects.

• These drugs may increase the effectiveness of anticoagulants.

Food Interactions

Thyroid hormone replacements should be taken as a single dose, preferably before breakfast.

Usual Dose

Levothyroxine

Starting dosage—as little as 12.5 mcg a day, which is then increased in steps of 12.5–25 mcg once every 2–8 weeks depending upon response. Maintenance dosage—100–300 mcg a day. It is essential to take levothyroxine at the same time each day.

Liothyronine

Adult: 5–100 mcg a day.

Senior and Child: begin at the low end of the dosage range and increase slowly until the desired effect has been achieved.

Liotrix

Adult: a single "¼"–"2" tablet a day, depending on the condition being treated and your response to therapy. Liotrix tablets are rated according to their approximate equivalent to thyroid hormone.

Senior and Child: Begin at the low end of the dosage range and increase slowly until the desired effect has been achieved.

Thyroglobulin and Thyroid Hormone

Starting dosage—16–32 mg, or ¼–½ grain a day, which is then increased in 15-mg steps every 1–2 weeks until response is satisfactory. Maintenance dosage—30–160 mg a day.

Overdosage

Symptoms include headache; irritability; nervousness; sweating; rapid heartbeat with unusual stomach rumbling—with or without cramps; chest pain; heart failure; and shock. Take the victim to a hospital emergency room immediately. ALWAYS bring the prescription bottle or container.

Special Information

Thyroid hormone replacement therapy is usually a lifelong treatment. Take the drug as prescribed and do not stop taking it unless instructed by your doctor.

Do not switch brands, especially in the case of levothyroxine, without your doctor's or pharmacist's knowledge. Different brands of the same thyroid hormone replacement are not always equivalent.

Call your doctor if you develop nervousness, diarrhea, excessive sweating, chest pain, increased pulse rate, heart palpitations, and intolerance to heat—which are signs you may be taking too high a dose—or any bothersome or persistent side effect.

Children beginning thyroid hormone replacement therapy may lose some hair during the first few months but this is only temporary and the hair generally grows back.

If you forget a dose, take it as soon as you remember. If it is almost time for your next dose, skip the one you forgot and continue with your regular schedule. Do not take a double dose. Call your doctor if you miss 2 or more consecutive doses.

Special Populations

Pregnancy/Breast-feeding

Small amounts of these drugs enter the fetal bloodstream. These medications have not been associated with any problems when used to maintain normal thyroid function in the mother. Pregnant women who have been taking a thyroid hormone replacement should continue their treatment under medical supervision.

Small amounts of these drugs pass into breast milk. Nursing mothers who must take them should consider bottle-feeding.

Seniors

Seniors, who may be more sensitive to the effects of these drugs, generally require reduced dosage.

Generic Name

Tiagabine (tye-AG-a-bene)

Brand Name

Gabitril

The information in this profile also applies to the following drug:

Generic Ingredient: Gabapentin
Neurontin

Type of Drug

Anticonvulsant.

Prescribed For

Partial seizure. Gabapetin may also be used for tremors associated with multiple sclerosis, nerve pain, bipolar disorder, and for the prevention of migrane headaches.

General Information

The exact way in which tiagabine hydrochloride works is not known but may be related to its ability to improve the activity of GABA, the major inhibitor of nerve transmission in the brain and central nervous system (CNS). This means that tiagabine probably slows GABA-related nerve impulses that lead to a seizure. The medication achieves maximum blood levels in 45 minutes. It is broken down in the liver.

Cautions and Warnings

Do not take this drug if you are **sensitive** or **allergic** to it. Several people taking tiagabine have developed a **severe rash**.

People with **liver disease** should take this drug with caution and receive reduced dosages. People with **kidney disease** require reduced dosages of gabapentin.

Suddenly stopping any antiepileptic drug can increase the frequency of seizures. Dosage should be reduced gradually.

In studies, a small number of people **died suddenly** while taking gabapentin. It is not known if these deaths were caused by the drug.

A feeling of **severe weakness** has developed in a small number of people taking tiagabine. The weakness goes away when the medication is reduced or stopped.

Tiagabine may bind to parts of the eye. There is no evidence that this produces long-term effects. Tell your doctor if you experience any changes in vision.

Possible Side Effects

Tiagabine

▼ Most common: dizziness, sleepiness, confusion, depression, weakness, nervousness, and nausea.

▼ Common: poor concentration, speech or language problems, abdominal or other pain, tremor, sleeplessness, tiredness, diarrhea, vomiting, sore throat, and rash.

▼ Less common: forgetfulness, tingling in the hands or feet, emotional upset, walking unusually, hostility rolling of the eyeballs, agitation, hunger, mouth sores, cough, itching, and flushing.

Gabapentin

▼ Most common: tiredness, dizziness, weakness, peripheral edema, and abnormal eyeball movement.

▼ Common: fatigue, double vision, blurred vision, and tremors.

▼ Less common: weight gain, back pain, upset stomach, dry mouth or throat, constipation, dental problems, muscle aches, runny nose, sore throat, speech problems, memory loss, depression, abnormal thinking, twitching, itching, abrasions, and impotence.

▼ Rare: leg swelling, increased appetite, broken bones, poor coordination, low red- and white-blood-cell counts, and flushing.

Drug Interactions

• Taking tiagabine with other medications for seizure control, including carbamazepine, phenytoin, phenobarbital, and valproate may affect the amount of each in the blood. Dosage adjustments may be necessary.

• Antacids reduce the absorption of gabapentin; take these drugs at least 2 hours apart.

• Comgining gabapentin and hydrocodone may affect each other's blood levels.

• Morphine significantly increases blood levels of gabapentin.

Food Interactions

Take tiagabine with food but avoid high-fat meals, which slow its absorption. Gabapentin may be taken with or without food.

Usual Dose

Tiagabine
   Adult (age 19 and over): starting dosage—4 mg once a day. Dosage may be increased in steps of 4 or 8 mg to 56 mg a day. Higher amounts should be divided into 2 or 4 doses a day.
   Child (age 12–18): starting dosage—4 mg once a day. Dosage may be increased in steps of 4 or 8 mg to 32 mg a day. Higher amounts should be divided into 2 doses a day.

Gabapentin
   Adult and Child (age 12 and over): 300–600 mg 3 times a day. Dosage must be reduced in people with kidney disease.
   Child (age 3–12): 4.5–7 mg per pound a day in 3 divided doses to start, increasing gradually over a period of about 3 days to a maximum of 22 mg per pound a day in divided doses.
   Child (under age 3): not recommended.

Overdosage

Tiagabine: Symptoms include tiredness, loss of consciousness, agitation, confusion, difficulty talking, hostility, depression, weakness, and muscle spasm.

Gabapentin: Symptoms include double vision, slurred speech, drowsiness, diarrhea, lethargy, weakness, breathing difficulties, sedation, droopy eyelids, and excitation.

   Take the victim to a hospital emergency room. ALWAYS bring the prescription bottle or container.

Special Information

This drug may make you dizzy or tired, or interfere with your concentration. Be extremely careful when driving or performing any task that requires concentration. Avoid alcohol or other nervous system depressants because they increase these effects.

Tell your doctor if you experience changes in vision, rash, or any bothersome or persistent side effect.

If you forget a dose, take it as soon as you remember. If it is almost time for your next dose, take the dose you forgot and space the remaining daily dosage evenly throughout the day. Do not take a double dose.

Special Populations

Pregnancy/Breast-feeding

This medication causes birth defects in lab animals. Seizure disorder itself has been associated with an increased risk of birth defects. Discuss with your doctor the need to control seizure and the potential benefits and risks of taking this medication during pregnancy.

Tiagabine may pass into breast milk. It is not known if gabapentin does so. Nursing mothers who must take either drug should consider bottle-feeding.

Seniors

Seniors may take tiagabine without special precaution but may require reduced dosage of gabapentin.

Generic Name

Ticlopidine (tih-KLOE-pih-dene) Ⓖ

Brand Name

Ticlid

Type of Drug

Anticoagulant (blood thinner).

Prescribed For

Reducing risk of stroke; also used to treat intermittent claudication and chronic circulatory occlusion, and to reduce the damage caused by stroke. It is used before open heart surgery to reduce the expected drop in platelet count, during coronary artery bypass surgery or stent placement to improve the chance of success, in some forms of kidney disease to help improve kidney function, and in sickle cell disease to reduce the number and severity of sickle cell attacks.

General Information

Ticlopidine hydrochloride makes blood platelets less "sticky," reducing the risk of blood clotting and the possible consequences of clot formation. It interferes with the functioning of the platelet cell membrane, changing platelet cells irreversibly until they are replaced by new ones. Maximum effect (60% to 70% reduction in platelet function) is seen 8 to 11 days after administration of 250 mg of ticlopidine twice a day. In studies, people taking ticlopidine regularly for 2 to 5 years experienced a 24% reduction in incidence of stroke.

Cautions and Warnings

Ticlopidine can cause severe **reductions in white-blood-cell counts,** greatly increasing the risk of infection. Some cases have been fatal. Your doctor should take white-blood-cell counts 2 weeks after you begin taking ticlopidine and continue testing every 2 weeks for the first 3 months of treatment. Only people showing signs of infection need to be tested after that period. Blood counts usually return to normal 1 to 3 weeks after you stop taking the drug.

Blood-platelet counts can also be depressed, leading to spontaneous bruising or bleeding. **Gastrointestinal bleeding** can also worsen during use of ticlopidine.

Do not take this medication if you are **allergic** to it or have an **active bleeding site such as an ulcer, reduced blood-cell counts,** or severe **liver disease**.

Ticlopidine causes an 8% to 10% increase in blood **cholesterol** within a month after you start taking the drug.

People being switched from an anticoagulant or thrombolytic to ticlopidine should stop the former drug and allow it to clear the system before starting ticlopidine.

People with severe **kidney disease** may need less ticlopidine.

Possible Side Effects

Side effects occur in more than 50% of all people. About 21% of ticlopidine patients stop taking the drug because of gastrointestinal side effects.

▼ Most common: diarrhea, nausea, upset stomach, rash, and stomach pain.

Possible Side Effects *(continued)*

▼ Less common: reduced white-blood-cell counts, vomiting, bruising, gas, itching, dizziness, appetite loss, and liver function changes.

Drug Interactions

• Antacids reduce the absorption of ticlopidine. Separate doses by at least 1 hour.

• Taking cimetidine on a regular basis can reduce the clearance of ticlopidine from the body by 50%, increasing the risk of drug toxicity and side effects.

• Combining aspirin and ticlopidine may increase the risk of bleeding. Do not combine these drugs.

• Ticlopidine may slightly reduce blood levels of digoxin. This is not a problem for most people, but dosage adjustment may be needed.

• Ticlopidine reduces the body's clearance of theophylline; your doctor may need to reduce your theophylline dosage.

• Ticlopidine may increase the effects of phenytoin. Use caution if taking these drugs simultaneously.

Food Interactions

Ticlopidine should be taken with meals to reduce stomach upset and maximize absorption of the drug. Take it at the same time each day to gain maximum benefit.

Usual Dose

250 mg taken twice a day with food.

Overdosage

Overdose may lead to increased bleeding and liver inflammation. Other possible effects include stomach bleeding, convulsions, breathing difficulties, and low body temperature. Take the victim to a hospital emergency room. ALWAYS bring the prescription bottle or container.

Special Information

Call your doctor if you have fever, chills, sore throat, or other indication of infection; severe or persistent diarrhea; rash; bleeding under the skin; yellowing of the skin or whites of the eyes; dark urine; light-colored stools; or any bothersome or persistent side effect.

Bleeding may be more difficult to stop if you are taking ticlopidine. Be sure your doctor, dentist, and other health care professionals know that you are taking this medication.

If you miss a dose, take it as soon as you can. If it is 4 hours or less until your next dose, skip the missed dose and continue with your regular schedule. Do not take a double dose.

Special Populations

Pregnancy/Breast-feeding

The safety of using ticlopidine during pregnancy is not known. When this drug is considered crucial by your doctor, its potential benefits must be carefully weighed against its risks.

Ticlopidine may pass into breast milk. Nursing mothers who must take it should bottle-feed.

Seniors

Seniors may be more sensitive to the effects of ticlopidine.

Generic Name

Timolol (TIM-oe-lol) G

Brand Names

Blocadren

The information in this profile also applies to the following drugs:

Generic Ingredient: Nadolol G
Corgard

Generic Ingredient: Sotalol G
Betapace   Betapace AF

Type of Drug

Beta-adrenergic blocking agent.

Prescribed For

High blood pressure, abnormal heart rhythms, prevention of second heart attack or migraine, tremors, and stage fright and other anxieties.

General Information

Timolol is one of many beta-adrenergic blocking drugs, or beta blockers, that interfere with the action of a specific part of the nervous system. Beta receptors are found all over the body and affect many body functions. Each beta blocker has particular characteristics that make it more suitable for certain conditions or people. When applied as eyedrops, timolol reduces ocular pressure (pressure inside the eye) by reducing the production of eye fluids and by slightly increasing the rate at which these fluids flow through and leave the eye.

Cautions and Warnings

Do not take timolol if you are **allergic** to beta blockers.

You should be cautious about taking timolol if you have **asthma, severe heart failure,** a **very slow heart rate,** or **heart block** (disruption of the electrical impulses that control heart rate) because the drug may aggravate these conditions.

People with **angina** who take timolol for high blood pressure risk aggravating their angina if they suddenly stop taking the drug. These people should have their drug dosage reduced gradually over 1 to 2 weeks.

Timolol should be used with caution if you have **liver or kidney disease** because your ability to eliminate the drug from your body may be impaired.

People with **asthma** should use timolol with caution, as it may worsen asthma symptoms.

Solatol can increase the risk of **ventricular arrhythmias,** sometimes fatal.

Timolol reduces the amount of blood pumped by the heart with each beat. This reduction in blood flow may aggravate the condition of people with **poor circulation** or **circulatory disease**.

If you are undergoing **major surgery,** your doctor may want you to stop taking timolol at least 2 days before surgery.

Timolol eyedrops should not be used by people who cannot tolerate oral beta-blocking drugs, such as propranolol.

Possible Side Effects

Side effects are relatively uncommon and usually mild.

▼ Less common: impotence, unusual tiredness or weakness, slow heartbeat, heart failure, dizziness, breathing difficulties, bronchospasm, depression, confusion, anxiety, nervousness, sleeplessness, disorientation, short-term memory loss, emotional instability, cold hands and feet, constipation, diarrhea, nausea, vomiting, upset stomach, increased sweating, urinary difficulties, cramps, blurred vision, rash, hair loss, stuffy nose, facial swelling, aggravation of lupus erythematosus, itching, chest pain, back or joint pain, colitis, drug allergy (symptoms include fever and sore throat), and liver toxicity.

Drug Interactions

• Timolol may interact with surgical anesthetics to increase the risk of heart problems during surgery. Some anesthesiologists recommend gradually stopping the drug by 2 days before surgery.

• Timolol may interfere with the signs of low blood sugar and with the action of oral antidiabetes drugs.

• Timolol increases the blood-pressure-lowering effects of other blood-pressure-reducing agents, including clonidine, guanabenz, and reserpine; and calcium channel blockers such as nifedipine.

• Aspirin-containing drugs, indomethacin, sulfinpyrazone, and estrogen drugs may interfere with the blood-pressure-lowering effect of timolol.

• Cocaine may reduce the effectiveness of all beta blockers.

• Timolol may worsen the problem of cold hands and feet associated with ergot alkaloids, used to treat migraine. Gangrene is a possibility in people taking both an ergot and timolol.

• Timolol will counteract thyroid hormone replacements.

• Calcium channel blockers, flecainide, hydralazine, oral contraceptives, propafenone, haloperidol, phenothiazine tranquilizers (molindone and others) quinolone antibacterials, and quinidine may increase the amount of timolol in the bloodstream and lead to increased timolol effects.

• Timolol should not be taken within 2 weeks of taking a monoamine oxidase inhibitor (MAOI) antidepressant.

• Cimetidine increases the amount of timolol absorbed into the bloodstream from oral tablets.

• Timolol may interfere with the effectiveness of some anti-asthma drugs including theophylline and aminophylline, and especially ephedrine and isoproterenol.

• Combining timolol and phenytoin or digitalis drugs may result in excessive slowing of the heart, possibly causing heart block.

• If you stop smoking while taking timolol, your dose may have to be reduced because your liver will break down the drug more slowly afterward.

• Aluminum salts, barbituates, calcium salts, cholestyra-mine, colestipol, ampicillin, and rifampin may reduce the effectiveness of timolol.

Food Interactions

None known.

Usual Dose

Timolol
10–60 mg a day divided into 2 doses.

Nadolol
40–80 mg a day.

Sotalol
80 mg twice a day.

Overdosage

Symptoms include changes in heartbeat—unusually slow, unusually fast, or irregular—severe dizziness or fainting, breathing difficulties, bluish-colored fingernails or palms, and seizures. The victim should be taken to a hospital emergency room. ALWAYS bring the prescription bottle or container.

Special Information

Timolol is taken continuously. Do not stop taking this drug unless directed to do so by your doctor: Abrupt withdrawal may cause chest pain, breathing difficulties, increased sweating, and unusually fast or irregular heartbeat. When ending timolol treatment, dosage should be reduced gradually over a period of about 2 weeks.

Call your doctor at once if you develop back or joint pain, breathing difficulties, cold hands or feet, depression, rash, or changes in heartbeat. Timolol may produce an undesirable lowering of blood pressure, leading to dizziness or fainting; call your doctor if this happens to you. Call your doctor if you experience persistent or bothersome anxiety, diarrhea, constipation, impotence, headache, itching, nausea or vomiting, nightmares or vivid dreams, upset stomach, trouble sleeping, stuffy nose, frequent urination, unusual tiredness, or weakness.

Timolol can cause drowsiness, dizziness, light-headedness, or blurred vision. Be careful when driving or performing complex tasks.

It is best to take timolol at the same time each day. If you forget a dose, take it as soon as you remember. If you take timolol twice a day and it is within 4 hours of your next dose, skip the dose you forgot and continue with your regular schedule. Do not take a double dose.

If you forget a dose of timolol eyedrops, administer it as soon as you remember. If it is almost time for your next dose, skip the dose you forgot and continue with your regular schedule. Do not take a double dose.

Special Populations

Pregnancy/Breast-feeding
Infants born to women who took a beta blocker while pregnant had lower birth weights, low blood pressure, and reduced heart rates. Timolol should be avoided by pregnant women.

Timolol passes into breast milk. Nursing mothers who must use it should bottle-feed.

Seniors
Seniors may require less of the drug to achieve results. Seniors taking timolol may be more likely to suffer from cold hands and feet, reduced body temperature, chest pain, general feelings of ill health, sudden breathing difficulties, sweating, or changes in heartbeat.

Generic Name

Tizanidine (tih-ZAN-ih-dene)

Brand Name

Zanaflex

Type of Drug

Skeletal muscle relaxant.

Prescribed For

Spastic muscle movements.

General Information

Tizanidine hydrochloride is prescribed for people who suffer from uncontrolled muscle spasms usually associated with a nervous system condition. It is presumed to work on the central nervous system by affecting nerves that control major muscle systems; it has no direct effect on skeletal muscles. Tizanidine begins working between 1 to 2 hours after it is taken and lasts for 3 to 6 hours.

Cautions and Warnings

Do not take tizanidine if you are sensitive or **allergic** to it.

Tizanidine can cause **low blood pressure**. This effect usually begins within 1 hour after taking the drug and reaches its height after 2 to 3 hours. Low blood pressure triggered by tizanidine is associated with **slow heart rate, light-headedness,** and **dizziness** when rising from a sitting or lying position.

About 50% of people taking tizanidine experience some **sedation**. Sedation usually begins 30 minutes after taking the drug and continues to get worse for about 1 hour. Sedative effects usually start during the first week of treatment or do not occur at all.

Tizanidine may cause **liver injury**. About 1 of 20 people who take this drug experience some liver inflammation, although most cases resolve once the drug is stopped. Several people have died from liver failure after taking tizanidine; it should be avoided by people with liver disease.

People taking tizanidine have experienced **hallucinations, delusion,** and **psychotic symptoms**.

Tizanidine should be used with caution by people who have **reduced kidney function**. These people need smaller-than-usual doses.

Possible Side Effects

▼ Most common: dry mouth, sleepiness, tiredness, and weakness.

▼ Common: dizziness.

▼ Less common: uncontrolled muscle movement, nervousness, constipation, sore throat, vomiting, frequent urination, urinary infection, liver inflammation, double vision, flu symptoms, runny nose, speech disorders, fever, depression, anxiety, tingling in the hands or feet, rash, sweating, skin sores, diarrhea, abdominal pain, and upset stomach.

▼ Rare: Rare side effects can occur in almost any part of the body Contact your doctor if you experience any side effect not listed above.

Drug Interactions

• Avoid combining alcohol and tizanidine or increased sedation may result.

• Women who combine oral contraceptives and tizanidine should receive reduced dosages of the latter to avoid increased side effects.

• Tizanidine may increase the effects of blood-pressure-lowering drugs.

• Tizanidine may delay the effects of acetaminophen.

Food Interactions

Tizanidine may be taken without regard to food or meals, though it may work faster with food.

Usual Dose

Adult: 4–8 mg every 6–8 hours as needed, up to 3 doses a day. Do not exceed 36 mg a day.

Child: not recommended.

Overdosage

Little is known about the effects of tizanidine overdose, but it may lead to very slow breathing. Overdose victims should be taken to a hospital emergency room. ALWAYS bring the prescription bottle or container.

Special Information

People taking tizanidine should be careful not to exceed the prescribed dosage since little is known about using higher dosages over an extended period.

Be careful when driving or performing any task that requires concentration.

If you take tizanidine on a regular basis and forget a dose, take it as soon as you remember. If it is almost time for your next dose, skip the one you forgot and continue with your regular schedule. Do not take a double dose.

Special Populations

Pregnancy/Breast-feeding

Tizanidine should only be taken during pregnancy if absolutely necessary and after its potential benefits have been carefully weighed against its risks.

Tizanidine may pass into breast milk. Nursing mothers who must take this drug should consider bottle-feeding.

Seniors

Seniors should use tizanidine with caution.

Generic Name

Tocainide (toe-KAY-nide)

Brand Name

Tonocard

Type of Drug

Antiarrhythmic.

Prescribed For

Abnormal heart rhythms; also prescribed for muscular dystrophy and trigeminal neuralgia (tic douloureux).

General Information

Tocainide hydrochloride works in the same way as lidocaine, one of the most widely used injectable antiarrhythmic drugs. Tocainide slows the speed at which nerve impulses are carried through the heart's ventricle, helping the heart to maintain a stable rhythm by making heart muscle cells less easily excited. Tocainide affects different areas of the heart than do other widely used oral antiarrhythmic drugs. Tocainide is usually prescribed as a follow-up to intravenous lidocaine for people with life-threatening arrhythmias.

Cautions and Warnings

People taking tocainide may develop **bone-marrow depression,** a drastic **drop in white-blood-cell count, low platelet count,** or other **abnormalities of blood components**. Because these abnormalities happen most often during the first 3 months on tocainide, you should have weekly blood counts throughout that period.

This drug should not be used by people who are **allergic** to it, to lidocaine, or to local anesthetics.

Some people using tocainide may develop **respiratory difficulties,** including fluid buildup in the lungs, pneumonia, and irritation of the lungs. Immediately report any cough, wheezing, shortness of breath, or breathing difficulties to your doctor. Tocainide should not be used by people with **heart failure** because the drug can actually worsen that condition.

Like other antiarrhythmic drugs, tocainide may occasionally **worsen heart rhythm problems**. It has not actually been proven to help people live longer.

Possible Side Effects

▼ Most common: nausea, dizziness, fainting, tingling in the hands or feet, and tremors. These reactions are generally mild and short-lived, and usually go away when dosage is reduced or when you take tocainide with food.

▼ Less common: vomiting, reduced appetite, light-headedness, confusion, disorientation, hallucinations, nervousness, mood or self-awareness changes, poor muscle coordination, blurred or double vision, increased sweating, giddiness, restlessness, anxiety, low blood pressure, slowing of the heart rate, heart palpitations, chest pains, cold sweats, headache, drowsiness, lethargy,

---

Possible Side Effects *(continued)*

ringing or buzzing in the ears, visual disturbances, rolling of the eyes, diarrhea, unusual feelings of heat or cold, joint inflammation and pain, and muscle aches.

▼ Rare: Rare side effects can affect your mental state, breathing, taste, smell, memory, speech, stomach and intestines, blood, urinary tract, sexual function, blood flow to the arms and legs, and muscles and joints. Contact your doctor if you experience any side effect not listed above.

Drug Interactions

• Tocainide taken with metoprolol or other beta-blocking drugs may cause too rapid a drop in blood pressure and slow the heart.

• Tocainide may produce additive cardiac side effects if taken with other antiarrhythmic drugs.

• Tocainide may increase the effects of other drugs that depress bone-marrow function, leading to low levels of white blood cells and blood platelets.

• Cimetidine and rifampin reduce the amount of tocainide absorbed into the bloodstream. Ranitidine, which can be used instead of cimetidine, does not have this effect.

Food Interactions

None known.

Usual Dose

Adult: 1200–1800 mg a day in 2–3 doses. Seniors and people with kidney or liver disease usually require lower doses.

Overdosage

The first symptoms of tocainide overdose are usually tremors or other nervous system effects. Other, more serious, side effects may follow. Victims should be taken to an emergency room for treatment at once. ALWAYS bring the prescription bottle or container.

Special Information

Be sure to report any side effects to your doctor, particularly breathing difficulties after exertion, cough, wheezing, tremors, palpitations, rash, easy bruising or bleeding, fever, chills, sore throat or mouth, or mouth sores.

Tocainide can make you dizzy or drowsy. Be careful while driving or performing other complex tasks.

Do not take more or less of this drug than prescribed. If you forget a dose and remember within 4 hours of your regular time, take it right away. If you do not remember until later, skip the dose you forgot and go back to your regular schedule. Do not take a double dose.

Special Populations

Pregnancy/Breast-feeding

In animal studies, tocainide caused spontaneous abortions and stillbirths. When this drug is considered crucial by your doctor, its potential benefits must be carefully weighed against its risks.

Tocainide passes into breast milk. Nursing mothers who must take this drug should bottle-feed.

Seniors

Seniors are more sensitive to the side effects of this drug, especially dizziness and low blood pressure.

Generic Name

Tolcapone (TOL-kap-one)

Brand Name

Tasmar

Type of Drug

COMT inhibitor.

Prescribed For

Parkinson's disease.

General Information

Tolcapone is believed to block the effects of an enzyme known as COMT, which is found throughout the body. COMT is an essential part of the process by which natural stimulants or catecholamines, including L-DOPA, are eliminated. This extends levodopa's beneficial effect on Parkinson's disease.

Cautions and Warnings

Do not take this drug if you are **sensitive** or **allergic** to it. Tolcapone can cause **liver irritation, injury, and failure,** which may be fatal. Liver function should be evaluated every two weeks for the first year of therapy, then every 4–8 weeks. People with **cirrhosis of the liver** should receive about half the usual dose. Other forms of liver disease do not affect tolcapone dosage. People with **severe kidney disease** should also use tolcapone with caution.

Tolcapone increases levodopa side effects, including **low blood pressure, dizziness, or fainting,** and **uncontrolled muscle movements**.

Possible Side Effects

▼ Most common: abnormal muscle movements, sleep disturbances, stiffness, vivid dreams, tiredness, confusion, nausea, appetite loss, diarrhea, vomiting, muscle cramps, dizziness, and fainting.

▼ Common: hallucinations, constipation, dry mouth, abdominal pain, respiratory infections, sweating, falling, and fatigue.

▼ Less common: loss of balance, changes in muscular activity, tingling in the hands or feet, upset stomach, gas, arthritis, neck pain, chest pain, low blood pressure, chest discomfort, breathing difficulties, sinus congestion, flu-like symptoms, urine discoloration, and difficulty urinating,

▼ Rare: agitation, irritability, hyperactivity, minor skin bleeding, hair loss, a burning sensation, feeling unwell, fever, cataracts, and eye inflammation.

Drug Interactions

• Do not combine tolcapone and any monoamine oxidase inhibitor (MAOI) drug except selegiline.

• Tolcapone may increase the blood-thinning effects of warfarin; do not combine these drugs.

• Tolcapone increases levodopa side effects.

Food Interactions

Take this drug at least 1 hour before or 2 hours after meals.

Usual Dose

Adult: 100–200 mg 3 times a day.
Child: not recommended.

Overdosage

Common symptoms include nausea, vomiting, and dizziness. Take the victim to a hospital emergency room. ALWAYS bring the prescription bottle or container.

Special Information

Nausea, dizziness or fainting, hallucinations, and other side effects are more likely when you first start taking this drug. Call your doctor if you experience any bothersome or persistent side effect.

Tolcapone can make you tired and dizzy. Be careful when driving or performing any task that requires concentration.

Your doctor may reduce your dosage of levodopa or carbidopa when you begin taking tolcapone.

If you forget a dose, take it as soon as you remember. If it is almost time for your next dose, skip the forgotten dose and continue with your regular schedule.

Special Populations

Pregnancy/Breast-feeding

The safety of using tolcapone during pregnancy is not known, though there is a risk that it may be toxic to a pregnant woman. It is always prescribed with levodopa, which is known to cause birth defects. When tolcapone is considered crucial by your doctor, its potential benefits must be carefully weighed against its risks.

Tolcapone may pass into breast milk. Nursing mothers who must take it should consider bottle-feeding.

Seniors

Seniors may be more sensitive to side effects, especially hallucinations.

Generic Name

Tolterodine (tole-TER-oe-deen)

Brand Name

Detrol   Detrol LA

Type of Drug

Anticholinergic.

Prescribed For

Overactive bladder.

General Information

Tolterodine improves bladder control by interfering with nerve receptors that control bladder muscles. By dulling the response of these receptors to nervous system stimulation, tolterodine can prevent bladder muscle contractions and the resulting urgent need to urinate. Tolterodine does not work the same for everyone. Because most of this drug is broken down in the liver, drug response as well as dosage may depend on your degree of liver function. People with liver disease should not take more than 1 mg twice a day.

Cautions and Warnings

Do not take this drug if you are **sensitive** or **allergic** to it, are **retaining urine,** or have a **stomach obstruction** or **uncontrolled narrow-angle glaucoma**. People being treated for narrow-angle glaucoma should use tolterodine with caution.

People with **reduced liver function** should not take more than 1 mg twice a day. People with **reduced kidney function** should use tolterodine with caution.

Possible Side Effects

▼ Most common: dry mouth and headache.

▼ Common: dizziness, fainting, abdominal pain, constipation, diarrhea, upset stomach, nausea, and tiredness.

▼ Less common: sleepiness, visual problems, very dry eyes, bronchitis, coughing, sore throat, runny nose, sinus irritation, respiratory infection, painful urination,

---

Possible Side Effects *(continued)*

frequent urination, urinary retention, joint pain, back pain, chest pain, high blood pressure, fungus infections, flu-like symptoms, and weight gain.

▼ Rare: tingling in the hands or feet, nervousness, itching, rash, dry skin, gas, and vomiting.

Drug Interactions

• Fluoxetine may increase tolterodine blood levels and side effects.

• Erythromycin, clarithromycin, ketoconazole, itraconazole, and miconazole can interfere with the breakdown of tolterodine in the liver. People taking any of these drugs should take no more than 1 mg a day of tolterodine.

Food Interactions

Tolterodine can be taken with or without food.

Usual Dose

Adult: 1–2 mg 2 times a day.
Child: not recommended.

Overdosage

Symptoms may include dry mouth and other side effects. Take the victim to a hospital emergency room. ALWAYS bring the prescription bottle or container.

Special Information

This drug can blur your vision, or cause dizziness or drowsiness.

If you forget a dose, take it as soon as you remember. If it is almost time for your next dose, skip the forgotten dose and continue with your regular schedule. Do not take a double dose.

Special Populations

Pregnancy/Breast-feeding

Large dosages of tolterodine caused fetal harm and birth defects in animal studies. When this drug is considered crucial by your doctor, its potential benefits must be carefully weighed against its risks.

Tolterodine may pass into breast milk. Nursing mothers who must take it should bottle-feed.

Seniors

Seniors may take tolterodine without special precaution.

Topamax *see **Topiramate**, below*

Generic Name

Topiramate (toe-PI-ruh-mate)

Brand Name

Topamax   Topamax Sprinkle

Type of Drug

Anticonvulsant.

Prescribed For

Partial onset seizures, tonic-clonic seizures, cluster headaches, migraine prevention, infantile spasms, and Lennox-Gastaut syndrome.

General Information

Topiramate has a broad spectrum of antiepileptic activity. It inhibits nerve transmission in the brain and nervous system by blocking sodium channels and the neurotransmitter glutamate, and by increasing the effect of the neurotransmitter gamma-amniobutynic acid (GABA). Topiramate reaches peak blood levels within 2 hours. It passes out of the body through urine.

Cautions and Warnings

Do not take topiramate if you are **sensitive** or **allergic** to it. People who **suddenly stop taking topiramate** may worsen their seizures. Anticonvulsant drugs should be reduced gradually.

People with moderate to severe **kidney disease** should receive half the usual dose; other dosage adjustments may be needed. People with **liver disease** may clear topiramate from their bodies more slowly than others do, but the reasons for this are not well understood. About 1.5% of people taking topiramate develop **kidney stones**. This effect may be avoided by drinking several glasses of water a day during treatment.

Possible Side Effects

Side effects usually affect the central nervous system.

▼ Most common: slow reflexes; slow thought processes; difficulty concentrating; speech or language problems, especially word-finding; tiredness; dizziness; weakness; poor muscle coordination; tingling in the hands or feet; tremors; depression; nausea; respiratory infections; and visual disturbances, including double vision.

▼ Less common: back or chest pain, leg pain, hot flushes, body odor, swelling, abnormal coordination, agitation, mood changes, aggressive reactions, reduced touch sensation, apathy, emotional instability, depersonalization, itching, rash, upset stomach, appetite loss, abdominal pain, constipation, dry mouth, breast pain, menstrual disorders, painful menstruation, sore throat, sinus inflammation, breathing difficulties, eye pain, weight loss, loss of white blood cells, muscle ache, hearing loss, and aggravated convulsions.

▼ Rare: chills, sweating, gum irritation, blood in the urine, nosebleeds, and a decrease in sexual desire. Other rare side effects can occur in almost any part of the body. Contact your doctor if you experience any side effect not listed above.

Drug Interactions

• Certain other anticonvulsant drugs—phenytoin, carbamazepine, and valproic acid—reduce topiramate levels.

• Topiramate increases the depressive effect of alcohol and other nervous system depressants. Avoid these combinations.

• Combining topiramate with a carbonic-anhydrase inhibitor drug may increase your risk of kidney stones.

• Topiramate reduces the effect of oral contraceptive pills and digoxin.

• Combining metformin with topiramate may affect each other's effectiveness.

Food Interactions

None known.

Usual Dose

Adult (age 17 and over): starting dose—25–50 mg a day. Increase gradually to 200 mg twice a day. People with moderate to severe kidney failure should begin with ½ the usual dose.

Child (age 2–16): starting dose—0.5–1.4 mg per pound, up to 25 mg at night for 1 week. Increase gradually until an optimal response is achieved (2.3–4 mg per pound per day, divided into 2 doses).

Overdosage

Overdose is likely to cause nervous system depression. Overdose victims must be taken to a hospital emergency room immediately. ALWAYS bring the prescription bottle or container.

Special Information

Drink several glasses of water or other fluids every day to avoid developing kidney stones.

Sprinkle capsule may be swallowed as is or may be opened and sprinkled onto a teaspoon of soft food. The mixture should be swallowed at once without chewing.

Be careful when driving or performing any task that requires concentration.

If you forget a dose, take it as soon as you remember. If it is almost time for your next dose, skip the dose you forgot and continue with your regular schedule. Do not take a double dose.

Special Populations

Pregnancy/Breast-feeding

Animal studies indicate that topiramate may cause birth defects. When this drug is considered crucial by your doctor, its potential benefits must be carefully weighed against its risks.

Animal studies show that topiramate passes into breast milk. Nursing mothers who must take it should consider bottle-feeding.

Seniors
Lower dosage may be needed because of age-related kidney impairment.

Toprol-XL see *Metoprolol,* page 698

Generic Name

Tramadol (TRAM-uh-dol)

Brand Name

Ultram

The information in this profile also applies to the following drug:

Generic Ingredients: Tramadol + Acetaminophen
Ultracet

Type of Drug

Non-narcotic pain reliever.

Prescribed For

Mild to moderate pain.

General Information

Tramadol hydrochloride is a synthetic compound that works in the central nervous system (CNS) to relieve pain. The exact way in which this drug works is unknown, but it binds to opioid receptors and reduces the uptake of two important neurohormones, serotonin and norepinephrine, into nerves. Pain relief begins about an hour after you take a dose and reaches its maximum effect in 2 to 3 hours. Like the narcotic pain relievers, tramadol can cause dizziness, tiredness, nausea, constipation, sweating, and itching. Unlike the narcotics, normal doses cause little interference with breathing and do not cause histamine reactions. It has no effect on heart function.

Cautions and Warnings

Do not take this drug if you are **sensitive** or **allergic** to it or are **intoxicated** with drugs, alcohol, or narcotics. People who must take tranquilizers, sedatives, or other nervous system depressants should take reduced doses of tramadol.

Large dosages of tramadol may **interfere with breathing**, especially when combined with alcohol.

Tramadol use should be avoided in people who have had **abdominal conditions** or a **head injury** because the drug may interfere with diagnosing the injury or understanding its severity.

Seizure has occurred in people taking oral doses of 700 mg or intravenous doses of 300 mg.

People who are dependent on narcotics and take tramadol may experience **withdrawal symptoms**.

People with **reduced kidney function** or **liver disease** should receive reduced dosage.

Possible Side Effects

▼ Most common: dizziness or fainting, nausea, constipation, headache, tiredness, vomiting, itching, weakness, sweating, upset stomach, dry mouth, and diarrhea.

▼ Less common: feeling unwell, warmth and flushing, nervousness, anxiety, agitation, euphoria (feeling "high"), emotional instability, trouble sleeping, abdominal pain, appetite loss, gas, rash, visual disturbances, urinary difficulties, and symptoms of menopause.

▼ Rare: Rare side effects can affect your senses, mental state, heart, stomach and intestines, liver, blood, and urinary tract. Headaches, fainting, and allergies can also occur. Contact your doctor if you experience any side effect not listed above.

Drug Interactions

• Carbamazepine reduces tramadol's effectiveness. People taking this combination may need twice the usual dosage of tramadol.

• The combination of tramadol and monoamine oxidase inhibitor (MAOI) antidepressant and SSRIs may cause severe reactions and should be used with caution.

• Quinidine may slow the breakdown of tramadol. The full impact of this interaction is not known.

• Tramadol may increase the effects of warfarin and digoxin.

Food Interactions

None known.

Usual Dose

Adult and Child (age 16 and over): 25–100 mg every 4–6 hours; do not exceed 400 mg a day. People with cirrhosis should receive 50 mg every 12 hours. People with severe kidney disease should receive no more than 100 mg every 12 hours.

Senior: do not exceed 300 mg a day.

Child (under age 16): not recommended.

Overdosage

Overdose can be deadly. Symptoms include breathing difficulties and seizure. Take the victim to a hospital emergency room at once. ALWAYS bring the prescription bottle or container.

Special Information

Drowsiness may occur: Be careful when driving or performing any task that requires concentration.

Do not drink alcohol while taking tramadol. Hypnotics, opioids, and psychotropic drugs interact adversely with tramadol.

If you forget a dose, take it as soon as you remember. If it is almost time for your next dose, skip the one you forgot and continue with your regular schedule. Do not take a double dose.

Special Populations

Pregnancy/Breast-feeding

Tramadol is toxic to animal fetuses and passes into the fetal circulation in humans. When this drug is considered crucial by your doctor, its potential benefits must be carefully weighed against its risks.

This drug passes into breast milk. Nursing mothers who must take it should bottle-feed.

Seniors

Seniors may be more sensitive to side effects and should not take more than 300 mg a day.

Generic Name

Trandolapril (tran-DOE-luh-pril)

Brand Name

Mavik

Combination Products

Generic Ingredients: Trandolapril + Verapamil
Tarka

Type of Drug

Angiotensin-converting enzyme (ACE) inhibitor.

Prescribed For

High blood pressure.

General Information

Trandolapril and other ACE inhibitors work by preventing the conversion of a hormone called angiotensin I to another hormone called angiotensin II, a potent blood vessel constrictor. Preventing this conversion relaxes blood vessels, thus reducing blood pressure and relieving symptoms of heart failure. Trandolapril also affects the production of other hormones and enzymes that participate in the regulation of blood-vessel dilation.

Some people who start taking trandolapril after they are already on a diuretic (agent that increases urination) experience a rapid drop in blood pressure after their first doses or when their dosage is increased. To prevent this from happening, your doctor may tell you to stop taking your diuretic 2 or 3 days before starting trandolapril or to increase your salt intake during that time. The diuretic may then be restarted gradually.

Trandolapril is prescribed for high blood pressure alone or with hydrochlorthiazide or another blood-pressure-lowering drug. The brand-name product, Tarka, contains trandolapril and verapamil, a calcium channel blocker.

Cautions and Warnings

Do not take trandolapril if you are **allergic** to it. Trandolapril causes very **low blood pressure**.

Women who are **pregnant** should not use this drug.

Trandolapril may affect **kidney function,** especially if you have congestive **heart failure**. Your doctor should check your urine for protein content during the first few months of treatment. Dosage adjustment of trandolapril is necessary if you have reduced kidney function or liver cirrhosis.

Trandolapril may affect white-blood-cell count, possibly increasing your susceptibility to **infection**. Your doctor should periodically monitor your blood counts.

Trandolapril may cause serious injury or death to the fetus if taken during pregnancy. Pregnant women should not take trandolapril.

People with **impaired liver function** should use trandolapril with caution.

Possible Side Effects

▼ Most common: upset stomach, muscle pain, dizziness, fatigue, headache, nausea, and chronic cough. The cough usually goes away a few days after you stop taking the medication.

▼ Less common: chest tightness or pain, dizziness when rising from a sitting or lying position, fainting, abdominal pain, nausea, vomiting, diarrhea, bronchitis, urinary tract infection, breathing difficulties, weakness, and rash.

▼ Rare: Rare side effects can occur in almost any part of the body. Contact your doctor if you experience any side effect not listed above.

Drug Interactions

• The blood-pressure-lowering effect of trandolapril is additive with diuretic drugs and beta blockers. Any other drug that causes a rapid drop in blood pressure should be used with caution if you are taking trandolapril.

• Trandolapril may increase blood-potassium levels, especially when taken with Dyazide or other potassium-sparing diuretics.

• Trandolapril may increase the effects of lithium; this combination should be used with caution.

• Antacids and trandolapril should be taken at least 2 hours apart.

• Combining 325 mg a day or more with this drug carries a higher risk of death than taking lower doses (less than 160 mg a day). People taking aspirin to prevent a heart attack should use the lower dose.

• Capsaicin may trigger or aggravate the cough associated with trandolapril therapy.

• Indomethacin may reduce the blood-pressure-lowering effects of trandolapril.

• Phenothiazine tranquilizers and antiemetics may increase the effects of trandolapril.

• The combination of allopurinol and trandolapril increases the chance of side effects.

• Trandolapril increases blood levels of digoxin, which may increase the chance of digoxin-related side effects.

• Trandolapril may reduce the absorption of tetracycline by about ⅓.

Food Interactions

You may take trandolapril with food if it upsets your stomach.

Usual Dose

Trandolapril: 1 mg a day; 2 mg a day in African Americans. Daily dosage may be adjusted up to 8 mg a day. Daily dosages greater than 4 mg may be taken in 2 doses.

Trandolapril-Verapamil Combination: Dosage for adults age 18 and over is 1 tablet a day. This sustained-release combination is available in a variety of strengths.

Overdosage

The principal effect of trandolapril overdose is a rapid drop in blood pressure, as evidenced by dizziness or fainting. Take the overdose victim to a hospital emergency room immediately. ALWAYS bring the prescription bottle or container.

Special Information

Trandolapril may cause swelling of the face, lips, hands, or feet. This swelling may also affect the larynx (throat) or tongue and interfere with breathing. If this happens, go to a hospital emergency room at once. Call your doctor if you develop sore throat, mouth sores, abnormal heartbeat, chest pain, persistent rash, or loss of taste perception.

You may get dizzy if you rise too quickly from a sitting or lying position. Avoid strenuous exercise or very hot weather because heavy sweating or dehydration can cause a rapid drop in blood pressure.

While taking trandolapril, avoid over-the-counter diet pills, decongestants, and other stimulants that can raise blood pressure.

If you take trandolapril once a day and forget a dose, take it as soon as you remember. If it is within 8 hours of your next dose, skip the one you forgot and continue with your regular schedule. If you take trandolapril twice a day and miss a dose, take it right away. If it is within 4 hours of your next dose, take 1 dose immediately and another in 5 or 6 hours, then go back to your regular schedule. Never take a double dose.

Special Populations

Pregnancy/Breast-feeding

ACE inhibitors can cause fetal injury or death. Women who are or might be pregnant should not take ACE inhibitors. If you become pregnant, stop taking this drug and call your doctor immediately.

Relatively small amounts of trandolapril pass into breast milk, and the effect on a nursing infant is likely to be minimal. However, nursing mothers who must take this drug should consider bottle-feeding.

Seniors

Seniors may be more sensitive to the effects of this drug due to age-related losses in kidney or liver function.

Generic Name

Trastuzumab (tras-TUE-zue-mab)

Brand Name

Herceptin

Type of Drug

Antineoplastic.

Prescribed For

Breast cancer.

General Information

Trastuzumab, which works differently than chemotherapy or hormonal anticancer drugs, is used to treat breast cancer in women whose tumor cells produce excessive amounts of a protein called HER2, which stands for human epidermal growth factor receptor 2. This overproduction of the HER2 protein is believed to fuel the cancer's growth. Trastuzumab works by binding to particles of the HER2 protein on the surface of cancerous cells and blocking the protein's effect. This action can slow the growth of tumors or reduce their size. Trastuzumab can be used alone or, for women who have not received chemotherapy, combined with paclitaxel. Trastuzumab is prescribed for breast cancer that has metastasized (spread) to other parts of the body.

Cautions and Warnings

Do not use trastuzumab if you are **allergic** to it or benzyl alcohol.

Cardiac health must be periodically evaluated while you are taking this drug. Using trastuzumab can lead to **congestive heart failure** and serious **heart ventricle disorders**. People who develop these conditions while taking trastuzumab may have to stop taking it.

Trastuzumab can cause **anemia** and a **low white-blood-cell count**. Periodic blood tests are necessary.

People with **lung disease** may be at risk for severe lung problems when taking trastuzumab.

Possible Side Effects

▼ Most common: chills or fever during the first infusion of trastuzumab, nausea, vomiting, rash, diarrhea, dizziness, sleeplessness, appetite loss, cough, breathing difficulties, sore throat, runny nose, abdominal pain, weakness, back pain, headache, infection, and pain.

▼ Common: heart failure, rapid heartbeat, depression, tingling in the hands or feet, swelling in the arms or legs, fluid retention, sinus irritation, and flu-like symptoms.

▼ Less common: nerve pain or inflammation, anemia, low white-blood-cell count, acne, cold sores, bone pain, joint pain, and urinary infection.

Possible Side Effects *(continued)*

▼ Rare: Rare side effects can occur in almost any part of the body. Contact your doctor if you experience any side effect not listed above.

Drug Interactions

• Trastuzumab should not be combined with any other drugs during intravenous infusion, except paclitaxel.

Food Interactions

None known.

Usual Dose

Adult: 0.9–1.8 mg per lb. of body weight given weekly by IV infusion in a hospital or medical clinic or your doctor's office.

Child: not recommended.

Overdosage

Not much is known about trastuzumab overdose. Symptoms may include chills, shaking, fever, nausea, vomiting, pain, dizziness, fainting, difficulty breathing, headache, rash, and weakness. Medical attention is necessary.

Special Populations

Pregnancy/Breast-feeding

The safety of using trastuzumab during pregnancy is not known, though it is likely to affect the fetus. When this drug is considered crucial by your doctor, its potential benefits must be carefully weighed against its risks.

Trastuzumab passes into breast milk. Nursing mothers should not breast-feed during drug treatment or for 6 months after treatment is finished.

Seniors

Seniors are more likely to develop cardiac side effects.

Generic Name

Trazodone (TRAY-zoe-done) Ⓖ

Brand Names

Desyrel   Desyrel Dividose

Type of Drug

Antidepressant.

Prescribed For

Depression with or without anxiety, cocaine withdrawal, panic disorder, agoraphobia (fear of open spaces), insominia, and aggressive behaviors.

General Information

Trazodone hydrochloride is chemically different from other antidepressants. It is just as effective as other drugs in treating the symptoms of depression but may be less likely to cause side effects. Symptoms can often be relieved as early as 2 weeks after starting trazodone, but 4 or more weeks may be required to achieve maximum benefit.

Cautions and Warnings

Do not use trazodone if you are **allergic** to it. Do not use trazodone if you are recovering from a **heart attack**. People with a previous history of **heart disease** should not use trazodone because it may cause abnormal heart rhythms.

Though rare, **painful and sustained erections** have occurred with trazodone. If this happens, stop taking the drug and call your doctor. One-third of these cases may require surgery or may lead to a permanent inability to achieve erection.

Possible Side Effects

▼ Common: upset stomach; constipation; abdominal pains; a bad taste in the mouth; nausea; vomiting; diarrhea; palpitations; rapid heartbeat; rash; swelling of the arms or legs; blood pressure changes; feeling of paralysis

Possible Side Effects *(continued)*

of the body; breathing difficulties; dizziness; anger; hostility; nightmares; vivid dreams; confusion; disorientation; loss of memory or concentration; drowsiness; fatigue; light-headedness; difficulty sleeping; nervousness; excitement; headache; loss of coordination; tingling in the hands or feet; tremor of the hands or arms; ringing or buzzing in the ears; blurred vision; red, tired, and itchy eyes; stuffy nose or sinuses; loss of sex drive; muscle ache and pain; appetite loss; weight gain or loss; increased sweating; clamminess; and feeling unwell.

▼ Less common: drug allergy, chest pain, heart attack, delusions, hallucinations, agitation, difficulty speaking, restlessness, numbness, weakness, seizures, increased sex drive, reverse ejaculation, impotence, missed or early menstrual periods, gas, increased salivation, anemia, reduced levels of certain white blood cells, muscle twitches, blood in the urine, reduced urine flow, increased urinary frequency, and increased appetite. Trazodone may cause elevations in levels of body enzymes, which are used to measure liver function.

Drug Interactions

• Trazodone may increase digoxin or phenytoin blood levels and the risk of side effects.

• Trazodone may increase the effects of sedatives, tranquilizers, alcohol, and other drugs that depress the nervous system.

• Trazodone may cause a small reduction in blood pressure. Your dosage of high blood pressure medication may have to be reduced slightly when you start taking trazodone. Clonidine (a drug used to treat high blood pressure) may be inhibited by trazodone. These interactions must be evaluated by your doctor.

• Trazodone may interfere with the effectiveness of warfarin (an anticoagulant).

• Carbamazepine and phenothiazines can affects the concentration of trazodone in the bloodstream, producing various side effects or decreasing the effectiveness of the drug.

• Little is known about the potential interaction between trazodone and monoamine oxidase inhibitor (MAOI) antidepressants. It is usually recommended that one antidepressant be discontinued 2 weeks before taking another. Caution should be used when combining trazodone and an MAOI.

• Ritonavir, a protease inhibitor prescribed for AIDS and HIV, raises levels of trazodone in the blood, possibly increasing trazodone side effects.

Food Interactions

Take trazodone with food to increase effectiveness and reduce the risk of upset stomach, dizziness, and light-headedness.

Usual Dose

Adult: 150 mg a day with food, to start. This dose may be increased by 50 mg a day every 3–4 days, to a maximum of 400 mg a day. Severely depressed people may be prescribed as much as 600 mg a day. Trazodone can cause drowsiness, which may require the administration of the major portion of the daily dose near bedtime.

Overdosage

Drowsiness and vomiting are the most frequent symptoms of trazodone overdose. Others include very severe side effects, especially those affecting mood and heart function. Fever may be present at first, but as time passes body temperature will drop below normal. Victims must be taken to a hospital emergency room immediately. ALWAYS bring the prescription bottle or container.

Special Information

Be careful when driving or performing any task that requires concentration. Avoid alcohol or other depressant drugs while taking trazodone.

Call your doctor if you develop any side effect, especially blood in the urine, dizziness, or light-headedness. Trazodone may cause dry mouth, irregular heartbeat, nausea, vomiting, or breathing difficulties.

If you forget a dose, take it as soon as possible. If it is within 4 hours of your next dose, skip the dose you forgot and go back to your regular schedule. Do not take a double dose.

Special Populations

Pregnancy/Breast-feeding

Trazodone may damage the fetus and generally should not be taken by women who are or might be pregnant. When this drug is considered crucial by your doctor, its potential benefits must be carefully weighed against its risks.

Trazodone passes into breast milk. Nursing mothers who must take it should consider bottle-feeding.

Seniors

Seniors may be more sensitive to trazodone's effects and should start with lower doses.

Generic Name

Tretinoin (TRET-in-oin) Ⓖ

Brand Names

Avita   Retin-A Micro
Renova   Vesanoid
Retin-A

The information in this profile also applies to the following drug:

Generic Ingredients: Mequinol + Tretinoin
Solagé

Type of Drug

Anti-acne; and antiwrinkling agent and skin irritant.

Prescribed For

Acne and other skin conditions, skin cancer, acute promyelocytic leukemia (APL), wrinkling, and liver spots caused by chronic sun exposure.

General Information

Tretinoin, also known as retinoic acid or vitamin A acid, works against acne by decreasing the cohesiveness of skin cells, causing the skin to peel. Tretinoin is usually not effective in treating severe acne.

Medical research shows that regular application of tretinoin cream to aging skin prevents wrinkling and may even reverse the wrinkling process for some people. Tretinoin causes a temporary "plumping" of the skin when it is applied, peeling the outer layer. This gives the appearance of improved skin and reduced wrinkling. Some tretinoin—about 5%—is absorbed through the skin. When used to treat APL, a blood cancer, tretinoin causes the leukemia cells to mature and reduces the spread of APL cells; the exact way it works is not known.

Cautions and Warnings

Do not use tretinoin if you are **allergic** to it or any of its components.

Women who are **pregnant** should not use tretinoin due to the high risk of birth defects.

This drug may increase the **skin-cancer-causing effects** of ultraviolet light. If you apply this drug to your skin you should allow a "rest period" between uses of tretinoin and other skin irritants or peeling agents. You must also limit sun exposure to treated areas and avoid sunlamps. If you cannot avoid sun exposure, use sunscreen and protective covering.

Do not apply tretinoin close to your eyes, the sides of the nose, or to mucous membrane tissue.

People with APL are at high risk for severe side effects. About 25% of people with APL treated with tretinoin develop a group of symptoms called retinoic acid-APL syndrome. These symptoms include fever, breathing difficulties, weight gain, and fluid in the lungs. Low blood pressure and loss of heart function may also occur.

Forty percent of people who take oral tretinoin develop a rapid **increase in white-blood-cell count,** which is associated with greater risk of life-threatening complications. Sixty percent of people taking tretinoin develop **high blood-cholesterol or triglyceride levels**.

Retinoids such as tretinoin have been associated with **pseudotumor cerebri** (increased pressure in the brain), especially in children. Early signs of this problem include swelling in the eyes, headache, nausea, vomiting, and visual difficulties.

There is limited information on children's use of tretinoin, though children ages 1 to 16 have used this medication.

Possible Side Effects

Skin Products

▼ Most common: burning, stinging, tingling, itching, swelling, or blistering of the skin; formation of crusts on the skin near the application site; and temporary skin discoloration and greater sun sensitivity. All side effects disappear after the drug has been stopped.

▼ Common: skin irritation.

▼ Less common: dry skin, crusting, and rash.

Capsules

▼ Most common: headache, fever, weakness, and fatigue. These generally go away with time.

▼ Common: skin changes, dry skin and membranes, bone pain and inflammation, itching, sweating, visual disturbances and other eye problems, hair loss, earache or a feeling of fullness in the ears, not feeling well, shivering, bleeding, infection, swelling in the arms or legs, pain, chest discomfort, weight gain, breathing difficulties, pneumonia, wheezing, abdominal pain, diarrhea, constipation, upset stomach, abnormal heart rhythms, blood-pressure changes, vein irritation, dizziness, tingling in the hands or feet, sleeplessness, depression, confusion, and bleeding in the brain.

▼ Less common: muscle aches, pain in the side, skin irritation, facial swelling, loss of color, lymph system problems, asthma, swollen larynx, gas, swollen liver, hepatitis, ulcer, heart failure, heart attack, heart inflammation, kidney problems including kidney failure, painful urination, frequent urination, enlarged prostate, agitation, hallucination, an unusual walk, convulsions, coma, depression, paralysis of the face, and a variety of nervous system problems.

▼ Rare: hearing loss.

Drug Interactions

Skin Products

• Other skin irritants will cause excessive sensitivity, irritation, and side effects. Among the substances that cause this interaction are medications that contain sulfur in topical form, resorcinol, benzoyl peroxide, or salicylic acid; abrasive soaps or skin cleansers; cosmetics, creams, or ointments with a severe drying effect; and products with a high alcohol, astringent, spice, or lime content.

• Tretinoin increases the absorption of minoxidil through the skin when they are applied together, leading to lower blood pressure.

• Do not use tretinoin if you are also taking a drug that increases sensitivity to the sun, such as thiazides, tetracyclines, and fluroquinolone antibiotics.

Capsules

• Combining ketoconazole, and other drugs that affect systems in the liver that break down tretinoin, with tretinoin causes a substantial increase in tretinoin blood levels.

Food Interactions

Tretinoin capsules are better absorbed when taken with food.

Usual Dose

Skin Products: Wash the affected area thoroughly, then wait 20–30 minutes and apply a small amount of tretinoin at bedtime.

Capsules: Dosage is individualized for each person. Doses are calculated from height and weight.

Overdosage

Ingesting tretinoin is like taking vitamin A and can be extremely dangerous for pregnant women, who should not take more vitamin A than is contained in their prenatal vitamins. Infants who swallow tretinoin should be taken to a hospital emergency room for treatment. Symptoms of accidental ingestion include headache, facial flushing, abdominal pain, dizziness, and weakness. These symptoms have resolved without apparent aftereffects.

Special Information

Your acne may worsen during the first few weeks of treatment because the drug is acting on deeper, hidden lesions. This is beneficial and is not a reason to stop using tretinoin. Results should be seen in 2 to 3 weeks but may not reach maximum effect for 6 weeks; normal cosmetics can be used during this time.

Keep this drug away from your eyes, nose, mouth, and mucous membranes. Avoid skin exposure to sunlight or sunlamps.

Applying too much tretinoin will cause skin irritation and peeling but will not increase its effectiveness. Use your fingertip, a gauze pad, or a cotton swab when applying tretinoin to acne lesions to reduce the chances of applying too much medication.

You may feel warmth and slight stinging when you apply tretinoin. If you develop a burning sensation, peeling, redness, or are uncomfortable, stop using tretinoin for a short time.

Extreme weather or wind may cause severe irritation of skin treated with tretinoin.

If you forget a dose of tretinoin, do not apply the forgotten dose. Skip it and continue with your regular schedule. Do not apply a double dose.

Special Populations

Pregnancy/Breast-feeding

At very high doses, tretinoin causes birth defects in animals. A pregnant woman taking tretinoin capsules is likely to deliver a severely deformed infant. When applied to the skin, tretinoin is rapidly broken down. When this drug is considered crucial by your doctor, its potential benefits must be carefully weighed against its risks. Women who need to take tretinoin capsules should be tested for pregnancy before treatment is started. Use 2 reliable forms of contraception while you are taking tretinoin and for 1 month after treatment has ended.

It is not known if tretinoin passes into breast milk. Nursing mothers who must take tretinoin should bottle-feed.

Seniors

Seniors may use this product without special restriction.

Generic Name

Triazolam (trye-AY-zuh-lam) G

Brand Name

Halcion

The information in this profile also applies to the following drugs:

Generic Ingredient: Quazepam
Doral

Generic Ingredient: Temazepam Ⓖ
Restoril

Type of Drug

Benzodiazepine sedative.

Prescribed For

Insomnia and sleep disturbances.

General Information

Triazolam is a member of the group of drugs known as benzodiazepines. Benzodiazepines work by a direct effect on the
brain. They make it easier to go to sleep and decrease the
number of times you wake up during the night. Triazolam has
the shortest action of drugs in this class. While this virtually
eliminates "hangover," it may also cause some people to
wake up earlier than they would like because the drug has
stopped working. Temazepam is considered to be an intermediate-acting sedative and generally remains in your body
long enough to give you a good night's sleep with minimal
hangover.

Cautions and Warnings

Triazolam has been associated with **memory loss,** especially when higher doses are taken. This effect, known as
traveler's amnesia, is most common among people who
take this medication to adjust to time zone changes during
travel; it may be linked to the use of alcoholic beverages
and to attempts at starting daily activity too soon after waking up.

If you abruptly stop taking triazolam, you may experience
rebound sleeplessness, where sleeplessness is worse during
the first 1 to 3 nights after you stop the drug than it was
before you started it.

People with respiratory disease may experience **sleep
apnea** (intermittent cessation of breathing during sleep)
while taking triazolam. People who have sleep apnea should
not take triazolam.

People with **kidney or liver disease** should be carefully
monitored while taking triazolam. Take the lowest possible
dose to help you sleep.

Clinical **depression** may be increased by triazolam, which can depress the nervous system. Intentional overdose is more common among depressed people who take sleeping pills than among those who do not.

All benzodiazepines can be **addictive** if taken for long periods of time and can cause drug withdrawal symptoms if suddenly discontinued. Withdrawal symptoms include tremors, muscle cramps, insomnia, agitation, diarrhea, vomiting, sweating, and convulsions.

Possible Side Effects

▼ Common: drowsiness, headache, dizziness, talkativeness, nervousness, apprehension, poor muscle coordination, light-headedness, daytime tiredness, muscle weakness, slowness of movement, hangover, and euphoria (feeling "high").

▼ Rare: Rare side effects can affect your heart, stomach and intestines, urinary tract, blood, muscles, and joints. Contact your doctor if you experience any side effect not listed above.

Drug Interactions

• As with all benzodiazepines, the effects of triazolam are enhanced if it is taken with alcohol, antihistamines, tranquilizers, barbiturates, anticonvulsants, tricyclic antidepressants, or monoamine oxidase inhibitors (MAOIs).

• Oral contraceptives, cimetidine, disulfiram, itraconazole, ketoconazole, nefazadone, and isoniazid may increase the effect of triazolam by interfering with the drug's breakdown in the liver. Probenecid may also increase triazolam's effect.

• Cigarette smoking, rifampin, and theophylline may reduce the effect of triazolam.

• Triazolam decreases the effectiveness of levodopa.

• Triazolam may increase the amount of zidovudine (an AIDS drug—also known as AZT), phenytoin, or digoxin in your blood, increasing the chances of side effects.

• Combining clozapine and benzodiazepines has led to respiratory collapse in a few people. Triazolam should be stopped at least 1 week before starting clozapine treatment.

• The effects of triazolam may be increased by the macrolide antibiotics—azithromycin, erythromycin, and clarithromycin.

Food Interactions

Triazolam may be taken with food if it upsets your stomach.

Usual Dose

Quazepam

Adult (age 18 and over): 7.5–15 mg at bedtime. Dosage must be individualized for maximum benefit. Seniors should take the lowest effective dose.

Child (under age 18): not recommended.

Temazepam

Adult: 15–30 mg at bedtime. The dose must be individualized for maximum benefit.

Senior: starting dose—15 mg at bedtime. Dosage may be increased if needed.

Child (under age 18): not recommended.

Triazolam

Adult (age 18 and over): 0.125–0.5 mg about 30 minutes before sleep.

Senior: starting dose—0.125 mg, then increase in 0.125 mg steps until the desired effect is achieved.

Child (under age 18): not recommended.

Overdosage

The most common symptoms of overdose are confusion, sleepiness, depression, loss of muscle coordination, and slurred speech. Coma may also occur. Overdose victims must be made to vomit with ipecac syrup—available at any pharmacy—to remove any remaining drug from the stomach: Call your doctor or a poison control center before doing this. If 30 minutes have passed since the overdose was taken or if symptoms have begun to develop, the victim must immediately be taken to a hospital emergency room. ALWAYS bring the prescription bottle or container.

Special Information

Never take more triazolam than your doctor has prescribed.

Avoid alcohol and other nervous system depressants while taking triazolam.

Exercise caution while performing tasks that require concentration and coordination. Triazolam may make you tired, dizzy, or light-headed.

If you take triazolam daily for 3 or more weeks, you may experience some withdrawal symptoms when you stop taking it.

Benzodiazepines, including triazolam, can cause a morning-after hangover. Do not take triazolam unless circumstances will allow for a full night's sleep and some time before you need to be alert and active.

If you forget to take a dose of triazolam and remember within 1 hour of your regular time, take it as soon as you remember. If you do not remember until later, skip the dose you forgot and continue your regular schedule. Do not take a double dose.

Special Populations

Pregnancy/Breast-feeding
Triazolam should absolutely not be used by pregnant women.

Triazolam passes into breast milk. Nursing mothers who must take it should bottle-feed.

Seniors
Seniors are more susceptible to the effects of triazolam.

Type of Drug
Triazole Antifungals

Brand Names

Generic Ingredient: Fluconazole
Diflucan

Generic Ingredient: Itraconazole
Sporanox

Generic Ingredient: Ketoconazole
Nizoral

Generic Ingredient: Voriconazole
Vfend

Prescribed For

Fungus infections of the blood, mouth, throat, vagina, or central nervous system. Fluconazole and itraconazole can be used to treat opportunistic fungal infections that inflict many people with AIDS or cancer whose immune systems have been compromised.

General Information

Triazole antifungals are used to treat a variety of fungal organisms, including *Candida, aspergillus, cryptococcus, blastomycosis, fusarium, histoplasmosis,* and *Scedosporium.* They work by inhibiting important enzyme systems in the organisms they attack. These drugs are broken down in the liver.

Cautions and Warnings

Do not take these drugs if you are **sensitive** or **allergic** to them. People who are allergic to similar antifungals—ketoconazole and miconazole—may also be allergic to these drugs, but cross-reactions are not common and serious allergic reaction is rare.

Triazole antifungals can affect heart rhythm and should be used with caution if you have a **history of abnormal heart rhythms**.

At least one in every 10,000 people who take ketoconazole develop liver inflammation. The inflammation generally subsides when the drug is discontinued.

Rarely, triazole antifungals can cause **liver damage**. The drug should be used with caution in people with preexisting liver disease.

Voriconazole tablets contain lactose. They should not be taken by patients with rare hereditary problems of **galactose intolerance, Lapp-lactase deficiency,** or **glucose-galactose malabsorption**.

Rash may be an important sign of drug toxicity, especially in people with acquired immunodeficiency syndrome (AIDS) or others with compromised immune function. Report any rashes, especially ones that do not heal readily, to your doctor.

These drugs can have very serious effects if combined with other medicines. See "Drug Interactions" for specific information.

Possible Side Effects

Side effects are generally more common among people with AIDS.

Fluconazole

▼ Most common: nausea, headache, rash, vomiting, abdominal pain, and diarrhea.

▼ Less common: liver toxicity, as measured by increases in specific lab tests. These changes in lab values are more common in people with AIDS or cancer, who are more likely to be taking several drugs, some of which may also be toxic to the liver; these include rifampin, phenytoin, isoniazid, valproic acid, and oral antidiabetes agents.

▼ Rare: seizures and exfoliative skin disorders. People with AIDS or cancer who take fluconazole for fungal infections may develop severe liver or skin problems.

Itraconazole

▼ Most common: nausea, vomiting, and rash.

▼ Less common: diarrhea, abdominal pain, appetite loss, swelling in the legs or feet, fatigue, fever, feeling unwell, itching, headache, dizziness, reduced sex drive, tiredness, high blood pressure, liver or kidney function abnormalities, low blood potassium, and impotence.

▼ Rare: gas, sleeplessness, depression, ringing or buzzing in the ears, bronchitis, chest pain, coughing, and swollen or painful breasts in men or women.

Ketoconazole

▼ Common: Nausea, vomiting, upset stomach, abdominal pain or discomfort, itching, and swollen breasts in men. Most of these side effects are mild and only a small number of people—1.5%—have to stop taking the drug because of severe side effects.

Voriconazole

▼ Most common: visual disturbances.

▼ Common: fever, rash, nausea, blood infections, swelling in the arms or legs, and respiratory disorder.

▼ Less common: chills, headache, diarrhea, blood pressure changes, abnormal heart rhythms, abdominal pain, vomiting, abnormal liver function, dry mouth, hallucinations, dizziness, and itching.

Possible Side Effects *(continued)*

▼ Rare: chest pain, jaundice (symptoms include yellowing of the skin or whites of the eyes), changes in elements of the blood, and kidney dysfunction or failure.

Drug Interactions

• Cimetidine and rifampin may reduce blood levels of fluconazole and ketoconazole but the importance of these interactions is not known.

• Fluconazole and ketoconazole may increase the amount of the oral antidiabetes drugs tolbutamide, glyburide, and glipizide in the blood, causing low blood-sugar. Cyclosporine, phenytoin, theophylline, warfarin, and zidovudine (an AIDS drug—also known as AZT) are similarly affected. Dosage adjustments of these drugs may be required.

• Fluconazole and ketoconazole may interfere with oral contraceptive drugs. Use special precautions.

• Hydrochlorothiazide may increase blood levels of fluconazole up to 40%.

• People who have taken astemizole, pimozide, or terfenadine with itraconazole have experienced severe cardiac side effects. DO NOT MIX THESE MEDICINES.

• Itraconazole and ketoconazole increase the effects of benzodiazepine anti-anxiety and sedative drugs, buspirone, carbamazepine, cisapride, digoxin, dofetilide, felodipine, haloperidol, nisoldipine, pimozide, protease inhibitors, quinidine, rifabutin, rifampin, rifapentine, sulfonylurea-type antidiabetes drugs, tacrolimus, tolterodine, verapamil, warfarin, and zolpidem. Dosage adjustments may be required before you start taking itraconazole.

• Avoid combining itraconazole or ketoconazole and the calcium channel blockers amlodipine and nifedipine.

• Antacids interfere with the absorption of ketoconazole. Take antacids more than 2 hours after taking ketoconazole.

• Ketoconazole increases donepezil blood levels, possibly increasing side effects.

• Erythromycin and clarithromycin can increase blood levels of itraconazole.

• Rarely, people who combine itraconazole with a statin-type blood-fat-lowering drug experience muscle pain and destruction. Some people who have experienced this interaction were also taking cyclosporine. Cyclosporine dosages should be lowered when combined with itraconazole and an HMG-CoA inhibitor.

• Cimetidine, didanosine, famotidine, isoniazid, nizatidine, phenytoin, protease inhibitors, ranitidine, rifabutin, rifampin, and rifapentine may interfere with the effectiveness of itraconazole.

• Voriconazole increases blood levels of cisapride, ergot drugs for migraines, pimozide, quinidine, rifabutin, and drugs for transplant rejection including tacrolimus and sirolimus. Dosage adjustments are required.

• Voriconazole increases blood levels of benzodiazepine anti-anxiety and sedative drugs, calcium channel blockers, cyclosporine, sulfonylurea-type antidiabetes drugs, tacrolimus, statin-type drugs, vinca-type anti-cancer drugs and warfarin. Dosage adjustments of these drugs may be needed to avoid side effects. Voriconazole increases the blood level of prednisolone but no dosage adjustment is needed.

• Combining voriconazole and phenytoin can lead to lower voriconazole levels and possible phenytoin toxicity.

• The effects of voriconazole are reduced by carbamazepine, phenobarbital, rifampin, and rifabutin.

• Voriconazole's effects can be increased by cimetidine.

• Combining voriconazole with a proton pump inhibitor such as omeprazole, or a protease inhibitor (excluding indinavir) can result in increased blood levels of both drugs.

• Combining voriconazole with an NNRTI for AIDS can either increase or decrease blood levels of voriconazole and increase blood levels of the NNRTI. Drug side effects may occur.

• Ketoconazole may increase blood levels of AIDS drugs including protease inhibitors and didanosine (ddI).

Food Interactions

Take voriconazole at least 1 hour before or 2 hours after a meal. Take ketoconazole with food or meals.

Usual Dose

Fluconazole
   Adult and Child (age 14 and over): 100–400 mg once a day.
   Child: 1.3–5.5 mg per lb. of body weight once a day; no more than 400 mg a day.

Itraconazole
    Adult: 200–600 mg once a day.
    Child (age 3–16): 100 mg a day has been prescribed, but the long-term effects of itraconazole in children are not known.

Ketoconazole
    Adult: 200–400 mg once a day. Treatment may continue for several months, depending on the type of infection being treated.
    Child (age 2 and over): 1.5–3 mg per lb. of body weight once a day.
    Child (under age 2): not recommended.

Cream
Apply to affected and immediately surrounding areas 1–2 times a day for 14 days.

Voriconazole
    Adult: 100–300 mg every 12 hours.
    Child: not recommended.

Overdosage

Overdose is likely to result in exaggerated drug side effects. Take the victim to a hospital emergency room. ALWAYS bring the prescription bottle or container.

Special Information

When taking fluconazole, regular doctor visits are necessary to monitor liver function and general progress.

Call your doctor if you develop reddening, loosening, blistering, or peeling of the skin; darkening of the urine; jaundice (yellowing of the skin or whites of the eyes); loss of appetite; or abdominal pain, especially on the right side. Report other symptoms that are bothersome or persistent.

Itraconazole must be taken for at least 3 months to determine its effectiveness, otherwise the infection may return.

If you forget a dose of one of these medicines, take it as soon as you remember. If it is almost time for your next dose, skip the one you forgot and continue with your regular schedule. Do not take a double dose.

Special Populations

Pregnancy/Breast-feeding
Animal studies with these medicines show effects on the fetus that have not been seen in humans. Pregnant women

should not use triazole antifungals unless the possible bene-fits outweigh the risks.

These drugs pass into breast milk. Nursing mothers who must these drugs should bottle-feed.

Seniors
Seniors may require a reduced dosage of fluconazole due to loss of kidney function. No dosage adjustment are necessary with itraconazole or voriconazole.

Tricor *see Fenofibrate, page 474*

Type of Drug

Tricyclic Antidepressants

Brand Names

Generic Ingredient: Amitriptyline Ⓖ
Elavil   Endep

Generic Ingredients: Amitriptyline + Perphenazine Ⓖ
Etrafon   Etrafon-Forte
Etrafon-A   Triavil

Generic Ingredients: Amitriptyline + Chlordiazepoxide Ⓖ
Limbitrol   Limbitrol DS

Generic Ingredient: Amoxapine Ⓖ
Asendin

Generic Ingredient: Clomipramine Ⓖ
Anafranil

Generic Ingredient: Desipramine Ⓖ
Norpramin

Generic Ingredient: Doxepin Ⓖ
Sinequan

Generic Ingredient: Imipramine Ⓖ
Tofranil   Tofranil-PM

Generic Ingredient: Nortriptyline Ⓖ
Aventyl   Pamelor
Aventyl Pulvules

Generic Ingredient: Protriptyline [G]
Vivactil

Generic Ingredient: Trimipramine
Surmontil

Prescribed For

Depression, with or without symptoms of anxiety or sleep disturbance; chronic pain due to migraine, tension headache, diabetic disease, tic douloureux, cancer, herpes lesions, and arthritis; pathologic laughing or weeping caused by brain disease; bulimia; sleep apnea; peptic ulcer disease; cocaine withdrawal; panic disorder; eating disorder; premenstrual depression; and skin problems. Clomipramine is prescribed only for obsessive compulsive disorder (OCD).

General Information

Tricyclic antidepressants block the passage of stimulant chemicals—norepinephrine or serotonin—in and out of nerve endings, producing a sedative effect. They also counteract the effects of the neurohormone acetylcholine. Recent theory maintains that antidepressants work by causing long-term changes in the way nerve endings function. Tricyclic antidepressants can elevate mood, increase physical activity and mental alertness, and improve appetite and sleep patterns after 2 to 4 weeks of use.

Tricyclic antidepressants have been used in treating nighttime bed-wetting but do not produce long-lasting results. The combination of amitriptyline and perphenazine, a tranquilizer, is used to treat anxiety, agitation, and depression associated with chronic physical or psychiatric disease. The combination of amitriptyline and chlordiazepoxide, an antianxiety drug, is used to treat anxiety and depression. Tricyclic antidepressants are broken down in the liver.

Cautions and Warnings

Do not take one of these drugs if you are **allergic** or **sensitive** to any tricyclic antidepressant. These drugs should not be used if you are recovering from a **heart attack;** rapid heartbeat and fainting when rising from a sitting or lying position are problems associated with protryptiline.

These drugs should be taken with caution if you have a history of **epilepsy or other convulsive disorders; seizure,** which may be a special problem with clomipramine; **difficulty uri-nating; glaucoma; heart disease; liver disease;** or **hyperthy-roidism**. Antidepressants may aggravate the condition of people who are schizophrenic or paranoid and may cause people with **bipolar (manic-depressive) disorder** to switch phase. These reactions are also possible when changing or stopping antidepressants.

Suicide is always a risk in severely depressed people, who should only be allowed to have minimal quantities of med-ication in their possession.

Amoxapine may cause very **high fever, muscle rigidity, changes in mental state, irregular pulse or blood pressure, sweating, abnormal heart rhythms,** and **rapid heartbeat**. This group of symptoms is associated with neuroleptic malignant syndrome (NMS), which may be **fatal**. If these symptoms develop, stop taking your medication at once and call your doctor. Clomipramine may also cause very high fever, espe-cially when used with other drugs; this may also be a sign of NMS.

Amoxapine may increase the risk of potentially irreversible involuntary muscle movements associated with tardive dys-kinesia (symptoms include lip smacking or puckering, puffing of the cheeks, rapid or worm-like tongue movements, uncon-trolled chewing motions, and uncontrolled arm and leg movements). This condition is more common among the elderly, especially women.

Possible Side Effects

▼ Most common: sedation and anticholinergic effects including blurred vision; disorientation; confusion; hallu-cinations; muscle spasm or tremors; seizures or convul-sions; dry mouth; constipation, especially in older adults; difficulty urinating; worsening glaucoma; and sensitivity to bright light.

▼ Less common: blood-pressure changes, abnormal heart rate, heart attack, anxiety, restlessness, excitement, numbness and tingling in the extremities, poor coordina-tion, rash, itching, fluid retention, fever, allergy, changes in blood composition, nausea, vomiting, appetite loss, upset stomach, diarrhea, enlargement of the breasts in men and women, changes in sex drive, and blood-sugar changes.

Possible Side Effects *(continued)*

▼ Rare: Rare side effects can occur in almost any part of the body. Contact your doctor if you experience any side effect not listed above.

Drug Interactions

• Combining a tricyclic antidepressant with a monoamine oxidase inhibitor (MAOI) antidepressant may cause high fever, convulsions, and death. Do not take an MAOI until at least 2 weeks after amitriptyline has been discontinued. People who must take both an MAOI and a tricyclic antidepressant require close medical observation.

• Selective serotonin reuptake inhibitors (SSRIs) may increase blood levels of tricyclic antidepressants.

• Tricyclics interact with guanethidine and clonidine (drugs used to treat high blood pressure). Tell your doctor if you are taking any drug for high blood pressure.

• Tricyclics increase the effects of barbiturates, tranquilizers, alcohol, and other sedative drugs. Barbiturates may decrease the effectiveness of a tricyclic antidepressant.

• Combining a tricyclic antidepressant and a thyroid drug enhances the effects of both, possibly causing abnormal heart rhythms. The combination of reserpine and a tricyclic antidepressant may cause overstimulation.

• Oral contraceptives ("the pill") may reduce the effect of a tricyclic antidepressant, as may smoking. Charcoal tablets may prevent antidepressant absorption by the blood. Estrogen may increase or decrease the effect of a tricyclic antidepressant.

• Bicarbonate of soda, acetazolamide, quinidine, and procainamide increase the effect of a tricyclic antidepressant. Combining a tricyclic antidepressant and cimetidine, methylphenidate, or phenothiazine drugs such as thorazine and compazine may cause severe side effects.

• Bupropion, haloperidol, and histamine blockers may increase the effects of tricyclic antidepressants.

• Combining tricyclic antidepressants and carbamazepine may effect each other's blood levels.

• Valproic acid may increase the side effects of tricyclic antidepressants.

• Valproic acid and anticholinergics may increase tricyclic antidepressant side effects.

Food Interactions

You may take a tricyclic antidepressant with food if it upsets your stomach.

Usual Dose

Amitriptyline

Adult and Child (age 12 and over): 25 mg 3 times a day, increased to 150 mg a day if necessary.

Senior: lower dosages are recommended, generally 30–50 mg a day.

Child (under age 12): not recommended.

Amoxapine

Adult and Child (age 17 and over): 100–400 mg a day. Hospitalized patients may need up to 600 mg a day.

Senior: lower dosages are recommended. People over age 60 usually take 50–300 mg a day.

Child (under age 17): not recommended.

Clomipramine

Adult: 25–250 mg a day.

Child: 25–100 mg a day in divided doses.

This drug may be taken at bedtime to minimize daytime sedation.

Desipramine

Adult and Child (age 12 and over): 100–200 mg a day. People taking higher dosages should have regular heart examinations to check for side effects.

Senior and Child (age 12 and over): lower dosages are recommended, usually 25–100 mg a day.

Doxepin and Imipramine

Adult: start with about 25–75 mg a day in divided doses, then increase or decrease as needed. The final daily dosage may be less than 75 or up to 300 mg. Long-term depression may be treated with sustained-release medication taken daily at bedtime or several times a day.

Senior: starting dosage—30–40 mg a day. Maintenance dosage—usually less than 100 mg daily.

Child (doxepin: age 12 and over; imipramine: age 6 and over): 25 mg a day, given 1 hour before bedtime for nighttime bed-wetting. If bed-wetting does not cease within a week, daily dosage is typically increased to 50–75 mg depending on age—more than 75 mg a day increases side effects without increasing effectiveness. Doses are often taken in mid-afternoon and at bedtime. The dosage should be gradually reduced to help prevent bed-wetting from recurring. Doxepin concentrate should be diluted with about 4 oz. of milk, water, or juice just before it is taken. Do not mix with soda or grape juice.

Nortriptyline

Adult: 25 mg 3 or 4 times a day, increased to 150 mg a day if necessary.

Senior: lower dosages are recommended, generally 30–50 mg a day.

Child (age 6–17): 30–50 mg a day.

Child (under age 6): not recommended.

Protriptyline

Adult: 15–40 mg a day in 3–4 divided doses. Protriptyline must not be taken as a single bedtime dose because of its stimulant effect.

Senior and Child (age 13 and over): lower dosages are recommended, usually up to 20 mg a day. Seniors taking more than 20 mg a day should have regular heart examinations.

Trimipramine

Adult: 75 mg a day in divided doses to start, then increased as necessary to 150–200 mg. The entire daily dosage may be taken at bedtime or divided into several doses a day. Hospitalized adults may receive up to 300 mg a day.

Senior and Child (age 13 and over): starting dosage—50 mg a day. Maintenance dosage—up to 100 mg daily.

Child: not recommended.

Overdosage

Symptoms include confusion, inability to concentrate, hallucinations, drowsiness, lowered body temperature, abnormal heart rate, heart failure, enlarged pupils, convulsions, severely lowered blood pressure, stupor, and coma. Overdose victims should be taken to a hospital emergency room immediately. ALWAYS bring the prescription bottle or container.

Special Information

Avoid alcohol and other depressants while taking any tricyclic antidepressant. Do not stop taking your medication without your doctor's knowledge. Abruptly stopping a tricyclic antidepressant may cause nausea, headache, and feelings of ill health.

Tricyclic antidepressants may cause drowsiness, dizziness, and blurred vision. Be careful when driving or doing any task that requires concentration. Avoid prolonged exposure to the sun.

Call your doctor immediately if you develop seizure, breathing difficulties or rapid breathing, fever and sweating, blood-pressure changes, muscle stiffness, loss of bladder control, or unusual tiredness or weakness. Dry mouth may lead to an increase in dental cavities and gum bleeding and disease. Maintain good dental hygiene while taking a tricyclic antidepressant.

If your symptoms are unchanged after 6 to 8 weeks of treatment with an antidepressant, contact your doctor.

When used for nighttime bed-wetting, doxepin and imipramine are often ineffective.

If you forget a dose, skip it and go back to your regular schedule. Do not take a double dose.

Special Populations

Pregnancy/Breast-feeding
Tricyclic antidepressants cross into the fetal circulation. Birth defects including heart, breathing, and urinary problems have been reported when women took a tricyclic antidepressant during the first 3 months of pregnancy. When any of these drugs is considered crucial by your doctor, its potential benefits must be carefully weighed against its risks.

Small amounts of these drugs pass into breast milk. Nursing mothers who must take a tricyclic antidepressant should bottle-feed.

Seniors
Seniors are more sensitive to the effects of these drugs, especially abnormal heart rhythms and other cardiac side effects, and often require reduced dosage.

Type of Drug

Triptan-Type Antimigraine Drugs

(TRIP-tan)

Brand Names

Generic Ingredient: Almotriptan
Axert

Generic Ingredient: Eletriptan
Relpax

Feneric Ingredient: Frovatriptan
Frova

Generic Ingredient: Naratriptan
Amerge

Generic Ingredient: Rizatriptan
Maxalt   Maxalt-MLT

Generic Ingredient: Sumatriptan
Imitrex

Generic Ingredient: Zolmitriptan
Zomig   Zomig ZMT

Prescribed For

Migraine headache. Sumatriptan injection can be used for cluster headaches.

General Information

Triptan-type drugs are used to alleviate symptoms of migraine, which include severe headaches as well as nausea, vomiting, and increased sensitivity to light and sound. These drugs work by affecting specific serotonin (5HT) receptors in the brain. This action constricts (narrows) blood vessels in the brain, which are usually dilated (widened) during a migraine attack. Triptan-type drugs mainly interfere with one type of serotonin receptor, known as 5-HT$_{1B/1D}$, and do not affect other serotonin receptors. While these drugs can alleviate symptoms of migraine, they do not prevent attacks.

Triptan-type drugs are only recommended after analgesics (pain relievers)—such as aspirin, acetaminophen, and other nonsteroidal anti-inflammatory drugs (NSAIDs)—have failed to relieve symptoms. If you experience serious, incapacitating migraines more often than twice a month, your doctor may recommend taking other medications on a regular basis to reduce the number and severity of attacks including beta blockers, calcium channel blockers, tricyclic antidepressants, MAOIs, methysergide, and cyproheptadine. Triptan-type drugs generally start to relieve migraine symptoms in about 1 hour; rizatriptan works fastest. They are broken down partially in the liver.

Cautions and Warnings

Do not use these drugs if you are **allergic** to them.

These drugs should only be prescribed after you have been diagnosed with migraine (sumatriptan injection may be used for cluster headaches) because they are not effective in treating other types of headache or pain.

Zolmitriptan, eletriptan and naratriptan should not be used if you have uncontrolled **high blood pressure**.

It is strongly recommended that triptan-type drugs not be taken by **people who have or are at risk for heart disease,** as indicated by high blood pressure, high blood cholesterol, smoking, obesity, diabetes, and a family history of heart disease. If you have any of these risk factors, your doctor must evaluate you heart disease risk before prescribing one of these drugs. People who take triptan-type drugs regularly or who develop risk factors for heart disease should be reevaluated by their doctors. Rarely, serious cardiac problems have occurred after taking one of these drugs.

People have experienced **chest, neck, or jaw tightness and pain** after taking one of these drugs, but these sensations are rarely associated with heart problems.

Do not take these drugs if your **headache is different** in any way. A change in the characteristics of your headache may signal a much more serious problem. Call your doctor at once.

Strokes and some fatalities have occurred in people taking a triptan-type drug, though they may have happened because a stroke-related headache was treated with a triptan rather than as a symptom of stroke. People with migraine are more likely to have a stroke or bleeding in the brain. Sumatriptan has been associated with **seizures**.

Rizatriptan must be used with caution by people with severe **kidney problems** or moderate to severe **liver disease**.

People with severe kidney or liver disease should not take naratriptan, sumatriptan, or eletriptan.

Frovatriptan accumulates in people with mild to moderate **liver disease,** but blood levels in these people are similar to blood levels in seniors. No dosage adjustment is needed. There is no experience with frovatriptan in people with severe liver disease.

Eletriptan should not be taken by people with **liver** disease.

Do not use eletriptan within at least 3 days of taking clarithromycin, itraconazole, ketoconazole, nelfinavir, ritonavir, or troleandomycin.

These drugs can collect in the colored part of the eye and cause **eye disorders** if taken over a long period. Have your eyes checked regularly.

Possible Side Effects

Side effects are usually mild or moderate, do not last long, and are the same in men and women regardless of age. Some reported side effects (nausea, vomiting, dizziness, fainting, a feeling of ill health, drowsiness, and sedation) are also migraine symptoms. Side effects may increase with dosage, especially tingling in the hands or feet; chest, neck, jaw, or throat tightness or heaviness; dizziness; tiredness; weakness; and nausea. Rare side effects can affect the heart and blood vessels, nervous system, skin, stomach and intestines, urinary and reproductive systems, blood, muscles and bones, eyes, ears, nose, throat, and other parts of the body. Contact your doctor if you experience any side effect not listed below.

Almotriptan
▼ Common: nausea, tiredness, tingling in the hands or feet, dry mouth, and headache.

Eletriptan
▼ Common: weakness, dizziness, sleepiness, and nausea.
▼ Less common: chest tightness, dry mouth, upset stomach, flushing, tingling in the hands or feet, abdominal pain or discomfort, and difficulty swallowing.

Frovatriptan
▼ Common: dizziness, tiredness, and headache.

Possible Side Effects *(continued)*

▼ Less common: tingling in the hands or feet, dry mouth, upset stomach, flushing, skeletal pain, and hot or cold sensations.

▼ Rare: heart attack, chest pain, and abnormal heart rhythms. Other rare side effects can occur in almost any part of the body. Contact your doctor if you experience any side effect not listed above.

Naratriptan

▼ Less common: weakness, nausea; tingling in the hands or feet; dizziness; fatigue; drowsiness; pain or pressure in the neck, throat, or jaw; and generalized pain.

Rizatriptan

▼ Common: dizziness, tiredness, fatigue, and nausea.

▼ Less common: tingling in the hands or feet; headache; pain or pressure in the neck, throat, chest, or jaw; generalized pain; and dry mouth.

Sumatriptan

▼ Common: tingling and nasal discomfort.

▼ Less common: unusual sensations of warmth or cold, flushing, heart palpitations, heaviness, tightness, pressure, eye problems, and weakness. At high dosages, agitation, eye irritation, and painful urination may occur.

Zolmitriptan

▼ Most common: dizziness, weakness, sleepiness, tightness in the jaw or neck, tingling, a warm or burning sensation, tiredness, nausea, and fainting.

▼ Less common: diminished sensitivity to stimulation, heart palpitations, chest pain or pressure, sweating, and muscle aches.

Drug Interactions

• Do not take any of these drugs within 24 hours of each other.

• Oral contraceptives ("the pill") increase frovatriptan blood levels and the risk of side effects.

• Ergotamine and dihydroergotamine may add to the effects of triptan-type drugs. Allow at least 24 hours between taking these drugs. Ergotamine reduces the amount of frovatriptan in the blood by about 25%.

• Do not take more than one triptan-type drug at a time.

• Cimetidine significantly increases blood levels of zolmitriptan.

• Monoamine oxidase inhibitor (MAOI) drugs can increase blood levels of almotriptan, sumatriptan, zolmitriptan, and rizatriptan, and the risk of their side effects. Do not combine these drugs. Stop taking an MAOI at least 2 weeks before starting on sumatriptan, zolmitriptan, or rizatriptan.

• Propranolol may significantly increase frovatriptan, eletriptan, and zolmitriptan blood levels.

• Rarely, combining sumatriptan, zolmitriptan, or rizatriptan with a selective serotonin reuptake inhibitor (SSRI) antidepressant such as fluoxetine, fluvoxamine, or sertraline can cause weakness, overly sensitive reflexes, and poor coordination. This interaction does not occur with paroxetine.

• Delavirdine, indinavil, nelfinavir, ritonavir, saquinavir, amiodarone, cimetidine, ciprofloxacin, clarithromycin, diltiazem, erythromycin, fluconazole, fluvoxamine, itraconazole, ketoconazole, mifepristone, nefazodone, norfloxacin, mibefradil, and troleandomycin can increase the amount of a triptan drug in the blood by interfering with its breakdown in the liver.

Food Interactions

These drugs may be taken with or without food.

Usual Dose

Almotriptan

Adult (age 18 and over): 6.25–12.5 mg as soon as migraine symptoms begin or at any time during the attack. If symptoms do not abate, you may take another tablet in 2 hours, but take no more than 12.5 mg a day. The safety of taking more than 4 doses a month has not been established.

Child: not recommended.

Eletripan

Adult (age 18 and over): A single 20 or 40 mg tablet when migraine symptoms begin. Repeat again in 2 hours, if needed. Daily dose should not exceed 80 mg.

Child: not recommended.

Frovatriptan

Adult (age 18 and over): One 2.5 mg tablet when migraine symptoms begin. If you experience pain after the first dose has worn off, you may take another 2.5 mg tablet, but be sure you take the second dose at least 2 hours after the first dose. The safety of treating more than 4 migraines a month with frovatriptan has not been established.

Naratriptan

Adult (age 18 and over): 1–2.5 mg as soon as migraine symptoms begin or at any time during the attack. If symptoms do not go away, you may take another tablet in 4 hours. Do not take more than 5 mg a day.

Child: not recommended.

Rizatriptan Tablets

Adult (age 18 and over): 5–10 mg as soon as migraine symptoms begin or at any time during the attack. If symptoms do not go away, you may take another tablet in 2 hours. Do not take more than 30 mg a day. People also taking propranolol should take no more than 5 mg of rizatriptan at a time, up to 15 mg a day.

Child: not recommended.

Rizatriptan Tablets (Disintegrating)

Dosage is the same as for regular rizatriptan tablets, but these tablets can be taken without fluid. Do not take the tablet out of its protective packaging until just before you swallow it. Make sure your hands are dry and place the tablet on your tongue, where it will dissolve and be swallowed with your saliva. For people with phenylketonuria (PKU disease): orally disintegrating tablets have 1.05 mg of phenylalanine per 5 mg.

Sumatriptan Tablets

Adult (age 18 and over): 25, 50, or 100 mg as soon as migraine symptoms begin or at any time during the attack. If symptoms do not go away, you may take another dose every 2 hours. Do not take more than 200 mg a day. The safety of using sumatriptan for more than 4 headaches a month (on average) has not been established. People with liver disease should take the lowest effective dosage.

Child: not recommended.

Sumatriptan Nasal Spray

Adult (age 18 and over): 1–2 sprays of the 5 mg nasal spray or 1 spray of the 20 mg spray into 1 nostril only. Higher dosages may increase side effects. The dose may be repeated 2 or more hours later if symptoms return. Do not take more than 40 mg (8 sprays of the 5-mg or 2 sprays of the 20-mg) a day.

Sumatriptan Injection

Adult (age 18 and over): 6 mg as a subcutaneous injection. People not responding to 1 injection are not likely to respond to a second 6 mg injection. Do not take more than 12 mg a day. Single doses larger than 6 mg are not more effective and are not recommended.

Child: not recommended.

Zolmitriptan

Adult (age 18 and over): 1.25–2.5 mg as soon as migraine symptoms begin or at any time during the attack. If symptoms do not go away, you may take another tablet in 2 hours; do not take more than 10 mg a day. People with liver disease should take the lowest effective dosage.

Child: not recommended.

Overdosage

Overdose can be expected to cause sedation, convulsions, tremors, swelling, redness in the arms or legs, physical inactivity, slowed breathing, bluish discoloration of the lips or skin under the fingernails, weakness, dilated pupils, paralysis, increased blood pressure, light-headedness, neck tension, or poor coordination. Take the victim to a hospital emergency room. ALWAYS bring the prescription bottle or container.

Special Information

Tell your doctor if you have had a stroke or high blood pressure, heart disease or a history of heart disease, high cholesterol, circulation problems, diabetes, obesity, or a history of smoking.

Stop taking the drug and contact your doctor at once if you develop shortness of breath; wheezing; heart palpitations; swelling in the eyelids, face, or lips; rash; lumps; hives; severe tightness in the chest or throat; or sudden abdominal pain.

These drugs may make you tired or dizzy. Be careful when driving or performing any task that requires concentration.

These drugs can increase your sensitivity to the sun. Use sunscreen and wear protective clothing.

These drugs are meant only to treat migraine or cluster headaches. They do not work for all types of headache or pain.

Take your medication at the first sign of a migraine—usually pain or aura. You may enhance the effect of the drug if you lie down in a quiet, dark room.

Avoid alcohol because it can worsen your headaches.

Read and follow the product instructions.

Call your doctor if the usual dosage does not relieve 3 consecutive headaches, if your headaches become more frequent or worse, or if you develop chest pain; difficulty swallowing or breathing; high blood pressure; chest pressure, tightness, or heaviness; nausea; vomiting; or any bothersome or persistent side effect.

People taking one of these medicines should have their eyes checked periodically.

Special Populations

Pregnancy/Breast-feeding

Animal studies have shown possible toxic effects on the fetus. When any of these drugs is considered crucial by your doctor, its potential benefits must be carefully weighed against its risks.

Sumatriptan and eletriptan pass into breast milk. Animal studies show that some other triptan-type drugs may pass into breast milk. Nursing mothers who must take any of these drugs should consider bottle-feeding.

Seniors

Almotriptan, eletriptan, rizatripan, sumatriptan, and zolmitriptan may be taken without special precaution. Seniors are more likely to develop naratriptan side effects; this drug is not recommended for them. Frovatriptan can raise blood pressure in some seniors, but it generally returns to normal on its own. However, even small increases in blood pressure have been linked to serious risks and should not be ignored.

Brand Name

Trizivir

Generic Ingredients

Abacavir + Lamivudine + Zidovudine

Type of Drug

Antiviral combination.

Prescribed For

AIDS and HIV-1 infection.

General Information

This drug is a combination of 3 different nucleoside antiviral drugs that are available individually. It is useful for people who would normally take the 3 active ingredients included in this product. The 3 ingredients of Trizivir attack the HIV-1 virus in different ways: Abacavir interferes with the growth of viral DNA, and lamivudine and zidovudine interfere with viral DNA duplication.

Cautions and Warnings

Trizivir is associated with **fatal sensitivity reactions** (fever, skin rash, fatigue, nausea, vomiting, diarrhea, pain, sore throat, difficulty breathing, or cough). Call your doctor at once if you develop signs of a reaction. This combination drug should be discontinued and other treatment started immediately.

Trizivir is associated with **severe blood toxicity**. Frequent blood counts are recommended.

Trizivir is associated with **liver toxicity**. People with AIDS who also have chronic liver disease due to hepatitis B infection are especially likely to be affected.

In rare instances, people taking nucleoside-type antivirals have developed **lactic acidosis** (a potentially fatal metabolic imbalance). Symptoms of lactic acidosis may include unexplained rapid breathing, breathing difficulties, and reduced blood-bicarbonate levels, which your doctor can detect with a routine blood test.

Trizivir may cause **muscle irritation and abnormalities** similar to those caused by HIV infection.

People with **impaired kidney or liver function** should use this drug with caution.

There is a possibility that **cross resistance** can develop between Trizivir and other nucleoside antivirals, reducing the effectiveness of these drugs against the HIV-1 virus.

Possible Side Effects

Side effects are the same as can be expected from each of the 3 products individually.

▼ Most common: anemia, reduced white-blood-cell counts, chills, rash, nausea, vomiting, diarrhea, appetite loss, abdominal pain or cramps, nervous system problems, including tingling and poor coordination, sleeplessness, dizziness, depression, stuffy or runny nose, cough, muscle pain, fever, headache, feeling or being sick, and weakness.

▼ Common: sensitivity reaction (fever, skin rash, fatigue, and gastrointestinal symptoms, such as nausea, vomiting, diarrhea or abdominal pain, and respiratory symptoms such as sore throat, difficulty breathing, or cough), upset stomach, joint pain, tingling in the hands or feet, and sleep disturbances. Trizivir may affect the results of a variety of blood tests.

▼ Less common: blood infection, nervousness, and irritability.

▼ Rare: pancreas irritation, weight loss, seizures, heart failure and other cardiac abnormalities, blood in the urine, and bladder infections.

Drug Interactions

• Trizivir slows the elimination of alcohol from the body and can lead to a large increase of alcohol in the blood.

• Interferon beta-1b, methadone, aspirin, indomethacin, probenecid, trimethoprim/sulfamethoxazole (an anti-infective combination), trimethoprim, and valproic acid increase the amount of Trizivir in the blood and the risk of Trizivir side effects.

• Cigarette smoking, clofibrate, phenobarbital, liothyronine, isoniazid, acetaminophen, rifampin, and rifampicin may reduce the amount of Trizivir in the blood.

• Mixing Trizivir with anti-cancer drugs or drugs that suppress the immune system increases the risk of blood toxicity.

• Mixing clarithromycin or fluconazole with Trizivir can increase the amount of Trizivir in the blood, but the importance of this interaction is not known.

• Atovaquone increases the amount of Trizivir in the blood by interfering with its breakdown in the liver. Trizivir dosage reduction may be necessary.

• Combining Trizivir with other drugs that can damage your kidneys, including pentamidine, dapsone, amphotericin B, flucytosine, vincristine, vinblastine, adriamycin, and alfa- and beta-interferon, increases the risk of loss of some kidney function.

• Trizivir can increase blood levels of acetaminophen, amitriptyline, bumetanide, chloral hydrate, chlorpheniramine, chlorpromazine, chlorzoxazone, dapsone, doxepin, fluconazole, imipramine, ketoconazole, labetalol, lamotrigine, miconazole, morphine, naloxone, non-steroidal anti-inflammatory drugs (NSAIDs), oxazepam, promethazine, propofol, and propranolol.

• Combining Trizivir and isoniazid may increase isoniazid levels in the blood.

• Acyclovir is used in combination with Trizivir to combat opportunistic infections in AIDS patients; however, this combination may cause severe drowsiness or lethargy.

• Other drugs that can cause anemia, including alfa-interferon, ganciclovir, and zalcitabine, should be used carefully in combination with Trizivir because of the risk of worsening drug-related anemia.

• Taking phenytoin and Trizivir together may affect the amounts of both drugs in the blood, usually increasing the amount of Trizivir. The effect on phenytoin blood levels varies. This combination can result in either too much phenytoin—leading to increased phenytoin side effects—or too little phenytoin—leading to a possible increase in the number of seizures. Your doctor should check your phenytoin levels if you are also taking Trizivir.

Food Interactions

You may take this product with food if it upsets your stomach.

Usual Dose

Adult (88 lbs. or over): 1 tablet two times a day.
Adult (less than 88 lbs.): not recommended.

Child (age 13 and over, and 88 lbs. and over): 1 tablet two times a day.

Child (age 13 and over, but under 88 lbs.): not recommended.

Child (under age 13): not recommended.

Overdosage

Overdose symptoms are usually mild. However, overdose victims should be taken to a hospital emergency room. ALWAYS bring the prescription bottle or container.

Special Information

Trizivir does not cure AIDS. It will not decrease the risk of your transmitting the HIV virus to another person; you must still practice safe sex. Trizivir may not prevent some illnesses associated with AIDS or AIDS-related complex (ARC) from continuing to develop.

Stop taking this drug and call your doctor at the first sign of allergy or drug sensitivity (symptoms include fever, rash, fatigue, nausea, vomiting, diarrhea, and abdominal pain).

See your doctor if any significant change in your health occurs. Periodic blood counts are very important while taking Trizivir to detect possibly serious side effects.

People taking Trizivir must take especially good care of their teeth and gums to minimize the risk of developing oral infections.

If you miss a dose of Trizivir, take it as soon as possible. If it is almost time for your next dose, skip the dose you forgot and continue with your regular schedule. Call your doctor if you forget 2 or more doses in a row. Do not take more Trizivir than your doctor prescribed.

Special Populations

Pregnancy/Breast-feeding

There are no studies of Trizivir use in pregnant women. However, in animal studies all 3 ingredients harmed developing fetuses. Pregnant women should only take this combination after discussing the possible risks and benefits with a doctor. Notify your doctor at once if you do become pregnant.

This drug passes into breast milk. It is recommended that mothers who are HIV-positive should bottle-feed their babies to avoid transmitting the virus.

Seniors

Seniors may take this product without special restriction.

Brand Name

Tussionex Pennkinetic Ⓐ

Generic Ingredients

Hydrocodone + Chlorpheniramine

Other Brand Names

S-T Forte 2

Type of Drug

Cough suppressant and antihistamine.

Prescribed For

Cough and other symptoms of a cold or other respiratory condition.

General Information

Tussionex Pennkinetic is one of many cough suppressant-antihistamine combinations that may be prescribed to treat a cough or congestion that has not responded to other medication. The narcotic cough-suppressant ingredient in this combination, hydrocodone, is more potent than codeine.

Cautions and Warnings

Do not use Tussionex Pennkinetic if you are **allergic** to any of its ingredients. Those allergic to codeine may also be allergic to Tussionex Pennkinetic. Chronic (long-term) use of this drug may lead to drug dependence or **addiction**. Tussionex Pennkinetic may cause **drowsiness, tiredness,** or **loss of concentration**. Use with caution if you have a history of **convulsions, glaucoma,** stomach **ulcer, hypertension** (high blood pressure), **thyroid disease, heart disease,** or **diabetes**.

Possible Side Effects

▼ Most common: light-headedness, dizziness, sleepiness, nausea, vomiting, increased sweating, itching, rash, sensitivity to bright light, chills, and dryness of the mouth, nose, or throat.

▼ Less common: euphoria (feeling "high"), weakness, agitation, uncoordinated muscle movement, disorientation and visual disturbances, minor hallucinations, appetite loss, constipation, facial flushing, rapid heartbeat, palpitations, feeling faint, urinary difficulties, reduced sexual potency, low blood sugar, anemia, yellowing of the skin or whites of the eyes, blurred or double vision, ringing or buzzing in the ears, wheezing, and nasal stuffiness.

Drug Interactions

• Do not use alcohol or other depressant drugs because they increase the depressant effect of Tussionex Pennkinetic.

• This drug should not be combined with monoamine oxidase inhibitor (MAOI) antidepressants.

Food Interactions

Take Tussionex Pennkinetic with food if it upsets your stomach.

Usual Dose

1 tsp. every 12 hours.

Overdosage

Symptoms include depression, slowed breathing, flushing, and upset stomach. Take the victim to a hospital emergency room. ALWAYS bring the prescription bottle or container.

Special Information

This drug causes sedation. Be careful when driving or doing any task that requires concentration.

If you forget a dose, take it as soon as you remember. If it is almost time for your next dose, skip the one you forgot and continue with your regular schedule. Do not take a double dose.

Special Populations

Pregnancy/Breast-feeding

Antihistamines pass into the circulation of the fetus but have not caused birth defects. Taking narcotics during pregnancy may lead to drug dependency in newborns or breathing difficulties if narcotics are used just prior to delivery. When this drug is considered crucial by your doctor, its potential benefits must be carefully weighed against its risks.

The ingredients in this product pass into breast milk and may affect an infant's breathing if abused. Nursing mothers who must take this drug should consider bottle-feeding.

Seniors

Seniors are more likely to be sensitive to both ingredients in Tussionex Pennkinetic and to experience depressant effects; dizziness, light-headedness or fainting when rising suddenly from a sitting or lying position; confusion; difficult or painful urination; feeling faint; dry mouth, nose, or throat; nightmares; excitement; nervousness; restlessness; or irritability.

Brand Name

Tussi-Organidin NR Ⓢ

Generic Ingredients

Codeine Phosphate + Guaifenesin Ⓖ

Other Brand Names

Cheracol	Halotussin AC Ⓢ Ⓐ
Gani-Tuss NR	Mytussin AC
Guiatuss AC	Robafen AC
Guiatussin with Codeine	Robitussin A-C Ⓢ

Type of Drug

Cough suppressant and expectorant.

Prescribed For

Cough due to a cold or other upper respiratory infection.

General Information

In Tussi-Organidin NR, codeine is the ingredient that suppresses cough. Guaifenesin, an expectorant, increases the production of mucus and other bronchial secretions, making coughs more productive. Many experts question the effectiveness of guaifenesin, especially for removing the mucus that accumulates during serious respiratory conditions such as bronchitis, bronchial asthma, emphysema, cystic fibrosis, or chronic sinusitis. Drinking plenty of fluid works as well as any expectorant for the average cold or upper-respiratory cough. Expectorants do not suppress your cough.

Cautions and Warnings

Do not take Tussi-Organidin NR if you are **allergic** or **sensitive** to any of its ingredients. Chronic (long-term) use of codeine may lead to drug dependence or **addiction**.

Possible Side Effects

▼ Most common: light-headedness, dizziness, sedation or sleepiness, nausea, vomiting, diarrhea, stomach pain, and sweating.

▼ Less common: euphoria (feeling "high"), weakness, headache, agitation, uncoordinated muscle movement, minor hallucinations, disorientation and visual disturbances, dry mouth, appetite loss, constipation, facial flushing, rapid heartbeat, palpitations, feeling faint, urinary difficulties or hesitancy, reduced sex drive or potency, itching, rash, anemia, lowered blood sugar, and yellowing of the skin or whites of the eyes. Narcotic analgesics (pain relievers) such as codeine may aggravate convulsions in those who have had them.

Drug Interactions

• Codeine has a general depressant effect and may affect breathing. Tussi-Organidin NR should be taken with extreme care in combination with alcohol, sedatives, tranquilizers, antihistamines, or other depressant drugs.

Food Interactions

Tussi-Organidin NR should be taken with a full glass of water or other fluid.

Usual Dose

2 tsp. every 4 hours as needed for cough relief.

Overdosage

Symptoms include breathing difficulties, pinpointed pupils, lack of response to pain stimulation, cold or clammy skin, slow heartbeat, low blood pressure, convulsions, heart attack, or extreme tiredness progressing to stupor and then coma. Take the victim to a hospital emergency room immediately. ALWAYS bring the prescription bottle or container.

Special Information

Codeine is a respiratory depressant and affects the central nervous system (CNS), producing sleepiness, tiredness, or an inability to concentrate. Be careful when driving or doing any task that requires concentration. Report persistent or bothersome side effects to your doctor.

If you take Tussi-Organidin NR 3 or more times a day and forget a dose, take it as soon as you remember. If it is almost time for your next dose, take 1 dose right away and another in 3 or 4 hours, then go back to your regular schedule. Do not take a double dose.

Special Populations

Pregnancy/Breast-feeding

Taking narcotics during pregnancy may lead to drug dependency in newborns or breathing difficulties if narcotics are used just prior to delivery. When Tussi-Organidin NR is considered crucial by your doctor, its potential benefits must be carefully weighed against its risks.

Codeine passes into breast milk and may affect an infant's breathing if abused. Nursing mothers who must take Tussi-Organidin NR should consider bottle-feeding.

Seniors

Seniors are more sensitive to the effects of codeine.

Ultracet   see *Tramadol,* page 1087

Generic Name

Valacyclovir (val-ay-SYE-kloe-vere)

Brand Name

Valtrex

Type of Drug

Antiviral.

Prescribed For

Herpes zoster (shingles) and recurrent genital herpes.

General Information

Valacyclovir hydrochloride is rapidly converted to the antiviral acyclovir in the liver and intestine after it is absorbed into the blood. Acyclovir, the form valacyclovir takes in order to work, fights the herpes virus by inhibiting and inactivating an enzyme that is key to viral reproduction and by affecting the growing viral DNA chain.

Cautions and Warnings

Do not take valacyclovir if you are **allergic** to it, acyclovir, or any component of the tablet.

Some people with advanced **HIV disease,** or who have had a **bone marrow transplant** or an **organ transplant,** developed a potentially fatal condition known as TTP (blood-clotting disorder) while taking valacyclovir. This drug should not be taken by anyone with **AIDS** or a **compromised immune system.**

People with **kidney disease** should use caution when taking valacyclovir, and may require a reduced dosage.

Possible Side Effects

▼ Most common: headache, diarrhea, dizziness, weakness, constipation, abdominal pain, appetite loss, nausea, and vomiting.

▼ Less common: aching joints, tingling in the hands or feet, stomach gas, fatigue, rash, not feeling well, leg pain, sore throat, a bad taste in the mouth, sleeplessness, and fever.

Drug Interactions

• Cimetidine and probenecid slow the rate at which valacyclovir is converted to acyclovir, but this does not change valacyclovir's effectiveness. No adjustments in valacyclovir dosage are necessary.

• Cimetidine and probenecid may decrease acyclovir elimination from your body and increase drug blood levels, raising the risk of side effects.

• Combining acyclovir and zidovudine (an AIDS drug—also known as AZT) may lead to severe drowsiness or lethargy.

Food Interactions

None known.

Usual Dose

Adult: shingles—1000 mg 3 times a day for 7 days. Genital herpes—1000 mg twice a day for 10 days for initial outbreak, preferably within 48 hours; 500 mg twice a day for 3 days for recurrent outbreaks; and 500 mg a day for prevention of outbreaks. Dosage is reduced in people with kidney disease.

Child (age 12 and under): not recommended.

Overdosage

Little is known about the effects of valacyclovir overdose. It may lead to kidney damage due to deposits of drug crystals in the kidney. Call your local poison control center for more information.

Special Information

Treatment with valacyclovir must be started as soon as possible after shingles is diagnosed. All information on the effectiveness of this drug was gathered from cases in which treatment was begun within 72 hours of diagnosis.

Women with genital herpes have an increased risk of cervical cancer. Check with your doctor about the need for an annual Pap smear.

Herpes may be transmitted even if you do not have symptoms of active disease. To avoid giving the condition to a sexual partner, do not have intercourse while visible herpes lesions are present. A condom should protect against transmission of the herpes virus, but spermicidal products or diaphragms do not. Valacyclovir alone will not prevent herpes transmission.

Call your doctor if valacyclovir does not relieve your symptoms, if side effects become severe, or if you become pregnant or want to begin breast-feeding.

Check with your dentist or doctor about how to take care of your teeth if you notice swelling or tenderness of the gums.

If you forget a dose of valacyclovir, take it as soon as you remember. If it is almost time for your next dose, skip the dose you forgot and continue with your regular schedule. Do not take a double dose.

Special Populations

Pregnancy/Breast-feeding
Acyclovir crosses into the circulation of the fetus. Animal studies have shown that large doses of acyclovir—up to 125 times the human dose—cause damage to both mother and fetus. When this drug is considered crucial by your doctor, its potential benefits must be carefully weighed against its risks.

Acyclovir passes into breast milk. Nursing mothers who must take it should consider bottle-feeding.

Seniors
People age 50 and over with shingles tend to have more severe attacks and respond best to valacyclovir treatment if the drug is started within 48 to 72 hours of the first sign of rash. Seniors with reduced kidney function should receive lower dosages.

Generic Name

Valproic Acid (val-PROE-ik) Ⓖ

Brand Names

Depacon	Depakote ER
Depakene	Depakote Sprinkle
Depakote	

Type of Drug

Anticonvulsant and antimanic.

Prescribed For

Petit mal and absence seizures and bipolar (manic-depressive) disorder; also prescribed for grand mal, myoclonic, and other seizures; prevention of fever convulsions in children; migraine; anger management; and anxiety or panic attacks.

General Information

Valproic acid is chemically unrelated to other drugs used in the treatment of seizure disorders. It may work by increasing levels of gamma-aminobutyric acid (GABA) and improving its effects in the brain. Valproic acid also has a stabilizing effect on cell membranes within the brain, which may account for some of the drug's other effects. It is broken down in the liver. The information in this profile applies to both forms of the drug: valproic acid (Depakene) and its related compound, divalproex sodium (Depakote). Divalproex sodium is made up of equal quantities of valproic acid and sodium valproate.

Cautions and Warnings

Do not take valproic acid if you are **sensitive** or **allergic** to it.

Use this drug with caution if you have a history of **liver problems**. Liver failure, sometimes resulting in death, has occurred in people taking valproic acid. **Children under age 2** are at increased risk for liver failure associated with valproic acid, especially if they are also taking other anticonvulsants or have congenital disorders of metabolism, severe seizure disorders, mental retardation, or organic brain disease. After age 2, the risk of a fatal liver reaction decreases sharply. Ammonia in the bloodstream, another factor that worsens liver disease, may also occur with valproic acid.

If it is going to occur, serious liver disease usually develops during the first 6 months of valproic acid treatment and is often preceded by feeling unwell, weakness, tiredness, facial swelling, appetite loss, yellowing of the skin or whites of the eyes, vomiting, and loss of seizure control. Your doctor should check your liver function before beginning valproic acid treatment and periodically thereafter.

Children and adults taking valproic acid have rarely developed cases of life-threatening **pancreatitis** (inflammation of the pancreas). **Abdominal pain, nausea, vomiting,** or **appetite loss** can be signs of pancreatitis and require immediate medical attention. Valproic acid can affect **platelet function,** leading to **bruising, bleeding,** or changes in **blood-clotting** function.

Possible Side Effects

Side effects worsen as dosage increases.

▼ Most common: nausea, vomiting, diarrhea, abdominal pain, dizziness, indigestion, sedation or sleepiness, weakness, rash, weight gain, emotional upset, depression, psychosis, aggression, hyperactive behavior, and changes in blood components.

▼ Less common: stomach cramps, constipation, increased or decreased appetite, hair loss, change in menstrual periods, headache, loss of eye-muscle control, drooping eyelids, double vision, spots before the eyes, loss of muscle control or coordination, and tremors.

Drug Interactions

• Valproic acid may increase the depressive effects of alcohol, sleeping pills, anti-anxiety drugs, tranquilizers, phenobarbital, primidone, and other depressant drugs. It may slightly decrease blood levels of clozapine or zidovudine (an AIDS drug also known as AZT).

• Valproic acid may increase the side effects of tricyclic antidepressants and their concentration in the blood.

• Dosages of carbamazepine, clonazepam, ethosuximide, lamotrigine, and phenytoin may have to be adjusted when you begin taking valproic acid.

• Valproic acid may affect oral anticoagulant (blood-thinning) drugs; your anticoagulant dose may have to be adjusted.

• Aspirin, cimetidine, chlorpromazine, erythromycin, and felbamate may increase the risk of valproic acid side effects by increasing the amount of valproic acid in the blood.

• Rifampin may reduce the amount of valproic acid in the blood.

• Valproic acid may increase the need for levocarnitine.

• Valproic acid may increase the risk of bleeding or bruising if combined with other drugs that affect platelet "stickiness." These include aspirin, which also increases valproic acid side effects, and other nonsteroidal anti-inflammatory drugs (NSAIDs), dipyridamole, sulfinpyrazone, and ticlopidine.

• Valproic acid may cause false-positive reactions in the urine ketone tests used in diabetes.

• Charcoal tablets interfere with the absorption of valproic acid.

Food Interactions

Food slows the absorption of valproic acid slightly, but you may take it with food if it upsets your stomach. The syrup form can be mixed with food to improve its taste.

Depakote Sprinkle can be taken whole or mixed with 1 tsp. of pudding, applesauce, or other soft food. Swallow the mixture promptly—do not chew.

Usual Dose

7–27 mg per lb. a day. Valproic acid is best taken in 1 dose at bedtime to minimize sedative effects. Daily dosages greater than 250 mg should be split into 2 or more doses a day. The dosage of divalproex sodium is measured in terms of the equivalent dosage of valproic acid.

Overdosage

Overdose may result in restlessness, hallucinations, flapping tremors of the hands, coma, and death. Call your local poison control center or take the victim to a hospital emergency room immediately. ALWAYS bring the prescription bottle or container.

Special Information

This medication may cause drowsiness: Be careful while driving or performing any task that requires concentration.

Call your doctor at once if you develop nausea, vomiting, abdominal pain, or loss of appetite.

Do not chew or crush the capsules or tablets.

Do not switch brands of valproic acid without your doctor's knowledge. In at least 1 case, seizures resulted when a person was switched to a new product after 3 seizure-free years on another brand of valproic acid.

Valproic acid can cause mouth, gum, and throat irritation or bleeding, and increased risk of mouth infections. Maintain good dental hygiene while taking this drug. Dental work should be delayed if your blood counts are low.

People with a seizure disorder should carry special identification indicating their condition and any drugs being taken.

If you take valproic acid once a day and forget a dose, take it as soon as possible. If you do not remember until the next day, skip the dose you forgot and continue with your regular schedule. If you take valproic acid 2 or more times a day and forget a dose, take it as soon as possible if you remember within 6 hours of your regular time. Take the remaining daily dosage at evenly spaced intervals. Go back to your regular schedule the next day. Never take a double dose.

Special Populations

Pregnancy/Breast-feeding

Taking valproic acid during the first 3 months of pregnancy may increase the risk of birth defects. Pregnant women should take valproic acid only after discussing with their doctors its potential benefits and risks.

Valproic acid passes into breast milk and may affect a nursing infant. Nursing mothers who must take this drug should consider bottle-feeding.

Seniors

Seniors are more likely to experience side effects due to reduced kidney or liver function and may require lower dosage.

Valtrex *see Valacyclovir, page 1137*

see Valacyclovir, page 1137

Generic Name

Venlafaxine (ven-luh-FAX-ene)

Brand Names

Effexor   Effexor XR

Type of Drug

Antidepressant.

Prescribed For

Depression and generalized anxiety disorder.

General Information

Chemically different from other antidepressant drugs, venlafaxine may work by inhibiting the ability of nerve endings in the brain to absorb serotonin, norepinephrine, and dopamine. Venlafaxine passes out of the body primarily via the urine.

Cautions and Warnings

Do not use venlafaxine if you are **allergic** to it. People with severe **kidney or liver disease** may require reduced dosages.

Venlafaxine can raise **blood pressure**. If this happens, your dosage of venlafaxine may have to be reduced. Venlafaxine has not been fully studied in people with recent **heart attack** or unstable **heart disease**, although a small study revealed no unusual changes in their cardiograms.

Possible Side Effects

Side effects increase with dosage.

▼ Most common: blurred vision, tiredness, dry mouth, dizziness, sleeplessness, nervousness, tremors, weakness, sweating, nausea, constipation, appetite loss, vomiting, impotence, and abnormal ejaculation.

▼ Less common: changes in sense of taste, ringing in the ears, dilated pupils, high blood pressure, rapid heart beat, anxiety, reduced sex drive, agitation, chills, yawning, and inability to experience orgasm.

▼ Rare: Rare side effects can occur in almost any part of the body. Contact your doctor if you experience any side effect not listed above.

Drug Interactions

• Taking venlafaxine within 2 weeks of taking a monoamine oxidase inhibitor (MAOI) antidepressant may cause severe and sometimes fatal reactions including high fever, muscle rigidity or spasm, mental changes, and fluctuations in pulse, temperature, or breathing rate. People stopping venlafaxine should wait at least 1 week before starting an MAOI.

• Cimetidine can increase blood levels of venlafaxine, desipramine, and haloperidol, although the effect on the body may be minimal.

• Cimetidine can interact with trazodone to produce changes in serotonin levels.

• Clozapine levels may be increased if taken with venlafaxine, with the potential for increased side effects including seizures.

• Venlafaxine increases blood levels of despiramine and haloperidol significantly.

• Sibutramine, sumatriptan, trazodone, and St. John's wort may cause a "serotonin syndrome," including shivering, spasm, or altered consciousness, if these drugs are taken with venlafaxine.

• Venlafaxine may increase the effects of warfarin.

• Combining venlafaxine and propafenone for severely abnormal heart rhythms may cause psychotic symptoms due to abnormally high levels of venlafaxine in the blood.

Food Interactions

Take each dose with food.

Usual Dose

Adult: 37.5–225 mg a day, divided into 2–3 doses. Some people may benefit from doses up to 375 mg a day. People with severe kidney or liver disease should receive half the usual daily dosage. Those with moderate kidney disease may need their daily dosage reduced by only 25%.

Child (under age 18): not recommended.

Overdosage

Symptoms may include tiredness, mild convulsions, and cardiac effects. Contact your local poison control center or a hospital emergency room for more information. Overdose victims should be taken to a hospital emergency room. ALWAYS bring the prescription bottle or container.

Special Information

Call your doctor if you develop rash, hives, or any other allergic-type reaction.

Venlafaxine may make you tired; be careful when driving or performing any task that requires concentration. Avoid alcohol.

If you forget a dose, take it as soon as you remember. If it is almost time for your next dose, skip the dose you forgot and continue with your regular schedule. Do not take a double dose.

Do not suddenly stop taking this drug. Venlafaxine dosage should be gradually reduced over a 2-week period.

Special Populations

Pregnancy/Breast-feeding

Animal studies of venlafaxine suggest that it may cause low birth weight and other problems. When this drug is considered crucial by your doctor, its potential benefits must be carefully weighed against its risks.

Venlafaxine passes into breast milk. Nursing mothers who must take this drug should consider bottle-feeding.

Seniors

Seniors may be more sensitive to side effects.

Generic Name

Verapamil (vuh-RAP-uh-mil) G

Brand Names

Calan	Isoptin SR
Calan SR	Verapamil Extended Release
Covera HS	Verelan
Isoptin	Verelan PM

Type of Drug

Calcium channel blocker.

Prescribed For

Angina pectoris and Prinzmetal's angina, high blood pressure, abnormal heart rhythm, asthma, cardiomyopathy, migraine, nighttime leg cramps, and bipolar (manic-depressive) disorder.

General Information

Verapamil hydrochloride is one of many calcium channel blockers available in the U.S. These drugs block the passage of calcium, an essential factor in muscle contraction, into the heart and smooth muscles. Such blockage of calcium interferes with the contraction of these muscles, which in turn dilates (widens) the veins and vessels that supply blood to them. This dilating effect reduces blood pressure, the amount of oxygen used by the heart muscle, and the risk of blood vessel spasm. Verapamil is therefore useful in treating not only high blood pressure but also angina pectoris (brief attacks of chest pain), a condition related to poor oxygen supply to the heart muscle.

Verapamil affects the movement of calcium only into muscle cells; it has no effect on calcium in the blood.

The sustained-release brands of verapamil should be used only for high blood pressure.

Cautions and Warnings

Do not take this drug if you have had an **allergic reaction** to it.

Verapamil may cause **low blood pressure** in some people.

People taking a beta-blocking drug who begin taking verapamil may develop **heart failure**.

Verapamil may cause **angina** when treatment is first started, when dosage is increased, or if the drug is rapidly withdrawn. This can be avoided by reducing dosage gradually.

People with **heart problems** such as severe congestive heart failure should not take verapamil.

Studies have shown that people taking calcium channel blockers—usually those taken several times a day, not those taken only once daily—have a greater risk of having a **heart attack** than do people taking beta blockers or other medication for the same purposes. Discuss this with your doctor to be sure you are receiving the best possible treatment.

In small numbers of people, verapamil can lead to an unusual **slowing of heart rate**.

People with **hypertrophic cardiomyopathy** (progressive weakening and destruction of heart muscle) who are receiving up to 720 mg a day of verapamil are at risk of developing severe cardiac side effects. Most of these effects respond to dosage reduction, and people generally may continue on verapamil at a lower dosage.

People with **kidney disease** or severe **liver disease** should use this drug with caution and may require dosage adjustments.

Verapamil may slow the transmission of nerve impulses to muscle in people with **Duchenne's muscular dystrophy,** possibly causing respiratory muscle failure.

Possible Side Effects

Verapamil generally causes fewer side effects than other calcium channel blockers.

▼ Most common: rash; low blood pressure; slowed heartbeat; heart failure or lung congestion marked by coughing, wheezing, or breathing difficulties; tiredness or weakness; swelling of the ankles, feet, or legs; upper respiratory infection; flu-like symptoms, headache; dizziness; light-headedness; constipation; and nausea.

▼ Rare: chest pain, rapid or irregular heartbeat, unusual production of breast milk, bleeding or tender gums, fainting, flushing, and feeling warm. Other rare side effects can occur in almost any part of the body. Contact your doctor if you experience any side effect not listed above.

Some people taking verapamil have experienced heart attack and abnormal heart rhythm, but the occurrence of these effects has not been directly linked to verapamil.

Drug Interactions

• If you take verapamil for long periods of time, your dosage of digoxin will have to be lowered by your doctor.

• Disopyramide should not be taken within 48 hours of taking verapamil.

• People taking verapamil together with quinidine may experience very low blood pressure, slow heartbeat, and fluid in the lungs.

• Verapamil's effectiveness and its side effects may be reversed by taking calcium products, including antacids.

• Amiodarone should be used with verapamil with caution.

• Verapamil may increase the effects of benzodiazepines, buspirone, certain statin drugs, imipramine, and prazosin.

• Verapamil should not be taken with dofetilide.

• Verapamil may interact with beta-blocking drugs to cause heart failure, very low blood pressure, or increased angina. Low blood pressure can also result from taking verapamil with fentanyl (a narcotic pain reliever).

• Verapamil may cause unexpected blood pressure reduction in patients also taking other medication to control their high blood pressure.

• Cimetidine and ranitidine increase the amount of verapamil in the blood and may account for a slight increase in its effect.

• The combination of dantrolene and verapamil may lead to high blood-calcium levels and heart muscle depression. If you are taking dantrolene, a calcium channel blocker other than verapamil should be prescribed by your doctor.

• Verapamil may increase the effects of carbamazepine, cyclosporine, and theophylline products, increasing the chance of side effects with those drugs.

• Verapamil may decrease the amount of lithium in your body, leading to a possible loss of antimanic control, lithium toxicity, and psychotic symptoms.

• Rifampin, barbiturates, phenytoin and similar antiseizure medicines, vitamin D, and sulfinpyrazone may decrease verapamil's effects.

Food Interactions

Take immediate-release products at least 1 hour before or 2 hours after meals. Take sustained-release products with food if they upset your stomach. Avoid grapefruit juice.

Usual Dose

120–480 mg a day, according to your needs.

Overdosage

Overdose of verapamil can cause low blood pressure. Symptoms are dizziness, weakness, and slowed heartbeat. If you have taken an overdose of verapamil, call your doctor or go to an emergency room. ALWAYS bring the prescription bottle or container.

Special Information

Call your doctor if you develop abnormal heart rhythm, swelling in the arms or legs, breathing difficulties, increased heart pain, dizziness, light-headedness, or low blood pressure. Do not stop taking verapamil abruptly.

If you forget to take a dose of verapamil, take it as soon as you remember. If it is almost time for your next dose, skip the one you forgot and continue with your regular schedule. Do not take a double dose.

Special Populations

Pregnancy/Breast-feeding

Verapamil may cause birth defects or interfere with fetal development. When this drug is considered crucial by your doctor, its potential benefits must be carefully weighed against its risks.

Verapamil passes into breast milk. Nursing mothers who must take this drug should bottle-feed.

Seniors

Seniors are more sensitive to side effects, especially low blood pressure.

Viagra *see Erectile Dysfunction Drugs, page 430*

Vioxx *see Rofecoxib, page 951*

Generic Name

Warfarin (WOR-far-in) Ⓖ

Brand Name

Coumadin

The information in this profile also applies to the following drugs:

Generic Ingredient: Anisindione
Miradon

Generic Ingredient: Dicumarol Ⓖ
Only available in generic form.

Type of Drug

Oral anticoagulant (blood thinner).

Prescribed For

Blood clots or coagulation; also prescribed for reducing the risk of small cell carcinoma of the lung, recurrent heart attack or stroke, and transient ischemic attack (TIA).

General Information

Warfarin prevents the formation of blood clots or coagulation by suppressing the body's production of vitamin-K-dependent factors essential to the coagulation process. If you are taking warfarin, you must take it exactly as prescribed. Notify your doctor at the earliest sign of unusual bleeding or bruising; blood in your urine or stool; or black, tarry stools. Warfarin may be affected by many other drugs, and these interactions may be dangerous (see "Drug Interactions"). Warfarin may also be extremely dangerous if not used properly. Periodic tests to monitor blood clotting are required for proper control of warfarin therapy.

Cautions and Warnings

Do not take warfarin if you are **allergic** to it. Anisindione is usually reserved for people allergic to warfarin.

Warfarin must be taken with care if you have any **blood-clotting disease**. Use of warfarin may be dangerous and should be discussed with your doctor if you have: **cramp-like pains and minor vaginal bleeding** that may or may not be followed by a spontaneous abortion during the first 20 weeks of pregnancy; past or planned eye or nervous system surgery; protein C deficiency—a hereditary condition; **liver inflammation or disease; kidney disease;** any **infection** being treated with an antibiotic; active **tuberculosis;** severe or prolonged **dietary deficiencies; stomach ulcer or bleeding; bleeding from the genital or urinary areas; high blood pressure;** severe **diabetes; vein irritation; disease of the large bowel, such as diverticulitis or ulcerative colitis;** and subacute bacterial **endocarditis**.

People with **congestive heart failure** may be more sensitive to dicumarol than to other anticoagulants.

Anisindione can cause **hepatitis** and **agranulocytosis** (condition characterized by a reduction in the number of white blood cells).

Anticoagulant therapy may increase the release of **microplaques** into the bloodstream. These microplaques may block very small blood vessels, leading to purple toe syndrome (condition that occurs when pressure exerted by normal walking leads to bleeding into the skin of your toes). This usually goes away when anticoagulant treatment is stopped but it may be a sign of a more serious problem present in another part of your body.

Women taking anticoagulants may be at risk of **ovarian bleeding** when they ovulate.

People taking warfarin must be extremely careful to **avoid cuts, bruises, or other injuries** that may cause internal or external bleeding.

Possible Side Effects

Warfarin and Dicumarol

▼ Most common: bleeding, which may occur with usual dosages and even when the results of blood tests used to monitor anticoagulant therapy are normal. If you bleed abnormally while you are taking anticoagulants, call your doctor immediately.

▼ Less common: abdominal cramps, nausea, vomiting, diarrhea, fever, anemia, adverse effects on blood components, hepatitis, jaundice (symptoms include yellowing of the skin or whites of the eyes), itching, rash, hair loss, sore throat or mouth, red or orange urine, painful or persistent erection, and purple toe syndrome.

Anisindione

▼ Common: rash.

▼ Less common: headache, sore throat, blurred vision, hepatitis, liver or kidney damage, jaundice (symptoms include yellowing of the skin or whites of the eyes), red or orange urine, and changes in blood components.

Drug Interactions

Anticoagulants may have more drug interactions than any other kind of medication. Your doctor and pharmacist should keep records of all drugs you take in order to anticipate possible interactions. It is essential that your doctor and pharmacist know about every medication you are taking including over-the-counter (OTC) drugs containing aspirin.

• Drugs that may increase the effect of warfarin include the following: acetaminophen; aminoglycoside antibiotics; amiodarone; androgen; aspirin and other salicylate drugs; beta blockers; cephalosporin antibiotics; chloral hydrate; chloramphenicol; chlorpropamide; cimetidine; clofibrate; corticosteroids; cyclophosphamide; dextrothyroxine; diflunisal; disulfiram; erythromycin; fluconazole; gemfibrozil; glucagon; hydantoin antiseizure drugs—blood levels of the hydantoins may also be increased in this interaction; ifosfamide (an influenza virus vaccine); isoniazid; ketoconazole; leflunomide, loop diuretics; lovastatin; metronidazole; miconazole; mineral oil; moricizine; nalidixic acid; nonsteroidal anti-inflammatory drugs (NSAIDs); omeprazole; orlistat, penicillin; phenylbutazone; propafenone; propoxyphene; quinidine; quinine; quinolone antibacterials; sulfa drugs; sulfinpyrazone; tamoxifen; tetracycline antibiotics; thioamines; thyroid hormones; and vitamin E.

• Some drugs decrease the effect of warfarin and the interaction may be just as dangerous. Some examples are alcohol, aminoglutethimide, ascorbic acid (vitamin C), barbiturates, carbamazepine, cholestyramine, dicloxacillin, glutethimide, ethchlorvynol, etretinate, meprobamate, griseofulvin, estrogen, oral contraceptives ("the pill"), chlorthalidone, nafcillin, rifampin, spironolactone, sucralfate, thiazide-type diuretics, trazodone, and vitamin K.

• Warfarin should not be combined with any anticoagulant supplements, including garlic, ginko biloba, chamomile, and ginseng.

Food Interactions

Warfarin is best taken on an empty stomach because food slows the rate at which it is absorbed by the blood. Vitamin K counteracts the effects of warfarin. Avoid eating large quantities of vitamin-K-rich foods, such as spinach and other green, leafy vegetables. Any change in dietary habits or alcohol intake may affect warfarin's action.

Usual Dose

Warfarin: 2–10 mg on the first day, 2–15 mg or more a day thereafter; dosage must be individualized.

Anisindione: 300 mg the first day, 200 mg the second day, 100 mg the third day, and 25–250 mg daily thereafter.

Dicumarol: 200–300 mg the first day, then 25–200 mg a day.

Overdosage

The primary symptom is bleeding. Bleeding may make itself known by the appearance of blood in the urine or stool, an unusual number of black-and-blue marks, oozing of blood from minor cuts, or bleeding from the gums after brushing the teeth. If bleeding does not stop within 10 to 15 minutes, call your doctor. Your doctor may tell you to skip a dose of warfarin or go to a hospital or doctor's office for blood evaluations, or may give you a prescription for vitamin K, which antagonizes the effect of warfarin. This last approach has some dangers because it may complicate subsequent anticoagulant therapy.

Special Information

Do not change warfarin brands without your doctor's knowledge. Different brands may not be equivalent.

Do not stop taking warfarin unless directed to do so by your doctor.

Do not stop or start ANY other medication without your doctor's or pharmacist's knowledge. Avoid alcohol, aspirin and other salicylates, and drastic changes in your diet, since all of these may affect your response.

Call your doctor if you develop unusual bleeding or bruising, red or black tarry stool, or red or dark-brown urine.

Warfarin may turn your urine a red or orange color. This is different from blood in the urine—which causes urine to appear red or brownish in color—and generally happens only if your urine has less acid in it than normal.

If you forget a dose, take it as soon as you remember, then continue with your regular schedule. If you do not remember until the next day, skip the missed dose and continue with your regular schedule. Do not take a double dose. Call your doctor if you miss a dose.

Special Populations

Pregnancy/Breast-feeding

Warfarin is not considered safe for use during pregnancy. It passes into the fetal circulation and causes bleeding, brain and other abnormalities, and stillbirth in 30% of fetuses. In some pregnant women, the benefits of taking warfarin may outweigh its risks, but the drug should not be used during the first 3 months of pregnancy. Pregnant women who need an anticoagulant are often given heparin because it does not cross into the fetal bloodstream.

Warfarin and dicumarol pass into breast milk in an inactive form. Full-term babies are not affected by warfarin but dicumarol may affect a nursing child. The effect on premature babies is not known. Nursing mothers who must take dicumarol should bottle-feed.

Seniors
Seniors may be more sensitive to the effects of warfarin and obtain maximum benefit with smaller dosages.

Wellbutrin SR   *see Bupropion, page 175*

Xalatan   *see Prostaglandin Agonists, page 903*

Type of Drug
Xanthine Bronchodilators   (ZAN-thene)

Brand Names

Generic Ingredient: Aminophylline G
Phyllocontin   Truphylline

Generic Ingredient: Dyphylline G
Dilor   Lufyllin-400
Dilor-400   Neothylline
Lufyllin

Generic Ingredient: Oxtriphylline G
Choledyl SA

Generic Ingredient: Theophylline G
Accurbron   Lanophyllin
Aerolate*   Quibron-T Dividose
Aquaphyllin   Quibron-T/SR Dividose
Asmalix   Respbid
Bronkodyl   Slo-bid Gyrocaps
Elixomin   Slo-Phyllin
Elixophyllin   Slo-Phyllin Gyrocaps

Sustaire
T-Phyl
Theo-24
Theo-Dur
Theo-Sav
Theo-X
Theobid Duracaps
Theochron
Theoclear-80

Theoclear L.A.
Theocron
Theolair
Theolair-SR
Theospan-SR
Theostat-80
Theovent
Uni-Dur
Uniphyl

*Some products in this brand-name group are alcohol- or sugar-free. Consult your pharmacist.

Prescribed For

Asthma and bronchospasm associated with emphysema, bronchitis, and other diseases; also prescribed for essential tremors and chronic obstructive pulmonary disease (COPD).

General Information

Xanthine bronchodilators are a mainstay of therapy for bronchial asthma and similar diseases. Although the dosage of each of these drugs is different, they all work by relaxing bronchial muscles and helping to reverse spasms. The exact way in which they work is not known.

Some xanthine bronchodilators are sustained-release products that act throughout the day. These minimize potential side effects by avoiding the peaks and valleys associated with immediate-release xanthine drugs. They also allow you to reduce the total number of daily doses.

Initial treatment with a xanthine bronchodilator requires your doctor to take blood samples to assess how much of the drug is in your blood. Dosage adjustments may be required based on these blood tests and on your response to the therapy. Because dyphylline is not eliminated by the liver, it is not subject to many of the drug interactions or limitations placed on the other xanthine bronchodilators.

Cautions and Warnings

Do not use a xanthine bronchodilator if you are **allergic** or **sensitive** to any of these medications. If you have a **stomach ulcer,** congestive **heart failure, heart disease, liver disease, low blood-oxygen levels,** or **high blood pressure,** or are an **alcoholic,** you should use this drug with caution. People with **seizure disorders** should not take a xanthine bronchodilator unless they are receiving appropriate anticonvulsant medicines. Theophylline may cause or worsen preexisting **abnormal heart rhythm**. Any change in heart rate or rhythm warrants your doctor's immediate attention.

Status asthmaticus, a medical condition in which the breathing passages are almost completely closed, does not respond to oral bronchodilators. Victims of this condition must be taken to a hospital emergency room at once for treatment.

Serious side effects, including convulsions, serious arrhythmias, and death, may be among the initial signs of drug toxicity. Periodic monitoring by your physician is mandatory if you are taking one of these drugs.

Dosage of dyphylline must be altered in the presence of **kidney failure**.

Possible Side Effects

Side effects are directly related to the amount of drug in your blood. As long as you stay in the proper range—below 20 mcg per ml of blood—you should experience few, if any, problems.

▼ Most common: nausea; vomiting; stomach pain; diarrhea; irritability; restlessness; difficulty sleeping; rectal irritation or bleeding, especially with suppositories; and rapid breathing.

▼ Less common: excitability, heartburn, high blood sugar, muscle twitching or spasms, heart palpitations, seizures, brain damage, or death. These effects are more likely when drug levels reach 35 mcg per ml or more.

▼ Rare: vomiting blood, regurgitating stomach contents while lying down, fever, headache, rash, hair loss, and dehydration.

Drug Interactions

• Taking two xanthine bronchodilators together may increase side effects.

• Xanthine bronchodilators are often given in combination with a stimulant drug such as ephedrine. Such combinations can cause excessive stimulation and should be used only as your doctor specifically directs.

• Reports have indicated that combining erythromycin, flu vaccine, allopurinol, beta blockers, calcium channel blockers, cimetidine—and, rarely, ranitidine—oral contraceptives, corticosteroids, disulfiram, ephedrine, interferon, mexiletine, quinolone antibacterials, or thiabendazole with a xanthine bronchodilator will increase blood levels of the xanthine bronchodilator. Higher blood levels mean the possibility of more side effects. Tetracycline may also increase the risk for xanthine bronchodilator side effects.

• The following drugs may decrease theophylline levels: aminoglutethimide, barbiturates, charcoal, ketoconazole, rifampin, sulfinpyrazone, sympathomimetic drugs, and phenytoin and other hydantoin anticonvulsants. The hydantoin level may also be reduced.

• Smoking cigarettes or marijuana makes xanthine bronchodilators less effective by increasing the rate at which your liver breaks them down. This does not apply to dyphylline.

• Drugs that may either increase or decrease xanthine bronchodilator levels include carbamazepine, isoniazid, and furosemide and other loop diuretics. Persons combining a xanthine bronchodilator with one of these drugs must be evaluated individually. Again, consult your doctor when combining xanthine bronchodilators with any of these drugs.

• People with an overactive thyroid clear xanthine bronchodilators faster and may require a larger dose. People with an underactive thyroid have the opposite reaction. Correcting thyroid function through medical or surgical treatment will normalize your response to a xanthine bronchodilator.

• A xanthine bronchodilator may counteract the sedative effect of valium and other benzodiazepine tranquilizers.

• Xanthine bronchodilators may interfere with or interact with a number of different drugs used during anesthesia. Your doctor may temporarily alter your bronchodilator dose or change drugs to avoid this problem.

• Blood lithium levels may be lowered by xanthine bronchodilators.

• Probenecid may increase the effects of dyphylline by interfering with its removal from the body through the kidneys.

• Xanthine bronchodilators may counteract the sedative effects of propofol.

Food Interactions

To obtain a consistent effect from your medication, take it at the same time each day on an empty stomach, at least 1 hour before or 2 hours after meals.

Theophylline is eliminated from the body faster if your diet is high in protein and low in carbohydrates. Eating charcoal-broiled beef also aids theophylline elimination. Conversely, the rate at which your body eliminates theophylline is reduced by a high-carbohydrate, low-protein diet. You may take some food with a liquid or immediate-release xanthine bronchodilator if it upsets your stomach. Dyphylline is not affected in this way.

Caffeine—a xanthine derivative—may add to the side effects of the xanthine bronchodilators, except dyphylline. Avoid large amounts of caffeine-containing products, such as coffee, tea, cola, cocoa, and chocolate, while taking one of these drugs.

Usual Dose

Aminophylline
  Adult (age 16 and over): 100–200 mg every 6 hours. Sustained-release—200–500 mg a day in 1–3 doses.
  Child (under age 16): 50–100 mg every 6 hours, or 1–2.5 mg per lb. of body weight every 6 hours.

Dyphylline
  Adult: up to 7 mg per lb. of body weight every 6 hours. Dosage is reduced when kidney failure is present.

Oxtriphylline
  Adult: about 2 mg per lb. of body weight every 6 hours. Sustained-release—400–600 mg every 12 hours.
  Child (age 1–9): 2.8 mg per lb. of body weight every 6 hours.

Theophylline
  Adult: up to 6 mg per lb. of body weight a day, in divided doses at 6– or 8–hour intervals, to a maximum daily dose of 900 mg. Sustained-release—same dosage, but taken 1–3 times a day.
  Child (age 12–16): up to 8.1 mg per lb. of body weight a day.
  Child (age 9–11): up to 9 mg per lb. of body weight a day.
  Child (age 1–8): up to 10.8 mg per lb. of body weight a day.
  Infant (6–52 weeks): Your doctor will calculate total daily dosage in mg by a formula that factors in age and weight. Under 6 months, give ⅓ the total daily dosage every 8 hours; age 26 weeks–1 year, give ¼ the total daily dosage every 6 hours.

Premature Infant (25 days and over): 0.68 mg per lb. of body weight every 12 hours.

Premature Infant (under 24 days): 0.45 mg per lb. of body weight every 12 hours.

Dosage of xanthine bronchodilators is often calculated on the basis of theophylline equivalents, and must be tailored to your specific condition. The best dose is the lowest that will control your symptoms. Children break down xanthine bronchodilators faster than adults and usually require more drug per lb. of body weight.

Overdosage

The first symptoms of overdose are loss of appetite, nausea, vomiting, nervousness, difficulty sleeping, headache, and restlessness. These symptoms are followed by rapid or abnormal heart rhythm, unusual behavior, extreme thirst, delirium, convulsions, very high temperature, and collapse. These serious toxic symptoms are rarely experienced after overdose by mouth, which generally produces loss of appetite, nausea, vomiting, and stimulation. The overdose victim should be taken to a hospital emergency room immediately. ALWAYS bring the prescription bottle or container.

Special Information

Do not chew or crush coated or sustained-release capsules or tablets. Doing so could result in the immediate release of large amounts of the drug, possibly causing serious side effects.

To ensure consistent effectiveness, take your medication at the same time and in the same way, with or without food, every day.

Call your doctor if you develop nausea, vomiting, heartburn, sleeplessness, jitteriness, restlessness, headache, rash, severe stomach pain, convulsions, or a rapid or irregular heartbeat. Acute drug toxicity may descend abruptly, with little or no warning; serious side effects such as convulsions, life-threatening arrhythmias, and death may result. Periodic monitoring by your physician is mandatory if you are taking a xanthine bronchodilator.

Do not change xanthine bronchodilator brands without notifying your doctor or pharmacist. Different brands of the same bronchodilator may not be identical in their effect on your body.

If you forget to take a dose of your xanthine bronchodilator, take it as soon as you remember. If it is almost time for your next dose, skip the one you forgot and continue with your regular schedule. Do not take a double dose.

Special Populations

Pregnancy/Breast-feeding

Xanthine bronchodilators pass into the fetal circulation. They do not cause birth defects, but they may produce dangerous drug levels in a newborn's bloodstream. Babies born to women who take one of these drugs may be nervous, jittery, and irritable, and may gag or vomit when fed. Pregnant women who must use a xanthine bronchodilator to control asthma or other conditions should talk with their doctors about the risks of this medication.

These drugs pass into breast milk and may cause a nursing infant to be nervous and irritable or to have difficulty sleeping. Nursing mothers who must use one of these drugs should bottle-feed.

Seniors

Seniors, especially men age 55 and over, may take longer to clear the xanthine bronchodilators from their bodies. Seniors with heart failure or other cardiac conditions, chronic lung disease, a viral infection with fever, or reduced liver function may require a lower dosage of this medication to account for the clearance effect.

Yasmin *see Contraceptives, page 290*

Generic Name

Zalcitabine (zal-SYE-tuh-bene)

Brand Name

Hivid

Type of Drug

Antiviral.

Prescribed For

Human immunodeficiency virus (HIV) infection, either alone or in combination with zidovudine (AZT).

General Information

Zalcitabine, also known as ddC or dideoxycytidine, was first approved for use in multiple-drug treatment of acquired immunodeficiency syndrome (AIDS), but it can be used alone in people who cannot tolerate AZT or whose disease has progressed while taking AZT. Zalcitabine interferes with the reproduction of the HIV virus by interrupting its internal DNA manufacturing process. DNA carries the essential genetic messages that direct all life processes; by acting on the DNA of HIV, zalcitabine interferes with the life of the HIV virus. Zalcitabine was originally approved because of its ability to increase levels of CD4 cells in the blood. CD4 cells represent the level of immune function and are considered an important indicator of the severity of an HIV infection.

Zalcitabine has been compared with didanosine (ddI) as a single-drug treatment for HIV infection. In these studies, both drugs were equally effective in prolonging the time to the next AIDS-defining event, but survival comparisons favored zalcitabine. When zalcitabine was given with AZT to people who had not previously received AZT, the combination was better than AZT alone. People who had been taking AZT and then added zalcitabine did not benefit more than people who took either drug alone.

Cautions and Warnings

Zalcitabine has caused **severe, potentially fatal side effects**. Although it is rare, people taking zalcitabine, AZT, or didanosine can develop lactic acidosis (a potentially fatal metabolic imbalance) along with an enlarged liver and liver failure.

Between 22% and 35% of people taking zalcitabine experience **nervous system inflammation**, which is generally signaled by numbness and burning pain in the hands and feet. These symptoms may be followed by sharp shooting pains or a severe and continuous burning pain. If the drug is continued, these pains may become permanent. People who already have signs of this kind of nerve damage should not take zalcitabine. Stop taking zalcitabine if the numbness, burning, and pain become moderately uncomfortable. If the symptoms improve on their own after you stop taking the drug, you may, after consultation with your doctor, start taking zalcitabine again in a smaller dosage.

Fatal inflammation of the pancreas has occurred in less than 1% of people taking zalcitabine. People with a history of pancreatic inflammation should take this drug only after careful consideration. Symptoms of inflammation of the pancreas include major changes in blood-sugar levels, rising blood levels of triglycerides, a drop in blood calcium, nausea, vomiting, and abdominal pain. People who develop pancreatic inflammation must stop taking zalcitabine.

Mouth ulcers developed in about 3% of people taking zalcitabine during clinical studies. Infrequently, people taking zalcitabine develop **ulcers of the esophagus**. People taking zalcitabine may develop heart failure. People who already have **heart failure** should take this drug only after careful consideration.

Zalcitabine can cause reductions in white- and red-blood-cell counts and should be taken with caution by people with **bone marrow disease**.

Do not take zalcitabine if you are **allergic** to it or any ingredient in the zalcitabine tablet. Zalcitabine may worsen the condition of people with **liver disease**. Death from liver failure may also occur with zalcitabine. **Alcohol abuse** aggravates the liver problems associated with zalcitabine.

Possible Side Effects

▼ Most common: peripheral neuropathy, diarrhea, abnormal liver function, mouth sores, nausea and vomiting, appetite loss, abdominal pain, itching, rash, headache, muscle ache, joint pain, tiredness, sore throat, fever, chest pain, and weight loss.

▼ Less common: swallowing difficulties, constipation, stomach irritation and ulcers, night sweats, and foot pain.

▼ Rare: Rare side effects can occur in almost any part of the body. Contact your doctor if you experience any side effect not listed above.

Drug Interactions

• Chloramphenicol, cisplatin, dapsone, didanosine, disulfiram, ethionamide, glutethimide, gold, hydralazine, iodoquinol, isoniazid, metronidazole, nitrofurantoin, phenytoin, ribavirin, vincristine, and other drugs that can cause nervous system inflammation should be avoided while taking zalcitabine.

• Drugs such as probenecid, foscarnet, cimetidine, amphotericin, and aminoglycoside-type antibiotics may interfere with the elimination of zalcitabine from the kidneys, increasing the risk of side effects.

• Drugs that may cause inflammation of the pancreas—including intravenous pentamidine—should not be taken with zalcitabine.

• Taking metoclopramide together with zalcitabine moderately reduces the amount of zalcitabine absorbed into the blood.

• Aluminum- and magnesium-based antacids may reduce the effectiveness of zalcitabine. Do not take these drugs with zalcitabine.

Food Interactions

Food interferes with the amount of zalcitabine absorbed and the speed at which it is absorbed into the blood. Take zalcitabine on an empty stomach, or 1 hour before or 2 hours after meals.

Usual Dose

Adult and Child (age 13 and over): 0.75 mg every 8 hours, usually in combination with other antiretroviral drugs. For people with poor kidney function, dosage may be reduced to 0.75 mg once or twice a day.

Overdosage

Zalcitabine overdose victims generally experience side effects of the drug, especially inflammation of the nervous system. Victims should be taken to a hospital emergency room for testing and monitoring. ALWAYS bring the prescription bottle or container.

Special Information

Zalcitabine is not an AIDS cure. It will not prevent you from transmitting the HIV virus to another person; you must still practice safe sex. Patients may still develop AIDS-related opportunistic infections while taking this drug.

Zalcitabine may cause anemia and affect other components of the blood. Your doctor should perform blood tests to check for any changes.

People taking zalcitabine must take care of their teeth and gums to minimize the risk of oral infections.

Call your doctor if you develop any of the following symptoms of zalcitabine toxicity: numbness and burning pain in the hands and feet; sharp, shooting pains or a severe and continuous burning pain; nausea; vomiting; or abdominal pain.

If you forget to take a dose of zalcitabine, take it as soon as you remember. If it is almost time for your next dose, allow 2 to 4 hours to pass between the dose you took late and your next dose, and then continue with your regular schedule. Do not take a double dose. Call your doctor for more specific advice if you forget to take several doses.

Special Populations

Pregnancy/Breast-feeding

In animal studies, zalcitabine causes the development of malformed fetuses. When this drug is considered crucial by your doctor, its potential benefits must be carefully weighed against its risks. Use effective contraception while taking zalcitabine.

It is not known if zalcitabine passes into breast milk. Nursing mothers who are HIV positive should always bottle-feed, regardless of whether they take this drug, to avoid transmitting the virus.

Seniors

People with reduced kidney function, including older adults, should receive smaller doses of zalcitabine than those with normal kidneys.

Generic Name

Zaleplon (zah-LEP-lon)

Brand Name

Sonata

Type of Drug

Hypnotic.

Prescribed For

Insomnia.

General Information

Zaleplon works on the same nerve receptors as the benzodi-azepine-type drugs, though it is chemically different from them. Zaleplon usually works within an hour. It is removed from the body relatively quickly and causes little or no "morning-after hangover" effect, which may occur with other sleeping pills. Zaleplon is broken down in the liver.

Cautions and Warnings

People with moderate **liver disease** should take the lowest effective dosage.

Take zaleplon just before you go to bed. Taking it during the day causes **tiredness** and an **inability to concentrate** and may interfere with normal activities.

People taking zaleplon nightly for an extended period of time may become **anxious** and have **trouble sleeping** when they stop the drug.

The effect of zaleplon in people with **respiratory illness** is not known.

Possible Side Effects

In studies, side effects were similar in people taking za-leplon and those taking a placebo (sugar pill).

▼ Most common: headache.

▼ Common: abdominal pain, weakness, muscle aches, memory loss, dizziness, and tiredness.

▼ Less common: fever, difficulty swallowing, tingling in the hands or feet, tremors, eye pain, unusually sensitive hearing, changes in sense of smell, and painful menstrual periods.

▼ Rare: anxiety, feeling unwell, fainting, nosebleeds, visual problems, ear pain, loss of a sense of reality or sense of self, hallucinations, reduced sensitivity to stimulation, increased sensitivity to the sun, appetite loss, and

---

Possible Side Effects *(continued)*
colitis. Other rare side effects can occur in almost any part of the body. Contact you doctor if you experience any side effect not listed above.

Drug Interactions

A number of drug interactions are possible, some of which may not appear below.

• Do not combine zaleplon and diphenhydramine (an over-the-counter antihistamine and sleeping pill).

• Zaleplon increases the depressant effects of alcohol and other nervous system depressants, imipramine, and thioridazine.

• Rifampin reduces zaleplon's effect.

• Combining zaleplon and cimetidine can almost double zaleplon blood levels. People taking cimetidine regularly for heartburn, ulcers, or stomach acid reduction should begin with the lowest effective dosage of zaleplon.

Food Interactions

Take this drug on an empty stomach, at least 2 hours after meals. High-fat meals can reduce its effectiveness.

Usual Dose

Adult: 5–10 mg at bedtime.
Senior: begin with 5 mg nightly and increase if needed.
Child: not recommended.

This medication is usually taken for 7–10 days, and rarely longer than 2–3 weeks.

Overdosage

Symptoms include dizziness, tiredness, an inability to concentrate or perform complicated tasks and can lead to coma. Take the victim to a hospital emergency room. ALWAYS bring the prescription bottle or container.

Special Information

Sleeping pills sometimes cause memory loss of events that occur during the several hours after a dose. Call your doctor if this happens.

If you see no improvement with this drug in 7 to 10 days, call your doctor.

Taking zaleplon during the day will make you drowsy and interfere with your concentration and coordination. Use it just before bedtime.

If you find that you need a larger dose of zaleplon to help you sleep, you may be developing a tolerance to the drug.

Sometimes, people who stop taking zaleplon after using it for 2 weeks or more have difficulty sleeping or become anxious. These are drug withdrawal symptoms and usually go away after 1 or 2 nights. More severe symptoms are rare.

Special Populations

Pregnancy/Breast-feeding
Taking zaleplon in the weeks just before delivery may cause tiredness or listlessness in newborns. Zaleplon should not be taken during pregnancy.

Small amounts of zaleplon pass into breast milk. Nursing mothers who must take it should bottle-feed.

Seniors
Seniors may be more sensitive to side effects.

Generic Name

Zanamivir (zuh-NAM-ih-veer)

Brand Name

Relenza

Type of Drug

Antiviral.

Prescribed For

Influenza A or B viral infection (type A or B flu).

General Information

Zanamivir is the first antiviral agent to be approved for treating flu symptoms. It must be inhaled within 2 days of the beginning of symptoms. It is inhaled directly into the nose and throat, where the influenza virus typically takes hold. Studies of zanamivir in people age 12 and over (average age was 34) suggest that people using this product feel better about 1 day sooner. Zanamivir is used to treat uncomplicated cases of the flu and is not intended for flu prevention.

Cautions and Warnings

Do not use zanamivir if you are **sensitive** or **allergic** to any ingredients in the inhalation. Stop taking zanamivir if you develop a skin rash or other signs of allergy.

People with **chronic lung problems** like asthma may not benefit from zanamivir inhalations. Also, zanamivir can cause **bronchospasm** (breathing difficulty) in a small number of people with asthma.

People using this drug are still contagious and should be careful about spreading the virus to others.

Individual virus particles can become **resistant** to zanamivir, but it is not yet known if virus infections will become resistant to zanamivir.

The safety of zanamivir in people with **severe liver disease** and in **children under age 12** is not known.

Possible Side Effects

▼ Less common: headache; diarrhea; nausea; vomiting; stuffy nose; nasal irritation; bronchitis; cough; sinus irritation; ear, nose, and throat infections; and dizziness.

▼ Rare: feeling unwell, tiredness, fever, abdominal pain, muscle aches, joint pain, and itching.

Drug Interactions

None known.

Food Interactions

Do not have any food in your mouth when you use this product.

Usual Dose

Adult and Child (age 12 and over): 2 inhalations 2 times a day for 5 days. Make sure to take 2 doses on your first day of treatment, even if they are only 2 hours apart.

Child (under age 12): consult your doctor.

Overdosage

Little is known about the effects of zanamivir overdose or accidental ingestion. Call your local poison control center or a hospital emergency room for more information.

Special Information

Make certain to complete the full 5-day course of zanamivir treatment, even if you start to feel better sooner.

Ask your doctor or pharmacist to instruct you on how to use the Diskhaler device that comes with each 5-day package of zanamivir. The drug comes in a small blister pack that is inserted into the Diskhaler. The blister pack is punctured inside the device and the powdered medication inside is drawn into the throat and nasal passages when you inhale through the Diskhaler.

Make certain that you do not have any food in your mouth when you use this product.

Special Populations

Pregnancy/Breast-feeding

Zanamivir may pass into the fetal circulation in extremely small amounts. When this drug is considered crucial by your doctor, its potential benefits must be carefully weighed against its risks.

It is not known if this drug passes into breast milk. Nursing mothers using zanamivir should consider bottle-feeding.

Seniors

Seniors may use this product without special restriction.

Zetia *see Ezetimibe, page 460*

Generic Name

Zidovudine (zih-DOE-vuh-dene) Ⓖ

Brand Name

Retrovir

Type of Drug

Antiviral.

Prescribed For

Human immunodeficiency virus (HIV) infection.

General Information

Zidovudine, also known as azidothymidine or AZT, was the first drug approved for treating HIV infection. Over the years, zidovudine use has been expanded from adults to children to the prevention of HIV transmission between a pregnant woman and her developing fetus. Zidovudine is a nucleoside reverse transcriptase inhibitor (NRTI). It works by linking itself to the HIV genetic material so the virus cannot copy itself into the cell's genetic material. Typically, antiviral treatment is first prescribed when CD4 cells—a key part of the immune system—drop to between 200 and 350.

AZT must be combined with other anti-HIV drugs. Typical drug cocktails or combinations include AZT, another nucleoside, and a protease inhibitor. Or, two nucleoside drugs can be combined with nevirapine or delavirdine. Drug combinations have become the standard of care because they can slow the progression of the disease and raise CD4 counts.

Cautions and Warnings

AZT may cause severe reductions in white- and red-blood-cell counts and should be taken with caution by people with **bone-marrow disease** or those whose bone marrow has already been compromised by other treatments. Your doctor should take a blood count every 2 weeks; if problems develop, the dosage should be reduced.

In rare instances, people taking AZT or other nucleoside-type antivirals have developed **lactic acidosis** (a potentially fatal metabolic imbalance), along with **enlargement of the liver.** Symptoms of lactic acidosis may include unexplained rapid breathing, breathing difficulties, and reduced blood-bicarbonate levels—which your doctor can detect with a routine blood test.

People with **impaired kidney or liver function** should use this drug with caution.

Prolonged use of AZT may cause **muscle irritation and abnormalities** similar to those caused by HIV infection.

Possible Side Effects

Adults

▼ Most common: anemia, reduced white-blood-cell counts, headache, fatigue, loss of appetite, vomiting, nausea, sleeplessness, and muscle aches.

▼ Less common: Less common side effects can occur in almost any part of the body. Contact your doctor if you experience any side effect not listed above.

Children

▼ Most common: anemia, reduced white-blood-cell counts, vomiting, abdominal pain, fever, cough, liver enlargement, skin rash, diarrhea, nausea, and sleeplessness.

▼ Less common: headache, blood infection, nervousness, and irritability.

▼ Rare: weight loss, seizures, heart failure and other cardiac abnormalities, blood in the urine, and bladder infections.

Drug Interactions

• Combining AZT with other drugs that can damage your kidneys, including pentamidine, dapsone, amphotericin B, flucytosine, vincristine, vinblastine, adriamycin, alfa- and beta-interferon and some experimental nucleoside analog drugs, increases the risk of loss of some kidney function.

• Avoid using AZT with stavudine, ribavirin, and doxorubicin.

• Probenecid may reduce the rate at which your body eliminates AZT, increasing the amount of the drug in your blood and the risk for side effects. Other drugs that can reduce the liver's ability to break down AZT are acetaminophen, aspirin, indomethacin, and trimethoprim; combining any of these drugs with AZT may lead to increased side effects.

• Acyclovir is often used in combination with AZT to combat opportunistic infections in AIDS patients; however, this combination may cause lethargy or seizures.

• Other drugs that can cause anemia, including ganciclovir or zalcitabine, should be used carefully in combination with AZT because of the risk of worsening drug-related anemia.

• Taking AZT together with rifampin or rifampicin may reduce the amount of AZT absorbed into the blood.

• Taking phenytoin and AZT together may affect the amounts of both drugs in the blood, usually increasing the amount of AZT. The effect on phenytoin blood levels varies. This combination can result in either too much phenytoin (leading to phenytoin side effects) or too little phenytoin (leading to a possible increase in the number of seizures). Your doctor should check your phenytoin levels if you are also taking AZT.

• Atovaquone, methadone, probenecid, trimethoprim, and valproic acid may increase blood levels of AZT.

Food Interactions

AZT is best taken on an empty stomach, but you may take it with food if it upsets your stomach.

Usual Dose

Adult: symptomatic AIDS—100 mg every 4 hours around the clock, even if sleep must be interrupted. Dosage may be reduced if side effects develop. Asymptomatic AIDS—100 mg every 4 hours during waking hours. Combination therapy with zalcitabine—200 mg of AZT with 0.8 mg of zalcitabine every 8 hours.

Pregnancy: AZT is used to prevent transmission of HIV infection to the fetus. After 14 weeks of pregnancy—100 mg 5 times a day, until labor starts. During labor and delivery—intravenously, until the umbilical cord is clamped.

Child (age 3 months–12 years): up to 100 mg every 6 hours.

Infant: about 1 mg per lb. of body weight every 6 hours by mouth, starting within 12 hours of birth and continuing through 6 weeks of age. The drug may be given intravenously if necessary.

Overdosage

The most serious effect of AZT overdose is suppression of bone marrow and its ability to make red and white blood cells. Take the victim to a hospital emergency room at once. ALWAYS bring the prescription bottle or container.

Special Information

AZT does not cure AIDS. It will not decrease the risk of your transmitting the HIV virus to another person; you must still practice safe sex. AZT may not prevent some illnesses associated with AIDS or AIDS-related complex (ARC) from continuing to develop.

See your doctor if any significant change in your health occurs. Periodic blood counts are very important while taking AZT to detect possibly serious side effects. Avoid acetaminophen, aspirin, and other drugs that may increase AZT toxicity.

Be sure to take this drug exactly as prescribed—around the clock if needed, even though it will interfere with your sleep. Do not take more AZT than your doctor has prescribed.

People taking AZT must take especially good care of their teeth and gums to minimize the risk of developing oral infections.

If you miss a dose of AZT, take it as soon as possible. If it is almost time for your next dose, allow 2 to 4 hours to pass between the dose you took late and your next dose, and then continue with your regular schedule. Do not take a double dose.

Protect AZT capsules and liquid from light.

Special Populations

Pregnancy/Breast-feeding

If you are HIV-positive and pregnant, talk to your doctor about taking or continuing your AZT. AZT treatment in HIV-positive women who are pregnant has been shown to sharply reduce the risk of transmitting the HIV virus to babies. Treatment should begin by the 14th week of pregnancy and continue through delivery. The baby should also be given AZT for the first 6 weeks of life. Studies have shown that the risk of birth defects is not increased by taking AZT during pregnancy.

It is not known if AZT passes into breast milk. Nursing mothers with HIV should always bottle-feed, regardless of whether they take this drug, to avoid transmitting the virus.

Seniors

Seniors may be at a greater risk of side effects due to reduced kidney function.

Generic Name

Ziprasidone (zih-PRAS-uh-done)

Brand Name

Geodon

Type of Drug

Antipsychotic.

Prescribed For

Schizophrenia.

General Information

Ziprasidone may be prescribed for people who have not been helped by other antipsychotics or for whom other antipsychotics have stopped working. Ziprasidone affects the neurotransmitters serotonin and dopamine in the brain, normalizing their chemical balance and relieving symptoms of schizophrenia.

Cautions and Warnings

Do not take ziprasidone if you are **sensitive** or **allergic** to it.

Ziprasidone can affect **heart function,** leading to potentially fatal abnormal heart rhythms called *torsade de pointes.* Ziprasidone may affect the heart more acutely than other antipsychotic medicines. The chances of developing this abnormal heart rhythm increase if your blood potassium or magnesium levels are too low.

Sudden unexplained death has occurred with ziprasidone, as it has with other antipsychotic drugs.

Neuroleptic malignant syndrome (NMS), a potentially fatal group of symptoms associated with ziprasidone and other psychiatric drugs, can occur. NMS consists of very **high fever, muscle rigidity, mental changes, irregular pulse or blood pressure, rapid heartbeat, sweating, and abnormal heart rhythm**. NMS is potentially fatal and requires **immediate medical attention**.

Ziprasidone may produce **extrapyramidal side effects,** including spasm of the neck muscles, rolling back of the eyes, convulsions, difficulty swallowing, and symptoms associated with Parkinson's disease. These side effects usually disappear after the drug has been stopped, although symptoms affecting the face, tongue, or jaw may persist for as long as several years, especially in older adults with a history of brain damage. Contact your doctor if you experience any of these side effects.

Antipsychotic drugs, including ziprasidone, may cause **involuntary movements** of the face and tongue called tardive dyskinesia, which may become permanent. Contact your doctor if you develop any of these side effects.

Possible Side Effects

▼ Most common: sleepiness and nausea.

▼ Common: itching, weakness, rapid heartbeat, dizziness, constipation, upset stomach, diarrhea, inability to remain in a sitting position, restlessness and a feeling of muscular quivering, extrapyramidal symptoms (see "Cautions and Warnings"), and respiratory conditions.

▼ Less common: accidental injury, rash, fungus infection of the skin, dry mouth, appetite loss, muscle aches, abnormal muscle tone, rigid muscles, runny nose, coughing, and abnormal vision.

▼ Rare: fainting and seizures. Other rare side effects can occur in almost any part of the body. Contact your doctor if you experience any side effect not listed above.

Drug Interactions

• Do not mix ziprasidone with other drugs that can affect the heart. Some drugs to avoid are quinidine, dofetilide, pimozide, sotalol, thioridazine, moxifloxacin, and sparfloxacin.

• Ziprasidone can increase the effects of sedatives, tranquilizers, and other nervous system depressants.

• Ziprasidone may increase the effect of drugs that lower blood pressure.

• Delavirdine, indinavir, nelfinavir, ritonavir, saquinavir, amiodarone, ciprofloxacin, clarithromycin, diltiazem, erythromycin, fluconazole, fluvoxamine, itraconazole, ketoconazole, mifepristone, nefazodone, norfloxacin, mibefradil, and troleandomycin may increase the amount of ziprasidone in the blood by interfering with its breakdown in the liver.

• Carbamazepine, phenobarbital, phenytoin, rifampin, and rifampicin may reduce ziprasidone blood levels.

Food Interactions

Grapefruit juice may interfere with the breakdown of ziprasidone. Take this drug with food.

Usual Dose

Adult: 20–100 mg twice a day. The lowest effective dose is recommended.

Child: not recommended.

Overdosage

In one person who overdosed, the only side effects that developed were minimal sedation, slurring of speech, and a rise in blood pressure that decreased with time. Overdose victims should be taken to a hospital emergency room at once for monitoring and treatment. ALWAYS bring the prescription bottle or container.

Special Information

Avoid alcohol when taking ziprasidone, as with other antipsychotics.

Ziprasidone may take a few weeks to work. Keep taking this drug for as long as your doctor instructs. Do not stop taking ziprasidone if you are feeling better.

Be sure to notify your doctor if you have or had heart disease.

Call your doctor if you become dizzy, faint or have heart palpitations (signs of torsade de pointes), very high fever, muscle rigidity, mental changes, irregular pulse or blood pressure, rapid heartbeat, sweating, or abnormal heart rhythms (signs of NMS).

Rash is common with ziprasidone and may be a sign of a more serious illness. Call your doctor at once if a rash develops.

Some antipsychotics like ziprasidone can interfere with the body's temperature-regulating mechanism. Avoid extreme heat when taking this drug.

Ziprasidone can make you sleepy. Be careful driving and engaging in activities that require coordination and concentration, especially when you first start taking ziprasidone.

If you forget to take a dose of ziprasidone and it is within 2 hours of your next dose, take the dose you forgot. Otherwise, skip the dose you forgot and continue with your regular schedule. Do not take a double dose.

Special Populations

Pregnancy/Breast-feeding

Ziprasidone may make it more difficult for women to become pregnant. Animal studies suggest that ziprasidone can cause birth defects and fetal death. When this drug is considered crucial by your doctor, its potential benefits must be weighed against its risks.

It is not known if ziprasidone passes into breast milk. Nursing mothers who must take this drug should bottle-feed.

Seniors

Seniors may take this medicine without special restriction. Older adults may experience more side effects.

Zithromax see Azithromycin, page 131

Zocor see Statin Cholesterol-Lowering Agents, page 987

Zoloft see Selective Serotonin Reuptake Inhibitors (SSRIs), page 965

Generic Name

Zolpidem (ZOLE-pih-dem)

Brand Name

Ambien

Type of Drug

Sedative.

Prescribed For

Insomnia.

General Information

Zolpidem is a nonbenzodiazepine sleeping pill that works in the brain in much the same way as do benzodiazepine sleeping pills and tranquilizers. Unlike the benzodiazepines, however, zolpidem has little muscle-relaxing or antiseizure effects. It is meant for short-term use—7 to 10 days—and should not be taken regularly for longer than that without your doctor's knowledge. Unlike a benzodiazepine, zolpidem causes little or no "hangover," and there are no rebound effects after stopping the drug. Zolpidem is broken down in the liver.

Cautions and Warnings

Sleeping problems often result from a **physical or psychological illness**. Zolpidem does not affect the underlying causes of insomnia. It should be taken only with your doctor's knowledge. If you cannot sleep after 7 to 10 days of taking zolpidem, contact your doctor.

Zolpidem has caused **amnesia** (memory loss), but this happens mostly at dosages larger than 10 mg a night.

Suddenly stopping zolpidem after having taken it for some time may produce **drug withdrawal** (symptoms include fatigue, nausea, flushing, light-headedness, crying, vomiting, stomach cramps, panic, nervousness, and general discomfort). People with a history of substance abuse may be more likely to develop **drug dependence** on zolpidem.

Zolpidem is a nervous system depressant and may cause **loss of coordination and concentration**. It should be taken just before bedtime. Zolpidem may interfere with normal activities the next day, especially if taken with alcohol.

People with **liver disease** require reduced dosage. People with severe **kidney disease** should be monitored for side effects.

Zolpidem should be avoided in the presence of severe **depression,** severe **lung disease, sleep apnea** (condition characterized by intermittent cessation of breathing during sleep), and **drunkenness** or you run the risk of increasing the depressive effects of zolpidem or worsening your overall condition.

Possible Side Effects

Short-Term Use (10 Days or Less)

▼ Most common: headache, drowsiness, dizziness, nausea, and diarrhea.

▼ Less common: chest pain, fatigue, unusual dreams, memory loss, anxiety, nervousness, difficulty sleeping, appetite loss, vomiting, and runny nose.

▼ Rare: Rare side effects can occur in almost any part of the body. Contact your doctor if you experience any side effect not listed above.

Long-Term Use

▼ Most common: headache, dizziness, nausea, drowsiness, and a feeling of being drugged.

▼ Common: allergy symptoms, back pain, flu-like symptoms, lethargy, sensitivity to light, depression, upset stomach, constipation, abdominal pain, muscle and joint pain, upper respiratory infection, sinus irritation, sore throat, rash, urinary infection, heart palpitations, and dry mouth.

Drug Interactions

• Avoid combining zolpidem with alcohol and other nervous system depressants including tranquilizers, narcotics, barbiturates, antidepressants, and antihistamines. Taking a benzodiazepine such as diazepam with zolpidem may result in excessive depression, tiredness, sleepiness, breathing difficulties, or similar symptoms.

Food Interactions

For the most rapid and complete effect, take zolpidem on an empty stomach at least 2 hours after a meal.

Usual Dose

Adult (age 18 and over): 10 mg immediately before bedtime. Zolpidem can act very quickly.

Senior: 5 mg immediately before bedtime.

Child: not recommended.

People with liver disease should take 5 mg.

Overdosage

Overdose results in excessive nervous system depression, from unconsciousness to light coma. Combining zolpidem with alcohol or other nervous system depressants may be fatal or affect other body organs. Take the victim to a hospital emergency room at once. ALWAYS bring the prescription bottle or container.

Special Information

Zolpidem may cause tiredness, drowsiness, and an inability to concentrate. Be careful when driving or performing any task that requires concentration on the day following a dose.

People taking zolpidem on a regular basis may develop a drug withdrawal reaction if the medication is stopped suddenly (see "Cautions and Warnings").

If you forget a dose, take it as soon as you remember. If it is almost time for your next dose, skip the forgotten one and continue with your regular schedule. Do not take a double dose.

Special Populations

Pregnancy/Breast-feeding

Animal studies with large dosages show that zolpidem may affect the fetus. When this drug is considered crucial by your doctor, its potential benefits must be carefully weighed against its risks.

Small amounts of zolpidem pass into breast milk. Nursing mothers who must take this drug should bottle-feed.

Seniors

Seniors, who are likely to be more sensitive to zolpidem and its side effects, should take the lowest effective dosage.

Generic Name

Zonisamide (zoh-NIS-uh-mide)

Brand Name

Zonegran

Type of Drug

Anticonvulsant.

Prescribed For

Partial seziures.

General Information

Zonisamide was available in Japan for 11 years before it was approved for sale in the U.S. The exact way that this drug works is unknown, but studies suggest it may affect sodium and calcium flow in and out of nerve cells. It does not affect the neurotransmitter GABA, unlike some other anticonvulsant medicines.

Cautions and Warnings

Do not take zonisamide if you are **sensitive** or **allergic** to it or to **sulfa drugs**.

Zonisamide has been associated with **central nervous system** side effects, including depression, psychosis, sleepiness, psychomotor slowing, and difficulty concentrating.

People with severe **kidney disease** may accumulate ⅓ more zonisamide in their blood than others. Lower dosages may be required.

Unexplained skin rash may be a sign of a severe reaction that can be fatal. Contact your doctor immediately if you experience this side effect.

Possible Side Effects

▼ Most common: sleepiness, appetite loss, dizziness, headache, nausea, agitation, and irritability.

▼ Common: anxiety, poor muscle coordination, confusion, depression, difficulty concentrating, memory problems, sleeplessness, abdominal pain, and double vision.

▼ Less common: kidney stones, mental slowing, tiredness, unusual eye movements, tingling in the hands or feet, psychotic behavior, constipation, diarrhea, upset stomach, verbal difficulty, taste changes, dry mouth, easy bruising, flu symptoms, rash, runny nose, and weight loss.

▼ Rare: Rare side effects can occur in almost any part of the body. Contact your doctor if you experience any side effect not listed above.

Drug Interactions

Some drugs can increase the amount of zonisamide in the blood by inhibiting enzymes that break it down in the liver. They include delavirdine, indinavir, ritonavir, saquinavir, amiodarone, cimetidine, ciprofloxacin, clarithromycin, diltiazem, erythromycin, fluconazole, fluvoxamine, itraconazole, ketoconazole, mifepristone, nefazodone, norfloxacin, mibefradil, and troleandomycin.

• Some drugs may reduce the amount of zonisamide in the blood by stimulating enzymes that break it down in the liver. They include efavirenz, nevirapine, carbamazepine, corticosteroids, modafinil, phenobarbital and other barbiturates, phenytoin, pioglitazone, and rifampin.

Food Interactions

Zonisamide may be taken with or without food. Avoid drinking grapefruit juice with zonisamide because it can interfere with enzymes that break down the drug.

Usual Dose

100–400 mg a day. Most people taking zonisamide do well with doses in the 100–200 mg range. Higher doses may offer some additional benefit, but they are also associated with an increase in drug side effects.

Overdosage

Overdose symptoms primarily affect the central nervous system, including very low heart rate, coma, low blood pressure, and difficulty breathing. Take the victim to a hospital emergency room. ALWAYS bring the prescription bottle or container.

Special Information

Call your doctor at once if you develop an unexplained skin rash. This may be a sign of a severe reaction.

Sudden back pain, abdominal pain, and blood in the urine may be signs of a kidney stone. Drink plenty of water every day to avoid this problem. Contact your doctor if you experience any of these side effects.

Fever, sore throat, ulcers, and easy bruising can be signs of a blood problem related to zonisamide. Contact your doctor if any of these symptoms develop.

Zonisamide may make you drowsy. Be careful while driving or performing any tasks that require coordination and alertness.

If you forget a dose of zonisamide, take it as soon as you remember. If it is almost time for your next dose, skip the dose you forgot and continue with your regular schedule. Do not take a double dose.

Special Populations

Pregnancy/Breast-feeding

Animal studies of zonisamide have shown it can cause birth defects. Seizure disorder itself has been associated with increased risk of birth defects. Discuss with your doctor the need to control seizure and the potential benefits and risks of taking this medication during pregnancy.

It is not known if zonisamide passes into breast milk. Women taking zonisamide should bottle-feed or talk to their doctor about switching to a different drug.

Seniors

Seniors may require a lower dose of zonisamide due to normal reductions in kidney or liver function.

Zyprexa   see *Olanzapine*, page 795

Zyrtec   see *Cetirizine*, page 216

Twenty Questions to Ask Your Doctor and Pharmacist About Your Prescription

Many pharmacies now routinely hand out prescription drug "fact sheets" when a medication is first prescribed. If your pharmacist does not provide you with one, ask him or her for a copy.

1. What is the name of this medication?

2. What results may be expected from taking it?

3. How long should I wait before reporting if this medication does not help me?

4. How does the medication work?

5. What is the exact dosage of the medication?

6. What time of day should I take it?

7. Do alcoholic beverages have an effect on this medication?

8. Do I have to take special precautions with this medication in combination with other prescription medications I am taking?

9. Do I have to take special precautions with this medication in combination with over-the-counter (OTC) medications?

10. Does food have any effect on this medication?

11. Are there any special instructions I should have about how to use this medication?

12. How long should I continue taking this medication?

13. Is my prescription renewable?

14. For how long a period may my prescription be renewed?

15. Which side effects should I report, and which ones may I disregard?

16. May I save any unused part of this medication for future use?

17. How should I store this medication?

18. How long may I keep this medication without it losing its strength?

19. What should I do if I miss a dose of this medication?

20. Does this medication come in a less expensive, generic form?

Other Points to Remember for Safe Drug Use

- Store your medications in a sealed, light-resistant container to maintain maximum potency, and be sure to follow any special storage instructions listed on your prescription bottle or container, such as "refrigerate," "do not freeze," "protect from light," or "keep in a cool place." Protect all medications from excessive humidity; do not keep them in your bathroom medicine cabinet.
- Make sure each doctor you see knows about all the medications you use regularly, including prescription and over-the-counter (OTC) medications.
- Keep a record of any bad reaction you have had to a medication.
- Fill each prescription you are given. If you do not fill a prescription, make sure your doctor knows you are not taking the medication.
- Try to fill your prescriptions at the same pharmacy each time. Your pharmacist will keep a record of all your prescription and OTC medications. This listing, called a *Patient Drug Profile,* is used to check for potential problems. You may want to keep your own drug profile and take it to your pharmacist for review whenever a new medication is added.
- Do not take extra medication without consulting your doctor or pharmacist.
- Follow the label instructions exactly. If you have any questions, call your doctor or pharmacist.
- Report any unusual symptoms that develop after taking any medication.
- Always read the label before taking your medication. Do not trust your memory.

- Do not share your medication with anyone. Your prescription was written for you and only you. Do not use a prescription medication unless it has been specifically prescribed for you.
- Be sure the label stays on the container until the medication is used or destroyed.
- Keep the label facing up when pouring liquid medication from the bottle so that it is not obscured by spilled medicine.
- For liquid medication, do not forget to shake the bottle, unless directed otherwise.
- If you move to another city, ask your pharmacist to forward your prescription records to your new pharmacy. Carry important medical facts about yourself in your wallet. Such things as drug allergies, chronic diseases (e.g., diabetes), and special requirements may be very useful. Whenever you travel, carry your prescription in its original container.

Safe Use of Eyedrops

To administer eyedrops, lie down or tilt your head back. Hold the dropper above your eye, gently squeeze your lower lid to form a small pouch, and release the drop or drops of medication inside your lower lid while looking up. Release the lower lid, keeping your eye open. Do not blink for 40 seconds. Press gently on the bridge of your nose at the inside corner of your eye for 1 minute to help circulate the drug in your eye. To avoid infection, do not touch the dropper tip to your finger, eyelid, or any other surface. Wait at least 5 minutes before using another eyedrop or eye ointment.

Safety Tips for Self-Injectables

Syringe Storage, Disposal, and Safety
- Store your syringes and needles where others do not have access to them. Some medicines come in prefilled syringes. Store them according to label directions.
- Do not reuse needles or syringes.

- After you have finished using a syringe and needle, cut the needle off and dispose of the needle and syringe in a puncture-resistant, non-see-through container used only for this purpose. Containers specifically designed for needle and syringe disposal can be obtained from a pharmacy.
- Most needles have a device built in so that you may safely cut the needle off. If you do not have one of these devices, you can break the needle off by covering the needle with its protective sheath and working it back and forth until it breaks. Broken needles should be discarded in your disposal device or plastic container.
- Keep containers in areas that are child- and animal-proof.
- When the container is full, seal it securely and throw the entire container away with your regular garbage. Do not throw loose syringes into the garbage.
- Do not put containers filled with used syringes in your recycling bin.
- Do not throw loose needles or lancets into the recycling bin or trash.
- Do not put needles and syringes in soda cans or bottles, glass containers, or milk cartons.
- Do not flush needles or lancets down the toilet.

Choosing an Injection Site
Choose an area for injection (site) where the skin is loose and soft (flabby), away from joints, nerves, and bones. Try to avoid the panty or belt line at the waist and the seat portion of your buttocks, as daily activity may irritate these areas.

Good places to use for subcutaneous (under the skin) injection include:
- Arms (outer and upper back portion)
- Abdomen (except around navel and waistline)
- Buttocks (upper outer area)
- Thighs (front and sides except at groin and knee)

Rotating Injection Sites
Change the site where you inject your medicine each time. This helps prevent reactions at the injection site. It also gives the site time to heal from the last injection. Keep a record of where and when you last gave yourself an injection to make sure you do not use the same site too often. If your regular injection areas become tender, talk to your doctor about other possible injection sites.

Self Injection and Administering Injections to Another Person

- Before you begin, gather your needle and syringe, medicine, alcohol swabs and cotton balls, or gauze pad. Be sure you also have your needle disposal container nearby.
- Do not use an injection solution if it has particles floating in it.
- Certain injection mixtures should not be shaken. Refer to your product patient information for specific instruction.
- Wash your hands.
- Choose an area for injection. Use a different site each day. Do not use any area in which you feel lumps, bumps, firm knots, or pain. Do not use any area in which the skin is discolored, depressed, scabbed, or has broken open.
- You may use an alcohol swab to clean the skin at the injection site. Let the area air dry. Discard the wipe. Uncap the needle.
- Slowly draw the exact amount of drug prescribed into the syringe being careful to avoid air bubbles in the solution to be injected.
- Pinch up the skin to prevent injecting the drug into a muscle and pull back slightly on the plunger to make sure you have not entered a vein.
- Hold the syringe like a pencil or dart and insert the needle at a 45° angle to the skin.
- If blood enters the syringe, remove it and throw it away.
- If no blood enters the syringe, slowly depress the syringe plunger until the contents have been completely injected.
- Hold another alcohol swab on the injection site. Remove the needle from the skin. Gently massage the injection site with a dry cotton ball or gauze pad.
- You may ice the area before and after injection to reduce pain and inflammation.
- If injecting into the leg, extend your leg out to reduce the chance of injecting into a muscle.
- Your doctor, nurse, or pharmacist can help you master this procedure.

Complications of Self-Injection

- You may notice bruising around the injection. This is due to the piercing of tiny blood vessels and is generally not a problem.
- Sometimes harmless but unsightly lumpy areas develop at injection sites. This is due to an increase in fatty tissue

at the site of injection, especially when injecting daily insulin. Avoid injecting into these fatty lumps.

- Visible depressions in the skin may develop due to a loss of fat tissue at the injection site.
- To avoid infection at injection sites, always wash your hands before you begin the procedure, do not touch the bare needle before the actual injection, and do not reuse or share needles with another person.
- Call your doctor if an injection site becomes infected. Signs of infection include redness, pain, swelling, and possible oozing. You may apply a non-prescription antibiotic cream or ointment to that area, but your doctor should be aware of this complication.

Medicine and Money

- Make sure you tell the doctor everything that is wrong. More information allows your doctor to provide the most effective treatment.
- Do not hesitate to discuss the cost of medical care with your doctor or pharmacist.
- Generic drugs are usually less expensive than brand-name drugs, whether you pay for them out-of-pocket or have a co-pay with your insurance company. A drug often becomes available generically when its patent has expired, typically 20 years after the patent was granted.
- If you suffer from a chronic condition, you will probably save money by buying in larger quantities.
- Prescription prices vary from pharmacy to pharmacy; it may be worthwhile to comparison shop for the more expensive medications. Internet pharmacies may also have low-cost prescription drugs available, although you must allow additional time for delivery. Many pharmacies will match internet prices, if requested.
- Some insurance companies offer discounted quantities of prescription drugs through a mail-order pharmacy program. Most mail order programs will fill a three-month supply of medication and only charge the co-pay for a two-month supply. Again, extra time must be factored in for delivery.

THE TOP 200 PRESCRIPTION DRUGS IN THE UNITED STATES

RANKED BY NUMBER OF PRESCRIPTIONS DISPENSED FROM JANUARY TO DECEMBER 2003

(Note: Generic drugs by different manufacturers have been combined.)

1. Hydrocodone with APAP
2. Lipitor
3. Synthroid
4. Atenolol
5. Albuterol
6. Furosemide
7. Lisinopril
8. Hydrochlorothiazide
9. Amoxicillin
10. Norvasc
11. Zoloft
12. Alprazolam
13. Toprol-XL
14. Zocor
15. Prevacid
16. Propoxyphene-N with APAP
17. Zithromax Z-Pak
18. Premarin
19. Triamterene with hydrochlorothiazide
20. Zyrtec
21. Cephalexin
22. Metformin
23. Levoxyl
24. Celebrex
25. Prednisone
26. Ambien
27. Metoprolol
28. Fluoxetine
29. Fosamax
30. Allegra
31. Nexium
32. Lorazepam
33. Potassium chloride
34. Vioxx
35. Singulair
36. Ortho Tri-Cyclen
37. Neurontin
38. APAP with codeine
39. Ranitidine
40. Effexor XR
41. Protonix
42. Celexa
43. Plavix

44. Paxil
45. Warfarin
46. Viagra
47. Wellbutrin SR
48. Amitriptyline
49. Pravachol
50. Ibuprofen
51. Trimox
52. Clonazepam
53. Advair Diskus
54. Trazodone
55. Lexapro
56. Flonase
57. Amoxicillan with potassium clavulanate
58. Enalapril
59. Levaquin
60. Sulfamethoxazole with trimethoprim
61. Accupril
62. Naproxen
63. Cyclobenzaprine
64. Zithromax
65. Altace
66. Diovan
67. Omeprazole
68. Diazepam
69. Coumadin
70. Lotrel
71. Isosorbide mononitrate
72. Glucotrol XL
73. Risperdal
74. Diflucan
75. Verapamil SR
76. Tramadol
77. Zyprexa
78. Clarinex
79. Glyburide
80. Bextra
81. Digitek
82. Allopurinol
83. Penicillin VK
84. Actos
85. Carisoprodol
86. Cozaar
87. Oxycodone with APAP
88. Clonidine
89. Doxycycline
90. Avandia
91. Folic acid
92. Diovan HCT
93. Aspirin
94. Promethazine
95. Paxil CR
96. Flomax
97. Lisinopril with hydrochlorothiazide
98. Ortho Evra
99. Cipro
100. Methylprednisolone
101. Aciphex
102. Seroquel
103. Lotensin
104. Nasonex
105. Glucophage XR
106. Evista
107. Actonel
108. Xalatan
109. OxyContin
110. Lanoxin
111. Allegra-D
112. Spironolactone
113. Levothroid
114. Amaryl
115. Doxazosin
116. Tricor
117. Hyzaar
118. Combivent
119. Depakote
120. Estradiol
121. Amoxil
122. Temazepam
123. Flovent
124. Concerta
125. Glucovance
126. Metoclopramide
127. Prilosec
128. Gemfibrozil

129. Famotidine
130. Adderall XR
131. Hydroxyzine
132. Metronidazole
133. Acetaminophen
134. Yasmin
135. Valtrex
136. Imitrex
137. Detrol LA
138. Meclizine
139. Aricept
140. Docusate sodium
141. Lantus
142. Coreg
143. Avapro
144. Prempro
145. Bisoprolol
     fumarate with
     hydrochlorothiazide
146. Glipizide
147. Promethazine with
     codeine
148. Buspirone
149. Endocet
150. Duragesic
151. Ultracet
152. Topamax
153. Nystatin
154. Minocycline
155. Humulin
156. Clindamycin
157. Klor-Con
158. Zetia
159. Terazosin
160. Cartia XT
161. Skelaxin
162. Monopril
163. Propranolol
164. Macrobid

165. Ferrous sulfate
166. Dilantin
167. Butalbital with APAP
     and caffeine
168. Rhinocort Aqua
169. Nasacort AQ
170. Medroxyprogesterone
171. Carbidopa with
     levodopa
172. Omnicef
173. Augmentin ES
174. Lovastatin
175. Acyclovir
176. Captopril
177. MiraLax
178. Guaifenesin/CD
179. Bactroban
180. Ditropan XL
181. Paroxetine
182. Aviane
183. Timolol
184. Cefzil
185. Clotrimazole with
     dexamethasone
186. Patanol
187. Triamcinolone
188. Methotrexate
189. Nortriptyline
190. Biaxin XL
191. Ciprofloxacin
192. Quinine
193. Zyrtec-D
194. Humalog
195. Miacalcin
196. Biaxin
197. Phenobarbital
198. Nitroglycerin
199. Niaspan
200. Inderal LA

Source: IMS Health, 2004.

Index of Generic and Brand-Name Drugs

A

Abacavir, 3, 1128
Abilify, 108, plate A
Acarbose, 6
Accolate, 617, plate A
AccuNeb, 38
Accupril, 912, plate A
Accurbron, 1155
Accuretic 10/12.5, 912

Accuretic 20/12.5, 912
Accutane, 595, plate A
Acebutolol, 9
Aceon, 913
Acephen, 13
Aceta, 13
Acetaminophen, 13, 254, 480,
    832, 833, 895, 1087
Acetaminophen Uniserts, 13
Aceta with Codeine, 833
Acetazolamide, 16
Acetohexamide, 1003
Achromycin V, 1044
Aciphex, 906, plate A
Acitretin, 19
Aclovate, 317
Acrivastine, 94
Acticin, 844
Acticort 100, 318
Actiq Lozenge on a Stick, 282
Activella, 445
Actonel, 159, plate A
Actos, 526, plate A
Acular Eyedrops, 599
Acyclovir, 23
Adalat, 775
Adalat CC, 775, plate A
Adapalene, 26
Adderall, 29, plate A
Adderall XR, 29
Adefovir, 32
Adoxa, 1043
Adprin-B, 111
Advair Diskus, 958
Advicor, 987, plate A
Advil, 549
AeroBid, 303
AeroBid-M, 303
Aerolate, 1155
Aeroseb-Dex, 317
Agenerase, 72
Aggrenox, 35, plate A
Agrylin, 77
Airet, 38

AK Beta, 148
AK-Dex, 300
Akne-mycin, 437
AK-Pred, 300
AK-Spore, 759
AK-Spore H.C. Otic, 322
Ak-Zol, 16
Ala-Cort, 318
Alamast, 819
Ala-Scalp, 318
Ala-Tet, 1044
Alavert, 651
Albuterol, 38
Albuterol Sulfate, 585
Alclometasone Dipropionate,
    317
Aldactazide, 393, plate A
Aldactone, 42
Aldara, 559
Aldomet, 688
Aldosterone Blockers, 42
Alendronate, 158
Alesse, 289
Aleve, 748
Alferon N, 578
Alfuzosin, 51
Alinia, 783
Alitretinoin, 45
Alka-Seltzer with Aspirin, 111
Allay, 833
Allegra, 216, plate A
Allegra-D, 96, plate B
Allergen Ear Drops, 129
AllerMax, 369
Allopurinol, 48
Almotriptan, 1120
Alocril, 328
Alomide Eyedrops, 603
Alora Transdermal System, 445
Alosetron, 90
Alpha Blockers, 51
Alphagan, 173
Alphagan P, 173
Alphatrex, 317

Alprazolam, 55
Alprostadil, 58
Alrex, 300
Altace, 913, plate B
Altocor, 986
Alupent, 680
Amaphen, 483
Amaryl, 1003, plate B
Ambien, 1178, plate B
Amcinonide, 317
Amen, 664
Amerge, 1120
Amiloride, 393
Aminolevulinic Acid, 61
Aminophylline, 1155
Amiodarone, 63
Amitriptyline, 1113
Amlexanox, 67
Amlodipine, 69, 653
Amodopa, 688
Amoxapine, 1113
Amoxicillin, 825, 906
Amoxil, 825, plate B
Amphetamine Aspartate, 29
Amphetamine Sulfate, 29
Ampicillin, 825
Amprenavir, 72
Amvaz, 69
Anafranil, 1113
Anagrelide, 77
Anakinra, 79
Analpram-HC, 318
Anamine, 95
Anamine T.D., 95
Anaplex, 95
Anaprox, 748
Anaprox DS, 748
Anaspaz, 381
Anastrozole, 82
Anatuss LA, 421
Ancobon, 492, plate B
**Androderm Transdermal
    System**, 1039
Androgel, 1039

Android, 1040
Anexsia 5/500, 833
Anexsia 7.5/650, 833
Anexsia 10/660, 833
Angiotensin II Blockers, 84
Anisindione, 1150
Anoquan, 483
Ansaid, 550, plate B
Anspor, 211
Antagon, 659
Antibiotic, 322
Antiemetics (5HT3 Type), 90
Antihistamine-Decongestant
    Combination Products, 94
Antihistamine Eyedrops, 99
Antipyrine, 129
Antivert, 366, plate B
Antivert 25, 366
Antrizine, 366
Anucort-HC, 318
Anumed HC, 318
Anusol-HC, 318
Anzemet, 90
Apacet, 13
Aphthasol, 67
Apraclonidine, 102
Aprepitant, 105
Apresoline, 544
Apri, 290
Aquaphyllin, 1155
Aquatab, 421
Aquatensen, 1053
Arava, 615
Arestin, 1043
Aricept, 239, plate B
Arimidex, 82
Aripiprazole, 108
Aristocort, 311, 319
Aristocort A, 319
Armour Thyroid, 1059
Aromasin, 458
**Arthritis Foundation Pain
    Reliever**, 111
Arthritis Pain Formula, 111

Arthrotec, 550, plate C
Asacol, 169
Ascriptin, 111
Asendin, 1113
Asmalix, 1155
A-Spas S/L, 381
Aspergum, 111
Aspirin, 35, 111, 427, 483, 486, 837, 895, 987
Aspirin Free Anacin Maximum Strength, 13
Aspirin Free Pain Relief, 13
Asprimox, 111
Astelin, 216
Atacand, 84, plate C
Atapryl, 971
Atarax, 547, plate C
Atazanavir Sulfate, 115
Atenolol, 119
Ativan, 347, plate C
Atolone, 311
Atomoxetine, 123
Atorvastatin, 986
Atovaquone, 126
Atretol, 193
Atridox, 1043
Atrohist Pediatric, 95, 96
Atromid-S, 259
Atropine Sulfate, 381, 733
Atrovent, 584
A/T/S, 437
Augmented Betamethasone Dipropionate, 317
Augmentin, 825, plate C
Augmentin ES-600, 825
Augmentin XR, 825, plate C
Auralgan Otic, 129
Auroto Otic, 129
Avage, 1019
Avalide, 84, plate C
Avandamet, 526
Avandia, 526, plate C
Avapro, 84, plate C
Avelox, 495, plate D

Aventyl, 1113
Aventyl Pulvules, 1113
Aviane, 289
Avita, 1099
Avodart, 477
Avonex, 581
Axert, 1120, plate D
Axid, 793, plate D
Axid AR, 793
Aygestin, 664
Azatadine, 95
Azatadine Maleate, 225
Azelastine, 99, 216, 800
Azithromycin, 131
Azmacort, 303
Azopt, 196
Azulfidine, 998
Azulfidine EN-Tabs, 998

B

Bacampicillin, 825
Baclofen, 134
Bactine Hydrocortisone, 318
Bactocill, 825
Bactrim, 974
Bactrim DS, 974, plate D
Bactrim Pediatric, 974
Bactroban, 735
Balsalazide, 169
Bancap HC, 833
Banophen, 369
Barbidonna, 381
Bayer, 111
Bayer Select Pain Relief Formula, 549
Becaplermin, 137
Beclomethasone Dipropionate, 302, 306
Beclovent, 302
Beconase AQ, 306
Beepen-VK, 826
Belladonna Alkaloids, 381
Bellatal, 381, 851

Bemote, 351
Benadryl Allergy, 369
Benazepril, 139
Benazepril Hydrochloride, 653
Bendroflumethiazide, 1052
Benicar, 85
Benicar HCT, 85
Bentyl, 351, plate D
Benzamycin, 437
Benzocaine, 129
Bepridil, 142
Betaderm, 317
Betagan, 148
Betaine, 145
Betamethasone, 310, 317
Betamethasone Dipropionate, 657
Betapace, 1069
Betapace AF, 1069
Betapen-VK, 826
Betaseron, 581
Betatrex, 317
Beta-Val, 317
Betaxolol, 147, 154
Betaxon, 148
Betimol, 148
Betoptic, 147
Betoptic S, 147
Bextra, 206, plate D
Biaxin, 250, plate D
Biaxin Filmtabs, 250
Biaxin XL, 250, plate D
Bicalutamide, 151
Bimatoprost, 902
Biohist-LA, 95
Bio-Tab, 1043
Bismuth Subsalicylate, 540
Bisoprolol, 154
Bisphosphonates, 158
Bitolterol, 164
Blocadren, 1069, plate D
Bonine, 366
Bonviva, 159
Bosentan, 167

Bowel Anti-Inflammatory Drugs
  (5-ASA Type), 169
Brethaire, 1031
Brethine, 1031, plate E
Brevicon, 290
Brexin L.A., 95
Bricanyl, 1031
Brimonidine, 173
Brinzolamide, 196
Bristacycline, 1044
Brofed Liquid, 95
Bromfed, 95
Bromfed-PD, 95
Bromfenex, 95
Bromfenex PD, 95
Brompheniramine, 95
Broncholate, 422
Bronkaid Dual Action, 422
Bronkodyl, 1155
Budesonide, 303, 306, 310
Buffered Aspirin, 111
Bufferin, 111
Buffex, 111
Bumetanide, 644
Bumex, 644, plate E
Bupropion, 175
BuSpar, 179, plate E
BuSpar Dividose, 179
Buspirone, 179
Butalbital, 480, 483, 486
Butalbital Compound, 483
Butal Compound, 483
Butenafine, 182
Butoconazole, 707
Byclomine, 351

C

Caffeine, 480, 483, 486, 837, 895
Calan, 1146, plate E
Calan SR, 1146, plate E
Calcimar, 184
Calcitonin, 184
Calm-X, 366

Cama Arthritis Pain Reliever, 111
Camila, 291
Canasa, 169
Candesartan, 84
Capecitabine, 186
Capital with Codeine, 833
Capoten, 189, plate E
Capozide, 189, plate E
Captopril, 189
Carafate, 996
Carbamazepine, 193
Carbatrol, 193
Carbenicillin Indanyl Sodium, 825
Carbex, 971
Carbidopa, 983
Carbinoxamine, 95
Carbiset, 95
Carbiset TR, 95
Carbodec, 95
Carbodec TR, 95
Carbonic-Anhydrase Inhibitors, Eyedrops, 196
Carbonyl Iron, 588
Cardec-S, 95
Cardene, 766
Cardene SR, 766
Cardiem LA, 362
Cardioquin, 916
Cardizem, 362, plate E
Cardizem CD, 362, plate E
Cardizem SR, 362, plate F
Cardura, 384, plate F
Carteolol, 148, 199
Cartia XT, 363, plate F
Cartrol, 199, plate F
Carvedilol, 202
Casodex, 151
Cataflam, 550
Catapres, 265, plate F
Catapres-TTS-1, 265
Catapres-TTS-2, 265
Catapres-TTS-3, 265

Caverject, 58
Ceclor, 210, plate F
Ceclor CD, 210
Ceclor Pulvules, 210
Cedax, 211
Cefaclor, 210
Cefadroxil, 210
Cefdinir, 210
Cefditoren Pivoxil, 210
Cefixime, 211
Cefpodoxime Proxetil, 211
Cefprozil, 211
Ceftibuten, 211
Ceftin, 211, plate F
Cefuroxime Axetil, 211
Cefzil, 211, plate F
Celebrex, 206, plate F
Celecoxib, 206
Celestone, 310
Celexa, 965, plate F
CellCept, 741, plate F
Cena-K, 872
Cenestin, 445
Centany, 735
Centrax, 347
Cephalexin, 211
Cephalexin Hydrochloride, 211
Cephalosporin Antibiotics, 210
Cephradine, 211
Cerebyx, 854
Cetacort, 318
Ceta-Plus, 833
Cetirizine, 216
Cetrorelix, 659
Cetrotide, 659
Cevimeline, 219
Cheracol, 1134
Chibroxin, 495
Children's Advil, 549
Children's Motrin, 549
Childrens' Pain Reliever, 13
Chlorafed H.S. Timecelles, 95
Chlorafed Timecelles, 95
Chlordiazepoxide, 222, 1113

Chlordrine SR, 95
Chlorothiazide, 1053
Chlorotrianisene, 445
Chlorphedrine SR, 95
Chlor-Phen, 225
Chlorpheniramine, 1132
Chlorpheniramine Maleate, 95,
   96, 225
Chlorpheniramine Tannate, 96
Chlorpromazine, 229
Chlorpropamide, 1003
Chlorthalidone, 119, 1053
Chlor-Trimeton, 225
Chlorzoxazone, 233
Choledyl SA, 1155
Cholestyramine, 235
Cholinesterase Inhibitors, 239
Cialis, 430, plate F
Ciclopirox, 242
Cilostazol, 244
Ciloxan, 495
Cimetidine, 246
Cipro, 495, plates F & G
Ciprofloxacin, 495
Cipro XR, 495, plate G
Citalopram, 965
Claravis, 595
Clarinex, 651, plate G
Clarinex RediTabs, 651
Clarithromycin, 250, 906
Claritin, 651
Claritin-D 12-Hour, 96
Claritin-D 24-Hour, 96
Claritin Reditabs, 651
Clemastine, 254
Cleocin, 256
Cleocin T, 256
Climara, 445
**Climara Pro Transdermal
   System**, 445
Clinda-Derm, 256
Clindagel, 256
ClindaMax, 256
Clindamycin, 256

Clindets, 256
Clinoril, 550, plate G
Clobetasol Propionate, 317
Clobex, 317
Clocortolone Pivalate, 317
Cloderm, 317
Clofibrate, 259
Clomipramine, 1113
Clonazepam, 262
Clonidine, 265
Clopidogrel, 270
Clopra, 695
Clorazepate, 272
Clotrimazole, 276, 657
Cloxacillin Sodium, 825
Cloxapen, 825
Clozapine, 278
Clozaril, 278, plate G
Codeine, 282
Codeine Phosphate, 486, 833,
   837, 890, 891, 1134
Codimal L.A., 95
Co-Gesic, 833
Cognex, 239
Colazal, 169, plate G
Colchicine, 286
Coldmist, 421
Colesevelam, 235
Colestid, 236
Colestipol, 236
Colfed-A, 95
Colocort, 311
CombiPatch, 445
Combivent, 585
Combivir, 608
Comhist, 96
Comhist LA, 96
Commit, 770
Compazine, 886, plate G
Compazine Spansule, 886,
   plate G
Compro, 886
Comtan, 418, plate G
Concentraid, 344

Concerta, 691, plate G
Condylox, 869
Congess, 421
Congestac, 421
Conjugated Estrogens, 445
Contraceptives, 289
Contuss, 421
Copaxone, 523
Cophene No.2, 95
Cordarone, 63, plate G
Cordran, 318
Cordran SP, 318
Cordran Tape, 318
Coreg, 202
Corgard, 1069, plate G
Cormax, 317
CortaGel, 318
Cortaid Intensive Therapy, 318
Cortaid with Aloe, 318
Cortatrigen Ear Drops, 322
Cort-Dome, 318
Cortef, 311
Cortenema, 311, 318
Corticosteroids, Eye Products,
    300
Corticosteroids, Inhalers, 302
Corticosteroids, Nasal, 306
Corticosteroids, Oral, 310
Corticosteroids, Topical, 317
Cortifoam, 311, 318
Cortisone Acetate, 311
Cortisporin Otic, 322
Cortizone-5, 318
Cortizone-10, 318
Cortone, 311
Cortril, 318
Cosopt, 324
Cotrim, 974
Cotrim DS, 974
Cotrim Pediatric, 974
Coumadin, 1150, plate H
Covera HS, 1146, plate H
Cozaar, 84, plate H
Crestor, 987

Crinone, 664
Crixivan, 562
Crolom, 328
Cromolyn, 328
Cromoptic, 328
Cryselle, 290
Curretab, 664
Cutivate, 318
Cyanocobalamin, 871
Cyclessa, 291
Cyclobenzaprine, 332
Cyclocort, 317
Cyclosporine, 335
Cycrin, 664
Cylert, 820
Cyproheptadine Hydrochloride,
    225
Cystadane, 145
Cytomel, 1058
Cytospaz, 381
Cytotec, 724
Cytovene, 514

D

Dallergy-JR, 95
Dalmane, 504, plate H
Dapacin, 13
Darron Pulvules, 894
Darvocet-N 50, 895
Darvocet-N 100, 895, plate H
Darvon, 894
Darvon Compound, 895
Darvon-N, 895
Daypro, 551, plate H
Daypro ALTA, 551
Dayto Sulf, 999
Dazamide, 16
DDAVP, 344
Decadron, 300, 311, 317
Decaspray, 317
Declomycin, 1043
Deconamine, 95
Deconamine SR, 95, plate H

Deconsal II, 421
Deconsal Sprinkle, 422
Defen LA, 421
Delavirdine, 341
Delcort, 318
Del-Mycin, 437
Deltasone, 311, plate H
Delta-Tritex, 319
Demadex, 644
Demeclocycline, 1043
Demerol, 674, plate H
Demulen 1/35, 290
Demulen 1/50, 290
Denavir, 823
Depacon, 1139
Depakene, 1139
Depakote, 1139, plate H
Depakote ER, 1139, plate H
Depakote Sprinkle, 1139,
  plate H
Deponit, 788
Depo-Provera, 664
Dermabet, 317
Dermacort, 318
Derma-Smoothe/FS, 318
Dermatop, 319
Dermatop E Emollient, 319
Dermolate, 318
Dermol HC, 318
Dermtex HC with Aloe, 318
Desenex Max, 1028
Desipramine, 1113
Desloratadine, 651
Desmopressin, 344
Desogen, 290
Desonide, 317
DesOwen, 317
Desoximetasone, 317
Desyrel, 1096, plate H
Desyrel Dividose, 1096, plate I
Detrol, 1082, plate I
Detrol LA, 1082, plate I
Dexameth, 311
Dexamethasone, 300, 311, 317

Dexaphen-SA, 95
Dexbrompheniramine, 95
Dexchlorpheniramine Maleate,
  225
Dexedrine, 29
Dexmethylphenidate, 692
Dexone, 311
Dextroamphetamine
  Saccharate, 29
Dextroamphetamine Sulfate, 29
Dextromethorphan
  Hydrobromide, 890
Dextrostat, 29
DiaBeta, 1003, plate I
Diabinese, 1003, plate I
Diamox, 16
Diamox Sequels, 16
Diastat, 347
Diazepam, 347
Diazepam Intensol, 347
Diclofenac, 550
Dicloxacillin Sodium, 825
Dicumarol, 1150
Dicyclomine, 351
Didanosine, 354
Didronel, 158
Dienestrol, 445
Difenoxin, 733
Differin, 26
Diflorasone Diacetate, 318
Diflucan, 1107, plate I
Diflunisal, 550
Digitek, 358
Digoxin, 358
Dihydrocodeine Bitartrate, 837
Dilacor XR, 363, plate I
Dilantin, 854, plate I
Dilantin Kapseals, 854
Dilatrate-SR, 591
Dilor, 1155
Dilor-400, 1155
Diltia XT, 363
Diltiazem, 362
Dimenhydrinate, 366

Dimetabs, 366
Diovan, 85, plate I
Diovan HCT, 85, plate J
Dipentum, 169
Diphen AF, 369
Diphenhist, 369
Diphenhydramine
   Hydrochloride, 369
Diprolene, 317
Diprolene AF, 317
Diprosone, 317
Dipyridamole, 35
Dirithromycin, 372
Disobrom, 95
Disopyramide, 374
Di-Spaz, 351
Ditropan, 812, plate J
Ditropan XL, 812, plate J
Diucardin, 1053
Diurese, 1053
Diurigen, 1053
Diuril, 1053, plate J
Docetaxel, 815
Dofetilide, 378
Dolacet, 833
Dolasetron, 90
Dolene, 894
Dolobid, 550
Donepezil, 239
Donnamar, 381
Donnapine, 381
Donnatel Extencaps, 381
Dopar, 626
Doral, 1103, plate J
Doryx, 1043
Dorzolamide, 196, 324
Doxazosin, 384
Doxepin, 1113
Doxercalciferol, 387
Doxy Caps, 1043
Doxychel Hyclate, 1043
Doxycycline, 1043
Dramamine, 366
Drisdol Liquid, 387

Drixomed, 95
Dronabinol, 390
Drotic, 322
Duagen, 477
Duocet, 833
DuoNeb, 585
Duragesic (Patch), 282
Duralex, 95
Durasal II, 421
Dura-Tap/PD, 95
Duratuss, 421
Duricef, 210, plate J
Dutasteride, 477
Dyazide, 393, plate J
Dycill, 825
Dymelor, 1003
Dynabac, 372, plate J
Dynacin, 1043
DynaCirc, 775, plate J
DynaCirc CR, 775
Dynafed, 13
Dynafed Asthma Relief, 422
Dynapen, 825
Dynex, 421
Dyphylline, 1155
Dytuss, 369

E

Ear-Eze, 322
Easprin, 111
E-Base, 437
EC-Naprosyn, 748
Econazole, 396
Econopred, 300
Econopred Plus, 300
Ecotrin, 111
Ed A-Hist, 96
Edecrin, 644
Edex, 58
ED-IN-SOL, 588
E.E.S. 200, 437
E.E.S. 400, 437, plate J
Efalizumab, 398

Efavirenz, 401
Effer-K, 873
Effexor, 1143, plate J
Effexor XR, 1143, plate K
Eflornithine, 404
Elavil, 1113
Eldecort, 318
Eldepryl, 971
Elestat, 99
Eletriptan, 1120
Elidel Cream, 859
Elimite, 844
Elixomin, 1155
Elixophyllin, 1155
Elmiron, 830, plate K
Elocon, 319
Embeline, 317
Embeline E, 317
Emedastine, 99
Emend, 105
Emgel, 437
EMLA, 406
Empirin, 111
**Empirin with Codeine
  No. 3**, 837
**Empirin with Codeine
  No. 4**, 837
Emtricitabine, 409
Emtriva, 409
E-Mycin, 437
Enalapril, 412, 629
Enbrel, 452
Endafed, 95
Endal, 422
Endal-SR, 421
Endep, 1113
Endocet, 832
Endocodone, 282
Endolor, 483
Enduron, 1053
Enfuvirtide, 416
Enoxacin, 495
Enpresse, 291
Entacapone, 418

Entex LA, 422
Entex PSE, 421
Entocort EC, 310
Ephedrine, 422
Epicort, 318
Epinastine, 99
Epitol, 193
Epivar, 99
Epivir, 608
Epivir-HBV, 608
Eplerenone, 42
Epoetin, 425
Epogen, 425
Epromate-M, 427
Eprosartan, 84
Equagesic, 427
Equanil, 677
Erectile Dysfunction Drugs, 430
Ergamisol, 621
Ergoloid Mesylates, 435
Errin, 291
Ertaczo Cream, 276
Eryc, 437
Erycette, 437
Eryderm, 437
Erygel, 437
Erymax, 437
EryPed, 437
EryPed 200, 437
EryPed 400, 437
EryPed Drops, 437
Ery-Tab, 437, plate K
Erythra-Derm, 437
Erythrocin Stearate, 437,
  plate K
Erythromycin, 437
Erythromycin DR, 437
Erythromycin ES, 437
Erythromycin Estolate, 437
Erythromycin Ethylsuccinate,
  437
Erythromycin Filmtabs, 437
Erythromycin Stearate, 437
Eryzole, 437

Escitalopram, 965
Esclim, 445
Esgic, 480
Esgic-Plus, 480
Esidrix, 1053
Eskalith, 639, plate K
Eskalith CR, 639, plate K
Esomeporazole
  Magnesium, 906
Estazolam, 441
Esterified Estrogens, 445
Estinyl, 446
Estrace, 445, plate K
Estraderm, 445
Estradiol, 445
Estrasorb, 445
Estratab, 445
Estratest, 445, plate K
Estratest HS, 445
Estring, 445
Estrogen, 289, 290, 291, 445
Estropipate, 446
Estrostep 21, 291
Estrostep Fe, 291
Etanercept, 452
Ethacrynic Acid, 644
Ethinyl Estradiol, 446
Ethotoin, 854
Etidronate, 158
Etodolac, 455
Etrafon, 1113
Etrafon-A, 1113
Etrafon-Forte, 1113
Eulexin, 507, plate K
Evista, 919, plate K
Evoxac, 219
Exelon, 239, plate K
Exemestane, 458
Ezetimibe, 460
Ezide, 1053

F

Factive, 495
Famciclovir, 463

Famotidine, 465
Famvir, 463, plate K
Fansidar, 998
Fareston, 1014
Fedahist Expectorant, 421
Fedahist Gyrocaps, 95
Fedahist Timecaps, 95
Felbamate, 468
Felbatol, 468
Feldene, 865, plate K
Felodipine, 412, 471, 629
Femara, 82
Femcet, 480, 483
Femhrt, 446
Femiron, 588
FemPatch, 445
Femring, 445
Femstat, 707
Fenofibrate, 474
Fenoprofen, 550
Fentanyl, 282
Fentanyl Oralet (Lozenge), 282
Feosol, 588
Feostat, 588
Feratab, 588
Fer-Gen-Sol, 588
Fergon, 588
Fer-In-Sol, 588
Ferretts, 588
Ferrex 150, 589
Ferrous Fumarate, 588
Ferrous Gluconate, 588
Ferrous Sulfate, 588
Feverall, 13
Fexofenadine, 96, 216
Finasteride, 477
Fioricet, 480, plate L
Fiorinal, 483
Fiorinal with Codeine, 486
Fiorital, 483
Fiorpap, 480
Flagyl, 703, plate L
Flagyl ER, 703
Flarex, 300

Flecainide, 489
Flexeril, 332, plate L
Flomax, 1016, plate L
Flonase, 306
Florone, 318
Florone E, 318
Florvite, 871
Flovent, 303
Flovent Diskus, 303
Flovent Rotadisk, 303
Floxin, 495, plate L
Floxin Otic, 495
Fluconazole, 1107
Flucytosine, 492
Flumadine, 940
Flunisolide, 303, 306
Fluocinolone Acetonide, 318
Fluocinonide, 318
Fluonex, 318
Fluonid, 318
Fluorometholone, 300
Fluor-Op, 300
Fluoroquinolone Anti-
 Infectives, 495
Fluoxetine, 965
Fluoxymesterone, 501
Fluphenazine Hydrochloride,
 229
Flurandrenolide, 318
Flurazepam, 504
Flurbiprofen, 550
Flurosyn, 318
Flutamide, 507
Flutex, 319
Fluticasone, 958
Fluticasone Propionate, 303,
 306, 318
Fluvastatin, 986
Fluvoxamine, 965
FML, 300
FML Forte, 300
FML-S, 300
Focalin, 692
Folic Acid, 871

Foradil Aerolizer, 164
Foromoterol, 164
Forteo, 1036
Fortovase, 961
Fosamax, 158, plate L
Fosamprenavir, 73
Fosfomycin, 509
Fosinopril, 511
Fosphenytoin, 854
Frova, 1120
Frovatriptan, 1120
FS Shampoo, 318
Fungoid, 276
Furadantin, 785
Furosemide, 644
Fuzeon, 416

G

Gabapentin, 1063
Gabitril, 1063
Galantamine, 239
Ganciclovir, 514
Ganirelix, 659
Gani-Tuss NR, 1134
Gantanol, 998
Gantrisin, 998
Gastrocrom, 328
Gatifloxacin, 495
Gefitinib, 517
Gemfibrozil, 520
Gemifloxacin, 495
Genahist, 369
Genapap, 13
Genebs, 13
Gengraf, 335
Gen-K, 872
Genpril, 549
Genprin, 111
Gen-Xene, 272
Geocillin, 825
Geodon, 1175, plate L
Gerimal, 435
GFN/PSE, 421

Glatiramer, 523
Gleevec, 556, plate L
Glimepiride, 1003
Glipizide, 1003
Glitazone Antidiabetes Drugs, 526
Glucophage, 685, plate L
Glucophage XR, 685, plate L
Glucotrol, 1003, plate M
Glucotrol XL, 1003, plate M
Glucovance, 529, plate M
Glyburide, 529, 1003
Glycerin, 129
Glynase PresTab, 1003, plate M
Glyset, 714
GP-500, 421
Gramicidin, 759
Granisetron, 90
Guaifed, 421
Guaifed-PD, 421
Guaifenesin, 421, 422, 1134
Guaifenex GP, 421
Guaifenex PSE, 421
Guaifenex RX, 421
Guaimax-D, 422
Guaimax-S, 422
Guaipax PSE, 422
Guaitab, 422
Guaitex PSE, 422
Guaituss PE, 422
Guai-Vent PSE, 422
Guanabenz, 534
Guiatuss AC, 1134
Guiatussin with Codeine, 1134
Gynecort, 318
Gyne-Sulf, 999
Gynodiol, 445

H

Habitrol, 770
Halazepam, 347
Halcinonide, 318
Halcion, 1103, plate M

Haldol, 536
Halenol, 13
Halfprin, 111
Halobetasol Propionate, 318
Halog, 318
Halog-E, 318
Haloperidol, 536
Halotestin, 501, plate M
Halotussin AC, 1134
Haltran, 550
1% HC, 318
Heartline, 111
Hectorol Capsules, 387
Helidac, 540
Hemocyte, 588
Hemril HC Uniserts, 318
Hepsera, 32
Heptogesic, 427
Herceptin, 1093
Hexadrol, 311
Hi-Cor 1.0, 318
Hi-Cor 2.5, 318
Histalet, 95
Histalet X, 422
Histor-D, 96
Hivid, 1161, plate M
HMS, 300
H 9600 SR, 422
Humalog, 572
Humalog Mix 50/50, 572
Humalog Mix 75/25, 572
Humulin 50/50, 572
Humulin 70/30, 572
Humulin L, 572
Humulin N, 572
Humulin R, 572
Humulin U, 573
Hycort, 318
Hydergine, 435
Hydergine LC, 435
Hydralazine, 544
Hydrocet, 833

Hydrochlorothiazide, 84, 85, 139, 154, 189, 393, 412, 511, 636, 730, 898, 912, 1053
Hydrocodone, 1132
Hydrocodone Bitartrate, 833, 837
Hydrocort, 318
Hydrocortisone, 311, 318, 322
Hydrocortone, 311
HydroDIURIL, 1053
Hydroflumethiazide, 1053
Hydrogesic, 833
Hydromox, 1053
Hydro-Par, 1053
HydroTex, 318
Hydroxyzine, 547
Hygroton, 1053
Hyonatal, 381
Hyoscyamine Sulfate, 381
Hyosol, 381
Hyosophen, 381
Hyosyne, 381
Hy-Phen, 833
Hytinic, 589
Hytone, 318
Hytrin, 51, plate M
Hyzaar, 84, plate M

I

Ibandronate, 159
IBU, 550
Ibuprin, 550
Ibuprofen, 549, 837
Ibuprohm, 550
Icar, 588
Iletin II, 572
Ilosone, 437
Ilosone Pulvules, 437
Ilotycin, 437
Imatinib, 556
Imdur, 592, plates M & N
Imipramine, 1113
Imiquimod, 559

Imitrex, 1120, plate N
Imodium, 648
Imodium A-D, 648
Indapamide, 1053
Inderal, 898, plate N
Inderal LA, 898, plate N
Inderide, 898, plate N
Inderide LA, 898
Indinavir, 562
Indochron E-R, 566
Indocin, 566, plate N
Indocin SR, 566, plate N
Indomethacin, 566
Infants' Motrin, 550
Infants' Pain Reliever, 13
Infergen, 578
Infliximab, 570
Innofem, 445
Innopran XL, 898
Inspra, 42
Insulin, 572
Insulin Aspart, 572
Insulin Glargine, 572
Insulin Lispro, 572
Intal, 328
Interferon Alfa, 578
Interferon Alfa-2b, 928
Interferon Beta, 581
Intron A, 578
Invirase, 961
Iopidine, 102
Iosal II, 422
Ipratropium, 584
Ipratropium Bromide, 585
Irbesartan, 84
Ircon, 588
Iressa, 517
Iron Supplements, 588
ISMO, 592
Isocet, 480
Isochron, 591
Isoniazid, 934
Isoptin, 1146
Isoptin SR, 1146

Isordil Tembids, 591
Isordil Titradose, 591, plate N
Isosorbide Dinitrate, 591
Isosorbide Mononitrate, 592
Isotrate ER, 592
Isotretinoin, 595
Isradipine, 775
Itraconazole, 1107

J

Jolivette, 291

K

K + 8, 873
K + 10, 873
Kaletra, 947, plate N
Kaochlor 10%, 872
Kaochlor S-F, 872
Kaon, 872
Kaon-Cl-10, 873
Kaon-Cl 20%, 872
Kariva, 290
Kay Ciel, 872, 873
Kaylixir, 872
K+Care, 872
K + Care ET, 873
K-Dur 10, 873
K-Dur 20, 873, plate O
Keflet, 211
Keflex, 211, plate O
Keftab, 211
Kenacort, 311
Kenalog, 319
Kenalog-H, 319
Kenonel, 319
Keppra, 624
Kerlone, 154, plate O
Kesso-Gesic, 894
Ketoconazole, 1107
Ketoprofen, 550
Ketorolac, 599
Ketotifen, 603

K-G Elixir, 872
Kineret, 79
K-Lease, 873
Klerist-D, 95
Klonopin, 262, plate O
K-Lor, 873
Klor-Con, 873, plate O
Klor-Con 8, 873
Klor-Con 10, 873
Klor-Con/25, 873
Klor-Con/EF, 873
Klorvess, 872, 873
Klotrix, 873
K-Lyte, 873
K-Lyte/Cl, 873
K-Lyte/Cl 50, 873
K-Lyte DS, 873
K-Norm, 873
Kolyum, 872, 873
Kronofed-A, 95
Kronofed-A Jr., 95
K-Tab, 873, plate O
K-Vescent, 873
Kytril, 90, plate O

L

Labetalol, 605
LactiCare-HC, 318
Lamictal, 611, plate O
Lamictal CD, 611
Lamisil, 1028
Lamisil AT, 1028
Lamivudine, 608, 1128
Lamotrigine, 611
Lanacort-5, 318
Lanacort-10, 318
Lanophyllin, 1155
Lanorinal, 483
Lanoxicaps, 358, plate O
Lanoxin, 358, plates O & P
Lansoprazole, 906
Lantus, 572
Larodopa, 626

Larotid, 825
Lasix, 644, plate P
Latanoprost, 903
LazerSporin-C, 322
Ledercillin VK, 826
Leflunomide, 615
Lente Iletin II, 572
Lente Insulin, 572
Lescol, 986, plate P
Lescol XL, 986
Lessina, 289
Letrozole, 82
Leukotriene
  Antagonists/Inhibitors, 617
Levalbuterol, 38
Levamisole, 621
Levaquin, 495, plate P
Levatol, 698, plate P
Levbid, 381
Levetiracetam, 624
Levitra, 430, plate P
Levlen, 290
Levlite, 289
Levobetaxolol, 148
Levobunolol, 148
Levocabastine, 99, 800
Levodopa, 626, 983
Levofloxacin, 495
Levonorgestrel, 445
Levora, 290
Levotabs, 1058
Levothroid, 1058
Levothyroxine Sodium, 1058
Levoxyl, 1058, plate P
Levsin, 381
Levsinex Timecaps, 381
Levulan Kerastick, 61
Lexapro, 965, plates P & Q
Lexiva, 73
Lexxel, 412, 629, plate Q
Librium, 222, plate Q
Lidex, 318
Lidex-E, 318
Lidocaine, 406

Limbitrol, 1113
Limbitrol DS, 1113
Linezolid, 633
Lioresal, 134
Liothyronine Sodium, 1058
Liotrix, 1058
Lipitor, 986, plate Q
Liquibid, 422
Liquid Pred, 311
Liquiprin, 13
Lisinopril, 636
Lithane, 639
Lithium Carbonate, 639
Lithium Citrate, 640
Lithobid, 639
Lithonate, 639
Lithotabs, 639
Livostin, 99, 800
LoCHOLEST Light, 235
LoCHOLEST Prevalite, 235
Locoid, 318
Lodine, 455, plate Q
Lodine XL, 455, plate Q
Lodosyn, 983
Lodoxamide, 603
Lodrane LD, 95
Loestrin 1.5/30, 290
Loestrin 1/20, 290
Loestrin 21 1.5/30, 290
Loestrin 21 1/20, 290
Loestrin Fe 1/20, 290
Lofibra, 474
Lomefloxacin, 495
Loniten, 717
Loop Diuretics, 644
Lo/Ovral, 290
Loperamide, 648
Lopid, 520, plate Q
Lopinavir, 947
Lopressor, 698, plate Q
Loprox, 242
Lorabid, 211, plate Q
Loracarbef, 211
Loratadine, 651

Lorazepam, 347
Lorazepam Intensol, 347
Lorcet 10/650, 833
Lorcet-HD, 833
Lorcet Plus, 833, plate Q
Lortab, 833
Lortab 2.5/500, 833
Lortab 5/500, 833
Lortab 7.5/500, 833
Lortab 10/500, 833
Losartan Potassium, 84
Lotemax, 300
Lotensin, 139, plate Q
Lotensin HCT, 139, plate Q
Loteprednol Etabonate, 300
Lotrel, 653, plate R
Lotrimin, 276
Lotrisone, 657
Lotronex, 90
Lovastatin, 986, 987
Low-Ogestrel, 290
Lozol, 1053, plate R
Ludiomil, 721
Lufyllin, 1155
Lufyllin-400, 1155
Lumigan, 902
Luteinizing Hormone Inhibitors, 659
Luvox, 965, plate R
Luxiq, 317

M

Macrobid, 785, plate R
Macrodantin, 785, plate R
Magnaprin, 111
Malathion, 661
Mapap, 13
Maprotiline, 721
Maranox, 13
Marcillin, 825
Margesic, 483
Margesic H, 833
Marinol, 390

Mavik, 1090
Maxair, 38
Maxalt, 1120
Maxalt-MLT, 1120
Maxaquin, 495, plate R
Maxidex, 300
Maxifed, 422
Maxifed G, 422
Maxiflor, 318
Maximum Strength Cortaid, 319
Maximum Strength Cortaid-Faststick, 319
Maximum Strength KeriCort-10, 319
Maxivate, 317
Maxolon, 695
Maxzide, 393
Maxzide-25, 393
Meclan, 1043
Meclizine, 366
Meclocycline Sulfosalicylate, 1043
Meclofenamate, 550
Meclomen, 550
Meda Cap/Tab, 13
Medigesic, 483
Medispaz, 381
Medrol, 311
Medroxyprogesterone, 445
Medroxyprogesterone Acetate, 664
Med-RX, 422
Medrysone, 300
Mefenamic Acid, 550
Mellaril, 229, plate R
Mellaril-S, 229
Meloxicam, 668
Memantine, 671
Menadol, 550
Menest, 445
Meni-D, 366
Mentax, 182
Mentax-TC, 182

Meperidine, 674
Mephenytoin, 854
Meprobamate, 427, 677
Meprogesic, 427
Meprogesic Q, 427
Mepron, 126
Meprospan, 677
Mequinol, 1099
Meridia, 980, plate R
Mesalamine, 169
Mesantoin, 854
Mesoridazine Besylate, 229
Metadate, 692
Metadate CD, 692
Metadate ER, 692
Metaglip, 1003, plate R
Metahydrin, 1053
Metaproterenol, 680
Metaxalone, 682
Metformin, 526, 529, 685, 1003
Methyclothiazide, 1053
Methyldopa, 688
Methylin, 692
Methylin ER, 691
Methylphenidate, 691
Methylprednisolone, 311
Methyltestosterone, 445, 1040
Meticorten, 311
Metipranolol, 148
Metoclopramide, 695
Metolazone, 1053
Metoprolol, 698
Metric 21, 703
MetroCream, 703
MetroGel, 703
MetroLotion, 703
Metronidazole, 540, 703
Mevacor, 986, plate R
Miacalcin, 184
Micardis, 85
Micardis HCT, 85
Miconazole, 706
Micrainin, 427
Microgestin Fe 1.5/30, 290

Microgestin Fe 1/20, 290
Micro-K Extencaps, 873, plate R
Micro-K 10 Extencaps, 873
Micro-K LS, 873
Micronase, 1003, plate R
Microzide, 1053
Midodrine, 709
Midol, 550
Midol-IB, 550
Mifeprex, 711, plate S
Mifepristone, 711
Miglitol, 714
Miltown, 677
Minipress, 879, plate S
Minipress XL, 879
Minirin, 344
MiniThin Asthma Relief, 422
Minitran, 788
Minizide, 879, plate S
Minocin, 1043, plate S
Minocycline Hydrochloride,
    1043
Minoxidil, 717
Miradon, 1150
Mirapex, 876, plate S
Miraphen PSE, 422
Mircette, 290
Mirena, 292
Mirtazapine, 720
Misoprostol, 550, 724
Mobic, 668, plate S
Modafinil, 727
Modicon, 290
Moduretic, 393, plate S
Moexipril, 730
Mometasone Furoate, 319
Mometasone Furoate
    Monohydrate, 307
Monistat, 706
Monodox, 1043
Monoket, 592
Monopril, 511, plate S
Monopril HCT, 511
Montelukast, 617

Monurol, 509
Motofen, 733
Motrin, 550
Motrin IB, 550
Moxifloxacin, 495
M-Oxy, 282
Mupirocin, 735
Muromonab-CD3, 738
Muse, 58
Mycelex, 276
Mycophenolate, 741
Mykrox, 1053
Mylaramine, 225
Mymethasone, 311
Mytussin AC, 1134

N

Nabumetone, 745
Nadolol, 1069
Nafcillin, 825
Nalfon, 550, plate T
Naloxone, 837
Namenda, 671
Naprelan, 748
Naprosyn, 748, plate T
Naproxen/Naproxen Sodium, 748
Naqua, 1053
Naratriptan, 1120
Nardil, 846
Nasabid, 422
Nasabid-SR, 422
Nasacort AQ, 307
Nasalcrom, 328
Nasalide, 306
Nasarel, 306
Nasatab LA, 422
Nasonex, 307
Nateglinide, 931
Naturetin, 1052
ND Clear, 95
Necon 1/35, 290
Necon 1/50, 290

Necon 7/7/7, 291
Necon 10/11, 291
Nedocromil, 328
Nefazodone, 752
Nelfinavir, 755
Neocon 0.5/35, 290
Neomycin Sulfate, 322, 759
Neopap, 13
Neoral, 335
Neosporin Ophthalmic, 759
Neothylline, 1155
Nephro-Fer, 588
Nesstab LA, 422
Neuramate, 677
Neurontin, 1063, plate T
Nevirapine, 761
Nexium, 906, plate T
Niacin, 764, 871, 987
Niacor, 764
Niaspan, 764
Nicardipine, 766
Nicoderm, 770
Nicoderm CQ, 770
Nicolar, 764
Nicorette, 770
Nicorette DS, 770
Nicotine, 770
Nicotinex, 764
Nicotrol, 770
Nicotrol Inhaler, 770
Nicotrol NS, 770
Nifedical XL, 775
Nifedipine, 775
Nifeditab CR, 775
Niferex, 589
Niferex-150, 589
Nilandron, 152
Nilutamide, 152
Nimodipine, 780
Nimotop, 780
Nisoldipine, 775
Nitazoxanide, 783
Nitrek, 788
Nitro-Bid, 788

Nitrocine, 789
Nitro-Derm, 789
Nitrodisc, 789
Nitro-Dur, 789
Nitrofurantoin, 785
Nitrogard, 789
Nitroglycerin, 788
Nitroglyn, 789
Nitrol, 789
Nitrolingual, 789
Nitrong, 789
NitroQuick, 789
Nitrostat, 789
Nitro Tab, 789
Nitro-Time, 789
Nix, 844
Nizatidine, 793
Nizoral, 1107, plate T
Nolvadex, 1013, plate T
Nora-BE, 291
Norco, 833
Nordette, 290
Norethindrone Acetate, 445,
 446, 664
Norfloxacin, 495
Norgestimate, 445
Norinyl 1 + 35, 290
Norinyl 1 + 50, 290
Noritate, 703
Normodyne, 605
Noroxin, 495, plate T
Norpace, 374, plate T
Norpace CR, 374, plate T
Norplant II, 291
Norpramin, 1113, plate T
Nor-Q.D., 291
Nor-Tet, 1044
Nortrel 0.5/35, 290
Nortrel 1/35, 290
Nortriptyline, 1113
Norvasc, 69, plate T
Norvir, 947
Norwich, 111
Novafed A, 95

Novolin 70/30, 572
Novolin L, 572
Novolin N, 572
Novolin R, 572
Novolog, 572
Novolog Mix 70/30, 572
NPH Iletin II, 572
NPH Insulin, 572
Nu-Iron, 589
Nu-Iron 150, 589
NuLev, 381
Nuprin, 550
Nutracort, 319
NuvaRing, 291, 445

O

Octamide, 695
Octicair, 322
Ocuflox Eyedrops, 495
Ocupress, 148
Ofloxacin, 495
Ogen, 446
Ogestrel, 290
Olanzapine, 795
Olmesartan, 85
Olopatadine, 99, 799
Olsalazine, 169
Olux, 317
Omeperazole, 906
Omnicef, 210, plate T
Omnipen, 825
Ondansetron, 90
Onxol, 815
Opticrom, 328
Optimine, 225
Optipranolol, 148
Optivar, 99, 800
Oraphen-PD, 13
Oraprel, 311
Orasone, 311
Oretic, 1053
Oreton Methyl, 1040
Orinase, 1003

Orlistat, 802
Ortho-Cept, 290
Orthoclone OKT3, 738
Ortho-Cyclen, 290
Ortho Dienestrol, 445
Ortho-Est, 446
OrthoEvra, 291
Ortho-Micronor, 291
Ortho-Novum 1/35, 290
Ortho-Novum 1/50, 290
Ortho-Novum 7/7/7, 291
Ortho-Novum 10/11, 291
Ortho-Prefest, 445
Ortho Tri-Cyclen, 291
Ortho Tri-Cyclen Lo, 291
Orudis, plate T
Orudis KT, 550
Oruvail, 550, plate T
Oseltamivir, 805
Otic-Care, 322
Otocalm Ear, 129
Otocort, 322
Otomycin-HPN Otic, 323
Ovcon-35, 290
Ovcon-50, 290
Ovide, 661
Ovral, 290
Ovrette, 291
Oxacillin, 825
Oxazepam, 347
Oxcarbazepine, 807
Oxiconazole, 810
Oxistat, 810
Oxtriphylline, 1155
Oxybutynin, 812
Oxycodone Hydrochloride, 282,
    832, 833, 837
Oxycodone Terephthalate, 837
OxyContin, 282, 833
Oxydose, 282
OxyFAST, 282
OxyIR, 282
Oxytetracycline, 1043
Oxytrol, 812

P

Pacerone, 63
Paclitaxel, 815
Pamelor, 1113, plate U
Panacet 5/500, 833
Panadol, 13
Panasol-S, 311
Pandel, 319
Panixine Disperdose, 211
PanMist-Jr., 422
PanMist LA, 422
PanMist Syrup, 422
Panmycin, 1044
Panretin, 45
Pantoprozole, 906
Paraflex, 233
Parafon Forte DSC, 233, plate U
Parnate, 846
Paroxetine, 965
Patanol, 99, 799
Pathocil, 825
Paxil, 965, plate U
Paxil CR, 965, plate U
Paxipam, 347
PBZ, 225
PBZ-SR, 225
PCE, plate U
PCE Dispertab, 437
Pediacare Fever, 550
Pediamycin, 437
Pediapred, 311
Pediazole, 437
Pediotic, 323
Peganone, 854
PegIntron, 578
PemADD, 820
Pemirolast, 819
Pemoline, 820
Penbutolol, 698
Penciclovir, 823
Penecort, 319
Penetrex, 495

Penicillin Antibiotics, 825
Penicillin G, 826
Penicillin V, 826
Penicillin VK, 826
Penlac Nail Lacquer, 242
Pentasa, 169
**Pentazine VC with Codeine
Liquid,** 890
Pentazocine, 833, 837
Pentosan Polysulfate
Sodium, 830
Pen-Vee K, 826
Pepcid, 465, plate U
Pepcid AC, 465
Pepcid Complete, 465
Pepcid RPD, 465
Percocet, 832
Percodan, 837
Percodan-Demi, 837
Percolone, 282, 833
Pergolide, 841
Periactin, 225
Perindopril, 913
Periostat, 1043
Permax, 841
Permethrin, 844
Permitil, 229
Perphenazine, 1113
Pfizerpen, 826
Phenameth DM Syrup, 890
**Phenaphen with Codeine
No. 2,** 833
**Phenaphen with Codeine
No. 3,** 833
**Phenaphen with Codeine
No. 4,** 833
PhenaVent, 422
Phenelzine, 846
Phenergan, 890, plate U
Phenergan VC, 96
Phenergan VC Syrup, 891
**Phenergan VC with Codeine
Syrup,** 891

**Phenergan with Codeine
Syrup,** 890
**Phenergan with
Dextromethorphan Syrup,**
890
Phenobarbital, 381, 851
Phenylephrine, 422
Phenylephrine Hydrochloride,
96, 891
Phenylephrine Tannate, 96
Phenyltoloxamine, 96
Phenytek, 854
Phenytoin, 854
Pherazine DM Syrup, 890
**Pherazine VC with Codeine
Syrup,** 891
**Pherazine with Codeine
Syrup,** 890
Phyllocontin, 1155
Pimecrolimus, 859
Pindolol, 861
Pioglitazone, 526
Pirbuterol, 38
Piroxicam, 865
Plan B, 292
Plavix, 270, plate U
Plendil, 471, plate U
Pletal, 244, plate V
Podofilox, 869
Polaramine Repetabs, 225
Polymyxin B Sulfate, 322, 759
Polysaccharide Iron Complex,
589
Polytabs-F, 871
Polythiazide, 879, 1053
Poly-Vi-Flor, 871
Ponstel, 550, plate V
Portia, 290
Potasalan, 872
Potassium Chloride, 872, 873
Potassium Clavulanate, 825
Potassium Gluconate, 872, 873
Potassium Replacements, 872

Potassium Salt Combination, 872, 873
Pramipexole, 876
Pramoxine HC, 319
Prandin, 931, plate V
Pravachol, 987, plate V
Pravastatin, 987
Pravigard PAC, 987
Prazepam, 347
Prazosin, 879
Precose, 6
Pred Forte, 300
Pred Mild, 300
Prednicarbate, 319
Prednicen-M, 311
Prednisolone, 300, 311
Prednisone, 311
Prednisone Intensol, 311
Prehist, 96
Prelone, 311
Premarin, 445, plate V
Premphase, 445
Prempro, 445
Prevacid, 906, plate V
Prevalite, 235
Preven, 292
Prevpac, 906
Prilocaine, 406
Prilosec, 906, plate V
Primatine, 422
Principen, 825
Prinivil, 636, plate V
Prinzide, 636
ProAmatine, 709, plate V
Probampacin, 825
Pro-Banthine, 381
Probate, 677
Probenecid, 825
Procainamide, 883
Procanbid, 883
Procan-SR, 883
Procardia, 775, plate V
Procardia XL, 775, plate V
Prochlorperazine, 886

Procort, 319
Procrit, 425
Proctocort, 319
Proctocream-HC, 319
Proctofoam-HC, 319
Profen II, 422
Progestasert, 292
Progesterone, 664
Progestin, 289, 290, 291, 292
Prograf, 1008, plate W
Pro-Hist-8, 225
Prolixin, 229, plate W
Promethacon, 890
Promethazine, 96, 890, 891
Promethazine VC, 96
Promethazine VC Plain, 96
Promethazine VC Plain
  Syrup, 891
Promethegen, 890
Promethist with Codeine
  Syrup, 891
Prometh Plain, 890
Prometh VC Plain, 96
Prometh VC Plain Liquid, 891
Prometh VC with Codeine
  Liquid, 891
Prometh with Codeine Syrup,
  890
Prometh with
  Dextromethorphan Syrup,
  890
Prometrium, 664, plate W
Promine, 883
Pronestyl, 883
Pronestyl-SR, 883
Propacet 100, 895
Propantheline, 381
Propecia, 477
Propoxyphene Hydrochloride,
  894, 895
Propoxyphene Napsylate, 895
Propranolol, 898
Proscar, 477, plate W
ProSom, 441

Prostaglandin Agonists, 902
ProStep, 770
Protonix, 906, plate W
Proton-Pump Inhibitors, 906
Protopic, 1008
Protostat, 703
Protriptyline, 1113
Proventil, 38
Proventil HFA, 38
Proventil Repetabs, 38
Provera, 664, plate W
Provigil, 727
Prozac, 965, plate W
Prozac Weekly, 965, plate W
Pseudoephedrine, 94, 95, 96,
    254, 421
Pseudovent, 422
Pseudovent-PED, 422
Psorcon E, 318
Psorion Cream, 317
Pulmicort Respules, 303
Pulmicort Turbohaler, 303
Pyrazinamide, 934
Pyridoxine, 871
Pyrilamine Tannate, 96
Pyrimethamine, 998

Q

Quazepam, 1103
Questran, 235
Questran Light, 235
Quetiapine, 909
Quibron-T Dividose, 1155
Quibron-T/SR Dividose, 1155
Quinaglute Dura-Tabs, 916
Quinalan, 916
Quinapril, 912
Quinethazone, 1053
Quinidex Extentabs, 916,
    plate W
Quinidine, 916
Quinora, 916
Quin-Release, 916

Quixin Eyedrops, 495
QVAR 40, 302
QVAR 80, 302

R

Rabeprazole, 906
Raloxifene, 919
Ramipril, 913
Ranitidine, 922
Ranitidine Bismuth Citrate, 925
Rapamune, 1009
Raptiva, 398
Rebetron, 928
Rebif, 581
Reclomide, 695
Redutemp, 13
Refenesen Plus, 422
Reglan, 695, plate W
Regranex, 137
Relafen, 745, plate W
Relenza, 1168
Relpax, 1120
Remeron, 720, plate W
Remeron SolTab, 720
Remicade, 570
Reminyl, 239, plate X
Remular-S, 233
Renagel, 978
Renese, 1053
Renova, 1099
Repaglinide, 931
Repan, 480
Requip, 955
Rescon, 95
Rescon ED, 95
Rescon JR, 95
Rescriptor, 341
Rescula, 903
Respahist, 95
Respaire, 422
Respaire-120 SR, 422
Respa-1st, 422
Respbid, 1155

Restoril, 1104, plate X
Retin-A, 1099
Retin-A Micro, 1099
Retrovir, 1170, plate X
Reyataz, 115
Rhinatate, 96
Rhinocort Aqua, 306
Ribavirin, 928
Riboflavin, 871
Rid, 844
Ridenol, 13
Rifadin, 934
Rifamate, 934
Rifampin, 934
Rifater, 934
Rilutek, 937
Riluzole, 937
Rimactane, 934
Rimantadine, 940
Rimexolone, 300
Rinade B.I.D., 95
Risedronate, 159
Risperdal, 943, plate X
Risperdal M-TAB, 943
Risperidone, 943
Ritalin, 692
Ritalin LA, 692
Ritalin-SR, 692, plate X
Ritonavir, 947
Rivastigmine, 239
Rizatriptan, 1120
Robafen AC, 1134
Robitussin A-C, 1134
Robitussin PE, 422
Rofecoxib, 951
Roferon-A, 578
Rogaine, 717
Rondec, 95
Rondec-TR, 95
Ropinirole, 955
Rosiglitazone, 526
Rosuvastatin, 987
Rowasa, 169
Roxicet, 832

Roxicet 5/500, 832
Roxicodone, 282, 833
Roxilox, 832
Roxiprin, 837
R-Tannamine, 96
R-Tannamine Pediatric, 96
R-Tannate, 96
Rum-K, 872
Ru-Tuss DE, 422
Ru-Vert-M, 366
Rymed, 422
Rynatan, 96
Rynatan Pediatric, 96
Rynatan-S Pediatric, 96

S

Salmeterol, 958
Saluron, 1053
Sandimmune, 335, plate X
Saquinavir Mesylate, 961
Sarafem, 965
Scalpicin, 319
Scopolamine Hydrobromide, 381
Sectral, 9, plate X
Selective Serotonin Reuptake Inhibitors (SSRIs), 965
Selegiline, 971
Semprex-D, 94
Septra, 974
Septra DS, 974, plate X
Serax, 347, plate X
Serentil, 229
Serevent, 958
Seroquel, 909, plate X
Sertaconazole, 276
Sertraline, 965
Serzone, 752, plate Y
Sevelamer, 978
Severent Diskus, 958
Sibutramine, 980
Siladryl, 369
Silapap, 13

Sildenafil Citrate, 430
Simvastatin, 987
Sinemet, 983, plate Y
Sinemet CR, 983
Sinequan, 1113
Singulair, 617, plate Y
Sinufed Timecelles, 422
Sinupan, 422
Sinuvent PE Tablets, 422
Sirolimus, 1009
Skelaxin, 682, plate Y
Skelid, 159
Slo-bid Gyrocaps, 1155
Slo-Niacin, 764
Slo-Phyllin, 1155
Slo-Phyllin Gyrocaps, 1155
Slow-FE, 588
Slow-K, 873, plate Z
Sodium Fluoride, 871
Solagé, 1099
Solareze Gel, 550
Solfoton, 851
Soluvite, 871
Sonata, 1165, plate Z
Sonazine, 229
Sorbitrate, 591, plate Z
Soriatane, 19
Sosol, 998
Sotalol, 1069
Sotret, 595
Sparfloxacin, 495
Spasdel, 381
Spasmolin, 381
Spectazole, 396
Spectracef, 210
Spectrobid, 825
Spiriva, 585
Spironazide, 393
Spironolactone, 42, 393
Spirozide, 393
Sporanox, 1107
Sprintec, 290
S-P-T, 1059

St. Joseph Adult Chewable Aspirin, 111
Stagesic, 833
Stamoist E, 422
Starlix, 931, plate Z
Staticin, 437
Statin Cholesterol-Lowering Agents, 986
Stavudine, 993
S-T Cort, 319
Stelazine, 229
Sterapred, 311
Sterapred DS, 311
S-T Forte 2, 1132
Stie-Cort, 319
Stimate, 344
Strattera, 123, plate Z
Striant, 1039
Strifon Forte DSC, 233
Sucralfate, 996
Sudal, 422
Sular, 775
Sulfabenzamide, 999
Sulfacetamide, 999
Sulfadiazine, 998
Sulfadoxine, 998
Sulfa Drugs, 998
Sulfamethizole, 998
Sulfamethoprim, 974
Sulfamethoprim DS, 974
Sulfamethoxazole, 974, 998
Sulfasalazine, 998
Sulfathiazole, 999
Sulfatrim, 974
Sulfisoxazole, 437, 998
Sulfonylurea Antidiabetes Drugs, 1003
Sulindac, 550
Sultrin, 999
Sumatriptan, 1120
Sumycin, 1044, plate Z
Suprax, 211
Surmontil, 1114, plate Z
Susano, 381

Sustaire, 1156
Sustiva, 401
Symax, 381
Synacort, 319
Synalar, 318
Synalar-HP, 318
Synalgos-DC, 837
Syn-RX, 422
Syntest DS, 445
Syntest HS, 445
Synthroid, 1058, plates Z & AA

T

TACE, 445
Tacrine, 239
Tacrolimus, 1008
Tadalafil, 430
Tagamet, 246, plate AA
Tagamet HB, 246
Talacen, 833
Talwin Compound, 837
Talwin Nx, 837, plate AA
Tambocor, 489
Tamiflu, 805
Tamoxifen Citrate, 1013
Tamsulosin, 1016
Tanafed, 96
Tannate, 96
Tanoral, 96
Tapanol, 13
Tarka, 1090
Tasmar, 1079
Tavist, 254
Tavist ND, 651
Taxol, 815
Taxotere, 815
Tazarotene, 1019
Tazorac, 1019
Taztia XT, 363
Tegaserod, 1021
Tegretol, 193, plate AA
Tegretol Chewable, plate AA
Tegretol-XR, 193, plate AA

Tegrin-HC, 319
Teladar, 317
Telmisartan, 85
Temazepam, 1104
Temodar, 1023
Temovate, 317
Temovate E, 317
Temozolomide, 1023
Tempra, 13
Ten-K, 873
Tenofovir, 1026
Tenoretic, 119
Tenormin, 119
Tequin, 495
Terazol 3, 1035
Terazol 7, 1035
Terazosin, 51
Terbinafine, 1028
Terbutaline, 1031
Terconazole, 1035
Teril, 193
Teriparatide, 1036
Terramycin, 1043
Testin, 1039
**Testoderm Transdermal
   System,** 1039
Testopel, 1039
Testosterone, 1039
Testred, 1040
Tetracap, 1044
Tetracycline, 540
Tetracycline Antibiotics, 1043
Tetracycline Hydrochloride,
   1044
Tetracyn, 1044
Tetralan, 1044
Teveten, 84
Teveten HCT, 84
Texacort, 319
T-Gesic, 833
Thalidomide, 1049
Thalitone, 1053
Thalomid, 1049
Theo-24, 1156

Theobid Duracaps, 1156
Theochron, 1156
Theoclear-80, 1156
Theoclear L.A., 1156
Theocron, 1156
Theo-Dur, 1156
Theolair, 1156
Theolair-SR, 1156
Theophylline, 1155
Theo-Sav, 1156
Theospan-SR, 1156
Theostat-80, 1156
Theovent, 1156
Theo-X, 1156
Theramycin Z, 437
Thiamine, 871
Thiazide Diuretics, 1052
Thioridazine Hydrochloride, 229
Thiosulfil Forte, 998
Thorazine, 229
Thorazine Spansules, 229
Thyrar, 1059
Thyroglobulin, 1059
Thyroid Hormone, 1059
Thyroid Hormone Replacements, 1058
Thyroid Strong, 1059
Thyrolar, 1058
Thyro-Tabs, 1058
Tiagabine, 1063
Tiamate, 363
Tiazac, 363, plate AA
Ticlid, 1066, plate AA
Ticlopidine, 1066
Tikosyn, 378
Tilade, 328
Tiludronate, 159
Time-Hist, 95
Timolol, 148, 324, 1069
Timoptic, 148
Timoptic-XE, 148
Tioconazole, 707
Tiotropium Bromide, 585

Tizanidine, 1074
TMP-SMZ, 974
Tocainide, 1076
Tofranil, 1113
Tofranil-PM, 1113
Tolazamide, 1003
Tolbutamide, 1003
Tolcapone, 1079
Tolectin, 550, plate AA
Tolectin DS, 550
Tolinase, 1003, plate AA, plate BB
Tolmetin Sodium, 550
Tolterodine, 1082
Tonocard, 1076
Topamax, 1084, plate BB
Topamax Sprinkle, 1084
Topicort, 317
Topicort LP, 317
Topicycline, 1044
Topiramate, 1084
Toprol-XL, 698, plate BB
Toradol, 599
Toremifene Citrate, 1014
Tornalate, 164, 680
Torsemide, 644
Totacillin, 825
Touro A & H, 95
Touro LA, 422
T-Phyl, 1156
Tracleer, 167
Tramadol, 1087
Trancot, 677
Trandate, 605
Trandolapril, 1090
Tranmep, 677
Transderm-Nitro, 789
Tranxene, 272
Tranxene-SD, 272
Tranxene T-Tab, 272, plate BB
Tranylcypromine Sulfate, 846
Trastuzumab, 1093
Travatan, 903
Travist, 254

Travoprost, 903
Trazodone, 1096
Tretinoin, 1099
Triacet, 319
Triad, 483
Triamcinolone, 311
Triamcinolone Acetonide, 303, 307, 319
Triamterene, 393
Triavil, 1113
Triazolam, 1103
Triazole Antifungals, 1107
Trichlormethiazide, 1053
Tricor, 474, plate BB
Tricyclic Antidepressants, 1113
Triderm, 319
Tridesilon, 317
Trifluoperazine Hydrochloride, 229
Tri-K, 872
Trileptal, 807, plate BB
Tri-Levlen, 291
Trimethoprim, 974
Trimipramine, 1114
Trimox, 825, plate BB
Trinalin Repetabs, 95
Tri-Norinyl, 291
Triostat, 1058
Triotann, 96
Tripelennamine Hydrochloride, 225
Triphasil, 291
Triple Sulfa, 999
Triptan-Type Antimigraine Drugs, 1120
Triptone, 366
Tritan, 96
Tri-Tannate, 96
Tri-Tannate Pediatric, 96
Tritec, 925
Trivora, 291
Trizivir, 1128, plate BB
Trovafloxacin, 495
Trovan, 495

Truphylline, 1155
Trusopt, 196
Trymex, 319
Trysul, 999
T Scalp, 319
T-Stat, 437
Tussionex Pennkinetic, 1132
Tussi-Organidin NR, 1134
Tuss-LA, 422
Tusstat, 369
Twin-K, 872
Tylenol, 13
Tylenol with Codeine No. 1, 833
Tylenol with Codeine No. 2, 833, plate BB
Tylenol with Codeine No. 3, 833, plate BB
Tylenol with Codeine No. 4, 833
Tylox, 832, plate BB

U

UAD, 323
ULTRAbrom, 95
ULTRAbrom PD, 95
Ultracet, 1087
Ultralente Insulin, 573
Ultram, 1087
Ultravate, 318
Uni-Ace, 13
Uni-Dur, 1156
Unipen, 825
Uniphyl, 1156
Uniretic, 730
Uniserts, 13
Unithyroid, 1058
Univasc, 730, plate CC
Unoprostone, 903
Uri-Tet, 1043
Uroxatral, 51

V

Vagifem, 445

Vagistat-1, 707
Valacyclovir, 1137
Valcyte, 514
Valdecoxib, 206
Valisone, 317
Valisone Reduced Strength,
317
Valium, 347, plate CC
Valnac, 317
Valproic Acid, 1139
Valrelease, 347
Valsartan, 85
Valtrex, 1137, plate CC
Vancenase AQ, 306
Vancenase Pockethaler, 302,
306
Vanceril, 302
Vanceril Double Strength, 302
Vaniqua, 404
Vantin, 211
Vardenafil, 430
Vascor, 142
Vaseretic, 412, plate CC
Vasotec, 412, plate CC
V-Cillin K, 826
V-Dec-M, 422
Vectrin, 1043
Veetids, 826, plate CC
Velosef, 211
Velosulin BR, 572
Venlafaxine, 1143
Ventolin, 38
Ventolin HFA, 38
Ventolin Nebules, 38
Ventolin Rotacaps, 38
Verapamil, 1090, 1146
Verapamil Extended Release,
1146
Verelan, 1146, plate DD
Verelan PM, 1146
Versacaps, 422
Vesanoid, 1099
Vexol, 300
Vfend, 1107

Viagra, 430, plate DD
Vibramycin, 1043, plate DD
Vibra-Tabs, 1043, plate DD
Vicodin, 833, plate DD
Vicodin-ES, 833, plate DD
Vicodin-HP, 833
Vicoprofen, 837
Vi-Daylin/F, 871
Videx, 354
Videx EC, 354
Vigamox Eyedrops, 495
Vioxx, 951, plate DD
Viracept, 755
Viramune, 761
Viread, 1026
Virilon, 1040
Visken, 861
Vistaril, 547
Vitamin A, 871
Vitamin B1, 871
Vitamin B2, 871
Vitamin B3, 871
Vitamin B6, 871
Vitamin B12, 871
Vitamin C, 871
Vitamin D, 871
Vitamin E, 871
Vitrasert, 514
Vitron-C, 588
Vivactil, 1113
Vivelle, 445
Vivelle-Dot, 445
Volmax, 38
Voltaren, 550
Voltaren-XR, 550
Voriconazole, 1107
V.V.S., 999

W

Warfarin, 1150
Welchol, 235, plate DD
Wellbutrin, 175, plate DD
Wellbutrin SR, 175, plate DD

Wellbutrin XL, 175, plate DD
Westcort, 319
Wygesic, 895
Wymox, 825
Wytensin, 534

X

Xalatan, 903
Xanax, 55, plate DD
Xanax XR, 55
Xanthine Bronchodilators, 1155
Xeloda, 186
Xenical, 802, plate EE
Xopenex, 38

Y

Yasmin, 290

Z

Zaditor Eyedrops, 603
Zafirlukast, 617
Zagam, 495
Zalcitabine, 1161
Zaleplon, 1165
Zanaflex, 1074, plate EE
Zanamivir, 1168
Zantac, 922, plate EE
Zantac 75, 922
Zantac EFFERdose, 922
Zaroxolyn, 1053, plate EE
Zebeta, 154, plate EE
Zelnorm, 1021
Zephrex, 422

Zephrex LA, 422
Zerit, 993, plate EE
Zerit XR, 993
Zestoretic, 636, plate EE
Zestril, 636, plate EE
Zetia, 460, plate FF
Ziac, 154, plate FF
Ziagen, 3
Zidovudine, 608, 1128, 1170
Zileuton, 617
Ziprasidone, 1175
Zithromax, 131, plate FF
Zocor, 987, plate FF
Zofran, 90
Zofran ODT, 90
Zolmitriptan, 1120
Zoloft, 965, plate FF
Zolpidem, 1178
Zomig, 1120, plate FF
Zomig ZMT, 1120
Zonegran, 1181
Zonisamide, 1181
ZORprin, 111
Zovia 1/35E, 290
Zovia 1/50E, 290
Zovirax, 23, plate FF
Zyban, 175, plate FF
Zydone, 833
Zyflo, 617
Zyloprim, 48
Zyprexa, 795, plate FF
Zyprexa Zydis, 795
Zyrtec, 216, plate FF
Zyrtec-D, 216, plate FF
Zyvox, 633, plate FF

ABOUT THE EDITOR

Educated at Columbia University, Dr. Harold Silverman has been a hospital pharmacist, author, educator, and pharmaceutical industry consultant. Currently he is Medical Director of the Global Healthcare Practice at Manning Selvage and Lee, a worldwide public relations and public affairs consulting firm. Professionally, Dr. Silverman seeks to help people understand why medicines are prescribed and how to get the most from them. In addition to *THE PILL BOOK,* Dr. Silverman is coauthor of *THE VITAMIN BOOK: A No-Nonsense Consumer Guide* and *The MED FILE Drug Interactions System*. He is also the author of *THE PILL BOOK GUIDE TO SAFE DRUG USE, THE CONSUMER'S GUIDE TO POISON PROTECTION, THE WOMAN'S DRUG STORE,* and *TRAVEL HEALTHY*. Dr. Silverman's contributions to the professional literature include more than 70 articles, research papers, and textbook chapters. He is a member of many professional organizations and has served as an officer for several, including the New York State Council of Hospital Pharmacists, for which he served as president. He has taught pharmacology and clinical pharmacy at several universities and won numerous awards for his work. Dr. Silverman resides in a Washington suburb with his wife, Judith Brown, and their son, Joshua.